AF615611

# EQUINE RESPIRATORY DISORDERS

# EQUINE RESPIRATORY DISORDERS

---

JILL BEECH, V.M.D.

*Associate Professor of Medicine*
*University of Pennsylvania*
*School of Veterinary Medicine*
*New Bolton Center*
*Kennett Square, Pennsylvania*

1991

LEA & FEBIGER • PHILADELPHIA • LONDON

Lea & Febiger
200 Chester Field Parkway
Malvern, Pennsylvania 19355-9725
U.S.A.
(215) 251-2230
1-800-444-1785

Lea & Febiger (UK) Ltd.
145a Croydon Road
Beckenham, Kent BR3 3RB
U.K.

**Library of Congress Cataloging-in-Publication Data**

Equine respiratory disorders / [edited] by Jill Beech.
p. cm.
ISBN 0-8121-1325X
1. Horses—Diseases. 2. Respiratory organs—Diseases. I. Beech. Jill.
SF959.R47E68 1991
636.1'089'62—dc20 90-5885
CIP



PRINTED IN THE UNITED STATES OF AMERICA

Print number: 5 4 3 2 1

Reprints of chapters may be purchased from Lea & Febiger in quantities of 100 or more.

THIS BOOK IS DEDICATED:

*To our equine patients.*

*To New Bolton Center's referring veterinarians, with appreciation and with hopes that they will find this book useful.*

*To Dr. C. W. Raker.*

# *Preface*

The aim of this book is to provide comprehensive coverage of equine respiratory tract disorders in a format usable in clinical medicine. Heretofore, there has been no such modern English language textbook which veterinarians could consult and it is hoped that this book will fill this void. I have divided the material in such a way that I hope will be most clear and allow readers to find most efficiently the information they seek. Although there is a chapter on applied physiology and details on anatomy in some of the chapters, the book is not meant to serve as a text in respiratory physiology or anatomy and the information presented is within the framework of clinical medicine.

Contributors were selected based on their expertise in their respective fields and ability to present the most current information available. I realize that, in a North American textbook, some areas of clinical medicine relevant elsewhere in the world potentially may not be addressed adequately; hopefully, that information may be found elsewhere. In Chapter 11 on viral diseases, some background information on laboratory testing is provided because I believe such information is not readily available to practitioners and may be of both interest and help in clinical practice. Technical information is also provided on staining for those interested in cytology. A chart on dosage regimens for commonly used antibiotics is included, but other medications (such as bronchodilators, mucolytics, etc.) are not listed because there is so little clinically validated information and dosages appear disparate among clinicians for different patients. The contributors attempted to present the most current information, realizing that this is likely to expand or change within the time span required for publication. As equine respiratory medicine progresses, I hope this book will serve as a foundation to which additional information will be added in the future.

I am grateful to all the secretaries who toiled on these manuscripts and for the numerous contributors' expertise and commitment. I would also like to recognize the many veterinarians in practice with whom I collaborate and who provide so much information but often are not acknowledged for their contributions.

I hope the book will be useful to students and veterinarians alike.

*Kennett Square, Pennsylvania* Jill Beech

# *Contributors*


JILL BEECH, V.M.D.
*Diplomate, ACVIM*
*Associate Professor of Medicine*
*University of Pennsylvania*
*School of Veterinary Medicine*
*New Bolton Center*
*Kennett Square, PA*

FREDERIK J. DERKSEN, D.V.M., PH.D.
*Diplomate, ACVIM*
*Professor of Medicine*
*Michigan State University*
*Veterinary Clinic Center*
*East Lansing, MI*

CHARLES S. FARROW, D.V.M.
*Diplomate, ACVR*
*Professor of Radiology*
*Western College of Veterinary Medicine*
*University of Saskatchewan*
*Saskatoon, Saskatchewan*
*Canada*

DAVID E. FREEMAN, M.V.B., M.R.C.V.S., PH.D.
*Diplomate, ACVS*
*Assistant Professor of Surgery*
*University of Pennsylvania*
*School of Veterinary Medicine*
*New Bolton Center*
*Kennett Square, PA*

DEBORAH M. GILLETTE, D.V.M., PH.D.
*Diplomate, ACVP*
*Assistant Professor of Pathology*
*University of Pennsylvania*
*School of Veterinary Medicine*
*New Bolton Center*
*Kennett Square, PA*

ANNE M. KOTERBA, D.V.M., PH.D.
*Diplomate, ACVIM*
*Associate Professor of Medicine*
*University of Florida*
*College of Veterinary Medicine*
*Gainesville, FL*

MICHAEL O'CALLAGHAN, M.R.C.V.S., PH.D.
*Associate Professor of Surgery*
*Tufts University*
*School of Veterinary Medicine*
*North Grafton, MA*

PAUL G. ORSINI, D.V.M.
*Lecturer in Surgery*
*University of Pennsylvania*
*School of Veterinary Medicine*
*New Bolton Center*
*Kennett Square, PA*

JOHN R. PASCOE, B.V.SC., PH.D.
*Diplomate, ACVS*
*Assistant Professor of Surgery*
*University of California*
*School of Veterinary Medicine*
*Davis, CA*

VIRGINIA B. REEF, D.V.M.
*Diplomate, ACVIM*
*Associate Professor of Medicine in the Widener Hospital*
*University of Pennsylvania*
*School of Veterinary Medicine*
*New Bolton Center*
*Kennett Square, PA*

James Robertson, D.V.M.
*Diplomate, ACVS*
*Associate Professor, Equine Surgery*
*The Ohio State University*
*College of Veterinary Medicine*
*Columbus, OH*

James R. Rooney, D.V.M.
*Diplomate, ACVP*
*Professor*
*J. Maxwell Gluck Research Center*
*Department of Veterinary Science*
*University of Kentucky*
*Lexington, KY*

Corinne R. Sweeney, D.V.M.
*Diplomate, ACVIM*
*Assistant Professor of Medicine*
*University of Pennsylvania*
*School of Veterinary Medicine*
*New Bolton Center*
*Kennett Square, PA*

# Contents

# CHAPTER 1

# APPLIED RESPIRATORY PHYSIOLOGY

*FREDERIK J. DERKSEN*

## Upper Airway

As air enters the lung to participate in gas exchange, it first traverses the upper respiratory system. This part of the respiratory system not only functions as a conduit for air during respiration, but it also has a role in olfaction, phonation, and filtering and conditioning the inspired air. In addition, the upper respiratory system is important in thermoregulation. The upper airway of the horse is unique because the horse can only breathe efficiently through the nares, and mouth breathing is used as a last resort. The obligate nasal breathing is the result of a tight seal that is formed between the soft palate and the laryngeal cartilages. This implies that upper airway obstruction involving the nasal passages is particularly important in this species, because the horse cannot bypass such an obstruction by mouth breathing.

Upper airway resistance is a significant portion of total resistance to airflow.[1] Some authors have indicated that as much as 70 to 85% of total respiratory resistance arises in the upper airway of normal horses,[2] whereas a lower percentage (<20%) is cited elsewhere.[1] It would probably be most accurate to state that approximately 30 to 50% of total air flow resistance is attributable to the upper airway. Measurements may differ because upper airway resistance is quite variable. The horse is able to decrease upper airway resistance markedly[3] by muscular dilatation of portions of the upper airway, especially the external nares and larynx, by straightening of the airway and by constriction of vascular sinuses located in the nasal mucosa. Within the upper airway resistance to flow is primarily at the external nares and at the larynx.[1] The nasal passages and pharynx have a relatively large cross-sectional area and therefore contribute little to airflow resistance. The location of high-resistance regions at the external nares and larynx implies that small strategically located lesions may significantly increase total resistance to airflow. Thus lesions in the pharynx or nasal passages are less likely to result in significant airway obstruction than lesions in the external nares or larynx.

On inhalation, pressure within the upper airway is negative relative to atmospheric pressure, while on exhalation, the pressure in the upper airway lumen is positive.[3] The majority of upper airway structures are rigidly supported by cartilage or bone and are unaffected by these pressure swings. However, structures supported by muscle, such as the external nares, pharyngeal walls, soft palate and arytenoid cartilages, are moved into the lumen on inhalation. These slight dynamic movements of the upper airway during quiet breathing may be visualized using a fiberoptic endoscope and explain why in the resting horse upper airway resistance on inhalation is approximately 50% greater than on exhalation.[3] During exercise, pressure swings in the upper airway are much greater than at rest and may be as high as 40 cm $H_2O$. Videoendoscopy of horses exercising on a treadmill shows that the soft tissue structures of the upper airway such as the pharyngeal walls and soft palate clearly move inward on inhalation and outward on exhalation. Therefore, during heavy exercise, inspiratory resistance may be twice as high as expiratory resistance.[3]

When the horse starts to exercise, air flow through the upper airway increases from approximately 4 L/sec at rest to more than 75 L/sec during exercise (unpublished data). The upper airway can accommodate this enormous increase in airflow by greatly reducing resistance to air flow. The normal horse achieves this by dilatation of structures supported by muscle (Fig. 1–1), straightening of the airway, and vasoconstriction of the vascular mucosa. In diseases of the upper airway, these functions may be interfered with and airflow obstruction results. Upper airway obstruction may be fixed or dynamic. Fixed obstructions such as pharyngeal cysts cause dyspnea on inhalation as well as exhalation. However, dynamic obstructions such as left laryngeal hemiplegia only cause airway obstruction during inhalation.[4] In normal horses, the tendency of soft tissue to collapse into the lumen of the upper airway is counteracted by muscular activity. In conditions where this muscular activity may be interfered with, such as left laryngeal hemiplegia or facial nerve paresis, dynamic collapse of unsupported soft tissue structures will cause inspiratory dyspnea and flow limitation. That is, flow rates become constant despite increasing inspiratory efforts. While dynamic obstructions of the upper airway cause airway obstruction on inhalation, exhalation is not interfered with because during exhalation, airway luminal pressures are positive relative to atmosphere and any unsupported structures are moved out of the lumen by this pressure.[4]

In many horses with dynamic upper airway lesions, upper airway luminal pressure swings are insufficient to cause dynamic collapse at rest. However, during exercise pressure swings in the upper airway are much greater than at rest; galloping horses with left laryngeal hemiplegia may generate tracheal pressures up to 60 cm $H_2O$ on inhalation, and severe dyspnea and flow limitation result[4] (Fig. 1–1). Similarly, many horses with dorsal displacement of the soft palate are asymptomatic at rest or during modest exercise. However, during heavy exercise the soft palate epiglottic seal is broken and the soft palate is sucked upward into the pharyngeal lumen.

## The Lung

The main functions of the lung are to supply oxygen for metabolism by tissues and to remove metabolic carbon dioxide. This gas exchange function involves delivering appropriate volumes of air to the alveolar surfaces by ventilation, matching of ventilation with pulmonary blood flow, and diffusion of gases to and from the blood. To accommodate metabolic needs, the horse lung has an enormous

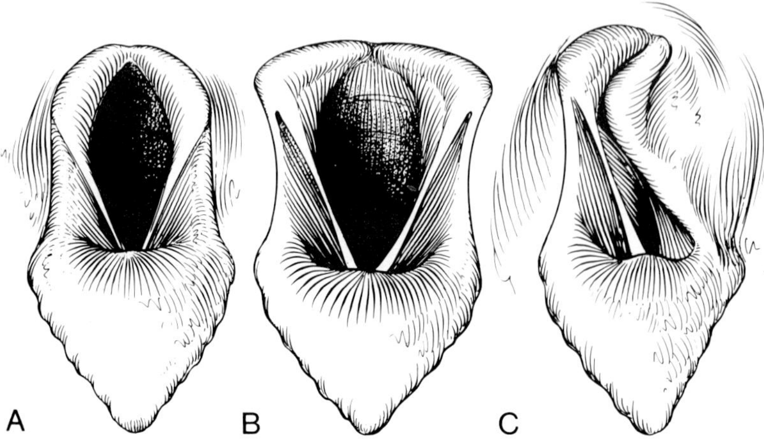


**FIG. 1–1.** Schematic endoscopic view of the larynx of a normal horse at rest, (A) and during exercise (B). Note that the arytenoid cartilages are abducted during exercise, reducing upper airway resistance to airflow. In a horse with left laryngeal hemiplegia, the affected arytenoid cartilage collapses into the airway during inhalation (C) but not during exhalation.

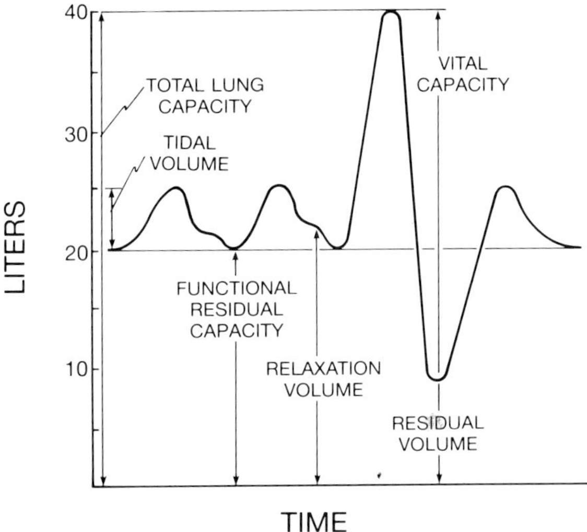


**FIG. 1–2.** Lung volumes of the horse. Note the pause in exhalation at the relaxation volume. In some horses, a similar pause is seen during inhalation.

surface area, estimated at more than 2000 m$^2$, exposed to the external environment.[5] This surface area, covered in most places by only a single layer of epithelial cells, is constantly challenged by dust particles, viruses, bacteria, and allergens. Complex defensive strategies have been devised to fend off these challenges. These pulmonary defenses were probably adequate when the horse lived on wide open grassy plains. However, domestication has resulted in many of our horses being kept under crowded conditions, in poorly ventilated barns, and being fed fodder containing up to 5,000 respirable particles/mg of feed.[6] Consequently, horses commonly suffer from respiratory disease ranging from viral and bacterial infections to heaves and exercise-induced pulmonary hemorrhage. Subclinical respiratory disease resulting in poor performance is probably even more common. To treat respiratory diseases of the horse effectively, the equine clinician must first understand the function of the lung in health and disease. This chapter discusses the gas exchange and metabolic functions of the normal and diseased lung and how the lung is defended against environmental challenges.

# Ventilation

Ventilation may be defined as the bulk movement of air into and out of the respiratory system.[7] The subdivisions of respiratory air are shown in Figure 1–2. Although the horse is able to breathe from total lung capacity at end inhalation to residual volume at end exhalation, the tidal volume that is chosen is usually much smaller and in a 500-kg horse is approximately 4 L. Inspired volume is slightly larger than expired volume because more oxygen is taken up by the tissues than $CO_2$ is released.[8] Multiplying tidal volume by respiratory frequency gives minute ventilation. Part of the minute ventilation is wasted or dead space ventilation because it is used to ventilate the conducting airways such as the upper airway, trachea, bronchi, and bronchioles. In large mammals such as the horse, the wasted or dead space ventilation at rest may be as large as 70% of the tidal volume.[9] Therefore, 30% of the tidal volume remains to ventilate the gas exchange regions of the lung and this portion of the tidal volume is called the alveolar ventilation.

When air enters the lung during inhalation, the muscles of respiration including the diaphragm and intercostal muscles exert the driving pressure (P) required. This pressure may be divided into pressure necessary to overcome the pulmonary elastic recoil, the resistance to air flow offered by the airways and lung tissues, and the inertial forces. This relationship is shown as follows:

$$P = P_E + P_R + P_I$$

where $P_E$ is pressure necessary to overcome elastic forces; $P_R$ is pressure necessary to overcome resistive forces; and $P_I$ is pressure necessary to overcome inertial forces.[10]

To understand mechanics of ventilation in health and disease it is useful to consider pulmonary elastic recoil, pulmonary resistance, and inertance separately.

## *Pulmonary Elastic Recoil*

The lung parenchyma contains elastin and collagen, which are the structural elements responsible for the pulmonary elastic recoil.[11]

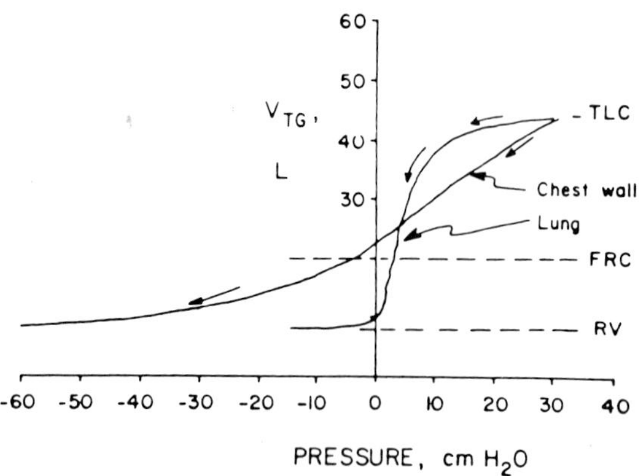


**FIG. 1–3.** Pressure-volume curves of the lung and chest wall of a normal horse (11 yrs old, 545 kg). (From Leith DE. Comparative mammalian respiratory mechanics. Physiologist, *19*:405, 1976.)

Over the tidal volume range the lung has a tendency to collapse. This tendency is resisted by the chest wall.[12] The elastic properties of the lung and the chest wall are best depicted by a pressure volume curve (Fig. 1–3). The curve is constructed by plotting the driving pressure necessary to inflate the lung versus lung volume. This pressure-volume curve shows several important concepts. At the lung volume labeled FRC, it can be seen that the tendency for the lung to collapse is equal and opposite to the tendency of the chest wall to expand. Most species choose this lung volume as the end of exhalation and it is called functional residual capacity (FRC) or the relaxation volume. Thus, in most species inhalation requires muscular activity, while exhalation is passive as lung volume decreases to FRC.[12] The adult horse, however, chooses a different breathing strategy.[13] When the horse reaches the relaxation volume, expiratory abdominal muscles are recruited to decrease lung volume even further. Therefore, the first part of inhalation is passive until the relaxation volume is reached. Subsequently, inspiratory muscles are recruited. Conversely the first part of exhalation is passive followed by recruitment of expiratory muscles. Recruitment of abdominal muscles during exhalation is often accentuated in lung disease and this clinical sign can give the clinician an indication of airway obstruction.

The pressure volume curve has additional clinical usefulness because the relationship between changes in volume ($\Delta V$) and changes in pressure ($\Delta P$) defines the compliance (C) or the elasticity of a structure.

$$C = \frac{\Delta V}{\Delta P}$$

Thus, compliance is the slope of the pressure volume curve at any point along its curve. Over the tidal volume range the pressure volume curve is approximately linear so that one value of compliance describes the elastic properties of the lung. However, as the lung volume approaches total lung capacity, the pressure volume curve flattens showing that the lung becomes less compliant at higher lung volumes. The compliance of the horse lung is altered in disease.[14,15] Measurement of compliance can give clues as to the type of pulmonary disease from which the horse is suffering. Restrictive lung diseases are characterized by a decrease in lung or chest wall compliance.[14] The stiffer lung results in increased work of breathing, exercise intolerance, and even dyspnea. Examples of restrictive pulmonary diseases in the horse include pulmonary fibrosis, interstitial pneumonia, and pulmonary edema. Pleural effusion, infectious pleuritis, and mediastinal masses are examples of nonpulmonary restrictive respiratory diseases. Increased pulmonary compliance in the horse is rare but may be caused by pulmonary emphysema.

The tendency for the inflated lung to recoil has two different origins. The elastic properties of the lung itself are in part responsible for this tendency, but surface tension forces are also a cause of elastic lung recoil. The effect of surface forces on elastic recoil were first described by Von Neergaard[16] in 1929 and can best be demonstrated by comparing pressure volume curves of an air filled and saline solution filled lung (Fig. 1–4). Filling the lung with saline solution eliminates the effect of surface forces of the air liquid interface and demonstrates the effect of surface forces on elastic lung recoil.[17] It can be seen that less pressure is required to maintain a given lung volume when saline solution is used to distend the lung instead of air. Thus, surface active forces contribute significantly to the lung elastic recoil. Yet, surface tension forces

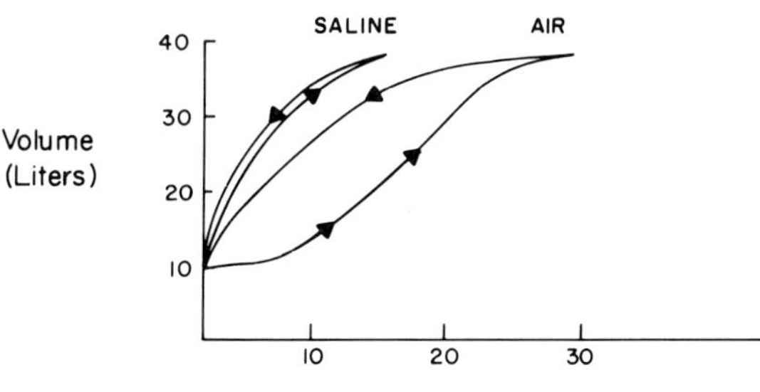


**FIG. 1–4.** Pressure-volume curves generated using excised lungs inflated with air and saline. Filling the lung with saline eliminates the effects of surface forces of the air-liquid interface and demonstrates the effect of surface forces on elastic lung recoil.

would be even greater without the presence of surfactant.[18]

## *Pulmonary Surfactant*

Pulmonary surfactant is a complex material composed mainly of lipids and proteins. The main constituents of lung surfactant are phospholipids.[19] Among the various species tested the make up of the various phospholipids is remarkably constant. Phosphatidylcholine is the predominant lipid making up approximately 50% of the total lipids and is largely responsible for surface activity.[20] Phosphatidylethanolanine makes up approximately 20% of the lipids, and three acidic phospholipids, phosphatidylinositol, phosphatidylserine, and phosphatidylglycerol constitute 12 to 15% of the total phospholipids. Numerous physiologic and physiochemical studies have shown that pulmonary surfactant is required to maintain alveolar stability and prevent atelectasis.[21,22] To maintain stability, pulmonary surfactant must lower alveolar surface tension to less than 10 dynes/cm.[20] Dipalmitoylphosphatidylcholine has the physiochemical properties needed to do this.[20]

Although lipids make up more than 80% of the surfactant, protein components also have a critical role in surfactant function.[23] The proteins most extensively studied, apoprotein A and B, are unique to the lung.[24] Their function is not clearly established, but early experiments have shown that they may accelerate adsorption of surfactant to the air-liquid interface.[23]

Pulmonary surfactant is produced by alveolar epithelial type II cells.[24] The sequence of intercellular storage release and adsorption to the air liquid interface is shown schematically in Figure 1–5. Surfactant is produced in the cytoplasm of alveolar type II cells and stored in folded layers in lamellar bodies. Subsequently lamellar bodies are released by membrane fusion and exocytosis into the overlying liquid subphase. The lamellar bodies then enfold and are transported in tubular myelin. The tubular myelin is finally incorporated in the monomolecular surface film probably with the help of the apoproteins.[24]

During fetal life, when there is no air liquid interface within the lung, surfactant is not required. However, an adequate supply of pulmonary surfactant must be present at birth to allow lung stability and prevent atelectasis after the first breath. In humans, at about 24 weeks of gestation surfactant production is under way, as evidenced by the presence of lamellar inclusion bodies in type II alveolar cells. In the foal, surfactant has been detected as early as 200 days of gestation,[25] but preliminary information suggests that pulmonary surfactant in the foal is insufficient to main lung stability before 300 days of gestation.[26] However, these numbers must be interpreted with caution because of the small number of

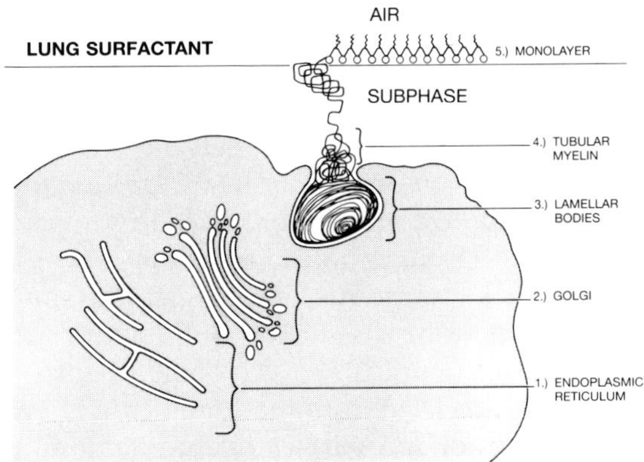


**FIG. 1–5.** Surfactant is produced in the cytoplasm of alveolar type II cells and stored in folded layers in lamellar bodies. The lamellar bodies are released into the liquid subphase, and form tubular myelin which in turn spreads as a monolayer at the air-liquid interface.

animals studied so far and the apparently large variability among individuals. If the production of surfactant is delayed or if the birth is premature, the neonatal foal is likely to suffer from neonatal respiratory distress syndrome. In human medicine, screening tests have been developed to detect the presence of surfactant material in amnionic fluid. One of these tests is the lecithin/sphingomyelin ratio.[27] Lecithin (phosphatidylcholine) concentrations in amnionic fluid increase as gestation progresses, while the sphingomyelin concentration stays relatively constant. Thus, high lecithin/sphingomyelin ratio suggests that the risk of neonatal respiratory distress syndrome is low.[27] The amnionic concentration of phosphatidylglycerol has also been used to assess surfactant production. Preliminary evidence in foals suggests that the results of these tests are highly variable and do not accurately predict the likelihood of development of neonatal respiratory distress syndrome.[28] In addition, amniocentesis is technically difficult to perform in the mare. Nonetheless, in the future more useful indices of pulmonary surfactant concentration may become available.

In most species, pulmonary surfactant has a half-life of approximately 14 hours. This means that surfactant must be produced constantly. Surfactant production may be reduced by a variety of metabolic disturbances including reduction in pulmonary blood flow as seen in hypovolemia, hypothermia, acidosis, or alkalosis. Thus, maintenance of homeostasis in neonatal foals is essential if pulmonary surfactant production is to be maintained and pulmonary atelectasis is to be prevented. Pulmonary surfactant production in late gestation may be enhanced by glucocorticoids. Thyroid hormones, beta receptor agonists, acetylcholine, prostaglandin, and estrogen may also enhance pulmonary surfactant production.[20,29–31] At present, glucocorticoids are used in human medicine to enhance pulmonary surfactant production in cases at risk for developing neonatal respiratory distress syndrome.[20] In veterinary medicine, much remains to be learned about the regulation of surfactant production before their use can be recommended. The most obvious therapy for neonatal respiratory distress syndrome is surfactant therapy. Several large studies in human beings using surfactant derived from bovine or ovine lung or human amnionic fluid have yielded conflicting results.[32–34] Synthetic surfactant is presently being evaluated in the treatment of neonatal respiratory distress syndrome.

## Pulmonary Resistance

In order for air to move in and out of the respiratory system, a force must be applied not only to overcome the elastic recoil of the lung, but also to generate air flow against the resistance of the airways and pulmonary tissues. In addition, during tidal breathing, air and lung tissues must be accelerated and decelerated and part of the forces generated by the respiratory muscles are used to overcome inertance. Inertial forces are negligible during tidal breathing[10] but become important when respiratory rate increases, as during exercise. Resistance (R) is calculated by measurement of driving pressure (P) and air flow rates ($\dot{V}$) using the general formula:

$$R = \frac{P}{\dot{V}}$$

Driving pressure may be measured using an esophageal balloon or by direct puncture of the pleural space,[35] while air flow rates may be evaluated using a pneumotachograph or other flow measuring device usually mounted on a face mask. In horses, the upper airway resistance is approximately one-half of the total resistance to air flow.[1] Within the lung the trachea and bronchi are the main contributors to air flow resistance.[36] An obstruction in these airways causes dyspnea. The resistance of the bronchioles is small and obstruction in these airways must be massive before dyspnea is encountered.[36]

The resistance of a cylindrical tube of a length (L) and radius (r) is given by the following formula:

$$R = \frac{8\mu L}{r^4}$$

were $\mu$ is the viscosity of the gas passing

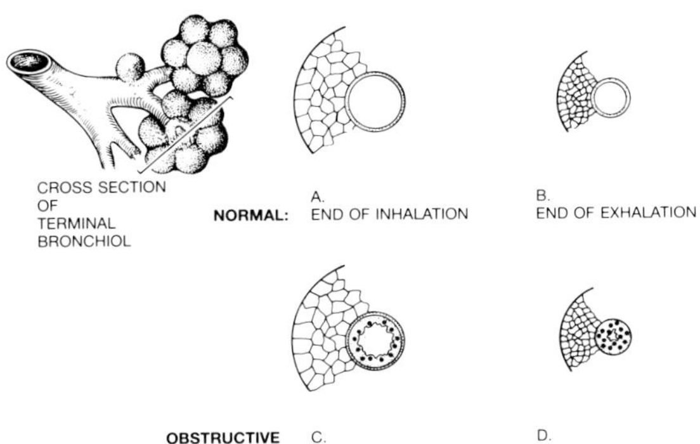


**FIG. 1–6.** Effects of lung volume on airway diameter. As the lung inflates, parenchymal attachments pull open airways (A). During exhalation, airway diameter decreases (B). Because inflammatory exudate and secretion decrease airway diameter (C), diseased airways may close at low lung volumes (D).

through the tube. This equation demonstrates that radius is a more important determinant of resistance than length. Doubling of the radius decreases resistance 16-fold. Because airway radius is the most important determinant of resistance to airflow in the lung, let us examine the factors that affect airway radius.

The airway radius may be changed passively as a result of changes in lung volume. As the lung inflates, parenchymal attachments pull open the airways, thereby reducing resistance to airflow[9] (Fig. 1–6). Conversely, during exhalation airway diameter decreases and some airways may even close at low lung volumes. Decreased airway diameter with decreased lung volumes explains why, in horses with partial airway obstruction, wheezes are loudest at end exhalation.

It also explains the recruitment of expiratory abdominal muscles seen in horses with small airway disease. In horses with conditions such as chronic obstructive pulmonary disease, the airway radius is reduced by inflammatory exudate, edema, and cellular infiltration.[37] At high lung volumes these bronchioles are kept open by the surrounding lung parenchyma. As lung volume decreases during tidal breathing, the inflamed bronchioles close and gas is trapped behind the closed airways. Affected horses attempt to reduce the thoracic lung volume actively by recruitment of expiratory muscles. In severe cases, the expiratory abdominal muscles hypertrophy and a "heave line" develops.

Because all conducting airways have smooth muscle in their walls, airway diameter may also be altered by smooth muscle contraction or relaxation. Airway smooth muscle tone may be altered directly through the effect of inflammatory mediators such as histamine, prostaglandins, or leukotrienes or indirectly by the action of the autonomic nervous system.[38]

## Autonomic Control of Airways

The autonomic innervation of the airways is shown in Figure 1–7. In all mammalian species studied, the most important division of the autonomic nervous system is the parasympathetic system.[39–41] Parasympathetic fibers travel in the vagus nerve and innervate the airways from the trachea to the bronchioles. In the horse, the distribution of parasympathetic innervation is not known.

Parasympathetic stimulation causes airway narrowing, especially of the bronchi. In normal horses, parasympathetic blockade using vagal cooling or atropine causes little bronchodilation; therefore, in normal horses there is little resting parasympathetic tone.[42] However, in disease, parasympathetic bronchoconstriction is a common mechanism resulting in poor performance, gas exchange impairment, or dyspnea. For example, in horses with recurrent airway obstruction (heaves), parasympathetic blockade using atropine results in bronchodilation, demonstrating an important role of parasympathetic bronchoconstriction in the pathogenesis of this disease.[43] A noncholinergic excitatory system with substance P as transmitter may also cause bronchoconstriction in some species but this system has not yet been identified in the horse.

The lung is richly supplied with adrenergic receptors,[44] especially $beta_2$ receptors. Most of these receptors are not innervated by sympathetic nerve fibers, and indeed the sympathetic innervation of the lung is rather sparse.[45] These receptors may be stimulated by circulating catecholamines released by the

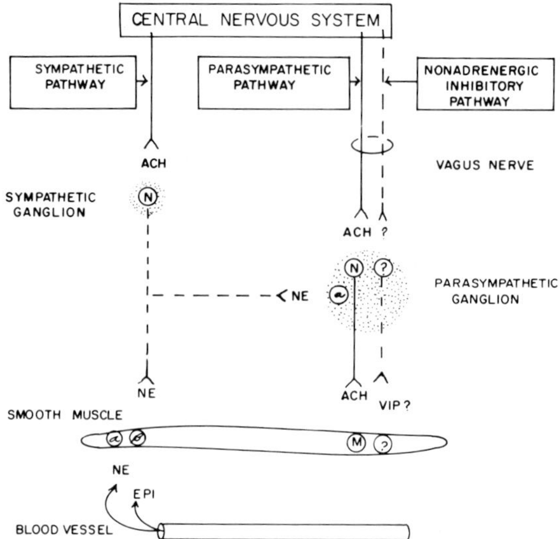


**FIG. 1–7.** Autonomic innervation of airway smooth muscle. The parasympathetic pathway consists of motor nerves traveling in the vagus nerve to parasympathetic ganglia, and they release acetylcholine (Ach). Postganglionic parasympathetic fibers also release Ach, which binds to muscarinic receptors (M) on smooth muscle causing contraction. The sympathetic pathway includes motor nerves which travel to sympathetic ganglia and release Ach, which stimulates nicotinic receptors (N) in the ganglia. Postganglionic sympathetic fibers may travel to parasympathetic ganglia, release norepinephrine (NE), and inhibit parasympathetic neurotransmission. Norepinephrine may also bind to β receptors (β) or α receptors (α) on smooth muscle and cause muscle relaxation or contraction, respectively. The nonadrenergic inhibitory pathway has not yet been identified in the horse. In the cat, fibers travel in the vagus nerve and release a neuropeptide, possibly vasoactive intestinal peptide (VIP) which causes smooth muscle relaxation. EPI, epinephrine. (From Nadel JA, Baines PJ, Holtzman MJ. Autonomic factors in hyperreactivity of airway smooth muscle. In: Handbook of Physiology. The Respiratory System. Vol III, Mechanics of Breathing. AP Fishman, PT Macklem, J Mead, et al (eds). Bethesda, MD, The American Physiological Society, 1986, pp 693–702.)

adrenal medulla or local release of norepinephrine from sympathetic nerve endings. Activation of $beta_2$ receptors causes bronchodilation. Although in the horse, as in humans, there appears to be little direct sympathetic pulmonary innervation,[45] sympathetic nerves may innervate parasympathetic ganglia and modulate release of acetylcholine.[46] Because normal horses, like other mammals studied, have little bronchomotor tone, $beta_2$ receptor stimulation does not increase airway caliber.[47,48] Airways must first be constricted with, for example, histamine before $beta_2$ receptor stimulation causes bronchodilation. Thus the sympathomimetic bronchodilators that have been examined have had little effect on airway caliber in normal horses.[47] However, when bronchoconstriction has occurred, either directly through smooth muscle inflammation or indirectly through parasympathetic nerve stimulation, $beta_2$ receptor stimulation causes airway smooth muscle relaxation.[49] In disease, $beta_2$ receptor activation by endogenous catecholamines may moderate bronchoconstriction. For example, in ponies with recurrent airway obstruction (heaves), beta receptor blockade increases airway resistance.[50] Thus beta receptors appear to act in a protective capacity, preventing excessive airway narrowing.

Alpha adrenergic receptors are also present in the lung. Although in normal animals alpha receptors are not as numerous as $beta_2$ receptors, alpha receptor numbers increase towards the smaller airways, and it has been shown in the ferret that in the terminal bronchioles α and β receptors may be equal in number.[51] Alpha-adrenergic receptor stimulation causes bronchoconstriction in ponies with recurrent airway obstruction (heaves), but not in normal ponies.[52] This suggests that, in the normal equine lung, α receptors play no important role in the regulation of bronchomotor tone, but that in disease α receptors may be upregulated, contributing to airway obstruction.

A nonadrenergic inhibitory system has been demonstrated in the cat.[53] This system courses in the vagus nerve and when stimulated causes airway dilation. The neurotransmitter of this system is not yet known but may be vasoactive intestinal peptide. Like the noncholinergic excitatory system, the nonadrenergic inhibitory system has not yet been identified in the horse.[45]

## Distribution of Ventilation

To allow gas exchange between the respired air and the blood, the inspired air must be distributed in the lung to match pulmonary blood flow. The main determinant of regional ventilation is the distribution of pleural surface pressure.[54] In the horse there is a vertical pleural pressure gradient so that the intrapleural pressure is most subatmospheric in the dorsal portions of the thorax.[35,55] Therefore, in the dorsal lung regions the lung is more distended and less compliant than in the ventral regions. This results in preferential ventilation of the ventral lung regions. The distribution of ventilation is determined not only by the regional distribution of pleural pressure, but also by the product of resistance and compliance. This product is called a time constant. When the time constant of a lung unit is long, it takes longer to ventilate this portion of the lung. In the normal lung, local airway resistance and compliance are relatively homogeneous. In lung disease the compliance and resistance of lung units may be greatly altered and these regional changes in time constants are likely to become important, contributing to severe maldistribution of ventilation, mismatching of ventilation and blood flow, and hypoxemia. Lung regions supplied by low resistant airways will receive preferential ventilation, while diseased lung regions supplied by partially obstructed airways will be underventilated. In the early stages of disease, during quiet breathing, the respiratory frequency may still be low enough to allow complete filling of the diseased region of the lung. However, as respiratory frequency increases, time constants of the diseased lung regions are too short to allow filling, and maldistribution of ventilation is exaggerated. This implies that the earliest signs of respiratory disease will be inability to perform during exercise when respiratory frequency is high. Only when respiratory disease progresses do clinical signs of lung disease become apparent at rest. In anesthetized horses, especially when positioned in dorsal recumbency, the weight of the animal and the abdominal content cause reduction in lung volume. Airway closure and marked uneven distribution of ventilation result.[56]

## Diffusion

In the gas exchange regions of the lung, $O_2$ and $CO_2$ are transported by diffusion. Diffusion is the passive tendency of molecules to move from a region of higher to one of lower concentration. As air enters the terminal bronchioles and alveolar ducts, bulk flow becomes so slow that it is superseded by diffusion. This process sets up a concentration gradient and a "stratified inhomogeneity" of $O_2$ concentration may result.[57] In the horse, with long terminal respiratory units, this inhomogeneity is probably of greater importance than in smaller animals and may be a limiting factor in maximal oxygen consumption during exercise.

Subsequently, oxygen molecules must pass through the air-blood barrier, which includes the fluid layer lining the alveoli, the alveolar

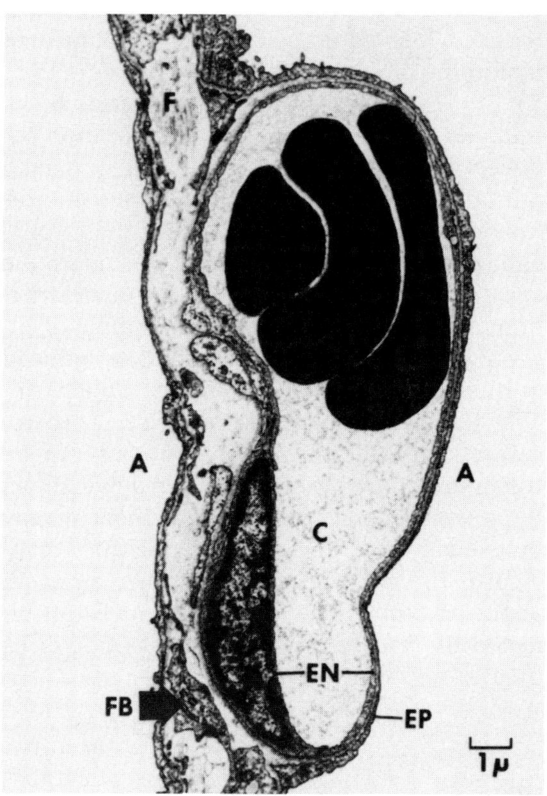


**FIG. 1–8.** Alveolar septum of human lung in thin section. Alveolar gases (A) diffuse into the capillary (C) through type I epithelium (EP) and endothelium (EN). On the left side the interstitium contains fibers (F) and fibroblast processes (FB); on the right side it is reduced to the fused basement membrane (Micrograph courtesy of Dr. E. Weibel). (From Weibel ER. Functional morphology of lung parenchyma. Handbook of Physiology. Vol III, part 1. Bethesda, MD, American Physiological Society, 1986, pp 89–111.)

epithelium, basement membrane and capillary endothelium (Fig. 1–8). Finally, once it is in the blood, the oxygen diffuses through the plasma and combines chemically with hemoglobin. The $CO_2$ diffuses in the opposite direction. Factors that determine the amount of gases diffusing per unit time are the concentration gradient between the alveolus and capillary blood, the physical properties of the gas, the surface area available for diffusion, and the thickness of the air blood barrier. It has been estimated that equilibration between alveolar and capillary oxygen tension occurs within one-third of the time pulmonary blood is in the capillaries and is available for gas exchange.[58] During exercise, however, pulmonary blood flow velocity increases and the oxygen tension in the mixed venous blood is reduced.[59] In addition, the hemoglobin content of the blood may be increased more than 50%.[59] Therefore, more oxygen needs to be transferred in less time, and equilibration between alveolar gas and capillary blood may not occur, resulting in hypoxemia. This diffusion limitation may account for the hypoxemia observed in normal horses during severe exercise. In lung diseases with tissue destruction, consolidation, atelectasis, filling of alveoli with exudate or edema fluid, or reduced perfusion pressures, the surface area available for gas exchange is reduced. This decreases the amount of oxygen that can be transported to the blood and may result in hypoxemia even at rest. Oxygen therapy may be used to treat these patients because it increases driving pressure of oxygen from alveolus to blood. The $CO_2$ transport is less affected by diseases of diffusion because of its greater solubility.

## The Pulmonary Blood Supply

The lung is supplied by two circulations, the pulmonary circulation and the bronchial circulation. The pulmonary circulation serves in gas exchange, filters venous blood, provides nutrients for the pulmonary parenchyma, and serves as a reservoir of blood for the left ventricle. In addition, in the pulmonary circulation the pharmacologic properties of many substances are altered and the pulmonary circulation provides a large surface area for liquid absorption. However, the chief function of the pulmonary circulation is to deliver blood to the terminal respiratory units so that gas exchange can occur. Anatomically, the pulmonary circulation is well suited for this function because it consists of inflow and outflow vessels that serve an extensive capillary network which provides an enormous surface area for gas exchange.[60] The pulmonary circulation accommodates almost the entire cardiac output. Yet, compared to the systemic circulation, the perfusion pressure is only about one-fifth of its systemic counterparts. The low pulmonary vascular resistance can be reduced even further because the pulmonary circulation can accommodate large increases in cardiac output with only small increases in pulmonary artery pressure. In humans, a three-fold increase in cardiac output during exercise raises pulmonary artery pressure only about 10 mmHg.[61] However, one report suggests that in the horse heavy exercise may increase pulmonary artery pressure up to 77 mmHg,[62] possibly because the cardiac output increases 7- to 8-fold during exercise. The consequences of this high pulmonary artery pressure during exercise are presently unclear, but it may predispose the horse to developing exercise-induced pulmonary hemorrhage. In most species, the pulmonary circulation is able to accommodate large increases in blood flow without concomitant large changes in perfusion pressure by recruitment of previously underperfused vessels and distension of other vessels.[63] In contrast to the systemic circulation the arterioles of the pulmonary circulation are not the main resistance vessels.[63] This results in pulsatile pulmonary capillary blood flow. Most of the resistance to pulmonary blood flow lies in the capillaries and the remainder resides in arterioles. There is negligible resistance to blood flow in the pulmonary venules.[63]

### *Distribution of Pulmonary Blood Flow*

In order for the lung to serve as an efficient gas exchange organ, the pulmonary blood flow must be distributed in the lung to match ventilation. Gravity significantly influences distribution of blood flow in a species with a large vertical lung height such as the horse. Amis et al. have calculated a vertical gradient of perfusion in the standing horse with the basal portion of the lung receiving more blood flow than the dorsal region.[64] As shown in Figure 1–9, the effect of gravity on distribution of pulmonary blood flow is influenced by pulmonary artery, pulmonary venous, and alveolar pressures.[63] In the dorsal region of the lung (zone 1), alveolar pressure is greater than both pulmonary artery and venous pressures and therefore there is no blood flow to this region. Because the vertical height of the equine lung is approximately 20 to 25 cm above the base of the heart and mean pulmonary artery pressure is approximately 20 to 25 cm of $H_2O$, the size of zone 1 in most horses is small, and in some horses zone 1 conditions may not exist. In zone 2, pulmonary artery pressure exceeds alveolar pressure, but alveolar pressure is greater than pulmonary venous pressure. In zone 2, pulmonary blood flow increases from no flow at the top of the zone to the level at which alveolar and pulmonary venous pressures are equal. Flow in this zone is determined by the difference in pressure between pulmonary artery and pulmonary alveolar pressure and is independent of venous pressure. In zone 3, pulmonary artery pressure is greater than pulmonary venous pressure and alveolar pressure. Blood flow increases from the top to the bottom of this zone because vessels are increasingly distended by hydrostatic pressure. In the most dependent lung region, zone 4, pulmonary blood flow decreases, probably as a result of increased interstitial pressure compressing the blood vessels.

As stated before, the pulmonary artery pressure and pulmonary venous pressure may change dramatically during exercise or with disease. If, during exercise, pulmonary artery pressure rises to up to 77 mmHg,[62] zone 1 conditions will not exist and all lung tissue will be well perfused. Conversely, in hypotensive shock, often seen in horses with colic or severe diarrhea, pulmonary artery pressure is insufficient to perfuse the most dorsal lung regions. Hypoxemia is likely to result.

Lung inflation has an important influence on pulmonary vascular resistance. As the lung inflates, large vessels distend and resistance is reduced. In contrast, capillaries in the alveolar walls are compressed by lung inflation increasing the resistance to blood flow. The net effect is that pulmonary vascular resistance is lowest at lung volumes near functional residual capacity and highest at residual volume and total lung capacity.[63] The effects of lung volume on pulmonary vascular resistance become of clinical importance during anesthesia. In adult horses, both recumbency and anesthesia reduce lung volume,[56] increase pulmonary vascular resistance, and decrease cardiac output. This is compounded

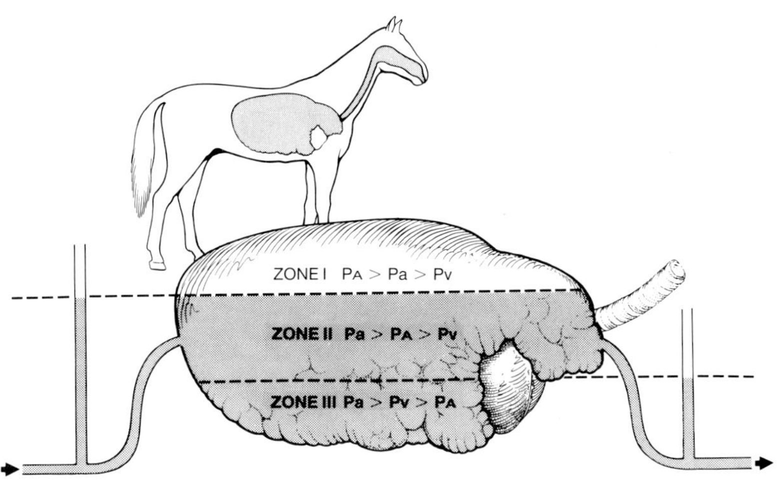


**FIG. 1–9.** Schematic illustration of the effect of gravity on distribution of pulmonary blood flow.

by positive pressure ventilation, which increases alveolar pressure and reduces pulmonary capillary perfusion.

## *Regulation of Pulmonary Vascular Resistance*

As discussed above, even in the normal lung ventilation and perfusion are not homogeneously distributed. Yet precise matching of ventilation and perfusion is necessary to obtain adequate gas exchange. The mechanisms the lung uses to match blood flow with ventilation are not well described. Although the pulmonary circulation receives both sympathetic and parasympathetic innervation, the autonomic nervous system plays only a minor role in the regulation of pulmonary vascular resistance.[63] Under most experimental conditions, parasympathetic stimulation causes vasodilation,[65] while sympathetic stimulation causes modest vasodilation or constriction depending on the presence of vascular tone.[66] Several humoral agents may cause vasoconstriction or vasodilation of the pulmonary vasculature. Angiotensin, histamine, prostaglandin $F_{2\alpha}$ and sulfidopeptide leukotrienes cause vasoconstriction, while prostacycline, isoproterenol, and acetylcholine cause vasodilation.[63,67–70] Yet the importance of these substances in regulating pulmonary vascular tone and matching ventilation with blood flow is unknown.

In contrast, alveolar hypoxia results in vigorous vasoconstriction.[63,71,72] Because alveolar hypoxia occurs in poorly ventilated lung regions, this response helps redistribute pulmonary blood flow to well-ventilated lung regions. The mechanism whereby hypoxia causes vasoconstriction of pulmonary vasculature is unknown, but it is independent of nerve supply because it is not attenuated in isolated perfused lungs.[63] Hypoxic vasoconstriction becomes even more important in disease. Lung regions that are atelectic or consolidated with pneumonia are poorly ventilated and become hypoxic. Hypoxic vasoconstriction redistributes blood flow to more normal regions of the lung.[73] This response explains why lung disease must be severe before arterial hypoxemia is observed.

## *The Bronchial Circulation*

The bronchial circulation receives less than 1% of the cardiac output and provides nutrient blood flow to the structural components of the lung, including the walls of the bronchi, large blood vessels, septa, and pleura.

Following its origin from the bronchoesophageal artery, the bronchial artery follows the tracheobronchial tree to the terminal bronchioles.[74] At the level of the bronchioles, vessels anastomose with the pulmonary circulation.[75] These anastomoses are numerous, especially at the capillary and venular levels. The bronchial circulation is drained via either the azygos or pulmonary veins.

Because of its small size, the bronchial circulation has generally been ignored. The suggestion that the bronchial circulation is unimportant in normal animals has been strengthened by experiments which have shown that ligation of the bronchial artery had no long-term demonstrable effects.[74] However, in disease the bronchial circulation may become important. It has been shown that gas exchange can be maintained when the pulmonary circulation is obstructed.[76] As the blood pressure in the pulmonary circulation decreases, blood is diverted from the bronchial circulation through the numerous pulmonary-bronchial anastomoses into the pulmonary circulation. In addition, the bronchial circulation is involved in repair of lung injury.[74] Following lung injury, the bronchial blood supply infiltrates the affected lung region, providing nutrients used in the healing process.[74] Recently extensive proliferation of the bronchial circulation has been described in the dorsal lung region of horses with exercise induced pulmonary hemorrhage (EIPH).[77] It was suggested that EIPH originates from the bronchial circulation.

## Evaluation of Oxygen Exchange in the Lung

In disease, strategies that the lung uses for efficient gas exchange are insufficient and hypoxemia results. For the equine clinician, measurement of arterial blood gas tension is the most practical method to assess ventilation and quantitatively evaluate the function of the horse lung. Therefore, it is important to understand how lung disease causes hypoxemia and how changes in ventilation alter blood gas tensions. When evaluating oxygen exchange, the clinician asks how effectively the lung is able to transfer oxygen from the alveolar air to the blood. This question can be answered if oxygen tension in the arterial blood ($Pa_{O_2}$) and oxygen tension in the alveolar air ($P_{AO_2}$) are known. If the difference between the $P_{AO_2}$ and $Pa_{O_2}$ is small, the lung is an efficient gas exchanger and unlikely to be affected by serious disease. However, if this difference is large, the lung functions inefficiently. Let us first look at the interpretation of arterial blood gas tensions and then relate this understanding to the $P_{AO_2}$.

For the equine clinician, the first step in evaluating gas exchange function of the lung is the measurement of oxygen tension ($Pa_{O_2}$) and carbon dioxide tension in the arterial blood ($Pa_{CO_2}$). In the adult horse, arterial blood may be collected from the common carotid or facial artery. In foals, the carotid artery or greater metatarsal artery is commonly used. Following collection in a heparinized syringe, all air should be expelled and the syringe sealed. The sample may be stored on ice for several hours before analysis.

The $Pa_{CO_2}$ does not yield information regarding gas exchange in the lung but instead is a measure of alveolar ventilation. The relationship between $Pa_{CO_2}$ and alveolar ventilation ($\dot{V}_A$) may be expressed by the following formula:[8]

$$\dot{V}_A = K \frac{\dot{V}_{CO_2}}{Pa_{CO_2}}$$

where $\dot{V}_{CO_2}$ is $CO_2$ production and K is a constant. Thus, the $Pa_{CO_2}$ is inversely related to alveolar ventilation. For example, if the alveolar ventilation is halved and $CO_2$ production remains unchanged, the $Pa_{CO_2}$ will double. The relationship between $Pa_{CO_2}$ and alveolar ventilation has great clinical significance because by measuring $Pa_{CO_2}$ alveolar ventilation can be assessed. Alveolar hypoventilation is encountered in cases of severe airway obstruction, central nervous system depression, or metabolic alkalosis. Alveolar hyperventilation is encountered with anxiety, high environmental temperatures, or metabolic acidosis.

The $Pa_{O_2}$ is determined by alveolar ventilation, inspired oxygen tension, and the gas exchange efficiency of the lung.[78] In normal horses breathing ambient air at sea level, the $Pa_{O_2}$ is 90 to 100 torr. When $Pa_{O_2}$ is decreased and alveolar ventilation is normal, it may be concluded that gas exchange efficiency of the lung has been impaired. Lung disease causes inefficient gas exchange mainly by mismatching of ventilation and perfusion.[78] For example, blood flow may persist through areas of lung consolidation where there is little ventilation. In extreme cases where blood flow passes through the lung without encountering alveolar gases, there is right-to-left shunting. Lastly, lung disease may cause hypoxemia by creating diffusion barriers. In clinical practice diffusion barriers are uncommon causes of hypoxemia. To distinguish between hypoxemia caused by hypoventilation or low inspired oxygen tension and hypoxemia caused by lung dysfunction, the $P_{AO_2}$ must be considered. Under most clinical conditions, the $P_{AO_2}$ can be estimated using the following formula:[78]

$$P_{AO_2} = P_{IO_2} - \frac{P_{ACO_2}}{R} + F$$

where $P_{AO_2}$ is alveolar oxygen tension, $P_{IO_2}$ is inspired oxygen tension, $P_{ACO_2}$ is alveolar carbon dioxide tension, R is the respiratory exchange ratio, and F is a small correction factor. Under most clinically relevant circumstances, the R is assumed to be 0.8, the alveolar $CO_2$ tension is assumed to equal arterial $CO_2$ tension, and F is ignored. At sea level, the $P_{IO_2}$ is approximately 150 torr. Using a normal $Pa_{CO_2}$ of 40 torr the $P_{AO_2}$ may be estimated.

$$P_{AO_2} = 150 - \frac{40}{0.8} = 100 \text{ torr}$$

Assuming a normal $Pa_{O_2}$ = 90 torr, the difference between alveolar and arterial oxygen tension [(A-a) $O_2$] may be calculated.

$$P_{AO_2} - Pa_{O_2} = 100-90 = 10 \text{ torr}$$

Thus, in a normal horse the (A-a)$O_2$ is between 0 to 10 torr. The (A-a)$O_2$ is only increased when gas exchange in the lung is impaired and it is not affected by changes in alveolar ventilation or changes in inspired oxygen tension. In clinical practice calculation of the (A-a)$O_2$ is particularly useful when there are concurrent changes in $Pa_{O_2}$ and $Pa_{CO_2}$ or when the inspired oxygen tension is changed, as is often the case during anesthesia.

# Control of Breathing

When observing a horse during its daily activity such as quiet standing, eating, whinnying, and exercising, it becomes readily apparent that the breathing pattern is highly variable. Yet when arterial blood gas tensions are evaluated, these values vary only slightly. This remarkable achievement indicates that at all times alveolar ventilation is tightly matched with metabolic activity. The matching of alveolar ventilation and metabolic rate is accomplished by a central controller, which receives feedback from peripheral receptors and activates the muscles of respiration.[79]

## *The Central Controller*

The breathing pattern is controlled by groups of neurons located in the pons and the medulla. The respiratory center located in the medulla is responsible for rhythmic respiration. Evidence for this stems from brainstem sectioning experiments which show that rhythmic respiration continues following transection of the brain at the pontal medullary junction and that transection below the medulla results in cessation of breathing.[80] The respiratory center in the medulla may be divided into two groups of neurons. The dorsal respiratory group of neurons located in the ventral lateral portion of the nucleus tractus solitarious is mainly inspiratory neurons. This dorsal respiratory group of neurons receives information from the ninth and tenth cranial nerves and passes on information to the muscles of respiration as well as a ventral respiratory group of neurons located near the nucleus ambiguous and nucleus retroambiguous. This group of neurons has both inspiratory and expiratory neurons. Axons from the ventral respiratory group of neurons project to the many accessory muscles of respiration. The activity of the respiratory neurons in the medulla is modulated by two respiratory centers in the pons. Neurons in the apneustic center located in the lower pons stimulate inspiratory neurons in the medulla.[81] In experimental animals, sectioning just above the apneustic center results in prolonged inspiratory gasps interrupted by transient expiratory efforts called apneustic breathing.[82] This breathing pattern may be observed in adult horses with central nervous system trauma such as skull fractures and in some foals with neonatal maladjustment syndrome.

The pneumotaxic center located in the upper pons switches off inspiration. This center receives afferent inputs from the vagus nerve and influences the response to hypoxia, hypercapnea, and lung inflation.[83]

## *Sensors*

In order for the horse's respiratory system to meet the ever-changing metabolic demands, sensors must be in place and able to give the respiratory control centers feedback about the results of adjustments in ventilation. The respiratory system is equipped with chemoreceptors in the arterial blood and mechanoreceptors in the lungs designed to give the needed feedback information. Peripheral chemoreceptors are located in the carotid bodies at the bifurcation of the common carotid arteries and in the aortic bodies near the aortic arch.[84] Each of these bodies is composed of receptor cells (Type 1 cells) and supporting cells (Type 2 cells).[84] Normally, the chemoreceptors are tonically active, sending afferent impulses to the respiratory control center via the glossopharyngeal and vagus nerves. Chemoreceptor activity is enhanced by hypoxemia, hypercapnea, and acidemia.

The response of these receptors to $Pa_{O_2}$ is alinear. As the inspiratory oxygen concentration decreases from 100 to 16%, there is little change in minute ventilation.[85] Only when the inspired oxygen content decreases below 15% and $PA_{O_2}$ below 60 torr is minute ventilation greatly enhanced. Peripheral chemoreceptor activity is not sensitive to oxygen content of the arterial blood, and hemoglobin concentration must fall to extremely low levels before they are activated.

The central chemoreceptors are located near the ventral aspect of the medulla.[86,87] Denervation of peripheral chemoreceptors abolishes the ventilatory response of hypoxia but only slightly attenuates the response to increased $Pa_{CO_2}$.[86] Thus, while the peripheral chemoreceptors are mainly responsible for increased ventilation in response to hypoxemia, the central chemoreceptors are most important in sensing changes in $Pa_{CO_2}$.[86,87] The central chemoreceptors are bathed in intracerebral interstitial fluid.[88] This fluid is separated from the blood by the blood brain barrier. This barrier is freely permeable to $CO_2$ and the response to $CO_2$ is probably through acidification of the intracerebral interstitial fluid. In contrast, hydrogen ions cannot easily cross the blood brain barrier. Therefore, acute changes in blood pH cannot be recognized by the central chemoreceptors and the ventilatory response to acute acidosis is attributed to the peripheral chemoreceptors. Acute changes in blood pH take several minutes to be manifested in cerebral interstitial fluid.[89] In the horse, conditions that result in acidosis, such as diarrhea, dehydration or colic, usually develop over several hours. This allows sufficient time for activation of the central chemoreceptors. Because the central chemoreceptors are more sensitive to pH changes than the peripheral chemoreceptors, the ventilatory response to metabolic acidosis in the horse is probably relayed mainly through central chemoreceptors.

Understanding of chemoreceptor function is particularly important when dealing with foals suffering from a combination of respiratory disease and acid base disturbances. Foals with severe respiratory disease commonly are hypoxemic, hypercapnic, and acidemic. Oxygen therapy alone not only will alleviate the hypoxemia, but also remove the hypoxemic respiratory drive. This results in a further increase in $Pa_{CO_2}$ and acidosis, and may decompensate the patient. In contrast, bicarbonate therapy alone increases peripheral blood pH, thereby reducing ventilatory drive as well. This results in worsening of the hypoxemia and hypercapnea. Thus, when treating horses with disturbances in gas exchange and acid base imbalances, therapy should be based on a working knowledge of chemoreceptor responses.

Within the lung there are three kinds of receptors that may influence respiration.[90] The pulmonary stretch receptor is located in the dorsal tracheal smooth muscle and in the smooth muscles surrounding the bronchi. Pulmonary stretch receptors have afferent myelinated nerve fibers traveling in the vagus nerve. Receptor activity is increased as the lung inflates, resulting in inhibition of further inspiratory activity.[91] Thus, pulmonary stretch receptors adjust the depth and consequently the rate of breathing so that the mechanical work of breathing is minimized. In the pony, cooling the vagus nerve results in slow, deep breathing, probably as a result of blockade of stretch receptors' nerve fibers.[92]

Irritant receptors and their myelinated nerve fibers are probably unimportant in regulation of breathing in a normal resting horse. However, they respond to a variety of stimulants such as inhalation of gaseous materials, dusts, immunologic reactions in the lung, and chemical mediators such as histamine and prostaglandins.[91,93] The reflex responses to stimulation of irritant receptors are tachypnea, bronchoconstriction, coughing, and increased mucus secretion. In experimental models of lung disease of the horse, such as ovalbumin-induced allergic lung disease and 3-methylindole induced pulmonary toxicosis, tachypnea caused by lung injury could be completely abolished by vagal blockade, suggesting the involvement of pulmonary receptors in the pathogenesis of the diseases.[15,42] In viral or bacterial pulmonary diseases of the horse tachypnea, bronchoconstriction and increased mucus production are common. It is likely that, in part, they are due to irritant receptor stimulation. Irritant receptors are located just below and between the epithelial cells lining the conducting airways.[91] Viral and bacterial infections that affect epithelium, or allergic conditions that expose irritant receptors may result in receptor stimulation, which persists long after the inciting agent(s) is (are) gone. This may explain, in part, the persistence of clinical signs of exercise intolerance, coughing, and excessive mucus production in many cases of seemingly uncomplicated viral infections.

C fiber receptors and their unmyelinated fibers are located in the pulmonary parenchyma, conducting airways, and blood vessels.[91,94] These receptors play no role in the control of breathing in normal animals, but respond to pulmonary edema, congestion and chemical mediators such as bradykinins. The importance of C fiber receptors in lung injury in horses is unknown.

## Lung Metabolism

The lung has enormous endothelial surface area, which is constantly in contact with the circulating blood. Endothelial cells not only function as a physical barrier, but also are active metabolically. In the last decade, it has become apparent that the lung serves important metabolic functions. As blood traverses through the lung, a large number of bioactive substances are removed. For example, serotonin, bradykinin, adenosine, prostaglandin $E_2$ and $F_{2\alpha}$ and leukotrienes are almost completely removed from the circulation after one passage through the lungs.[95–97] Other substances such as dopamine, histamine, and prostaglandin $A_2$ are unaffected by the pulmonary endothelium.[97–99]

The pulmonary endothelium may also convert a substrate to its biologically active form. For example, angiotensin I is converted to angiotensin II by angiotensin converting enzyme located in the pulmonary endothelium. Although some angiotensin converting enzyme may be found in systemic vascular endothelium, the majority is localized in the pulmonary endothelium.[100]

The lung with its large variety of cell types produces many substances important in local control of its function. These substances include histamine, vasoactive intestinal peptide, substance P and products of arachidonic acid metabolism. Little is known about the local metabolism of these products and their role in lung function in health and disease; however, because of their potential importance in the pathogenesis of a variety of lung diseases, some aspects of arachidonic acid metabolism in the lung warrant discussion.

## *Arachidonic Acid Metabolism in the Lung*

The cyclooxygenase and lipoxygenase pathways of arachidonic acid metabolism are shown in Figure 1–10. Arachidonate is released from the cell membrane by the action of phospholipases, especially phospholipase $A_2$.[101] Subsequently, a microsomal cyclooxygenase may generate the endoperoxide intermediates $PgG_2$ and $PgH_2$, which are then converted by enzymes into primary prostaglandins, thromboxane $A_2$ ($TxA_2$) or prostacycline.[102] Different cell types exhibit qualitative as well as quantitative differences in the biosynthesis of arachidonate metabolites, suggesting the existence of cell-specific metabolic pathways. For example, the predominant cyclooxygenase-derived product of mast calls and basophils is $PgD_2$, of neutrophils and mononuclear leukocytes $PgE_2$, and of vascular endothelium $PgI_2$.[103–105]

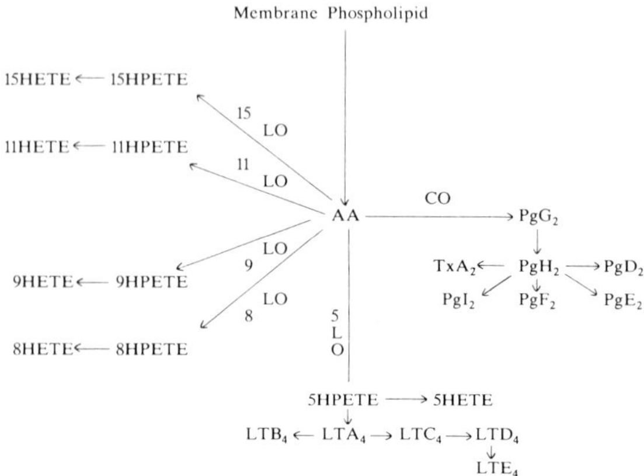


**FIG. 1–10.** Cyclooxygenase and lipoxygenase pathways of arachidonic acid metabolism.

The primary prostaglandins, including $PgE_2$, $PgD_2$ and $PgF_{2\alpha}$, are rapidly formed in the lung. Generally, the prostaglandins of the E series cause bronchodilation, while $PgD_2$ and the prostaglandins of the F series cause bronchoconstriction.[102,106] Thromboxane $A_2$ synthesis has also been demonstrated in the lung. In combination with potent vasopressor activity, $TxA_2$ administration results in marked bronchoconstriction. In ponies with recurrent airway obstruction (heaves), we recently demonstrated an increase in plasma thromboxane concentration during a time period when animals showed clinical signs of disease. However, pretreatment of these animals with flunixin meglumine, which blocked the rise in plasma thromboxane concentration, did not prevent airway obstruction or airway hyperresponsiveness. This suggests that cyclooxygenase products of arachidonic acid metabolism may not be important in the pathogenesis of heaves in horses.

Arachidonate may also be metabolized through the various lipoxygenase pathways, resulting in the biosynthesis of the hydroperoxyeicosatetraenoic acids (HPETE), the mono and dihydroeicosatetraenoic acids (HETE), and the leukotrienes.[107] These eicosanoids may be biosynthesized by a variety of cells including neutrophils, basophils, eosinophils, macrophages, and pulmonary epithelium. The 5-lipoxygenation of arachidonic acid is especially active in neutrophils producing 5-HPETE, which may be converted to 5-HETE or $LTA_4$. From $LTA_4$, subsequent pathways lead to $LTB_4$ or to the cystein-containing leukotrienes, including $LTC_4$, $LTD_4$, and $LTE_4$.[108] Leukotrienes $C_4$, $D_4$, and $E_4$ are now known to be the slow reacting substance of anaphylaxis (SRS-A).

The metabolic products of the 5-lipoxygenase pathways have been studied extensively. Numerous in vivo and in vitro studies have demonstrated that $LTB_4$ is a potent chemotactic agent.[109] While $LTC_4$, $LTD_4$, and $LTE_4$ are not important as chemotactic agents, they exert powerful effects on mucus secretion, lung mechanics, and gas exchange.[110] These sulfidopeptide leukotrienes are especially potent smooth muscle constricting agents, being up to $1000\times$ as potent as histamine.[110]

15-HETE, a product of 15-lipoxygenase, is a potent secretagogue and causes airway inflammation.[111] An increase in plasma 15-HETE concentration was recently demonstrated in ponies with recurrent airway obstruction during a period of exacerbation of lung disease.[112] The role of 15-HETE in the pathogenesis of COPD is presently under investigation.

The cyclooxygenase and lipoxygenase pathways of arachidonic acid metabolism are susceptible to pharmacologic blockade by a variety of drugs. Cyclooxygenase blockade may be produced by aspirin-like drugs such as phenylbutazone, flunixin meglumine, and indomethacin.[113] Specific lipoxygenase inhibitors are not available for use in horses, but several experimental compounds are presently under development. It appears likely that in the future lipoxygenase inhibitors will be part of the equine veterinarian's therapeutic arsenal.

## Pulmonary Defense Mechanisms

The respiratory system of the horse, with its enormous surface area, is constantly exposed to ambient air containing numerous potentially harmful particles including viruses, bacteria, allergens, chemical and physical agents. To prevent pulmonary injury, mechanisms have been devised to efficiently remove these agents from the lungs. Some of these clearance mechanisms are nonspecific and are able to remove particles regardless of their composition. Other clearance mechanisms are specific, and a recognition of the challenging agent is required before clearance is initiated.

Pulmonary diseases result when defensive mechanisms are overwhelmed and noxious agents are able to establish themselves in the lung. Conversely, once pulmonary disease has been established, defensive mechanisms may be affected by the disease process and lung disease may be exacerbated or prolonged. Because of their importance in disease, there is a clear need to understand how noxious agents are deposited in the lung and how the respiratory system handles airborne challenges.

## Aerosol Deposition in the Lung

Aerosols are groups of particles that, because of their low settling velocity, may remain suspended in air for a prolonged period of time. Large aerosol particles greater than 10 μ in size settle as a result of inertial impaction and are primarily filtered out in the upper respiratory system or at bifurcations in the large airways. Smaller particles settle by sedimentation which occurs in the region of the respiratory tract where linear airflow velocity is decreased—the small airways and gas exchange regions of the lung.[114] Particles less than 0.5 μ in size generally remain suspended in air and are exhaled. Thus, particles between 1 and 5 μ in size are able to penetrate deep within the lung and potentially cause disease in the bronchioles or gas exchange regions.[114] Other physical characteristics of particles in air affect their deposition in the lung. Some particles are hydrophilic, attract water as they travel in the airways, and are deposited in more central airways. Other particles are cigar-shaped and, in spite of a length greater than 10 μ, these particles' aerodynamic characteristics may allow deposition deep within the lung.

The pattern of breathing is of great importance in determining where aerosol is deposited on the respiratory mucosa. Rapid, shallow breathing favors deposition in the upper airway, while deep breathing encourages aerosol delivery to bronchioles and gas exchange regions of the lung.[115] Thus, exercising horses breathing polluted air are more likely to suffer respiratory injury than their sedentary counterparts.

It has been estimated that hay may contain up to 5000 respirable particles per mg.[6] Because of the horse's eating habits, which involve shaking the hay loose before eating, the respiratory tract of hay-fed horses is exposed to tremendous numbers of particles. Therefore it is not surprising that the incidence of respiratory disease in horses housed in barns and fed hay is particularly high.

## The Mucociliary System

The respiratory tract is covered with a double layer of mucus, a sol layer and a gel layer. This mucus is propelled toward the pharynx by ciliated cells[116] (Fig. 1–11). Any particle that deposits on the mucus is carried toward the pharynx and swallowed. All surfaces of the upper and lower respiratory tract are covered with ciliated epithelium except some portions of the nose, which have squamous epithelium, and the olfactory area, which has a specialized sensory epithelium.[117] The intrathoracic airways are ciliated to the respiratory bronchioles.[117]

Each ciliated cell has a diameter of approximately 5 μ and carries about 200 cilia at a density of 6 to 8/$\mu m^2$. The cilia are about 6 μ long in the large airways and length decreases to 5 μ in the bronchioles.[117] A cilium contains a central microtubular doublet and 9 surrounding pairs of microtubules (doublets). The doublets are linked by areas of nexin and have 2 dynein areas and 1 centrally directed spoke. The tip of the cilium supports 3 to 7 short claws 25 to 35 nm long.[117]

Impaired ciliary motion associated with ultrastructural defects has been described in man and dogs and predisposes to multiple respiratory infections.[118,119]

Cilia propel fluids because the cyclic movements they perform are asymmetric. During the effective stroke, the cilia remain fully extended and the sol layer is of such a depth that the tips of the cilia contact the gel layer. On the recovery stroke, a bend is propagated along the length of the cilium from base to tip so that the cilium swings back near the cell surface to reach the starting position for the next effective stroke. Cilia of adjacent cells appear to be coordinated so that waves of effective surface motion spread in the appropriate direction. How adjacent ciliated cells coordinate their movement is unknown.

The composition of respiratory tract mucus is critical for effective ciliary function. Respiratory mucus is a complex mixture of glycoproteins, proteoglycans, and lipids. The glycoproteins and proteoglycans associate closely to form the main structural component of the viscoelastic gel layer.[120] At the various

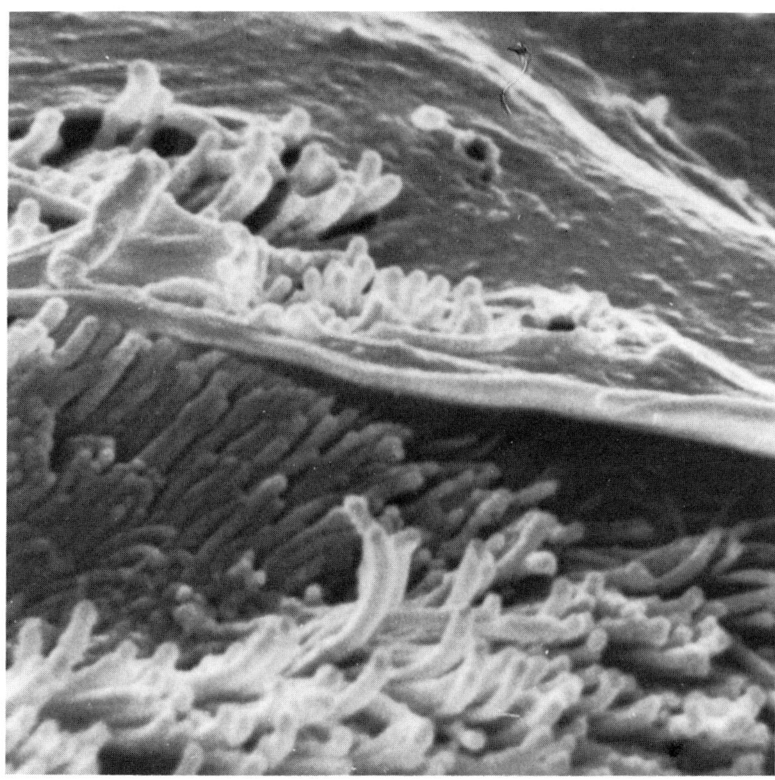

**FIG. 1–11.** Rabbit trachea showing details of the mucus blanket overlying the ciliated epithelium. Note that the mucus is clearly situated at the tip of the cilia (×13,270) (Micrograph courtesy of Dr. J.M. Sturgess; from Sturgess JM. The mucous lining of major bronchi in the rabbit lung. Am Rev Respir Dis, *115*:819, 1977.)

airway generations, different cells contribute to this fluid lining. In the terminal bronchioles and alveoli, the secretion is mainly serous in nature and may be in part produced by the clara cells.[121] Goblet cells first appear in the bronchioles and contribute a viscous secretion. This secretion forms a gel layer over the sol layer which traps particles and protects the sol layer from desiccation. In the central airways this gel is continuous, while in distal airways mucus rafts may float on the sol layer.[122] In the bronchi there are submucosal glands which are major contributors to the fluid lining of the airways. The submucosal glands contain both serous and goblet cells.[123] Myoepithelial cells, which are closely apposed to the secretory cells, aid the movement of secretions into the airway lumen.[123] In mammalian species that have been studied, goblet cells in the airway epithelium become more numerous with age, presumably in response to chronic irritation.[124]

The control of mucus secretion is poorly understood. It has been observed that if ciliated epithelium is left undisturbed, mucus secretion ceases and the cilia are left surrounded only by a low viscosity sol layer.[125] When a small particle is dropped onto the ciliated surface, mucus is secreted around the particle and it is carried away on a raft of mucus. Thus, mucus production may occur in response to mechanical stimulation, and this would explain the continuous blanket of mucus found in the central airways where more airborne particles are likely to impact, compared to more peripheral airways.[116]

Mucus secretion is increased by parasympathetic stimulation, whereas parasympatholytic agents like atropine decrease secretion.[126] Although parasympathetic stimulation has little effect on ciliary movement directly, cholinergic drugs stimulate mucociliary transport indirectly as increased mucus secretion stimulates ciliary motility.[117] Alpha adrenergic stimulation causes secretion from serous cells of the submucosal glands, while β stimulation increases mucus production. Beta adrenergic agonists stimulate ciliary movement directly.[127]

In disease the composition of mucus may be altered, thereby affecting mucociliary clearance and predisposing the lung to infections. Dehydration reduces the thickness of the sol layer, preventing effective ciliary motility. Infectious processes may increase the viscosity of the gel layer, making it more difficult for the cilia to propel.

## *Pulmonary Macrophages*

The most important clearance mechanism in the airways is the mucociliary transport system. The alveoli, however, have no ciliated cells. Particles deposited on the enormous alveolar surface are avidly phagocytosed and cleared by alveolar macrophages.[128] Alveolar macrophages may originate from the bone marrow and reach the lung via the blood as monocytes.[129] Within the pulmonary interstitium there is also a pool of cells from which macrophages may be derived.[130] The importance of this local production of macrophages in the dynamics of the pulmonary macrophage population is presently unknown. The mechanism whereby alveolar macrophages locate particles for phagocytosis is also unclear. Phagocytosis and killing of viable particles are facilitated by the presence of opsonins, lysozyme, interferon, and complement in the respiratory tract secretions.

Like other phagocytes, alveolar macrophages contain lysosomes which attach themselves to the phagosomal membrane surrounding the ingested pathogen. Subsequently the lysosomal membrane becomes continuous with the phagosomal membrane and the lysosomal enzymes enter the phagosome to kill and digest the organisms.

Among the enzymes known to be present in lysosomes are proteases, acid ribonuclease, β glucuronidase, acid phosphatase, lysozyme, β galactosidase, and phospholipases.[128] More important to the antimicrobial activity of macrophages than the lytic enzymes is the oxygen dependent cytotoxic system. Phagocytosis triggers increased oxygen consumption and the generation of oxygen radicals such as superoxide, hydroxyl radicals, singlet oxygen, and hydrogen peroxide. These oxygen radicals are potent toxins to lipids, proteins, and nucleic acids, thereby killing microorganisms.[128]

Once phagocytosed, particles may be digested by the macrophage or transported out of the lung. Most activated macrophages are removed via the mucociliary transport system. Some penetrate the alveolar interstitium and are removed via the lymphatic system.

Although macrophages located on the alveolar surface are most important, macrophages are also present in the airways, interstitium, and vasculature. Presumably, the role these macrophages play in the defense of the lung is similar to that of the alveolar macrophage.

Alveolar macrophage function may be depressed in disease. These highly specialized cells have become adapted to an oxygen rich environment. When portions of the lung become diseased, local areas of hypoxia commonly occur, and in these lung areas alveolar macrophage function is depressed. Alveolar macrophage function is also decreased by high levels of endogenous steroids produced by the horse in stressful situations such as athletic competition or shipping over long distances.[131] This may explain the high incidence of infectious pulmonary disease and subsequent pleuritis in horses exposed to these stresses. Exogenous steroid administration, virus infections, air pollution and inhalation of silica dust can also suppress macrophage function[132,133] and similarly predispose the horse to infectious pulmonary diseases.

Macrophages do not kill all organisms with the same efficiency. For example, Rhodococcus equi can remain viable in alveolar macrophages and thereby is protected against humoral immunity.[134] This explains why Rhodococcus equi pneumonia is resistant and why antibiotic therapy of Rhodococcus equi infection can be effective only if the antibiotic chosen efficiently penetrates this cell.

While alveolar macrophages are the most prominent phagocytic cell in the lung, there normally is also a population of neutrophils, eosinophils, and lymphocytes.[135] A dramatic increase in these cell types is a hallmark of pulmonary inflammation. In response to chemotactic agents, these inflammatory cells can quickly migrate into the pulmonary interstitium and air spaces and assist the alveolar macrophage in phagocytosis. In some cases the influx of inflammatory cells into the lung is inappropriate and proteolytic enzymes or toxic oxygen radicals released in the lung may actually be a cause of pulmonary injury.[136]

## *Specific Lung Defense*

In addition to nonspecific defenses, the lung has available immunologic responses that may be used to specifically select offending antigenic material and eliminate it. The alveolar macrophage is the link between the specific and nonspecific pulmonary defense mechanisms. The immune response, whether cellular or humoral, starts with the presentation of antigenic materials by the phagocytic cell to appropriate lymphocytes or plasma cells.

Lymphocytes and plasma cells are found in the walls and air spaces throughout the respiratory system. Collections of lymphoid tissues beneath the bronchial mucosa and covered by nonciliated epithelium is called bronchus-associated lymphoid tissue (BALT).[137] The BALT is strategically located near major airway bifurcations to sample antigenic material presented by alveolar macrophages and plays an important role in both humoral and cellular lung defenses.[138] Bronchus-associated lymphoid tissue is presented at birth, but it becomes more abundant with age, probably in response to cumulative antigenic stimulation. Smaller aggregates of lymphoid cells also populate the terminal and respiratory bronchioles. In addition, free lymphocytes can be harvested from the air spaces of the horse lung.[135] In other species most of these cells are T lymphocytes, but B lymphocytes capable of producing antibodies are also abundant.[139]

Secretions in horse airways contain all classes of immunoglobulin except IgM.[135] Secretory IgA is the predominant immunoglobulin in the upper respiratory tract.[140] Secretory IgA is a dimer of two serum IgA molecules, linked by a secretory component and a joining chain. Monomeric IgA and J chain are synthesized in the mucosa, and assembled and secreted into the airway lumen by epithelial cells.[141] Secretory IgA is of critical importance in local humoral defense of the respiratory tract and vaccine failure has been attributed to failure to induce local IgA production by the vaccine.

Immunoglobulin G and IgGT are abundant in bronchoalveolar lavage fluid of horses.[135] IgG is a potent opsonising antibody and may assist in bacterial killing by fixing of complement.

IgE molecules are attached to the surface of mast cells. In other species, the role of IgE in the development of allergic lung disease is well recognized. In the horse the involvement of IgE in disease processes is unclear as is its role in the defense of the normal lung.

Because most of the lymphocytes in the lung are T lymphocytes, it is likely that cell mediated immunity is critical to defense of the lung against invading organisms. Cytotoxic T cells specific for viral antigens have been described in the lungs of experimental animals. Little information is available about cell mediated immunity in the equine lung.

This chapter reviewed the mechanisms of airflow through the upper and lower respiratory tract, the production and function of surfactant, the autonomic control of airway caliber, the process of gas exchange, the control of breathing, lung metabolism, and pulmonary defense mechanisms. It is hoped that this will provide the reader with the working knowledge needed to understand the pathogenesis of respiratory diseases and therapeutic approaches described in the following chapters.

## References


1. Robinson NE, Sorenson PR. Pathophysiology of airway obstruction in horses: A review. J Am Vet Med Assoc, *172*:299, 1978.
2. Willoughby RA, McDonell WN. Pulmonary function testing in horses. Vet Clin N Am Symposium on Equine Respiratory Disease. Philadelphia, WB Saunders Co, *1*:171, 1979.
3. Derksen FJ, Stick JA, Scott EA, et al. Effect of laryngeal hemiplegia and laryngoplasty on airway flow mechanisms in exercising horses. Am J Vet Res, *47*:16, 1986.
4. Shappell KK, Derksen FJ, Stick JA, et al. Effect of ventriculectomy, prosthetic laryngoplasty and exercise on upper airway function in horses with left laryngeal hemiplegia. Am J Vet Res, *49*:1760, 1988.
5. Gehr P, Mwangi DK, Ammann A, et al. Design of the mammalian respiratory system v. scaling morphometric pulmonary diffusing capacity to body

mass: Wild and domestic mammals. Respir Physiol, *44*:61, 1981.
6. Clarke AF, Madelin T. Technique for assessing respiratory health hazards from hay and other source materials. Equine Vet J, *19*:442, 1987.
7. Murray JF. The Normal Lung. Philadelphia, WB Saunders Co, 1986, pp 83–119.
8. West JB. Respiratory Physiology—The Essentials. Baltimore, Williams & Wilkins, 1985, pp 15–20.
9. Derksen FJ, Robinson NE, Slocombe RF, et al. Pulmonary function in standing ponies: Reproducibility and effect of vagal blockade. Am J Vet Res, 43:598, 1982.
10. Mead J, Whittenberger JL. Physical properties of human lungs measured during spontaneous respiration. J Appl Physiol, *5*:779, 1953.
11. Weibel ER. Functional morphology of lung parenchyma. Handbook of Physiology, Vol III, Part 1. Bethesda, MD, American Physiological Society, 1986, pp 89–111.
12. Leith DE. Comparative mammalian respiratory mechanics. Physiologist, 19:405, 1976.
13. Koterba AM, Kosch PC, Beech J, et al. The breathing strategy of the adult horse (equus Caballus) at rest. J Appl Physiol, *64*:337, 1988.
14. Derksen FJ, Slocombe RF, Brown CM, et al. Chronic restrictive lung disease in a horse. J Am Vet Med Assoc, *180*:887, 1982.
15. Derksen FJ, Robinson NE, Slocombe RF, et al. 3-Methylindole-induced pulmonary toxicosis in ponies. Am J Vet Res, *43*:603, 1982.
16. Von Neergaard K. Neue Auffassungen über einen Grund-begriff der Atemmechanik. Die Retractionskraft der Lunge abhänging von der Oberflächenspannungen in den Alveolen. Z Gesamte Exp Med, *66*:373, 1929.
17. Brown ES, Johnson RP, Clements JA. Pulmonary surface tension. J Appl Physiol, *14*:717, 1959.
18. Clements JA, Nellenbogen J, Traham HJ. Pulmonary surfactant and evolution of the lungs. Science, *169*:603, 1970.
19. Goerke J, Clements JA. Alveolar surface tension and lung surfactant. Handbook of Physiology: The Respiratory System, Vol III, Part 1. Bethesda, MD, American Physiological Society, 1986, p 247.
20. Rooney SA. The surfactant system and lung phospholipid biochemistry. Am Rev Respir Dis, *131*:439, 1985.
21. Avery ME, Mead J. Surface properties in relation to atelectasis and hyaline membrane disease. Am J Dis Child, *97*:517, 1959.
22. Clements JA, Hustead RF, Johnson RP, et al. Pulmonary surface tension lining and alveolar stability. J Appl Physiol, *16*:444, 1961.
23. King RJ, Clements JA. Surface active materials from dog lungs. II Composition and physiological correlations. Am J Physiol, *223*:715, 1972.
24. King RJ, Clements JA. Lipid synthesis and surfactant turnover in the lungs. Handbook of Physiology: The Respiratory System, Vol 1. Bethesda MD, American Physiological Society, 1986, p 309.
25. Arvidson G, Astedt B, Ekelund L, et al. Surfactant studies in the fetal and neonatal foal. J Reprod Fert (suppl), *23*:663, 1975.
26. Pattle RE, Rossdale PD, Schock C, et al. The development of the lung and its surfactant in the foal and in other species. J Reprod Fert (suppl), *23*:651, 1975.
27. Gluck L, Kulovich MV, Borer RC, et al. The interpretation and significance of the lecithin/sphingomyelin ratio in amnionic fluid. Am J Obstet Gynecol, *120*:142, 1974.
28. Paradis MR. Lecithin/sphingomyelin ratios and phosphatidyl-glycerol in term and premature equine amnionic fluid. In: Proceedings of 5th American Veterinary Medical Forum, San Diego, 1987, p 789.
29. Rooney SA, Gobran LI, Mario PA, et al. Effects of betamethasone on phospholipid content composition and biosynthesis in the fetal rabbit lung. Biochem Biophys Acta, *572*:64, 1979.
30. Gross I, Dynia DW, Wilson CM, et al. Glucocorticoid-thyroid hormone interactions in fetal rat lung. Pediatr Res, *18*:191, 1984.
31. Khosla SS, Gobran LI, Rooney SA. Stimulation of phosphatidylcholine synthesis by 17β estradiol in fetal rabbit lung. Biochem Biophys Acta, *H617*:282, 1980.
32. Hallman M, Merritt TA, Schneider H, et al. Isolation of human surfactant from amnionic fluid and a pilot study of its efficacy in respiratory distress syndrome. Pediatrics, *71*:473, 1983.
33. Hallman M, Merritt TA, Jarvenpaa AL, et al. Exogenous human surfactant for the treatment of severe respiratory distress syndrome: A randomized prospective clinical trial. J Pediatr, *106*:963, 1985.
34. Kwong MS, Egan EA, Notter RH, et al. Double-blind clinical trial of calf lung surfactant extract for prevention of hyaline membrane disease in extremely premature infants. Pediatrics, *76*:585, 1985.
35. Derksen FJ, Robinson NE. Esophageal and intrapleural pressures in the healthy conscious pony. Am J Vet Res, *41*:1756, 1980.
36. Macklem PT, Mead J. Resistance of central and peripheral airways measured by retrograde catheter. J Appl Physiol, *22*:395, 1967.
37. Breeze RG. Heaves. The problem of disease definition. Vet Clin North Am, *1*:219, 1979.
38. Derksen FJ, Scott D, Robinson NE, et al. Intravenous histamine administration in ponies with recurrent airway obstruction (heaves). Am J Vet Res, *46*:774, 1985.
39. Woolcock AJ, Macklem PT, Hogg JC, et al. Effect of vagal stimulation on central and peripheral airways in dogs. J Appl Physiol, *26*:806, 1969.
40. Leff AR, Munoz NM, Tallet J, et al. Autonomic responses characteristics of porcine airway smooth muscle in vivo. J Appl Physiol, *58*:1176, 1985.
41. Barnes PJ. Neural control of human airways in health and disease. Am Rev Respir Dis, *134*:1289, 1986.
42. Derksen FJ, Robinson NE, Slocombe RF. Ovalbumin induced allergic lung disease in the pony: Role of vagal mechanisms. J Appl Physiol, *53*:719, 1982.

43. Broadstone RV, Scott JS, Derksen FJ, et al. Effects of atropine on lung function and airway reactivity in ponies with chronic airway disease. FASEB proceedings, 1988, p A1184.
44. Barnes PJ, Basbaum CB, Nadel JA, et al. Localization of beta-adrenoreceptors in mammalian lung by light microscopic autoradiography. Nature, *299*:444, 1982.
45. Mason DE, Muir WW, Olson LE. In vitro responses of equine trachealis muscle to electrical stimulation and exogenous acetylcholine. In: Proceedings of 5th Veterinary Respiration Symposium, Chicago, IL, 1987, p 7.
46. Danser AHJ, Van den Ende R, Lorenz RR, et al. Prejunctional $\beta_1$-adrenoceptors inhibit cholinergic transmission in canine bronchi. J Appl Physiol, *62*:785, 1987.
47. Derksen FJ, Scott JS, Slocombe RF, et al. Effect of clenbuterol on histamine-induced airway obstruction in ponies. Am J Vet Res, *48*:423, 1987.
48. Snapper JR, Braasch PS, Ingram RH, et al. Effects of beta adrenergic blockade on histamine and prostaglandin $F_{2\alpha}$ responsiveness in dogs. J Allergy Clin Immunol, *67*:199, 1981.
49. Russell JA. Differential inhibitory effect of isoproterenol on contractions of canine airways. J Appl Physiol, *57*:801, 1984.
50. Scott JS, Broadstone RV, Derksen RJ, et al. Beta adrenergic blockade in ponies with recurrent obstructive pulmonary disease. J Appl Physiol, *64*:2324, 1988.
51. Barnes PJ, Basbaum CB, Nadel JA. Autoradiographic localization of autonomic receptors in airway smooth muscle. Am Rev Respir Dis, *127*:758, 1983.
52. Scott JS, Garon HI, Broadstone RV, et al. Alpha 1 adrenergic induced airway obstruction in ponies with recurrent pulmonary disease. J Appl Physiol, *65*:687, 1988.
53. Irvin CG, Martin RR, Macklem PT. Nonpurinergic nature and efficacy of nonadrenergic bronchodilation. J Appl Physiol, *52*:562, 1982.
54. Milic-Emili J. Static distribution of lung volumes. In: Handbook of Physiology: The Respiratory System, Vol III, mechanics of breathing. AP Fishman, PT Macklem, J Mead, et al (eds). Bethesda, MD, American Physiological Society, 1986, pp 561–574.
55. Olson LE, Lai Fook SJ. Pleural liquid pressure measured with rib capsules in anesthetized ponies. J Appl Physiol, *64*:102, 1988.
56. Soronson PR, Robinson NE. Postural effects on lung volumes and asynchronous ventilation in anesthetized horses. J Appl Physiol, *48*:97, 1980.
57. Weibel ER, Taylor CR, Gehr P, et al. Design of the mammalian respiratory system IX. Functional and structural limits for oxygen flow. Respir Physiol, *44*:151, 1981.
58. West JB. Pulmonary Pathophysiology: The Essentials. Baltimore, Williams & Wilkins, 1977, pp 20–44.
59. Manchar M. Furosemide and systemic circulation during severe exercise. In: Equine Exercise Physiology 2, JR Gillespie, NE Robinson (eds). Ann Arbor, Edward Brothers, 1987, pp 132–147.
60. Fung YC, Sobin SS. Theory of sheet flow in alveoli. J Appl Physiol, *26*:472, 1969.
61. Gurtner HP, Walser P, Fassler B. Normal values for pulmonary hemodynamics at rest and during exercise in man. Prog Respir Res, *9*:295, 1975.
62. Erickson BK, Erickson HH, Landgren GL, et al. Cardiopulmonary dynamics and gas exchange during exercise-induced pulmonary hemorrhage in the horse. In: Proceedings of 5th Veterinary Respiratory Symposium, Chicago, IL, 1986, p 13.
63. Fishman AP. Pulmonary circulation. In: Handbook of Physiology, The Respiratory System, Vol 1, Circulation and Nonrespiratory Functions. Bethesda MD, American Physiological Society, 1986, pp 93–165.
64. Amis TC, Pascoe JR, Hornof W. Topographic distribution of pulmonary ventilation and perfusion in the horse. Am J Vet Res, *45*:1597, 1984.
65. Nandiwada PA, Hyman AL, Kadowitz PJ. Pulmonary vasodilator responses to vagal stimulation and acetylcholine in the cat. Cir Res, *53*:86, 1983.
66. Howard P, Barer GR, Thompson B, et al. Factors causing and reversing vasoconstriction in unventilated lung. Respir Physiol, *24*:325, 1975.
67. Bergofsky EH. Mechanisms underlying vasomotor regulation of regional pulmonary blood flow in normal and disease states. Am J Med, *57*:378, 1974.
68. Bergofsky EH. Humoral control of the pulmonary circulation. Annu Rev Physiol, *42*:221, 1980.
69. Fritts HW Jr, Harriw P, Clauss RM, et al. The effect of acetylcholine on the human pulmonary circulation under normal and hypoxic conditions. J Clin Invest, *37*:99, 1958.
70. Rubin LJ, Lazar JD. Nonadrenergic effects of isoproterenol in the dog with hypoxic pulmonary vasoconstriction. Possible role of prostaglandins. J Clin Invest, *71*:1366, 1983.
71. Ruiz AV, Bisgard GE, Tyson IB, et al. Regional lung function in calves during acute and chronic pulmonary hypertension. J Appl Physiol, *37*:384, 1974.
72. Nesarajah MS, Matalon S, Krasney JA, et al. Cardiac output and regional oxygen transport in acutely hypoxic conscious sheep. Resp Physiol, *53*:161, 1983.
73. Enjeti S, O'Neil JT, Terry PB, et al. Sublobar atelectasis and regional pulmonary blood flow. J Appl Physiol, *47*:1245, 1979.
74. Deffebach ME, Charan NB, Lakshminaryan S, et al. The bronchial circulation: Small, but a vital attribute of the lung. Am Rev Respir Dis, *135*:463, 1987.
75. Magno MG, Fishman AP. Origin, distribution and blood flow of bronchial circulation in anesthetized sheep. J Appl Physiol, *53*:272, 1982.
76. Lilker ES, Nagy EJ. Gas exchange in the pulmonary collateral circulation of dogs. Am Rev Respir Dis, *112*:615, 1975.
77. O'Callaghan MW, Pascoe JR, Tyler WS, et al. Exercise-induced pulmonary haemorrhage in the horse: Results of a detailed clinical, postmortem and imaging study v. microscopic observations. Equine Vet J, *19*:411, 1987.

78. West JB. Ventilation-perfusion relationships. In: Respiratory Physiology, The Essentials. Baltimore, Williams & Wilkins, 1985, pp 49–66.
79. Berger AJ, Mitchell RA, Severinghouse JW. Regulation of respiration. N Engl J Med, *297*:92, 1977.
80. Batsel HL. Location of bulbar respiratory center by microelectrode sounding. Exp Neurol, *9*:410, 1964.
81. Cohen MI. Central determinants of respiratory rhythm. Annu Rev Physiol, *43*:91, 1981.
82. Berger AJ, Mitchell RA, Severinghouse JW. Regulation of respiration. N Engl J Med, *297*:138, 1977.
83. Murray JF. Control of breathing. In: The Normal Lung. Philadelphia, WB Saunders Co, 1986, pp 233–260.
84. McDonald DM, Mitchell RA. The innervation of glomus cells, ganglion cells and blood vessels in rat carotid body. A quantitative ultrastructural analysis. J Neurocytol, *4*:177, 1975.
85. Muir WW, Moore CA, Hamlin RL. Ventilatory alterations in normal horses in response to changes in inspired oxygen and carbon dioxide. Am J Vet Res, *36*:155, 1975.
86. Leusen IR. Chemosensitivity of the respiratory center. Influence of $CO_2$ in the cerebral ventricles on respiration. Am J Physiol, *176*:39, 1954.
87. Mitchell RA, Loeschcke HH, Massion WH, et al. Respiratory responses mediated through superficial chemosensitive areas on the medulla. J Appl Physiol, *18*:523, 1963.
88. Fend V. Acid-base balance in cerebral fluids. In: Handbook of Physiology, The Respiratory System, Vol II, Control of Breathing. AP Fishman, NS Cherniak, JG Widdicombe, et al (eds). Bethesda, MD, American Physiological Society, 1966, p 115.
89. Davies DG, Nolan WF. Cerebral interstitial fluids acid-base status follow arterial acid-base perturbations. J Appl Physiol, *53*:1551, 1982.
90. Saint Ambragio G. Information arising from the tracheo-bronchial tree of mammals. Physiol Rev, *62*:531, 1982.
91. Coleridge HM, Coleridge JCG. Reflexes evoked from tracheobronchial tree and lung. In: Handbook of Physiology, The Respiratory System, Vol II, Control of Breathing. AP Fishman, NS Cherniack, JG Widdicombe, et al (eds). Bethesda, MD, American Physiological Society, 1986, pp 395–429.
92. Derksen FJ, Robinson NE, Stick JA. Technique for reversible vagal blockade in the standing conscious pony. Am J Vet Res, *42*:523, 1981.
93. Coleridge HM, Coleridge JCG, Ginzel KH, et al. Stimulation of 'irritant' receptors and afferent C fibers in the lungs by prostaglandins. Nature, *264*:451, 1976.
94. Paintal AS. Vagal sensory receptors and their reflex effects. Physiol Rev, *53*:159, 1973.
95. Thomas DP, Vane JR. 5-Hydroxytryptamine in the circulation of the dog. Nature, *216*:335, 1967.
96. Said SI. The lungs as a metabolic organ. N Engl J Med, *279*:1330, 1969.
97. Junod AF. 5-Hydroxytryptamine and other amines in the lungs. In: Handbook of Physiology, The Respiratory System, Vol 1, Circulation and Nonrespiratory Functions. AP Fishman, AB Fisher, SR Geiger (eds). Bethesda, MD, American Physiological Society, 1985, pp 337–349.
98. Boileau JC, Crexells C, Biron P. Free pulmonary passage of dopamine. Rev Can Biol, *31*:69, 1972.
99. Ferreira SH, Ng KK, Vane JR. The continuous bioassay of the release and disappearance of histamine in the circulation. Br J Pharmacol, *49*:543, 1973.
100. Ryan JW, Ryan US. Endothelial surface enzymes and the dynamic processing of plasma substrates. Int Rev Exp Pathol, *26*:1, 1983.
101. Hirata F, Axelrod J. Phospholipid methylation and biological signal transmission. Science, *209*:1082, 1980.
102. Bakhle YS, Ferreira SH. Lung metabolism of eicosanoids: Prostaglandins, prostacycline, thromboxane, and leukotrienes. In: Handbook of Physiology, The Respiratory System, Vol I, Circulation and Nonrespiratory Functions. AP Fishman, AB Fisher, SR Geiger (eds). Bethesda, MD, American Physiological Society, 1985, pp 365–386.
103. Lewis RA, Soter NA, Diamond PT, et al. Prostaglandin $D_2$ generation after activation of rat and human mast cells with IgE. J Immunol, *129*:1627, 1983.
104. Zurier RB, Sayadoff DM. Release of prostaglandins from human polymorphonuclear leukocytes. Inflammation, *1*:93, 1975.
105. Borgeat P, Samuelsson B. Arachidonic acid metabolism in polymorphonuclear leukocytes: Effects of ionophore A23187. Proc Natl Acad Sci (USA), *76*:2145, 1979.
106. Horton EW. Prostaglandins and smooth muscle. Br Med Bull, *35*:295, 1979.
107. Samuelsson B. Leukotrienes: A new class of mediators of immediate hypersensitivity reaction and inflammation. Adv Prostaglandin Thromboxane Leukotriene Res, *11*:1, 1983.
108. Borgeat P, Samuelsson B. Transformation of arachidonic acid by rabbit polymorphonuclear leukocytes. J Biol Chem, *254*:2643, 1979.
109. Palmer RMJ, Stepney RJ, Higgs GA, et al. Chemokinetic activity of arachidonic and lipoxygenase products on leukocytes of different species. Prostaglandins, *20*:411, 1980.
110. Dahlen SE, Hedqvist P, Hammarstrom P, et al. Leukotrienes are potent constrictors of human bronchi. Nature, *288*:484, 1980.
111. Johnson HG, McNee ML, Sun FF. 15-Hydroxyeicosatetraenoic acid is a potent inflammatory mediator and agonist of canine tracheal mucus secretion. Am Rev Respir Dis, *131*:917, 1985.
112. Gray PR, Derksen FJ, Robinson NE, et al. Increased plasma 15-hydroxyeicosatetraenoic acid (15-HETE) concentration during acute airway obstruction in ponies. FASEB J, A1184, 1988.
113. Vane JR. Inhibition of prostaglandin synthesis as a mechanism of action for aspirin-like drugs. Nature London New Biol, *231*:232, 1971.
114. Brain JD, Valberg PA. State of the art. Deposition of aerosol in the respiratory tract. Am Rev Respir Dis, *120*:1325, 1979.
115. Asmudsson T, Johnson RF, Kilbum KH, et al. Ef-

ficiency of nebulizers for depositing saline in human beings. Am Rev Respir Dis, *108*:506, 1973.

116. Sleigh MA, Blake JR, Lison N. State of the art. The propulsion of mucus by cilia. Am Rev Respir Dis, *137*:726, 1988.
117. Satin P, Dirksen ER. Function-structure correlations in cilia from mammalian respiratory tract. In: Handbook of Physiology, The Respiratory System, Vol I, Circulation and Nonrespiratory Functions. AP Fishman, AB Fisher, SR Geiger (eds). Bethesda, MD, American Physiological Society, 1985, pp 473–494.
118. Afzelius BA. The immotile-cilia syndrome and other ciliary diseases. Int Rev Exp Pathol, *19*:1, 1979.
119. Killingsworth CR, Slocombe RF, Wilsman NJ. Immotile cilia syndrome in an aged dog. J Am Vet Med Assoc, *190*:1567, 1987.
120. Coles SJ, Bhaskar KR, O'Sullivan DD, et al. Airway mucus: Composition and regulation of its secretion by neuropeptides in vitro. CIBA Found Symp, *109*:40, 1984.
121. Widdicombe JG, Pack RJ. The clara cell. Eur J Respir Dis, *63*:202, 1982.
122. Iravani J, Melville GN. Mucociliary function in the respiratory tract as influenced by physiochemical factors. Pharmacol Therapeutics—Part B, *2*:471, 1976.
123. Nadel JA, Davis B, Phipps RJ. Control of mucus secretion and ion transport in airways. Ann Rev Physiol, *41*:369, 1979.
124. Cosio MG, Hale KA, Niewoehner DE. Morphologic and morphometric effects of prolonged cigarette smoking on small airways. Am Rev Respir Dis, *122*:265, 1980.
125. Spungin B, Silberberg A. Stimulation of mucus secretion, ciliary activity, and transport in frog palate epithelium. Am J Physiol, *247*:C299, 1984.
126. Nadel JA. New approaches to regulation of fluid secretion in airways. Chest, *80*:849, 1981.
127. Verdugo P, Johnson NT, Tam PY. Beta adrenergic stimulation of respiratory ciliary activity. J Appl Physiol, *48*:868, 1980.
128. Brain JD. Macrophages in the respiratory tract. In: Handbook of Physiology, The Respiratory System, Vol I, Circulation and Nonrespiratory Functions. AP Fishman, AB Fisher, SR Geiger (eds). Bethesda, MD, The American Physiological Society, 1985, pp 447–471.
129. Godleski JJ, Brain JD. The origin of alveolar macrophages in mouse radiation chimeras. J Exp Med, *136*:630, 1972.
130. Bowden DH, Adamson IYR. Adaptive responses of the pulmonary macrophage system to carbon. I. Kinetic studies. Lab Invest, *38*:422, 1978.
131. Huston LJU, Bayly WM, Liggitt HD, et al. Alveolar macrophage function in Thoroughbreds after strenuous exercise. In: Equine Exercise Physiolgy 2. JR Gillespie, NE Robinson (eds). Davis, CA, ICEEP Publications, 1987, pp 243–252.
132. Liggett D, Huston L, Silflow R, et al. Impaired function of bovine alveolar macrophages infected with parainfluenza-3 virus. Am J Vet Res, *46*:1740, 1985.
133. Allison AC, Harington, JS, Birbeck M. An examination of the cytotoxic effects of silica on macrophages. J Exp Med *124*:141, 1966.
134. Johnson JA, Prescott JF, Markham RJ. The pathology of experimental corynebacterium equi infection in foals following intrabronchial challenge. Vet Pathol, *20*:440, 1983.
135. Derksen FJ, Miller DC, Scott JS, et al. Bronchoalveolar lavage in ponies with recurrent airway obstruction (heaves). Am Rev Respir Dis, *132*:1066, 1985.
136. Hogg JC. Neutrophil kinetics and lung injury. Physiol Rev, *67*:1249, 1987.
137. Bienenstock J, Johnston N. A morphologic study of rabbit bronchial lymphoid aggregates and lymphoepithelium. Lab Invest, *35*:343, 1976.
138. Bienenstock J, McDermott MR, Befus AD. The significance of bronchus-associated lymphoid tissue. Bull Eur Physiopathol Respir, *18*:153, 1982.
139. Hunninghake GW, Gadek JE, Kawanami O, et al. Inflammatory and immune processes in the human lung in health and disease—evaluation by bronchoalveolar lavage. Am J Pathol, *97*:149, 1979.
140. Kaltreider HB. State of the Art. Expression of immune mechanisms in the lung. Am Rev Respir Dis, *113*:347, 1976.
141. Tomari TBGR. Secretory immunoglobulins. N Engl J Med, *287*:500, 1972.
142. Nadel JA, Baines PJ, Holtzman MJ. Autonomic factors in hyperreactivity of airway smooth muscle. In: Handbook of Physiology, The Respiratory System. Vol III, Mechanics of Breathing. AP Fishman, PT Macklem, J Mead, et al (eds). Bethesda, MD, The American Physiological Society, 1986, pp 693–702.
143. Sturgess JM. The mucous lining of major bronchi in the rabbit lung. Am Rev Respir Dis, *115*:819, 1977.

## CHAPTER 2

# EXAMINATION OF THE RESPIRATORY TRACT

*JILL BEECH*

## History

The importance of an accurate history is widely accepted, yet frequently is one aspect of the examination that is overlooked. The exact complaint, duration and progression of signs, exposure to stresses such as transport, the vaccination and deworming program, medications, type of housing and availability of pasture, and health and performance of other horses in the same stable or trained or managed by the same person should be ascertained.

Age of the horse is important because certain diseases such as infections are more common in young horses and the incidence of chronic obstructive pulmonary disease (COPD) increases with age.

The type of environment, bedding, feed, etc. is important and one should carefully try to assess whether onset of signs was associated with any environmental or seasonal change. When one is presented with a chronically coughing horse, one should carefully question the owner about any change in feed, bedding, or pasture, change in origin of feeds or bedding, changes in weather, introduction of any new animals to the barn, or other differences. One should determine whether signs wax and wane and whether this follows any pattern or can be associated with any environmental or work factors. As certain conditions are more frequent in certain areas, one should determine whether the horse changed location. For example, lungworm infections would be unlikely in horses constantly kept in cold areas and certain fungal infections are more likely in warm or humid areas. COPD is reportedly rare in pastured animals although, in certain areas of the United States, a spring/summer pasture allergy occurs.

One should inquire about weight loss or anorexia. Horses with chronic bacterial infections or neoplasia usually lose weight even if their appetite remains fair. Horses with COPD may lose weight often because they decrease food intake due to dyspnea and coughing. Acute pharyngitis could also lead to anorexia because of soreness and dysphagia. Chronic bacterial infections may lead to severe weight loss and muscle wasting in mature horses and growth retardation in foals.

It is also important to determine how long the owner or trainer has had the horse and if it was acquired with a problem. Unknowingly, he or she may have acquired a horse with a chronic problem that may not be amenable to successful treatment. Likewise, one should try to determine if the horse has had any previous surgery for any respiratory tract abnormality.

## Physical Examination

A complete examination in a quiet area is essential. In some cases it may also be necessary to watch the horse exercise and examine it after exercise. Challenge exposure to certain environmental conditions may also be useful in selected cases. One should observe the horse at rest, noting its breathing pattern, effort and rate, how it stands, and whether it appears anxious or painful. Flared nostrils and an anxious expression can accompany some hypoxemic or painful conditions. Pleural pain should be suspected if the horse has restricted thoracic movement or a "catch" and hesitance to inspiration, muscle quivering over the thorax, abducted elbows, a short mincing forelimb gait, discomfort when lowering or raising its head and neck, if it grunts when it is touched over the thorax or moved or has a short soft hesitant cough. Horses with pleural pain may also be reluctant to lie down. They dislike going down an incline and if on uneven ground may choose to stand with their front limbs higher than their hind quarters. Nostril flaring is nonspecific and some horses with pleuritis "pinch" or constrict their nostrils. Fractured ribs may elicit signs of pleural pain.

If the horse has unrestricted inspiration but an increased abdominal expiratory effort, sometimes rather abrupt and jerking, causing a "two step" effort, one should suspect an obstructive airway disease. Foals with severe R. equi pneumonia may have a jerking double expiratory effort as well as an increased abdominal movement accompanying inspiration and decreased thoracic expansion. Decreased thoracic expansion without pain may accompany restrictive pneumonias, atelectasis and pneumothorax, and botulism. Severe respiratory efforts may be accompanied by pumping of the anus and some horses with COPD also have flatulence.

If a horse extends its head and neck to breathe and seems anxious, stenosis of the upper airway, especially of the pharynx or larynx, should be suspected. Stridor may occur during inspiration if there is upper airway obstruction and with severe obstruction it is also heard during expiration. It is a loud musical sound and is produced when the upper airway is narrowed to a point of closure and the opposite walls oscillate between the barely open and closed positions.

Respiratory rates above 18 to 20 breaths per minute are unusual in cool resting adult horses. If no cause for excitement, pain or metabolic dysfunction is found, inadequate gas exchange should be considered as a cause of tachypnea. Foals with pneumonia are more likely to have elevated respiratory rates than mature horses with pneumonia. Slow deep breathing may be seen if there is metabolic acidosis. One should always note if there is any ventral thoracic or abdominal or limb edema. A plaque of edema between the front limbs is common in horses with pleural effusion and their distal limbs may also develop edema.

One should note whether there is nasal exudate or exudate in the stall, in the feed, or in the water. Type of discharge should be noted. Increased serous nasal exudate usually suggests viral infection. It is not uncommon for normal horses to have slight serous discharge and this also may be increased in the presence of allergens or irritants. Whitish yellow mucopurulent discharge suggests (but is not diagnostic of) bacterial infection. Although nasal discharge may be profuse, the amount does not reflect the severity of pneumonia, as foals with severe R. equi abscesses in the lungs may have little discharge. Encapsulated lung abscesses may be present without any nasal exudate. Frequently, greyish white or greyish yellow/beige exudate is seen at the nostrils or in the trachea on endoscopic examination and interpreted as indicating septic bronchitis. However, many horses with COPD can have copious amounts of beige tinged white exudate and the latter is not diagnostic of a bacterial infection. In fact, cytologic examination of a transtracheal aspirate from many of these cases negates a primary bacterial disease and shows chronic active bronchitis with many macrophages and increased amounts of mucus with or without increased numbers of neutrophils.

One should note whether the discharge occurs only under certain conditions (lowering the head, in certain environments, etc.), whether it is consistently unilateral or bilateral, or whether there is any odor. Tissue necrosis or gas forming organisms such as anaerobes cause an odor. Inflammatory exudate due to COPD is not malodorous. It is also important to ascertain if the exudate ever contains any blood and, if so, whether it appears old (dark red brown) or fresh (bright red). Tissue necrosis often causes a foul smelling exudate with hemorrhage and may be associated with infections and accompanies many tumors. However, neoplasms such as hemangiosarcoma, and exercise induced pulmonary hemorrhage (EIPH) may cause significant bleeding without exudate or odor.

Any coughing should be characterized. Deep coughing usually indicates pulmonary origin; however, painful conditions such as pleuritis may attenuate this. Despite considerable exudate in the lower airways, coughing may appear nonproductive and it is likely that much of the exudate is swallowed and, therefore, not apparent to an observer. Paroxysms of coughing may occur with any airway irritation. Eating frequently precipitates coughing in horses with COPD or those with pharyngeal or laryngeal dysfunction. Absence of a cough, like absence of externally visible exudate, does not rule out the existence of exudate in the airways.

While observing the horse to evaluate breathing pattern, attitude and posture, presence of nasal exudate, or coughing, one can be obtaining a history. Closer examination can then follow and it is usually advisable to start at the horse's head.

Facial symmetry, nostril width, general attitude and expression, any nasal drainage and any cranial nerve dysfunction can be noted. One can check the nostrils and mouth for odor and also check each nostril for air flow to detect if it is equal. While standing at the head, one should listen to the horse breathing. Audible high pitched wheezing (especially expiratory) and sometimes "clicking" of mucus are not infrequent in severe cases of COPD. Obstructions in the upper airway usually cause a less musical, more snoring inspiratory wheeze. However, laryngospasm may create a characteristic high pitched squeaking, creaking, occlusive inspiratory sound. Grossly audible flutterings or gurgling sounds usually originate from exudate in the upper respiratory tract, but soft palate displacement may cause rattling. Pharyngeal narrowing due to collapsed walls, edema, cysts or distended guttural pouches may cause stertorous breathing. I have seen one foal with guttural pouch tympanitis that made a stertorous snoring noise from birth, yet never had externally distended guttural pouches; the diagnosis was based on endoscopic and radiographic examinations and its return to normal following surgery to correct the tympanitis. Nasal passage stenosis also may cause inspiratory snoring, but if it is unilateral one can detect decreased air movement on that side.

Sinuses should be percussed and each side compared. If one simultaneously opens the horse's mouth and gently pulls the tongue out to one side to keep the mouth open while percussing the sinuses, resonance will be greatly increased and subtle differences may be more apparent. One should also note whether the horse objects or seems painful when a particular sinus is percussed; consistent reaction to percussion of one area should lead one to suspect a focal problem.

Intermandibular lymph nodes and the parotid region can then be palpated. I then usually return to the horse's nose and palpate and directly visually examine the horse's distal nasal passages and false nostrils. Masses in the false nostrils such as atheromas may impair air flow during exercise. One can feel and see whether the nasal septum is thickened or deviated, the nasal meatus is narrowed, and the mucosa is normal. Although amyloidosis is rare in horses, the nasal passages are a common site and one should ensure there are no plaques or other lesions in the nasal mucosa. At the same time one can check that the nasal tear duct orifice is present near the mucocutaneous junction and oral and nasal mucous membrane color can also be evaluated. However, degree of mucosal pinkness is usually a poor indicator of ventilatory function; $Pa_{O_2}$ may drop as low as 40 mm Hg before the mucosa loses its pink color.

I then palpate the intermandibular space for width. A narrow intermandibular width has been associated with a narrow upper airway. One clinician has associated a wide intermandibular width with high performance and suggested that a horse with a wide jaw is more likely to have a healthy larynx than one with a narrow jaw (Cook, personal communication, 1988). The larynx can then be palpated. Primarily, the first two fingers (index and middle) are used. The sides and dorsum of the larynx should be felt for symmetry and any muscle atrophy. The muscular process of the arytenoid is distinctly palpable only when there is muscle atrophy. The "slap test" is advocated by some as a means of detecting laryngeal dysfunction. In order to do this correctly the horse must be relaxed and tranquilization with Xylazine* has been advocated (Cook, personal communication, 1988). The examiner palpates the arytenoids and an attendant slaps the horse behind the shoulder and withers over the dorsal thorax; the opposite cartilage should move, although in my experience in untranquilized horses, both may move. Both sides should be checked and if there is any question about abnormal function, the test should be repeated.

Endoscopic examination can be used later during the examination to directly observe arytenoid movement during the "slap test." On the basis of digital palpation, one examiner diagnosed left recurrent laryngeal nerve neuropathy in 73 to 100% of 784 Thoroughbreds and in not less than 81% of 54 nonsedated suckling Thoroughbred foals (Cook, personal communication, 1988). The larynx and cricotracheal space should be palpated for conformation. The skin and subcutis in this region should be examined for any scars. Previous laryngeal prosthesis placement often causes a palpable thickening over the area of placement in the larynx and the horse cannot move this arytenoid on a "slap test." The trachea can then be palpated for any anomalies such as fractured or irregular cartilage rings. With popularization of sternothyrohyoideus ("strap muscle") resection for palate displacement one should always palpate this region to detect if a myectomy has been performed.

One can also examine the jugular veins for patency and filling. Distended jugular veins and/or pulsation may accompany right heart failure, massive pleural effusion or masses obstructing blood flow returning to the heart.

One can then auscult the trachea and thorax. A quiet environment and good stethoscope are prerequisites that are sometimes overlooked. Normally, air movement in the trachea will sound clear and inspiratory air flow sounds will approximate expiratory sounds. Sounds may be referred from both the upper and lower respiratory tracts. The horse's body condition and hair coat are important factors when making a judgment about quality and loudness of lung (and heart) sounds. The normal soft air flow sounds may be difficult to hear in a fat animal but should be readily audible in a thin normal horse. Loud sounds in a fat horse and decreased sounds in a thin horse should alert one to the probable existence of lung disease. However, decreased air sounds may also be due to decreased breathing efforts for other reasons (such as botulism, metabolic factors, depression, or pain). One should always check that the breathing pattern and effort are not the cause of decreased air flow. Occasionally one is presented with a horse with suspected COPD showing marked dyspnea and an obstructive breathing pattern, yet lung sounds are greatly attenuated; presumably this is due to bronchoconstriction and decreased air flow as atropine usually reverses the condition. When air sounds are very quiet, it is usually necessary to use a rebreathing bag providing the horse will tolerate it and does not have a condition that would contraindicate its use. A large reservoir bag into which the horse can breathe and which will accumulate $CO_2$ and increase depth of breathing can be applied over the horse's lower face, taking care that it is not sucked up against the nostrils, occluding inspiration. This can be left on a variable period depending on the horse's condition and personality and the clinician's need. A subjective assessment can be made about the horse's tolerance and recovery. Normal horses will breathe quite easily, recover a normal breathing pattern rapidly, and will not cough. Those with reactive airway diseases such as COPD, and also pneumonia, often cough and the coughing may be so paroxysmal and severe that it prevents continued use of the rebreathing bag. Also, horses with pleuritis may not be candidates for its use because of the pain associated with the deep breathing. In horses in which the bag cannot be used, one may have to intermittently occlude the nostrils and listen to the deep breaths following release. In some cases it may be helpful to auscult the horse before

*Rompun, Haver, Miles Laboratories, Shawnee, Kansas.

and after exercise or before and after use of a bronchodilator.

In a normal horse the lung sounds are usually louder on the right side than on the left and usually louder over the carina area where large airways branch. Inspiration is always louder than expiration and the latter is usually very quiet, or in horses in good body condition often almost inaudible. If one listens to a thin horse and right lung sounds are significantly quieter than on the left which has audible inspiratory and expiratory air movement, one should suspect an abnormality on the right side. When expiratory sounds equal or exceed inspiratory sounds, one should suspect consolidation or effusion allowing transmission of large airway sounds because of loss of air filled alveoli. In a fat horse, the louder side is often the more abnormal side.

Soft air movement sounds may abruptly change and be replaced by loud sounds resembling air passing through large pipes (or tracheal sounds) when there is effusion or consolidation. The reader can simulate this type of sound by forcibly expiring with an open mouth. Expiration is usually louder than inspiration and there is frequently a pause between the two phases. It may be necessary to force the horse to breathe deeply to allow detection of these sounds.

Presence of intestinal sounds within the thorax as far cranially as the heart is common and may complicate interpretation of sounds. Some borborygmal sounds can mimic abnormal lung sounds, especially pleural rubs. To help differentiate between them one should try to determine whether the sound(s) consistently occur at one stage of breathing or whether they are random and whether they change with altered breathing pattern. Likewise, muscle quivering may hamper auscultation and can cause crackling type sounds. Obviously, subcutaneous emphysema or edema will dampen and affect lung sounds with the former creating many crackles under the stethoscope.

There has been a recent increase in interest in lung sound physiology especially as many of the details on generation of lung sounds are unknown.[1] In general, the terms crackles, rhonchi or wheezes, and rales are used.[1–3] Crackles are short explosive nonmusical sounds and usually are divided into "fine" and "coarse." Fine crackles sound like rubbing two hairs together or have a "velcro-like" character and occur during mid to late inspiration. In humans, they are heard primarily in dependent lung regions.[1] In horses, they also seem more common in the ventral and peripheral lung fields, although with certain conditions such as pulmonary edema and congestive heart failure they seem more diffuse. Coarse crackles are more popping, occur early in inspiration and may also be expiratory. They vary with the respiratory pattern. In humans the character of crackles has been associated with different diseases, many of which do not affect horses, and, such distinctions have not been made for horses. In equine COPD, crackles may be fine or coarse. Fine crackles are occasionally transiently heard in the "down" lung of foals when they first rise from recumbency even though there are no signs of pulmonary disease. Fine crackles may also be heard in healthy humans at the anterior bases during inspiration from a low lung volume.[1]

Rales refer to rattles that are nonmusical, often bubbling and moist. However, the term has been replaced by "crackles." The original idea that the lower and coarser the pitch, the larger the airway of origin has been disproved. Crackling due to bubbling secretions in airways occurs during both inspiration and expiration. When crackles are heard in the absence of secretions, they are generated by the explosive equalization of gas pressure between two compartments of the lung when a closed section of airway suddenly opens.[3]

Wheezes or rhonchi are musical sounds of varied pitch and duration and may be single or multiple. They indicate airway obstruction and may be exacerbated by deep breaths. The theory that higher pitched wheezes emanate from small airways and lower pitched rhonchi from larger airways has been disproved. High pitched wheezing may be generated from peripheral or central airways and may vary during a respiratory cycle. The pitch of a wheeze from a narrowed bronchus can vary greatly between inspiration and expiration.[3] The origin of wheezing is the oscillation of opposite walls of a bronchus when it is narrowed to the point of closure, analogous to the sound generated by a vibrating reed. The organ pipe model of sound generation has been shown to be incorrect.

Wheezes may be of a single musical tone (monophonic) or composed of several notes (polyphonic). Polyphonic wheezes can be heard in all obstructive lung diseases and are produced by compression of central bronchi. At least in those species studied, the number of wheezes heard does not indicate that this number was actually generated. An illusion of a great number may occur due to the wide transmission of a few loud wheezes having varying intensity relative to different areas on the thoracic wall.[3] They may be expiratory or inspiratory. High pitched wheezing may be heard at the nostrils of horses with COPD. Wheezing may also be heard when there is pneumonia and is not restricted to COPD. Also, in my experience some horses with COPD have more crackles than wheezes and others vice versa. In human asthmatics, loud high pitched expiratory wheezing and inspiratory wheezes reliably indicate severe airway obstruction and the absence of wheezing (with normal vesicular lung sounds) is not likely to occur if there is more than minimal obstruction.[1] When airway obstruction is functional and affected by exposure to dusts and/or allergens, wheezing may be variable and the same horse that is normal one morning may be wheezing in the afternoon. In horses suspected of having functional bronchoconstriction, multiple examinations or examination following allergen/dust provocation or exposure may be required to make a diagnosis.

If there is pleural inflammation, friction rubs may be auscultable. They are usually loudest at end inspiration/early expiration and location varies with the disease. However, the middle to ventral third of the thorax is frequently affected; pleural effusion can obscure the friction rubs, although they may still be audible dorsal to the effusion. Rubbing may sound like fine crackles, crunching sounds made when one walks through snow, a creaky old boat rocking in the waves and stretching its rope, or a creaking opening door. They may rapidly change in character even in a time span of a few hours.

Palpation and percussion of the thorax may be helpful. Both can reveal whether there is pleural pain. In some severe cases of pleuritis one can feel a reverberation by placing one's hand palm side against the thoracic wall. Especially in foals, palpation may give one a subjective impression of whether thoracic expansion is normal. Although percussion has now been replaced in many cases by ultrasonography, it can be helpful. It can be done with one's fingers and hand or using a plexor and pleximeter. When using one's hands, one hand's first two fingers serve as a pleximeter held flat on the thoracic wall in an intercostal space, and the other hand's first two fingers serve as a plexor to sharply tap the first hand's two fingers. The angle between the plexor and pleximeter should be kept constant as one progresses ventrally from the dorsalmost aspect of the lung. One can start cranially or caudally and cover each hemithorax. Percussion over a normal air filled lung sounds resonant and somewhat hollow; solid tissue or fluid sounds dull and flat. The lung's border is detected by a change in resonance, which over the caudal abdomen may actually sound more resonant if there is much gas distended intestine. The lung border runs in a curving line from the eighteenth rib with the following as approximate landmarks: seventeenth intercostal space level with the tuber coxae, sixteenth space level with the tuber ischii, thirteenth space level with the middle of the thorax, and eleventh with the point of the shoulder with a curving line going to the elbow level. On the left side, the area of cardiac dullness generally extends from the sixth rib at the sternum to approximately 1 to 2 inches above the sternum at the fifth space, then to the fourth rib about 5 inches above the sternal border and down to the third rib at the sternum. On the right side, the area of cardiac dullness is between the third and fourth intercostal spaces. Loss of air filled lung tissue near the pleural surface may be detected as dull areas, but consolidated or other nonaerated lesions deep to the lung surface cannot be detected. Ventral dullness often indicates pleural effusion or lung consolidation. If lung fields are expanded due to emphysema, percussion may detect the change. Focal areas of hyperresonance could suggest emphysematous bullae, and pneumothorax would sound hyperresonant. Accurate percussion is difficult if there is subcutaneous fluid or air, or the animal is very fat or is intolerant of the procedure. Normal horses do not cough when the chest is percussed and presence of coughing when a focal area is percussed may help localize the diseased area.

## Endoscopic Examination

This will be covered in another chapter. In cases where an upper respiratory tract lesion is suspected but not apparent at rest or after exercise, if a high speed treadmill is available, endoscopic examination of the horse at various stages of exercise may be helpful. Its use would also enable evaluation of the functional significance of results of laryngeal palpation and of endoscopic abnormalities seen with the horse at rest.

Electromyographic evaluation of the dorsal cricoarytenoid muscles has been reported for both normal horses and those with bilateral and unilateral laryngeal dysfunction.[4,5] In horses with laryngeal hemiplegia, the muscle on the affected side showed fibrillation potentials, frequently positive sharp waves, and occasionally bizarre high frequency discharges or reduced insertional activity.[5] Whether this technique will be useful for early detection of laryngeal paresis remains to be determined. As electromyography machines are expensive and expertise in performing and interpreting electromyograms is required, widespread use of this diagnostic approach is unlikely.

## Pulmonary Function Tests and Blood Gas Analysis

Pulmonary function testing (PFT) is widely applied in human clinical medicine but is not widely used in horses except for research. Many of the tests which are useful in detecting small airways dysfunction rely on patient cooperation and breathing maneuvers that are not possible in horses. Other deterrents to use are that equipment is expensive, horses may require training for even simple procedures if the tests are to be valid and repeatable, and trained personnel are needed. If PFTs were available for horses to detect minimal changes in lung function and small airways disease, they could be extremely helpful in evaluating horses suspected to be performing badly due to respiratory dysfunction, and in determining when a horse could safely return to work following respiratory illness.

Although most currently used methods for equine PFTs are not applicable to clinical practice, some basic information on some of the techniques is presented and a reference list is provided for interested readers.[6–28] The aims of PFTs in horses are the measurement of ventilation and gas flow, distribution of inspired air and alveolar capillary diffusion, lung volumes, and mechanical factors. It is possible to measure tidal volume ($V_T$), minute volume ($V_E$), resistance (R), flow volume curves, functional residual capacity (FRC), work of breathing, dead space ($V_D$), and alveolar ventilation. Gas distribution and diffusion tests as well as blood gas analysis can be performed (Table 2–1). To allow these measurements, integrated pneumotachography, spirometry, and plethysmography as well as gas analyzers have been employed. Any face mask that is used for pneumotachography must be well tolerated, air tight and snugly fitting, and have minimal dead space. Likewise dead space and resistance in all other tubing used must be minimized for accuracy.

Intrapleural pressure is usually measured by use of an esophageal balloon and less frequently by placing an intrapleural cannula for direct measurement. Use of an esophageal balloon eliminates possible complications of a pleural cannula, and measurements are similar for the two techniques. Some practice is required to place the esophageal balloon which entails passing a small bore tube with a balloon down the esophagus, then inflating the balloon to a set volume when it is located in the mid thoracic area. The balloon is attached to a pressure transducer external to the horse. Swallowing or peristaltic movements can be recognized and deleted from any measurements. The transpulmonary pressure can be calculated from the difference between atmospheric pressure, which is that

**TABLE 2–1.** ***Pulmonary Function Test Parameters and Their Definitions***

| *Term/Measurement* | *Definition* |
|---|---|
| Transpulmonary pressure | Difference in pressure between the inside and outside of the lung |
| Functional Residual Capacity (FRC) | Volume of gas remaining in the lungs at end expiration |
| Tidal Volume ($V_T$) | Volume of gas inspired or expired during each respiratory cycle |
| Minute Volume ($V_E$) | Total volume of gas inspired or expired in one minute |
| Respiratory Dead Space ($V_D$) | Volume of lungs that is ventilated but not perfused; it includes alveolar and airway (anatomic) dead space |
| Alveolar Ventilation ($V_A$) | Volume of gas that is used in gas exchange ($V_T - V_D$) |
| Compliance (C) | Volume change per unit of pressure |
| Resistance (R) | Pressure difference per unit of flow exchange |
| Conductance ($G_{AW}$) | Flow per pressure drop or 1/R airway |

measured at the face mask on the horse and esophageal pressure. Pressure volume loops can be derived relating changes in intrapleural pressure to tidal volume; the area within the loop corresponds to the nonelastic work of breathing.[25] Intrapleural pressure changes increase with obstructive lung disease and that measured during expiration may actually become positive.[17] Some investigators have used primarily intrapleural pressure changes and blood gas analysis for evaluating horses for COPD.[16] Concurrent use of a pneumotachograph and pulmonary function computer, and gas analyzers for measuring expired and inspired gases allows more critical and thorough evaluation.[11,18]

The pneumotachograph incorporated into a face mask allows one to measure flow signals and compute dynamic compliance, resistance, respiratory frequency, total volume, minute ventilation, peak gas flow, and work of breathing. The pneumotachograph system must be suitable for the horse and calibrated each time it is used.

Compliance refers to distensibility of the lung and includes static and dynamic components. Only the latter is measured in horses as the former requires patient cooperation and modified breathing patterns. Dynamic compliance is calculated by dividing the change in lung volume between end inspiration and end expiration by intrapleural pressure change. Because it is frequency dependent, its values will change with breathing rate. Any time there is increased compliance as in pulmonary emphysema there is impaired ability of the lung to passively recoil because of loss of stored elastic energy, and, in addition, the loss of elastic tissue supporting airways allows collapse during expiration and further impairment of lung emptying. Interstitial lung disease decreases compliance. Compliance is also decreased in COPD.

Resistance (airway and tissue) is calculated from the change in transpulmonary pressure (change in pleural pressure minus change in pressure at the face mask during a respiratory cycle) divided by air flow. It is increased whenever breathing effort is increased relative to flow, such as in conditions where there is bronchoconstriction. Resistance may be normal in horses with COPD when they are symptom free but markedly increases when they are exposed to allergens.[11] The work of breathing can be calculated as a product of volume ($V_T$) times transpulmonary pressure.

A plethysmograph suitable for standing awake horses has been developed.[24] Plethysmography involves placing the horse inside an airtight rigid box and having it breathe through a mouthpiece to the outside, allowing measurement of resistance, compliance, gas volumes, pulmonary blood flow and FRC. A pressure transducer inside the chamber external to the horse reflects volume changes in the box caused by changes in the horse's thoracic volume. A pressure transducer at the horse's mouthpiece reflects intrathoracic pressure when there is no air flow. The problems with gas distribution in the nitrogen washout and helium dilution techniques for FRC measurement are avoided by the use of plethysmography.

Tracheal pressure also has been measured

but, as it requires implanting a cannula in the trachea, it has been restricted to investigational use. Laryngeal and nasal resistance have also been determined both at rest and during exercise.[6,10,21]

A primary use for a spirometer is to enable measurement of functional residual capacity (FRC). The horse breathes helium in a closed circuit (with $CO_2$ removed to prevent its accumulation and oxygen added to maintain a constant concentration) and the percentage of helium in the gas mixture in the spirometer before and after re-breathing is measured and the FRC calculated from the equation FRC = V $(C_1 - C_2)/C_2$, where V is the initial known volume of gas in the spirometer, $C_1$ is the initial helium concentration and $C_2$ is the final helium concentration. FRC can also be calculated by measuring exhaled nitrogen in a nitrogen washout study. When this method is used, at end expiration the horse is changed to inhaling pure oxygen and all exhaled gas is collected over a set period of nitrogen washout. In order to compute the volume of exhaled nitrogen, the spirometer's nitrogen concentration and volume at the end are compared to those parameters at the beginning when it is flushed with oxygen. The FRC is then calculated by:

$$\text{FRC} = N_2 \text{ exhaled}/0.81 - \text{end tidal } N_2\% \text{ at end of washout or}$$

$$\text{FRC} = N_2 \text{ final} \times \text{expired volume}/\%\ N_2 \text{ alveolar}$$

Any contamination with room air (which contains 80% nitrogen) invalidates this technique. Also, in patients with abnormal distribution of ventilation a long time may be required for nitrogen (or helium) to be emptied from all parts of the lung and a falsely low FRC may be calculated. The FRC is the volume or level of inflation at the point when the tendency of the lungs to further passively collapse is equaled by the tendency of the thoracic wall to expand and it depends on elastic properties of the lungs and thoracic wall. The respiratory minute volume can also be measured during this spirometry and the alveolar ventilation calculated.

The simultaneous measurement of arterial blood gases and mixed exhaled oxygen and carbon dioxide plus measurement of tidal volume (VT) allows calculation of the dead space ventilation (VD). The VD/VT is important as an increase suggests nonuniform matching of blood flow with ventilation in this physiologic dead space.[23] The calculation requires expired gas be collected for at least 1 minute. An alternative way to estimate alveolar dead space would be to evaluate the end tidal $P_{CO_2}$ gradient ($Pa_{CO_2} - P_{ET}\ CO_2$).[25] When end tidal $CO_2$ is monitored one may use the equation:

$$V_A = \frac{V_{CO_2}}{\%\ \text{alveolar } CO_2 \times 100}$$

to approximate alveolar ventilation ($V_{CO_2}$ = volume of $CO_2$ expired over given interval). The $Pa_{CO_2}$ can be substituted for alveolar $CO_2$ if one uses the factor .863 for converting from fractional concentration to partial pressure. The VA and $V_{CO_2}$ must be converted to body temperature, saturated with water vapor, body pressure (BTPS). Alveolar ventilation is VT − VD and is important because it is that volume that participates in gas exchange. It is usually calculated per minute (VA = f [VT − VD]).

Lung scanning using radiolabeled materials for evaluating ventilation and perfusion is covered in Chapter 9. Use of devices such as magnetometers which measure changes in shape and diameter of the thorax and can then be calibrated to indicate volume events of breathing are unlikely to be applicable to mature horses because of the relatively rigid noncompliant thoracic wall. Their potential value in neonatal foals that have compliant thoracic walls remains unclear. An obvious advantage is that volume events can be measured without use of a face mask (except for calibration) or other equipment that would encumber a patient.

The technique of superimposing a low level oscillatory airflow on the animal's respiratory pattern and measuring impedance has recently been reported in ponies.[26] This is a rapid noninvasive method, requiring the patient to wear a face mask for a relatively short period of time. The measurement reflects resistance and compliance and allows detection of changes in both.

Blood gas analysis is applicable to many practice situations and may be helpful in some cases. Both $PaO_2$ and $PaCO_2$ provide a reliable index of gas exchange. Arterial, not venous samples should be collected. Various arteries such as the facial, submandibular, carotid, digital and great metatarsal arteries may be sampled. Collection should be performed aseptically and pressure applied over the artery for at least several minutes after collection. It is important that the patient is quiet during collection; if it struggles and hyperventilates, the $PaCO_2$ may be transiently decreased. One should use a heparinized (1000 IU/ml) small syringe (1 to 3 ml) and small (22 to 26 gauge) needle and ensure that all air is expelled from the syringe. For carotid artery sampling in a mature horse a 4.5-cm 20 to 18-gauge needle is used. Following collection the sample must be air free, sealed (a rubber stopper over the needle suffices), and kept in an ice bath or assayed right away. Samples can be kept in an ice water bath for up to 6 hours and still give accurate values.[27] However, it is best to analyze them as soon as possible, preferably within an hour. The patient's temperature should be recorded so that the measured blood gas values can be adjusted. This is especially important for the pH and $PaO_2$. Routine analysis at 37°C without adjustment can give falsely low $PaO_2$ and $PaCO_2$ and a high pH in a hyperthermic patient, and falsely increased values for a hypothermic patient.[28]

Normal mature horses at rest have a $PaO_2$ of at least 84 mm Hg. Hypoxemia is defined as a $PaO_2$ below 80 mm Hg and hypercapnea is a $PaCO_2$ above 45 mm Hg.[17] Older horses normally have a lower $PaO_2$ than young horses and altitude also exerts an effect.[17] The $PaCO_2$ is used to assess adequacy of ventilation. A low $PaO_2$ and normal $PaCO_2$ may occur with ventilation/perfusion mismatching and impaired gas diffusion and decreased lung volume. Hypoventilation increases $PaCO_2$ and decreases $PaO_2$. With ventilation perfusion abnormalities or right to left shunting the $PaO_2$ is decreased and $PaCO_2$ may be normal or elevated. Hyperventilation for any reason in normal horses decreases $PaCO_2$ as it increases $PaO_2$. Progression from normocarbic hypoxemia to hypercarbic (hypercapneic) hypoxemia indicates deteriorating gas exchange. Sequential blood gas analyses, therefore, can be helpful in evaluating a patient's progress and, in foals, deciding when ventilation may be needed. Although horses with COPD may be hypoxemic and hypercarbic, these values may be quite variable depending on the horses' environment; maintenance of abnormal values despite absence of allergen challenge would suggest chronic changes and a worse prognosis than if values return to normal when the horse is placed in a controlled environment.

## Testing for Allergies

Allergies are recognized as bona fide causes of respiratory disease, are sometimes suspected but not proven to be causes, and may in some cases be falsely blamed as causing respiratory disease and exercise intolerance. Except in horses that clearly respond to a challenge exposure, detecting whether a horse actually has allergic respiratory disease may be difficult. Allergen skin testing, bronchial provocation tests, and serology have been used.

Allergen skin testing has been widely used in human beings for many years, and when properly performed and interpreted with the clinical history has been considered reliable as a diagnostic test for allergic diseases. Results of skin testing in horses and the association with clinical disease have varied, with some clinicians believing they are helpful and others thinking they are invalid.[29–34] Some of the variation in results may reflect antigen variability, the horse's individual variability in disease and allergic threshold exposure potential, and variability in technique of testing and interpretation. Antigens vary geographically and what may be an important allergen in one location may be irrelevant or absent elsewhere. If a horse shows signs of COPD when pastured or only seasonally but the signs are not exacerbated by stabling or exposure to hay, allergen skin testing with barn allergens is not likely to be clinically relevant. As most horses with COPD have barn related allergies, it is barn related allergens, particularly molds, that have been most widely used for skin testing, and to my knowledge there has been relatively little investigation of plant allergens. Even when the same molds are used, the strains and antigenicity of the commercial preparations may be so dissimilar as to invalidate comparisons among different clinicians performing the tests unless the same preparations are used.

Allergen skin testing is easily performed and usually well tolerated. I recommend the intradermal technique. Occasional horses require use of a twitch or the administration of xylazine. An area approximately 20 × 25 cm (10″ × 8″) is clipped over the dorsal caudal/middle part of the neck (Fig. 2–1). Each injection site is spaced approximately 3 cm from another and marked with a dark marker below the point of injection. One tenth of 1 ml (0.1 ml) of each allergen (usually diluted to 1,000 PNU/ml) is injected intradermally using a TB syringe and a 25 to 26 gauge needle. It is important to make sure it is not injected subcutaneously. A positive control of histamine (1:1000) and negative control of saline solution are used. Although it has been suggested that codeine or morphine, which degranulate mast cells nonspecifically, would be more natural positive controls than histamine,[35,36] I know no one using these in horses. The injection sites are examined at 20 to 30 minutes for the immediate reaction and at 3 to 4 and 24 hours. Those relatively few horses showing 24-hour reactions are rechecked at 48 and 72 hours. It is important to measure the diameter and assess whether the reaction is raised, firm or soft, painful, or forms pseudopods. Each reaction should be compared with the positive and negative injections. Correct recording of the order of allergen injections is obviously critical.

False-positive skin test reactions may occur because of nonspecific irritation or irrelevant amounts of sensitization due to use of excess antigen, physical trauma to the site, or contaminants or preservatives in the solution. False-negative reactions may be caused by excessive dilution of antigens, loss of potency of allergens due to aging or incorrect storage and blocking effect of drugs, such as antihistamines, beta adrenergic drugs, theophylline, or antidepressants. In man certain areas are more sensitive than others and it is, therefore, advisable to maintain a consistent test site. In man immediate skin test reactions are more common in the evening than in the morning but it is unknown if this occurs in horses. Skin or systemic disease or variable skin thickness affects responses but this is probably of more concern in human beings. Psychologic/neurogenic influences are of unknown significance in horses but can eliminate reactions in man.

In order to minimize misinformation from skin testing it is advisable to identify a reputable commercial source of antigens, use only this source, and skin test normal horses to ascertain their responses. If the source of allergens must be changed or new allergens are added to those being tested, it is advisable

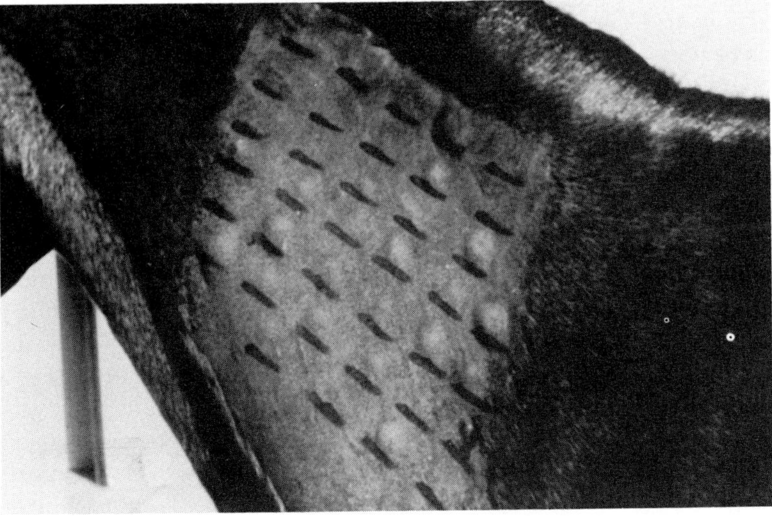

**FIG. 2–1.** Allergen skin test reactions in a horse.

to retest some control horses to evaluate the response to the new antigens. As there can be wide variation in the potency of extracts, the assessment of responses in normal horses is important. At present, even when the same source is used, it is not possible totally to eliminate variable antigenicity and quality control among different batches. In some situations an allergen suspected to be the cause of the horse's signs is not commercially available and it will be necessary to engage the help of an allergy clinic in trying to produce a suitable antigen solution. Standardization of such solutions may not be possible and it is often necessary to evaluate normal horses' responses and titrate the solution accordingly. Although the antigen solution should be sufficiently potent to elicit a reaction in allergic horses, it should not be so antigenic as to elicit large nonspecific reactions or adverse reactions (local or systemic). Allergen solutions should be kept cool and not diluted until close to time of use. The syringes should be dated and kept cool. Careful exact technique of injection at the same site in each horse is important and the time of day should be standardized as much as possible. The horse should be withdrawn from medications such as steroids, beta adrenergic agonists and antihistamines before the test. We use an arbitrary 10 to 14-day interval. People experienced with the technique should perform and interpret the test.

The type of skin test reactions (immediate or Type I, which is IgE and $IgG_4$ mediated; Type II or delayed IgG mediated Arthus reaction; and Type IV or cell mediated reaction) have been reviewed elsewhere.[29,35] It has become apparent that the late phase response that starts around 4 hours, maximizes at 6 to 12 hours, and lasts almost 24 hours is strongly dependent on the immediate response and in most allergic people not due to immune complex deposition.[37,38] As there is less emphasis on late phase or delayed reactions in people, it is impossible to compare the relative importance in horses and man. Delayed (3 to 4 hour) reactions are the most common in horses but as some horses show persistent delayed or cell mediated reactions even at 48 and 72 hours, it is important to check for the latter types of reactions.

Serology is used in human pulmonary medicine in the diagnosis of various fungal infections and allergic respiratory disease. Precipitating antibodies to Micropolyspora faeni and less frequently Thermoactinomyces vulgaris are found in sera from patients with farmer's lung disease. Serum levels of IgG and IgE (total and specific for individual antigens) are measured in human beings with suspected allergic respiratory disease. In type I reactions an antigen elicits a rise in IgE and in type 3 reactions antigens stimulate circulating IgG antibodies. There have been few published serologic studies in horses with respiratory disease.[31,32,39]

One study examined sera from horses with COPD and compared levels of precipitating antibodies to Micropolyspora faeni and Aspergillus fumigatus with those in unaffected horses.[31] Although antibodies were more frequent in horses with COPD, they were also found in some unaffected horses and horses with COPD without antibodies clinically worsened on inhalation challenge with these antigens.[31] Other studies also have shown a greater prevalence of precipitins against M. faeni in horses with COPD[34,39] (B. Pauli, H. Gerber and V. Schatzman, cited in [39]). In a report on chicken hypersensitivity pneumonitis in horses, normal as well as affected horses had precipitating antibodies to chicken serum.[32] As with allergen skin testing there is overlap in reactions. At the present time serologic techniques that can be accurately applied to clinical use in equine medicine are lacking. Tests specific for use in man cannot be applied indiscriminately to equine patients and until there is more information on basic equine immunology and antibody response to allergen exposure, serologic testing is not of great value to the practitioner.

Another serologic test which has been applied to horses is the serum $\alpha$-1-antitrypsin activity. This antiprotease is decreased in some human patients with emphysema and serves as a marker for the condition. Studies to determine whether horses with chronic pulmonary disease have a deficiency of this protein have shown no abnormality in serum levels compared to horses free from disease.[40] The test appears to have no value in clinical evaluation of horses with chronic respiratory disease.

## Bronchial Provocation Testing

Pulmonary function testing and blood gas analysis pre and post inhalation challenge with allergens has been used primarily in research in COPD. However, a less sophisticated approach using clinical evaluation and natural exposure could be used to identify whether a particular bedding, environment, or feedstuff was an inciting cause. This would necessitate having the horse in an asymptomatic drug free state prior to exposure, having a horse that shows unequivocal clinical signs of disease, being able to perform repeated exposures with different allergens, keeping accurate records for critical evaluation, and having an owner or trainer who will cooperate with such trials. Because feedstuffs such as hay contain large numbers of molds, a clinical reaction to hay exposure would not be specific. However, if the horse that reacted to alfalfa hay also reacted to alfalfa cubes, pellets or alfalfa HorseHage™ (TM Hillandale Farm, Pomfret, CT), then a true allergy to alfalfa could be suspected as the latter forms of alfalfa should not have the numbers or types of molds found in the loose hay.

## References


1. Kraman SS. Lung sounds for the clinician. Arch Intern Med, *146*:1411, 1986.
2. Cherniack RM, Cherniack L, Naimark A. The Manifestations of Pulmonary Disease. In: Respiration in Health and Disease. 2nd Ed. Philadelphia, WB Saunders Co, 1972, p 177.
3. Lehrer S. Understanding Lung Sounds. Philadelphia, WB Saunders Co, 1984, p 83.
4. Goulden BE, Barnes GRG, Quinlan TJ. Electromyographic activity of the intrinsic laryngeal muscles during quiet breathing in the anesthetized horse. NZ Vet J, *24*:157, 1976.
5. Moore MP, Andrews F, Reed SM, et al. Electromyographic evaluation of horses with laryngeal hemiplegia. G Pidgeon (ed). Madison, Omnipress, 1989. In: Proceedings of 7th ACVIM Forum, San Diego, 1989, p 1011.
6. Art T, Serteyn D, Lekeux P. Effect of exercise on the partitioning of equine respiratory resistance. Equine Vet J, *20*:268, 1988.
7. Art T, Lekeux P. A critical assessment of pulmonary function testing in exercising ponies. Vet Res Com, *12*:25, 1988.
8. Art T, Lekeux P. Pulmonary mechanics during treadmill exercise in race ponies. Vet Res Com, *12*:245, 1988.
9. Attenburrow DP, et al. Respiratory airflow and sounds intensity. In: Equine Exercise Physiology. DH Snow, SGB Persson, RJ Rose (eds). Cambridge, Granta Editions, 1983, pp 23–26.
10. Derksen FJ, Stick JA, Scott EA, et al. Effect of laryngeal hemiplegia and laryngoplasty on upper airway flow mechanics in exercising horses. Am J Vet Res, *47*:16, 1986.
11. Soma LR, Beech J, Gerber NH, Jr. Effects of Cromolyn in Horses with Chronic Obstructive Pulmonary Disease. Vet Res Com, *11*:339, 1987.
12. Derksen FJ, Scott D, Robinson NE, et al. Intravenous histamine administration in ponies with recurrent airway obstruction (heaves). Am J Vet Res, *46*:774, 1985.
13. Gillespie JR, Tyler WS, Eberly VE. Pulmonary ventilation and resistance in emphysematous and control horses. J Appl Physiol, *21*:416, 1966.
14. Derksen FJ, Robinson NE, Armstrong PJ, et al. Airway reactivity in ponies with recurrent airway obstruction (heaves). J Appl Physiol, *58*:598, 1984.
15. Derksen FJ, Robinson NE. Esophageal and intrapleural pressures in the healthy conscious pony. Am J Vet Res, *41*:1756, 1980.
16. McPherson EA, Lawson GHK. Some Aspects of Chronic Pulmonary Diseases of Horses and Methods used in their Investigation. Reprinted from: Equine Vet J, *6*:1–6. Presented at Annual Congress of British Equine Veterinary Association, Edinburgh, 1972.
17. Sasse HH. Some Pulmonary Function Tests in Horses. PhD Thesis, State University, Utrecht.
18. Willoughby RA, McDonell WN. Pulmonary Function Testing in Horses. Symposium on Equine Respiratory Disease. Vet Clin N Am [Large An], *1*:171, 1979.
19. Muylle E, Vanden Hende C, Oyaert W. Nitrogen clearance in horses as a respiratory function test. Zbl Vet Med A, *19*:310, 1972.
20. Muylle E, Oyaert W. Lung function tests in obstructive pulmonary disease in horses. Equine Vet J, *5*:37, 1973.
21. Robinson NE, Sorenson PR, Goble DO. Patterns of airflow in normal horses and horses with respiratory disease. Proc Am Assoc Eq Pract, *21*:11, 1975.
22. Spörri H, Leeman W. Zur Untersuchung der lungenmechanik bei grosstieren (Research on lung mechanics in large animals). Schw Arch Teir, *106*:699, 1964.
23. Spörri H, Zerobin K. Zur physiologic und methodik der lungenfunktionsprüfung (Toward a physiology and methodology of lung function tests). Tierärz Umschau, *19*:285, 1964.
24. Beadle R. Experiences with whole body plethysmography in horses with obstructive pulmonary disease. E Deegan (ed). Internat Symp, Hanover, 1985.

25. West JB. Respiratory Physiology—the essentials. 2nd Ed. Baltimore, Williams & Wilkins, 1979.
26. Young SS, Hall LW. A rapid noninvasive method for measuring total respiratory impedance in the horse. Equine Vet J, *21*:99, 1989.
27. Kosch PC, Koterba AM, Coons TJ, et al. Developments in management of the newborn foal in respiratory distress. Part I. Evaluation. Equine Vet J, *16*:312, 1984.
28. Guentner CA. Respiratory Function of the Lungs and Blood in Pulmonary Medicine. CA Guentner, MH Welch (eds). Philadelphia, JP Lippincott Co, 1977, pp 124–150.
29. Halliwell REW, Fleischman JB, Mackay Smith M, et al. The role of allergy in chronic pulmonary disease of horses. J Am Vet Med Assoc, *174*:277, 1979.
30. Hockenjos PH. The possible etiologic importance of hay mites in the development of allergic respiratory diseases in the horse (Zur moeglichin Aetiologischen Bedeutung von Heumilben fuer allergisch bedingte Lungenkiankheiten des Pferdes). Schweiz Arch Tierheilk, *123*:129, 1981.
31. Lawson GHK, McPherson EA, Murphy JR, et al. The prevalence of precipitating antibodies in the sera of horses with COPD. Equine Vet J, *11*:172, 1979.
32. Mansmann RA. Chicken hypersensitivity pneumonitis in horses. J Am Vet Med Assoc, *166*:673, 1975.
33. McPherson EA, Lawson GH, Murphy JR, et al. COPD in horses: Etiological studies. Responses to intradermal and inhalation antigen challenge. Equine Vet J, *11*:159, 1979.
34. Eyre P. Equine pulmonary emphysema: A bronchopulmonary mold allergy. Vet Rec, *91*:134, 1972.
35. Nelson HS. Diagnostic procedures in allergy. Allergy skin testing. Ann Allergy, *51*:411, 1983.
36. Knicker WT, Hales SW, Lee LK. Diagnostic methods to demonstrate IgE antibodies: Skin testing techniques. Bull NY Acad Med, *57*:524, 1981.
37. Solley GD, Gleich GJ, Jordon RE, et al. Late cutaneous reactions due to IgE antibodies. In: Asthma, Physiology Immunopharmacology and Treatment, Second International Symposium. New York, Academic Press, 1977, p 283.
38. Agarwall K, Zetterstiöm O. Diagnostic significance of late cutaneous allergic responses and their correlation with radioallergosorbent test. Clin Allergy, *12*:489, 1982.
39. Asmundrson T, Gunnarsson E, Johannesson T. "Haysickness" in Icelandic horses: Precipitin tests and other studies. Equine Vet J, *15*:229, 1983.
40. Breeze RG, Nicholls JM, Veitch J, et al. Serum antitrypsin activity in horses with chronic pulmonary disease. Vet Rec, *101*:146, 1977.

# CHAPTER 3

# TRACHEOBRONCHIAL ASPIRATES

*JILL BEECH*

## Techniques for Tracheobronchial Aspiration

Several methods of obtaining aspirates from the lower respiratory tract have been developed, each of which has its own advantages and disadvantages. With the advent of use of the fiber optic endoscope, passage of a catheter through the endoscope and into the lower trachea has become popular as it avoids the need for aseptic tracheal puncture and possible secondary complications. Transtracheal aspiration or tracheobronchial aspirates/ washings (TBA) obtained via tracheal puncture allows aseptic sampling and bypasses contamination from the upper airway which can occur when the endoscope is used. Many bacteria that populate the normal horse's pharynx are pathogenic in the lower respiratory tract and contamination of a tracheobronchial aspirate with any of these organisms could be diagnostically confusing.[1] Even the trachea of normal horses may harbor bacteria and fungi.[1–3] Streptococcal spp., Corynebacterium spp., Moraxella spp., Nocardia and many gram-negative microorganisms such as Pseudomonas spp., Enterobacter spp., Klebsiella spp. and anaerobes, including Clostridium spp., Bacteroides spp. Fusobacteria, and Peptostreptococcus spp. molds such as Aspergillus, Cladosporium, Mucor and Penicillium and also Mycoplasmas may be isolated from the pharynx.[1,2] Contamination is less likely when a pool of exudate can be seen in the trachea and the catheter tip directed into it for aspiration.

A disadvantage of tracheobronchial aspirates obtained via tracheal puncture is the rare secondary complication.[2,4] Even when strict asepsis is used and the technique is performed by an experienced clinician, an occasional horse will develop cellulitis at the site. This is usually localized but may extend along the entire ventral cervical region and dorsal to the jugular groove. Although this could be expected if the aspirate retrieved infectious exudate which could have contaminated the subcutaneous tissues, some cases have occurred when the aspirate has been noninflammatory in character and bacterial cultures have been negative. Tracheal cartilage laceration can result in chondromas and stenosis of the tracheal lumen; it is highly unlikely when the technique is performed by an experienced clinician using a small bore cannula, but was more likely when large 8- or 10-gauge needles were used. The possibility of the catheter breaking off in the tracheal lumen or in subcutaneous tissue is highly unlikely when the technique is performed correctly.

Techniques for transtracheal aspirates vary but aseptic technique is important in all of them. Most mature horses do not require sedation or additional restraint beyond that of the handler steadying the head and keeping the horse still. Occasionally a short acting tranquilizer such as xylazine* or use of a twitch is needed. Foals that are not severely ill or compromised usually require sedation or restraint to keep them still. Butorphanol†

*Rompum, Haver, Miles Laboratories, Shawnee, Kansas

†Stadol™, Bristol Laboratories, Syracuse, New York

(0.01 mg/kg IM or IV) can be given with xylazine if the latter is deemed inadequate. Use of a tranquilizer or twitch may help discourage some horses from coughing and dislodging the catheter retrograde into the pharynx. Local anesthesia at the site of puncture is not necessary providing that a small gauge (14 gauge) cannula is used.

The trachea should be palpated. A small area over the middle to lower third of the trachea where it is superficial and the cartilage rings are easily palpable should be aseptically prepared. The horse should be positioned so its neck is straight and landmarks are easily palpable. Heavy muscling of the neck may prevent using a site low in the neck. The person collecting the sample may easily perform the procedure alone, but some find it easier to have an assistant to handle the syringes. The latter person need not wear gloves but the person performing the technique should maintain asepsis. Following a surgical scrub the collector grasps the trachea with one gloved hand, palpates the tracheal rings, and selects a space between two rings for penetration (Fig. 3–1). No skin incision is needed as the cannula can be passed directly through the skin into the tracheal lumen. The skin should be tensed and the trachea stabilized so that the cannula will not slip off its side and potentially puncture tracheal rings or large vessels.

One method that works effectively uses a commercially available 16 gauge through the needle catheter* with a 58 cm (24″) tubing. The sterile catheter and needle come prepackaged and are convenient to use. They may be resterilized and used again if economically necessary. However, if the catheter is kinked or damaged by the needle, repetitive use increases the chance of poor sample collection due to narrowing of the catheter lumen, or breaking off the catheter in the patient. Alternatively, suitably sized polyethylene tubing may be cut into appropriate lengths, sterilized and packaged and then passed through a 14-gauge cannula.

Regardless of whether a commercially available catheter and cannula or "homemade" apparatus is used, care should be taken when passing the cannula so that the opposite tracheal wall is not struck and damaged. This is not likely in most mature horses but could easily happen in foals. Provided the cannula is sharp, penetration of the skin and trachea is usually easy and depth of penetration is easy to regulate. Old horses require more force for cannula penetration than foals. The cannula's bevel should always face downwards and the pointed end be uppermost to decrease the likelihood of cutting the catheter as it is passed down the trachea. Once the cannula is in the tracheal lumen the cannula should be directed downward and the hub upward, thereby directing the catheter down and not up the trachea. When the Intracath is used, prior to inserting the cannula it is important to ensure that the tip of the catheter does not extend beyond the cannula tip, thereby impeding the skin penetration. The entire outer sterile sleeve with the enclosed catheter may remain attached to the cannula's hub; this will ensure that the catheter remains sterile as it is passed down the cannula. However, it is sometimes cumbersome to do this and one may elect to loosen the outer sleeve prior to placing the cannula so that once the latter is in place the sleeve can easily be removed and the catheter passed. When polyethylene tubing is used, the cannula is usually placed by itself and then the tubing is passed through the hub and down the cannula. Some clinicians prefer to leave the cannula in place while performing the wash as they believe it decreases the likelihood of contaminating the soft tissues with secretions in or around the catheter as it is removed from the trachea, and because it decreases the likelihood of the horse coughing the catheter retrograde into the pharynx. Others prefer to remove the cannula once a suitable length of catheter is in the tracheal lumen as they believe leaving the cannula in place does not significantly decrease the chance of cellulitis and does increase the likelihood of the catheter being severed. When the cannula is removed from the neck, it should be pulled back near the adapter hub on the other end of the catheter so that if the horse or person moves suddenly it is not likely to sever the catheter near the exit site in the horse's neck. If the cannula is left in place, its sharp point

*Intracath, Deseret Co., Sandy, Utah

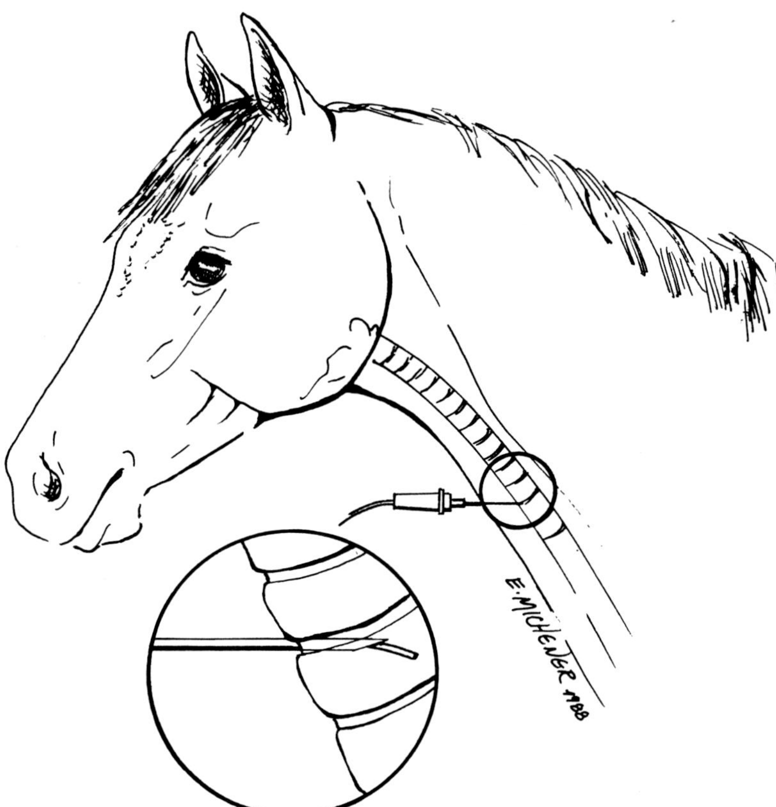


**FIG. 3–1.** Tracheobronchial aspiration. Placement of the catheter between two cartilage rings. Note the needle/cannula bevel facing downward so the sharp point will not lacerate the catheter as it is passed down the trachea. Retrograde catheter movement dorsal/cranial to the needle could result in catheter laceration.

should always be dorsal, the catheter should never be rapidly jerked back through the cannula, and the horse must be still. When an Intracath is used, the stylet within the catheter must be removed either prior to passage or when the catheter is in place. If there is resistance to one's pulling the stylet or the catheter back through the cannula, the latter should be immediately and smoothly removed to avoid cutting the catheter. Persistence in pulling the catheter back with the cannula in place can result in a severed catheter within the patient. Although one study in which stiff polyethylene catheters were deliberately severed in the horse's trachea showed that all horses coughed the tubing out within 15 minutes and were not distressed, this complication should be avoided as foreign bodies are not always expelled.[2] Also, if the catheter happens to have passed outside the trachea and down fascial planes and is cut off in the soft tissue, surgical removal will be necessary and may even require general anesthesia.

When the catheter has been passed down the trachea a sufficient length (to or past the thoracic inlet where the trachea becomes horizontal and secretions often pool), sterile 0.9% saline solution can be gently flushed in and aspirated. It is important to ensure that the saline solution does not contain a bacteriostatic agent as this could affect culture results. It is frequently necessary to detach the syringe and reaspirate several times. I prefer to start with 20 to 30 ml in a mature horse and will repeat flushing up to 100 ml if needed. In a 3- to 6-month old foal, 20 ml usually suffices and flushing and aspiration may be repeated several times. Small foals may require only half this volume. In my experience, if insufficient aspirate is obtained after 3 to 4 flushings, continued flushing is unlikely to be rewarding. One should not be too hasty to remove the catheter but should be patient when aspirating. If the patient's head is high, lowering it may increase the likelihood of retrieval of fluid. It is common and of no significance not to retrieve all the fluid injected. Excessive coughing is more likely with repeated flushing and makes adequate sample collection difficult as the catheter frequently is dislodged into the pharynx. However, coughing prior to the procedure or aspiration is often desirable as it would bring up material from deep within the respiratory tract. Exercise prior to aspiration may also help mobilize secretions. Aspiration from an area adjacent to the catheter tip does not yield a diagnostically valid sample if it is not representative of other regions of the airways.

Once the aspiration is finished, the catheter can be pulled from the neck. Maintaining suction may make leakage of catheter contents into soft tissues less likely. If the cannula has been left in place, the catheter should be removed slowly and then the cannula removed. Bleeding is usually minimal or nonexistent; gentle pressure with a sponge suffices if there is bleeding. Some clinicians inject gentamicin or other antibiotics into the soft tissue near the site of puncture as they believe it decreases the likelihood of an infectious cellulitis. I do not use this in routine cases, but it may be advisable if purulent or foul smelling material is retrieved. Penicillin should be injected if an anaerobic infection is suspected. In these cases, systemic antibiotic therapy is likely to be instituted and should decrease the likelihood of cellulitis.

If swelling does occur at the transtracheal puncture site, hot packing and local dimethyl sulfoxide (DMSO) application are helpful. If there is heat and one suspects a cellulitis is developing, it may be wise to open the area with a stab incision to allow drainage, inject nonirritant antibiotics locally, and institute systemic antibiotic medication. Drug selection should be based on Gram stain and culture results of the aspirate; if these are negative, broad spectrum coverage should be used. The horse's temperature should be monitored, although this will be lowered if nonsteroidal anti-inflammatory drugs are used to decrease pain and swelling.

When the aspirate is obtained with a flexible fiber optic endoscope, the only other materials required are a long polyethylene or Teflon catheter, an adapter hub, and syringes with sterile saline solution. The endoscope and its biopsy channel should be thoroughly cleaned with an appropriate antiseptic solution and flushed. A 0.13% glutaraldehyde-phenate bactericidal, virucidal, fungicidal, sporicidal and tuberculocidal solution* (10 minutes of contact time at room temperature) is commonly used to disinfect the biopsy channel. At present it is the preferred disinfectant as Pseudomonas spp. may remain viable in some disinfectants.[5–7] Although gas sterilization may be warranted if the endoscope has previously been used in horses with infectious disease, it is not used routinely. The same volumes (20 to 30 ml) of saline solution and flushing and aspiration technique as used in the transtracheal method usually suffice. The length of the catheter must be taken into account when aspirating samples, and patience and continued suction help. One hundred eighty cm is a workable length for the catheter. When a pediatric 9 mm diameter fiberscope is used, 180 to 240 cm (6 to 8 foot) of 190 PE tubing™† is passed into the biopsy channel. The same length of 240 PE tubing is used in the 11 mm diameter fiberscope. Although it is not necessary to wear gloves, direct handling of the portion of the catheter that will protrude into the trachea should be avoided to decrease chances of contamination. The catheter is passed into the biopsy channel until it is almost at the end of the endoscope and the latter is then passed in the routine manner. A twitch usually suffices for restraint. Occasional chemical restraint such as use of xylazine may be needed. The clinician can directly view the tip of the endoscope at the rima glottis and direct it through the opening down the trachea. It is helpful to have an attendant who can either hold or pass the endoscope or catheter under direction and flush and aspirate saline. When the endoscope's tip is in or beyond the mid-cervical trachea, the catheter is advanced from 20 to 50 cm and saline flushed in and aspirated. If exudate is present, the catheter can be directed into it. It is also possible to advance and retract the catheter. If indicated, the endoscope can be passed further into the trachea so that the carina is visible and one could perform unilateral flushing and aspiration of each mainstem bronchus. One

---

*Sporiciden, Sporiciden International, Washington, D.C.

†Clay Adams, Div. of Becton Dickinson Co., Parsippany, NJ

should perform the procedure as rapidly as possible to minimize the horse coughing and aspirating pharyngeal secretions, thereby contaminating the sample, and also to minimize tracheal and laryngeal trauma from the endoscope. Once the sample is obtained the catheter can be pulled back into the biopsy channel and the endoscope removed. The procedure is usually well tolerated in mature horses but if performed on weanlings or yearlings, chemical restraint is usually needed and a small diameter endoscope should be used. Several types of guarded endoscope tracheal swabs or brushes are commercially available* and have been reported to be reliable for obtaining cultures.[8,9] Each relies on a plugged catheter and sometimes an outer "guard" catheter. However, as isolation of upper airway contaminants or transient bacteria which are not causing inflammation is possible with any method of aspiration, it is always advisable to collect a sample that allows correlation of bacteriologic and cytologic findings.

## Sample Preparation

Several methods are available. If sufficiently cellular, the aspirate can be immediately smeared onto glass slides, the slides fixed with a commercial aerosol fixative such as Cytoprep† or air dried, and then stained. When a coating fixative is used, it should be applied to freshly prepared smears. The fixative should be removed prior to staining as it contaminates staining solutions; two washings (1 to 2 minutes each) in 80% ethyl alcohol suffice for most water soluble fixatives. Although air drying is frequently used in veterinary medicine, most human cytologists do not advocate its use due to difficulty in interpretation and potential error. This is more important when subtle cellular changes are being studied or one is trying to differentiate between benign and malignant processes. Because many samples are relatively acellular it is often necessary to centrifuge the sample 5 to 10 minutes in a centrifuge (conical) tube at 1500 × g, decant the supernatant, and then aspirate the mixed sediment to make cellular smears. Alternatively, the sample may be placed in a cytocentrifuge for 10 minutes at 75 RPM. Longer time periods (up to ½ hour) of 1500 RPM centrifuging of samples within 50 ml tubes are used in some laboratories.[10]

Regardless of how the slides are prepared in the laboratory, important cellular changes can occur in the interim. For that reason and because for many practitioners there is nearly always an unavoidable delay between obtaining the aspirate and processing it, wet fixation has been advocated. This entails adding an equal volume of 40 to 50% ethanol to the aspirate. This immediately prolongs degeneration, prevents maturation or phagocytosis, and preserves cellular detail.[11,12] One hundred ninety proof grain alcohol or other sources of pure ethanol can be appropriately diluted to 40% with sterile saline or distilled water. Ethanol fixed samples have frequently been stained with Sano's method for Pollack's trichrome stain using Mayer's or Gill's hematoxylin and cellular detail is excellent.[6,7] Air dried slides are not suitable for Romanovsky stains because of altered cell morphology. Concentration of ethyl alcohol should not exceed 50% when the sample is rich in protein as this excessively hardens the sediment. Smears can then be placed in 95% ethyl alcohol and left for several days if necessary. Gram stains can also be done. Details on commonly used stains are in Appendix 1. Commercial sources of ready made stains used for Papanicolaou staining are available.*

## Cytology

The cytology and bacterial isolates of TBA from normal horses and foals and those with various diseases have been reported (Table 4–1).[4,11–16] However, sampling technique can significantly affect cell numbers and even types of cells seen. A sample taken directly from an isolated pool of exudate in a trachea

*Darien microbiology aspiration catheter, Mill-Rose Laboratories, Inc., Mentor, OH 44060.

Guarded endoscopy culture swab, Harford Veterinary Supply Co., Potomac, MD 20854.

†Cytoprep fixative, Fisher Scientific, Pittsburgh, PA.

*Ortho Pharmaceutical Corp., Raritan, NJ Clay Adams, 141 E. 25th St., NY, NY.

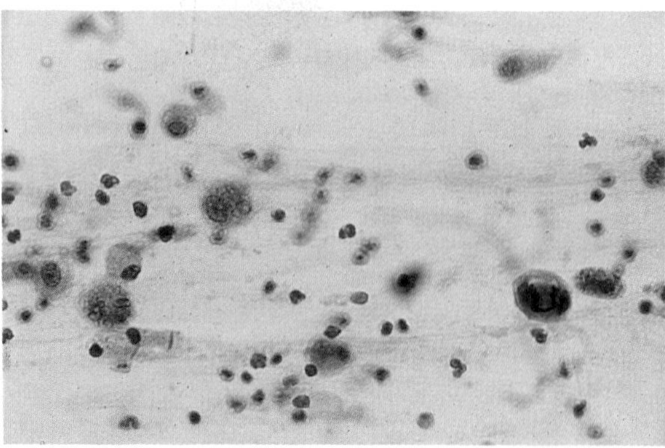

**FIG. 3–2.** Many macrophages, some containing green pigment (hemosiderophages or siderophages) and one on the right containing a pollen. There are several columnar epithelial cells with prominent terminal plates and cilia and scattered neutrophils and a few mucus strands in the background. Sano Trichrome stain. (From Beech J. Cytology of Tracheobronchial Aspirates in Horses. Vet Pathol, *12*:157, 1975.)

may look different from that obtained from flushing and aspirating from a larger area of the same trachea. If the horse coughs the catheter retrograde or if the procedure has to be abandoned for other reasons, an inadequate nonrepresentative sample may be obtained.

I do not advocate cell counts or differential cell counts on TBA specimens due to variability of volumes of fluid flushed and retrieved, failure to accurately determine the dilution factor, and variability in cellular distribution within and between smears from the same sample. Accurate counting of cells in clusters or in mucus plugs is not possible.

Normal horses have scant amounts of mucus and pulmonary alveolar macrophages (PAM) and epithelial cells predominate. Samples vary in their cellularity but are usually less cellular than those from diseased airways.

Pulmonary alveolar macrophages vary in size and shape but all have in common abundant cytoplasm and a vesicular nucleus (Fig. 3–2). Absence of PAM within the sample indicates the wash may not have retrieved adequate material from deep in the respiratory tract and hence may not accurately represent the lower airways.[10–12] The PAM nucleus is often bilobed and cells may be bi- or multinucleated. It has been suggested that the numbers of multinucleated macrophages increase when there is extracellular debris or chronic inflammation. However, multinucleated macrophages are also seen in normal horses, and in humans are often seen in sputum with no evidence of significant inflammation.[10] Percentage reported in normal horses varies according to investigator with some reporting up to 48% and others up to 68%. Frequently, racehorses with histories of chronic coughing and excess mucus in their tracheas have large numbers of active macrophages in a copious amount of mucus. In these horses the tracheal aspirate is often grossly mucoid and grey white giving the initial impression that there might be a bacterial infection and septic bronchitis, but cytology and culture results often show no evidence of sepsis or only the presence of secondary colonizers. The cytoplasm of the PAM is often finely vacuolated when there is alveolar edema or there may be large vacuoles and intracellular fungal or plant elements. Presence of ingested fungal elements does not indicate the horse has fungal pneumonia. Pigment granules may be seen. Iron pigment may vary from fine granular brownish gold material to larger irregular spheres. Aging of the pigment affects the refractile appearance and granularity. Hemosiderophages are commonly found in race horses or other horses in strenuous work[11,13] and indicate pulmonary hemorrhage or previous presence of blood in the airways (Fig. 3–2). They can be seen in healthy racehorses with no signs of respiratory disease, but are rarely seen in non-working, healthy horses. In one study of 24 normal horses, 18/19 (95%) in training had hemosiderophages but only 2/5 (40%) of nontraining horses had hemosiderophages. Also, the percent of hemosiderophages in horses known to have EIPH was less when the horses were not in active training.[13] In a study of 20 healthy foals between 1 and 6 months of age, no hemosiderophages were seen unless the foals had had repeated transtracheal aspirates.[16]

Other conditions (which cause hemorrhage into the airways) besides EIPH can result in hemosiderophages. As it is not possible to identify positively the source of iron in the macrophage, it has been suggested that the less specific term siderophage is more accurate than hemosiderophage.[17] Some authors point out that siderophages can occur in human lung when there are circulatory low flow states (such as in hemorrhagic shock), intravascular lysis of erythrocytes, and formation of abnormal heme. The iron could come from heme following hemorrhage or it could be picked up by macrophages after it has passed through cell membranes and then becomes bound by mucopolysaccharides from edema fluid or mucus.

Erythrophagocytosis may be seen if there has been fresh blood in the airways and is not pathognomonic for pulmonary hemorrhage. Also, if the aspirate contains erythrocytes secondary to bleeding associated with the procedure, viable macrophages within the aspirate can rapidly engulf the cells if the slides are not prepared or the aspirate fixed immediately following sample retrieval. In vitro studies have shown significant erythrophagocytosis can occur within 1 hour when macrophages are exposed to erythrocytes.[18] Nuclear debris may also be ingested by macrophages. Intracellular bacteria are not seen in normal horses.

Ciliated columnar epithelial cells form a significant proportion of cells retrieved from normal horses and may be more numerous in aspirates obtained via the endoscope.[11,13] When seen from the side the long cells have a nucleus at one end with finely granular chromatin and sometimes nucleoli, homogenous cytoplasm, a terminal plate, and well defined cilia (Fig. 3–2). When low columnar or cuboidal epithelial cells from the small airways are seen on end, little cytoplasm is visible around the nucleus and the cells are frequently in cohesive clusters. Presence of rounded ciliated cytoplasmic tufts lacking a nucleus in the presence of the basal fragment of the cell (ciliocytophthoria) is abnormal and in other species has been associated with viral infections (Fig. 3–3). The basal fragment has inclusions, pyknosis or karyorrhexis. Clinical and epidemiologic evidence has suggested but not proven a viral etiology in horses.[13,19] Ciliated tufts by themselves only indicate nonspecific cell fragmentation which commonly occurs with inflammation. Grouping of bronchiolar or bronchial epithelial cells indicates early squamous metaplasia, dysplasia, or hyperplasia.[10]

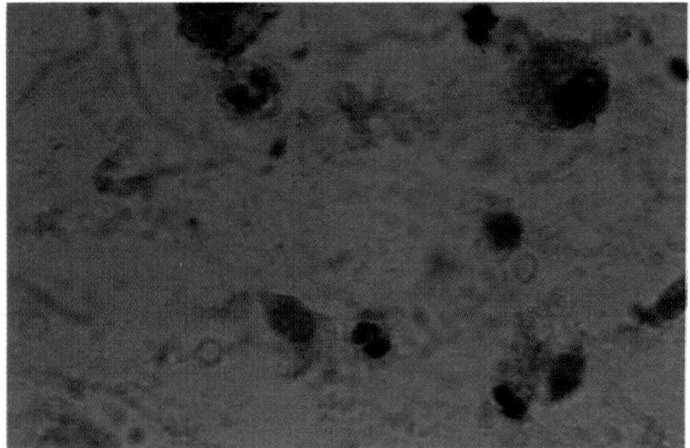

**FIG. 3–3.** Ciliated tuft. There is a macrophage in the top corner and several neutrophils. Sano Trichrome stain. (From Beech J. Cytology of Tracheobronchial Aspirates in Horses. Vet Pathol, *12*:157, 1975.)

Goblet cells are rare or absent in aspirates from normal horses.[11–13] An increase suggests metaplasia or hyperplasia secondary to chronic irritation. Their size varies according to their mucus content. They are nonciliated with a nucleus at one end and can be oval or more elongated.

Presence of squamous and superficial squamous epithelial cells usually indicates contamination from the upper respiratory tract and is more common in relatively acellular aspirates obtained via the endoscope. However, it may be difficult to distinguish pharyngeal squamous epithelial cells from those originating from squamous metaplasia lower in the respiratory tract and one should not assume they could only have originated from the upper airway if the cellular pattern and/or clinical signs suggest other possibilities. They also may be seen in aspirates retrieved from horses that are aspirating (Fig. 3–4). Stratified squamous epithelial cells and cuboidal nonciliated epithelial cells have been described in the trachea of a horse with COPD.[20] Early squamous metaplasia, dysplasia or hyperplasia of bronchiolar or bronchial cells has been described as a frequent abnormality in aspirates.[12] Such cells could be retrieved on a TBA from such horses. When pharyngeal or oral contamination occurs, squamous epithelial cells may be seen alone

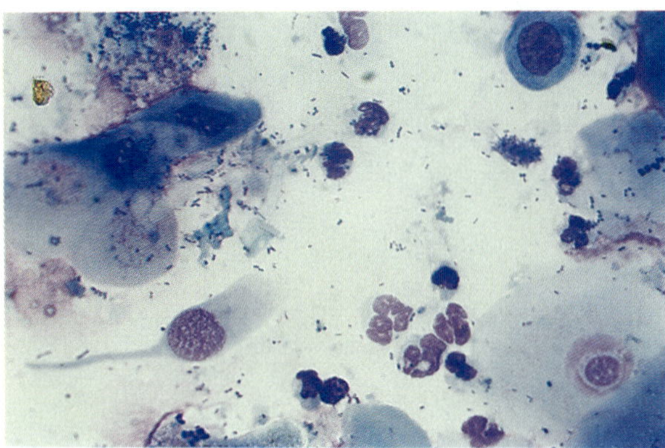

**FIG. 3–4.** Aspirate from a horse with aspiration pneumonia secondary to botulism. In the periphery are several squamous cells with surface bacteria. Neutrophils predominate and there is a damaged columnar epithelial cell which appears to have lost its terminal plate and cilia. Wright Giemsa stain.

or in groups and usually appear as large rectangular or trapezoidal cells with a small nucleus, homogeneous cytoplasm and frequently numerous small uniform pigment granules and/or surface bacteria. They also sometimes appear rolled up in cigar shapes.

Smaller squamous cells from parabasal layers may occasionally be seen even in normal horses, although their presence could indicate squamous metaplasia. They have relatively large nuclei and prominent chromatin granules and if in groups may have intercellular bridges.[13]

Presence of abnormal types of epithelial cells should alert one to the possibility of neoplasia or metaplasia, both of which are rare in equine lungs (Fig. 3–5). Neoplasia was diagnosed on the basis of an aspirate from a mare with an endometrial adenocarcinoma that had metastasized to the lungs. Extremely viscid copious secretions contained many sheets of abnormal epithelial cells, sometimes with abundant vacuolated cytoplasm and having varying nuclear size and sometimes many nuclei.[21]

The presence of other small nonciliated cuboidal or spherical cells of uncertain identification has been reported.[13] Creolar body type clusters have also been reported; they were rounded clusters of cuboidal epithelial cells with ill defined cilia.[13]

Neutrophils normally comprise a proportion of cells present even in normal horses but they are usually well preserved. As the lung is a normal site for removal of neutrophils, the presence of a few degenerate neutrophils is of no clinical significance. In one study in England on 42 normal horses and ponies, the percent neutrophils ranged from 0 to 21%.[14,15] In another study, mean percent neutrophils was $9 \pm 12\%$.[22] In contrast, a high percentage of neutrophils ($39.0 \pm 21.0$ sd or a range of 3 to 83%) was found in another study of histologically normal lung using both postmortem tracheobronchial lavage and antemortem transtracheal aspiration.[23] Similar findings were reported in another study on 10 clinically normal horses where mean percent neutrophils was $32 \pm 8.9$ SE; no postmortem confirmation of their status was available.[24] A study of transtracheal aspirates from 27 clinically normal horses with lungs that were grossly and histologically normal and 57 with respiratory tract disease suggested that more than 40% neutrophils was abnormal. In this study, four clinically and historically normal horses were found to have increased numbers of neutrophils and histologic evaluation revealed bronchiolitis.[11]

In a study of 20 clinically healthy foals between 1 to 6 months of age, 10 had more than 70% neutrophils in their transtracheal aspirates. Degenerate neutrophils were sometimes present and were more common when numbers of neutrophils were increased.

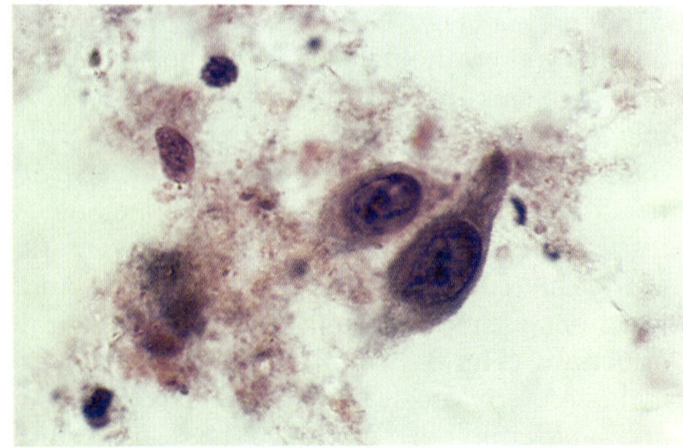

**FIG. 3–5.** Two large malignant cells with clumped chromatin in a transtracheal aspiration. Necropsy diagnosis was primary lung papillary adenocarcinoma. ×400 Sano Trichrome. (Courtesy Dr. J. Roszel.)

However, their presence was not significantly associated with the isolation of pathogenic bacteria.[16]

Usually, presence of degenerate neutrophils (karyolysis, hypersegmented or pyknotic nuclei, etc.) has been used as an indicator of sepsis and some people have used it to differentiate between horses with chronic nonseptic bronchiolitis or COPD and septic bronchitis. Nondegenerate neutrophils are greatly increased in horses with COPD and are usually the predominant cell type (Fig. 3–6).

Eosinophils are recognized by their characteristic granules or by multiple hollow spheres when degranulated (Fig. 3–7). They may be seen in low numbers in clinically normal horses. Percentages cited have usually been less than 3%.[14,15,22] Because eosinophils are frequently unevenly distributed in a smear and often grouped in mucus, other clinicians prefer to classify whether they are rarely or frequently seen.[11,12] It is important to look at several smears in their entirety, as cell differential counting in one area can be misleading. In one study, 1 out of 24 normal tracheal washes was reported to have significant numbers.[13] Five to 7% of normal horses in race training had eosinophils and 12% of horses with EIPH in race training were reported to have eosinophils. Interestingly, none of the 10 EIPH horses that were out of training had eosinophils.[13] In a study of 94

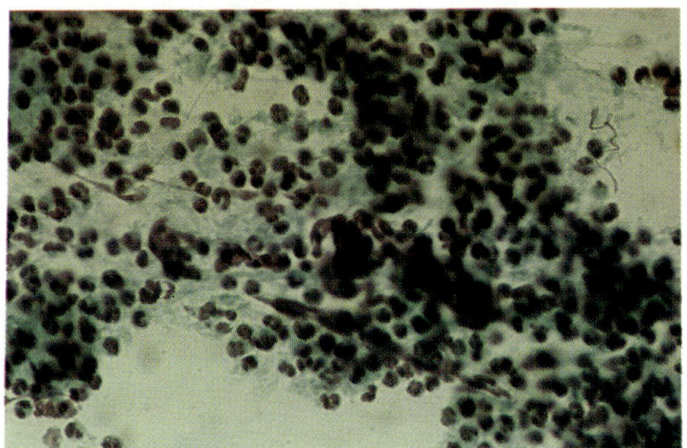

**FIG. 3–6.** Sheets of neutrophils in a proteinaceous background from a horse with COPD. A somewhat spiraling linear structure near the right margin resembles a Curshmann's spiral Sano Trichrome. (From Beech J. Cytology of Tracheobronchial Aspirates in Horses. Vet Pathol, *12*:157, 1975.)

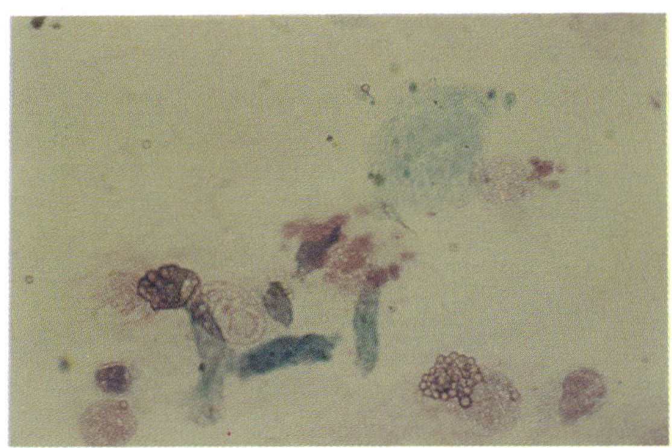

**FIG. 3–7.** Squamous cell contamination and eosinophils in an aspirate (DiffQuik™ stain). (Courtesy Dr. E. Ziemer.)

clinically normal racehorses stabled indoors at a racetrack, 45% had some eosinophils and they were more common in the 20 horses that had no evidence of EIPH (C.R. Sweeney, personal communication). Another study reported up to 8% eosinophils from normal washes; anthelminthic medication histories, parasite exposure or exposure to allergens were not reported.[20] It is probable that both environment and parasite exposure affect numbers seen. Age may also be important. A study on clinically normal foals showed that 14/20 initial aspirates had increased numbers of eosinophils and in 9 there were no other signs of inflammation. Aspirates performed at 3-week intervals on 9 of these foals showed the eosinophilia was maintained.[16] It is possible that ascarid migration was the cause of the eosinophils. Parasites are recognized potent sources of antigens and it is not surprising that young horses which are probably experiencing ascarid larval migration would have increased eosinophils in their aspirates. Increased numbers of eosinophils may be seen in horses with Dictyocaulus arnfieldi[13,15,25] (Fig. 3–8). Up to 36% of horses with chronic coughs have been reported to have eosinophils.[13] Most horses with COPD, however, have an overwhelming neutrophilia and eosinophils are not a predominant cell type.[11] A horse with eosinophilic infiltrates and granulomas was reported to have an increased eosinophilia in the tracheal wash.[13]

Lymphocytes have large nuclei and relatively small amounts of cytoplasm. They may

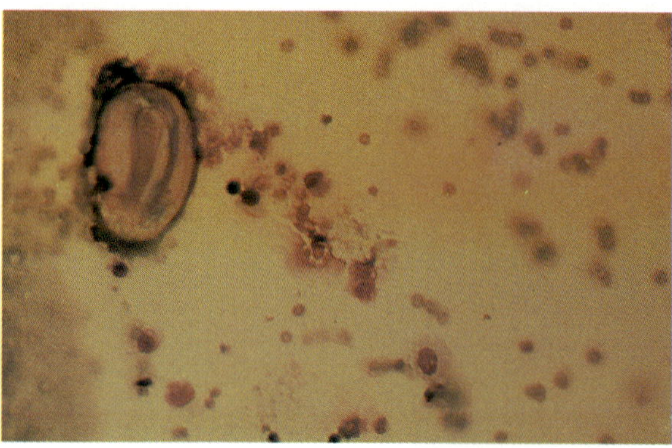

**FIG. 3–8.** Dictyocaulus arnfieldi (DiffQuik™ stain).

be difficult to differentiate from ciliated columnar epithelial cells seen "end-on" or small macrophages.

Basophils or plasma cells are rarely seen but were reported in a few chronically coughing horses.[13] Horses with diffuse eosinophilic lung changes were reported to generally have higher plasma cell and lymphocyte (as well as eosinophil) counts in their tracheobronchial lavages.[23]

Mast cells are not usually evaluated or quantified because stains commonly used (Diff-Quik, Gram stain)* do not identify them. Following fixation with a substance such as a Cytoprep fixative† slides should be stained with either Wright's stain or the quick toluidine blue method.[26] Mast cells are identified by their characteristic metachromatic staining granules. These granules contain both slowly and rapidly released preformed mediators which can generate immediate and late phase allergic reactions. Studies in other species have demonstrated their important role in allergic respiratory disease but there are scant data specific for the horse. They are either absent or present in low numbers in normal horse's tracheal or tracheobronchial aspirates.[14,22,23] In a study on 94 racehorses stabled indoors at a racetrack, mast cells were found in about 80% of the aspirates (CR Sweeney, personal communication). In a group of foals with eosinophils in their aspirates, mast cells were more frequently seen as percent eosinophils increased; however, this association was not statistically significant.[16]

Inclusions have been reported in epithelial cells and cells resembling histiocytes in bronchial aspirates from both healthy horses and those with respiratory disorders.[19] Inclusions are frequently used as an indicator of viral infections. However, they may be idiopathic due to deranged cell function or be part of nonspecific cell degeneration and death.[19] The ground glass appearing nuclei and nuclear inclusions were often surrounded by a clear halo and resembled those seen in equine herpesvirus type I infected tissue culture cells.[19]

Curschmann's spirals, which are casts of inspissated mucus plugs from small airways, are recognized by their coiled densely staining core and lighter periphery. They have been seen in horses with chronic lung diseases (Figs. 3–6 and 3–9).[11,12] Inspissated mucus may also form dark blobs. Lamellated purple round to oval structures have been seen in horses with severe purulent infections and may represent conglomerates of dead cells and/or inspissated partially mineralized exudate.[11] When Sano's trichrome stain is used, a pale watery blue background with precipitated granular material is compatible with pulmonary edema.[12]

It is not uncommon to find various plant spores and fungal elements in transtracheal aspirates. Their presence does not indicate fungal infection and probably reflects the horse's environment and mucociliary function. If bacteria are seen in the absence of

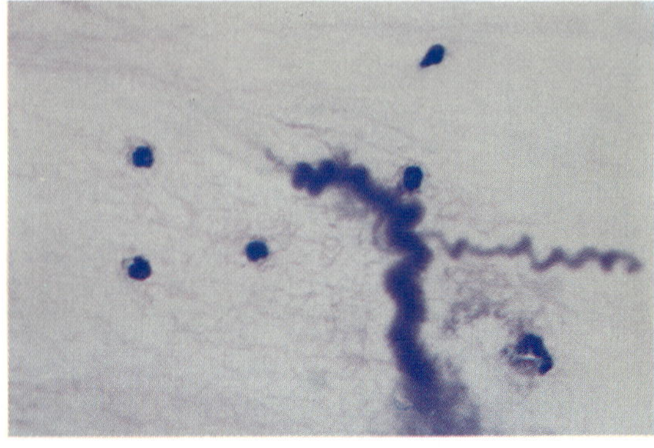

**FIG. 3–9.** Curshmann's spirals, Wright Giemsa stain. (Courtesy Dr. E. Ziemer.)

*Diff-Quik, Harleco, Gibbstown, NJ

†Cytoprep fixative, Fisher Scientific, Pittsburgh, PA

cytologic evidence of sepsis, it is unlikely they are the cause of the horse's respiratory ailment.

## Bacteriology

The portion of the sample that is to be submitted for culture and sensitivity should be processed rapidly to maximize accurate results. It is important to culture specimens rapidly as even nonbacteriostatic sterile saline solution reportedly may kill some organisms including S. pneumoniae.[27] Various commercial transport media are available. These media, such as Port-a-Cul,* are satisfactory for both aerobic and anaerobic isolation, but anaerobic isolation cannot be performed on samples not placed in the appropriate culture media specific for the procedure. The commonly used culture swabs within a plastic sheath are not suitable for anaerobic isolation.

Gram's staining should be performed promptly and will aid early antibiotic selection. On a Gram's stain, gram-positive bacteria will stain blue and gram-negative bacteria will stain red orange. Age of the bacteria can alter stain retention and intensity. Obviously, the numbers of bacteria present as well as cellular density and presence of pyknotic cellular debris or stain precipitate can affect interpretation of a Gram's stain. As mentioned previously if there is cytologic evidence of contamination from the upper respiratory tract, interpretation will be difficult. Also, the presence of bacteria, especially a mixed population with no evidence of septic cellular changes, should be cautiously interpreted.

In one study of 105 horses with historical and/or clinical evidence of bacterial pulmonary disease, gram-negative rods were seen in 55 and gram-positive cocci in 90.[28] Of the 55 specimens that had gram-negative organisms, 40 yielded one or more gram-negative bacterial rods on culture. Nineteen of the 105 aspirates that had no visible gram-negative rods yielded gram-negative anaerobes on culture, indicating a 68% cytologic prediction rate. Of the aspirates having gram-positive cocci, 72 yielded one or more aerobic gram-positive bacteria on culture, and the cytologic prediction rate was 94% as gram-positive bacteria were cultured from only five aspirates having no visible gram-positive bacteria. For R. equi the prediction was 83% as 5/6 aspirates from which it was cultured had gram-positive coccobacilli.[28]

One study determined bacterial isolates from the TBA of 36 healthy pastured nonexercising mature horses and 50 stabled healthy Thoroughbred race horses.[3] The TBA were obtained via an Intracath in 75% of the horses and via a large bore cannula and catheter in the others, and only samples determined to be normal cytologically were included. Aerobic pathogens were isolated with the same frequency (8%) from both racehorses and pastured horses. Most frequently isolated were Klebsiella pneumoniae, B hemolytic Streptococcus spp., Pasteurella spp. and Pseudomonas aeruginosa. Transient bacteria were isolated from 12/50 (24%) racehorses and 23/36 (64%) pastured nonexercising horses. Enterobacter agglomerans and hemolytic Streptococcus spp. and Bacillus spp. were most common in the pastured horses, whereas Staphylococcus epidermidis was most common in the racehorses. Enterobacter spp. are common in water and soil, Bacillus spp. are common in water, soil and air, and Staphylococcus epidermidis is common on skin and mucous membranes. Acinetobacter calcoaceticus and Pseudomonas stutzeri were other transient bacteria. Anaerobic culture of samples from 12 pastured horses yielded no isolates. Fungal growth was seen on the blood agar plates in 16% of both groups. Aspergillus predominated in nonracing horses, whereas Penicillium spp. and Mucor spp. predominated in racehorses. Nocardia was isolated in 19% of pastured horses but only 4% of racehorses. The higher number of pastured horses with positive cultures vs racing horses suggests that, as in other species, age, exercise and environment are important in determining equine mucociliary function and, therefore, bacterial presence in the lower respiratory tract.

Another study comparing 17 clinically normal horses in a new hospital with 17 clinically

*Port-a-Cul, Becton Dickinson, Cockeysville, MD 21030.

normal horses stabled in a wooden barn showed that twice the number of bacterial species were isolated from the former group and more than 7 times as many fungi were isolated from the latter.[2] No cytology was performed.

In mature horses with signs or histories of bacterial pneumonias, gram-positive bacteria most frequently cultured include Streptococcus spp. and, less frequently, Staphylococcus aureus. Commonly isolated gram-negative bacteria include Pasteurella spp., Escherichia coli, Enterobacter spp., Pseudomonas spp. and Klebsiella pneumonia. In addition to the above, in foals R. equi is an important isolate. Anaerobic bacteria that have been most frequently isolated include Bacteroides spp. and Clostridium spp.[29] Mycoplasmas have been reported in a small percentage of normal and diseased horses.[30,31] Their isolation requires use of special media.

In humans with chronic bronchitis and cystic fibrosis, colonization and infection with bacteria are common and some of these bacteria, especially Pseudomonas, can stimulate mucin secretion and exacerbate airway obstruction.[32] Whether this occurs in horses is unknown, but it is interesting that Pseudomonas is not an infrequent isolate from horses showing no signs of septic lung disease but having chronic excess mucus production.

As some veterinary laboratories may not routinely perform sensitivity testing on Streptococcal spp., if this need is anticipated, the request should accompany the sample. Recording sensitivity patterns may be helpful as it can reveal whether there are emerging resistance patterns and if it is necessary to alter antibiotics commonly prescribed for respiratory infections in situations where culture and sensitivity testing are not feasible.

Controversy exists over correlation of TBA cytology with lower respiratory tract disease with some investigators reporting good correlation and others not.[11,12,23] In my opinion the technique is useful for evaluating airway disease providing one is cognizant of the dynamic state of airways and the rapidity with which the cellular characteristics can change, and the possibility of sampling error. Also, smears must be examined for cytologic patterns and evaluated qualitatively. One cannot expect an inadequate or poorly handled aspirate to reflect accurately disease processes. I suspect that increased sophistication in cytologic interpretation of TBAs would greatly enhance their value in equine clinical medicine.

## References

1. Hoquet F, Higgins R, Lessard P, et al. Comparison of the bacterial and fungal flora in the pharynx of normal horses and horses affected with pharyngitis. Can Vet J, *26*:342, 1985.
2. Mansmann RA. Evaluation of transtracheal aspiration in the horse. J Am Vet Med Assoc, *169*:631, 1976.
3. Sweeney CR, Beech J, Roby KAW. Bacterial isolates from tracheobronchial aspirates of healthy horses. Am J Vet Res, *46*:2562, 1985.
4. Mansmann RA, Knight HD. Transtracheal aspiration in the horse. J Am Vet Med Assoc, *160*:1527, 1972.
5. Leach ED. A new synergized glutaraldehyde-phenate sterilizing solution and concentrated disinfectant. Infection Control, *2*:26, 1981.
6. Berkelman RL, Lewis S, Allen JR, et al. Pseudobacteria attributed to contamination of povidone-iodine with *Pseudomonas cepacia*. Ann Intern Med, *95*:32, 1981.
7. Nakahara H, Kozukue H. Isolation of chlorhexidine-resistant Pseudomonas aeruginosa from clinical lesions. J Clin Microbiol, *5*:166, 1982.
8. Sweeney CR, Sweeney RW, Benson CE. Bacteriology of guarded endoscope tracheal swabs compared to percutaneous tracheal aspirates in the horse. J Am Vet Med Assoc, *195*:1225, 1989.
9. Darien BJ, Brown CM, Walker RD, et al. A bronchoscopic technique to obtain uncontaminated lower airway secretions for bacterial culture. Poster Presentation. Proceedings of 7th Annual ACVIM, May, San Diego, 1989, p 1048.
10. Koss LG. Diagnostic Cytology and its Histopathologic Bases. 2nd Ed. Philadelphia, JB Lippincott Co, 1968.
11. Beech J. Cytology of tracheobronchial aspirates in horses. Vet Pathol, *12*:157, 1975.
12. Roszel JF, Freeman KP, Slusher SH. Equine pulmonary cytology. Proc 31st Annu Meet Am Assoc Equine Pract, 1985, p 171.
13. Whitwell KE, Greet TRC. Collection and evaluation of tracheobronchial washes in the horse. Equine Vet J, *16*:499, 1984.
14. Mair TS, Stokes CR, Bourne JR. Cellular content of secretions obtained by lavage from different levels of the equine respiratory tract. Equine Vet J, *19*:458, 1987.
15. Mair TS. Value of tracheal aspirates in the diagnosis of chronic pulmonary disease in the horse. Equine Vet J, *19*:463, 1987.
16. Crane SA, Ziemer EL, Sweeney CR. Tracheobron-

chial aspirates from clinically normal foals: Cytologic and bacteriologic evaluation. Am J Vet Res, *50*:2042, 1989.

17. Roszel JF, Freeman KP, Slusher SH, et al. Siderophages in pulmonary cytology specimens from racing and nonracing horses. In: Proceedings of 33rd Annual Meeting of American Association of Equine Practice, 1987, p 321.
18. Hand WL, King-Thompson NL. Effect of erythrocyte ingestion on macrophage antibacterial function. Infect Immun, *40*:917, 1983.
19. Freeman KP, Roszel JF, Slusher SH. Inclusions in equine cytologic specimens. J Am Vet Med Assoc, *184*:359, 1985.
20. Yamashiro S, Viel L, Bast T, et al. The morphological study of airways and cells recovered by bronchoalveolar lavage in a horse with chronic obstructive pulmonary disease (COPD). Anat Rec, *211*:219A, 1985.
21. Gunson DE, Gillette DM, Beech J, et al. Endometrial adenocarcinoma in a mare. Vet Pathol, *17*:777, 1980.
22. Nuytten J, Muylle E, Oyaert W, et al. Cytology bacteriology and phagocytic capacity of tracheobronchial aspirates in healthy horses and horses with chronic obstructive pulmonary disease (COPD). Zentbl Vet Med Assoc, *30*:114, 1983.
23. Larson VL, Busch RH. Equine tracheobronchial lavage: Comparison of lavage cytologic and pulmonary histopathologic findings. Am J Vet Res, *46*:144, 1985.
24. Derksen FJ, Brown CM, Sonea I, et al. Comparison of transtracheal aspirate and bronchoalveolar lavage cytology in 50 horses with chronic lung disease. Equine Vet J, *21*:23, 1989.
25. George LW, Tanner ML, Robertson EL, et al. Chronic respiratory disease in a horse infected with *Dictyocaulus arnfieldi*. J Am Vet Med Assoc, *179*:820, 1981.
26. Humason GT. Cytoplasmic elements. In: Animal Tissue Techniques. San Francisco, WH Freeman and Co, 1962, p 282.
27. Rein MF, Mandell GL. Bacterial killing by bacteriostatic saline solutions—potential for diagnostic error. N Engl J Med, *289*:794, 1973.
28. Morris DD. Equine tracheobronchial aspirates: Correlation of cytologic and microbiologic findings. J Am Vet Med Assoc, *184*:340, 1984.
29. Sweeney CR, Divers TJ, Benson CE. Anaerobic bacteria in 21 horses with pleuropneumonia. J Am Vet Med Assoc, *187*:721, 1985.
30. Allam WD, Powell DG, Andrews BE, et al. The isolation of *Mycoplasma spp* from horses. Vet Rec, *93*:402, 1973.
31. Windsor DG. The isolation of Mycoplasma from horses. Vet Rec, *93*:593, 1973.
32. Adler KB, Hendler D, Davis GS. Bacteria associated with obstructive pulmonary disease elaborate extracellular products that stimulate mucin secretion by explants of guinea pig airways. Am J Pathol, *125*:501, 1986.

# CHAPTER 4

# BRONCHOALVEOLAR LAVAGE

*CORINNE R. SWEENEY and JILL BEECH*

Bronchoalveolar lavage (BAL) is a diagnostic procedure which has become relatively widespread in human pulmonary medicine over the past 10 to 15 years[1] and its use is increasing in equine medicine. The aim of the procedure is to atraumatically instill fluid into the airways to collect epithelial lining fluid and cells from the alveoli and distal airways when this fluid is aspirated.

## Technique

There are several methods for BAL in the horse. Which method a veterinarian chooses may depend on the intended use of the BAL sample, the available equipment, and the need to know the lung location from which the BAL is collected. The two basic methods are the use of a flexible fiberoptic endoscope and the use of a blindly placed BAL tube.* Variations of these methods will be described.

Bronchoalveolar lavage is routinely done in the standing sedated horse. If large numbers of viable macrophages without blood contamination are necessary for macrophage function studies, general anesthesia may be required.[2] Five percent guaifenesin† and 0.2% thiopental‡ have been used following sedation with xylazine.§ Xylazine and ketamine|| anesthesia (1.1 mg/kg and 2.2 mg/kg respectively given slowly intravenously) has also been used. Standing sedation is the more frequently used method as it can readily be applied to clinical patients. In our experience, except for horses in profound respiratory distress, sedation had no negative influence on their welfare. In the standing horse, we recommend the use of xylazine (Rompun)* at 0.88 mg/kg (400 mg/450 kg horse) to help in successful lavage. Following placement of a nose twitch for restraint a ≥2 meter flexible fiberoptic endoscope is passed through the nasal passage to the carina and the distal end is then passed into a main stem bronchus. Obviously the diameter of the endoscope determines in what generation airway the tip will wedge. An 8 mm diameter endoscope will wedge in a fourth generation airway of a mature horse. The advantage of the flexible fiberoptic endoscope is that you can wedge the endoscope in a selected bronchus. This is particularly important if one is trying to lavage a specific area of the lung in a horse that has focal lung disease. Unfortunately, we have found from experience that even knowing the site that we "wish" to lavage has not always enabled us to lavage that exact lung segment. When the endoscope is passed into the proximal trachea the horse may cough mildly. When the endoscope passes the carina the horse may cough significantly. The coughing usually subsides once the endoscope is wedged and lavage fluid is infused. If violent coughing persists, the procedure should be stopped. To decrease this coughing many

*BAL Catheter, Bivona, Inc., Gary, Indiana.
†Byrnes Bio Tech, Omaha, Nebraska.
‡Biocentic Laboratory, Saint Joseph, Missouri.
§Haver Lockhart, Shawnee, Kansas.
||Ketamine, ABECO Co., Inc., Fort Dodge, Iowa.

*Haver Lockhart, Shawnee Mission, Kansas.

people like to infuse a dilute lidocaine solution ahead of the endoscope as they pass it by the carina and wedge it into a distal airway. The volume of the dilute lidocaine solution used is approximately 10 to 20 ml of a 0.4% solution. This may help in depressing the cough reflex but it is our impression that in horses with a particularly strong cough reflex, i.e. horses with COPD, the lidocaine solution only minimally depresses coughing. It is our recommendation that the horse be maximally sedated as this seems most beneficial in decreasing coughing during the procedure. The disadvantage of the use of the endoscope is the expense of the equipment, and use of a video endoscope decreases portability.

A BAL tube is inexpensive, can be purchased or homemade, is portable and is easily used in a "field setting." The commercially available BAL tube (equine bronchoalveolar lavage catheter*) is 3 m long with 10 mm external diameter and 2.5 mm internal diameter. Sedation and restraint are the same as when using the endoscope. The horse's head should be extended to facilitate passage of the tube blindly into the trachea. The tube is then passed down the trachea and wedged in a bronchus in a similar fashion to the endoscope. Unfortunately, as the wedging is done blindly, which lung and what site in the lung is being lavaged is not known. The commercially available BAL tube has an inflatable cuff at the distal end (where it is wedged into the lung) and although this cuff may be helpful we find we usually do the lavages without inflating this cuff. Just as with a nasogastric tube, the BAL tube should last for a long time unless used on the rare horse who coughs the tube retrograde and chews on it.

A "homemade" bronchoalveolar lavage tube can be made with a double lumen lavage device consisting of an equine nasogastric tube (10 mm outer diameter and 8 mm internal diameter) and a polyethylene tube (3.5 mm outer diameter and 2.7 mm internal diameter). The polyethylene tubing is threaded through the nasogastric tube so the tubing is flush with the end of the nasogastric tube distally and 15 cm of polyethylene tube extends out of the nasogastric tube proximally. A teat cannula is inserted into the 15 cm end of the polyethylene tubing and a three-way stopcock inserted into the cannula.

As there has not yet been standardization of BAL technique in horses the total volume of fluid infused and the size of the individual aliquots vary.[2–9] The volume used and the size of the aliquots may depend on the intended use of the BAL sample following collection. The optimal lavage volume must be sufficiently large to lavage more than just the airway where the distal end is wedged. Studies in both humans and horses suggested a volume must be greater than 50 ml. In horses, most investigators have used between 100 and 300 ml delivered in 100 ml aliquots. Lavages using these volumes are tolerated in both the normal adult horse and foal and equine patients with severe pneumonia. The method we prefer is a 300 ml lavage delivered in three 100 ml aliquots. Each 100 ml aliquot of solution is infused through the polyethylene tubing of the endoscope biopsy channel (or BAL tube) and aspirated immediately with a suction pump. Studies comparing delivering the 300 ml aliquot in one bolus and then aspirating versus 100 ml aliquots infused and aspirated and repeated three times has shown minimal difference in total cell count and differential cell counts in the lavage fluid recovered (Sweeney, C.R., unpublished data, 1989). We have found that when lavaging with a total volume of 300 ml, our fluid retrieval usually is approximately 75% of that infused, although it may range from 50 to 90% of the total volume initially infused. If the objective of the lavage is to obtain a large volume of viable alveolar macrophages rather than the determination of the total cell count and differential cell count in the epithelial lining fluid in one lung segment, much larger volumes of fluid can be delivered. A method previously described in the horse uses a 3 L reservoir of lavage fluid suspended above the thorax and a fluid administration set extended from it and its end wedged into the flanged outer end of the nasogastric tube (the "homemade" BAL tube).[2] A 60 ml syringe is attached to the 3-way stopcock which is attached to the polyethylene tubing protruding from the external flanged end. The lavage fluid is allowed to flow by gravity in 100 ml aliquots. Ten sec-

*Bivona, Inc., Gary, Indiana.

onds after each aliquot the lavage fluid is gently aspirated until no more can be retrieved. The stopcock valve can be adjusted to empty the fluid into sterile 50 ml plastic tubes. The lavage is repeated until about 300 ml of fluid is collected. A method using two polyethylene catheters within the nasogastric tube allows simultaneous infusion and aspiration but fluid recovery was low (9 to 30% of the infused fluid) and cell counts were not as high as in the previous method.[7] In humans, as long as lavage volumes were less than 300 ml the only undesirable side effect was fever and this was reported in only about 10% of the patients.[10] In performing large volume lavages (between 500 ml and 2 L) in mature horses we have not noticed any side effects.

Another variation in the technique is the method of suction. Gentle aspiration by hand is possible but yields a lower total volume of BAL fluid. Vacuum suction using 600 mm Hg is effective in removing large volumes of BAL fluid from the horse.

The type of solution used for BAL depends upon the intended use of the BAL sample. If routine analysis including total cell counts, differential cell counts, and cytologic examination is to be done, then sterile saline solution at room temperature is appropriate. Phosphate buffered saline solution may be needed for certain cell function analysis of the BAL fluid. Addition of 0.2% sodium EDTA to the PBSS has been advocated to chelate any $Ca^{+2}$ or $Mg^{2+}$, thus promoting detachment of alveolar surface macrophages.[11] In the early years of performing lavages in the horse it was felt that antibiotics should be contained in the lavage fluid. It is now a commonly accepted practice to infuse a sterile solution which does not contain any antibiotics. After doing BALs in a large number of both normal horses and horses with severe pulmonary disease, we feel that antimicrobials in the lavage fluid are not indicated. In our experience we have seen no side effects from lavage in either normal horses or horses with severe respiratory disease. No aftercare is necessary nor are systemic antibiotics indicated.

One objective of this chapter is to describe the variations that are possible in the technique of BAL. These could explain some of the differences in the BAL results reported for "normal" populations of horses. A standardized technique should be developed to facilitate interpretation and comparisons among clinicians.

Our standard technique is to use either the long flexible fiber optic endoscope (2 m) or the commercially available BAL catheter and perform the BAL in a heavily sedated horse. We deliver the sterile saline solution in three 100 ml aliquots and aspirate with a suction pump after the delivery of each 100 ml. We do not provide any routine aftercare other than observation.

## Sample Handling

The volume and the color of the recovered lavage fluid should be recorded. Previously it was recommended that the lavage fluid be filtered through 8 layers of thick gauze (surgical sponge) to remove the mucus from the fluid. From our experience it appears that this is unnecessary and may selectively eliminate some cells. In human beings the use of gauze to remove mucus has been reported to remove markers of contamination and result in preferential loss of significant numbers of bronchial epithelial cells.[12] Specimens for cytologic evaluation should be placed in 5 ml stopper bottles containing sodium EDTA or can be fixed in an equal volume of 40% ethanol. Cytologic specimens are usually prepared by cytocentrifugation and smears made from the mixed sediment. Air drying of the slides is unsatisfactory if Romanovsky stains are to be used but not if Wright Giemsa staining is performed. Millipore filters (5 μm) can be used combined with negative pressure (25 mm Hg) and the filters immediately fixed in 95% ethanol.[12] When cytocentrifugation was compared to filtration in processing human BALs it was found to falsely indicate the preparation was satisfactory and the authors suggested filtration was preferable.[13]

Total nucleated cell counts can be done manually using the Unopette microcollection system* and Nebauer hemocytometer.† The

*Becton-Dickinson and Co., Rutherford, NJ.

†Bright-Lime Hemocytometer, Reicher Scientific Instruments, Buffalo, NY.

Coulter counter should not be used for counting cells as it may significantly underestimate the number of cells. For differential cell counts, 200 cells from a representative area of a Wright-Giemsa or other suitably stained preparation should be examined. A toluidine blue stain preparation can be used to detect the presence of cells with metachromatic granules (predominantly mast cells). Cytologic examination should include a differential cell count, morphologic description of cells, and identification of pharyngeal contamination. For cell function studies the lavage fluid is centrifuged for 20 minutes at 400 times g, the supernatant decanted, and the cell pellet resuspended, pulled, and washed three times with PBS, balanced salt solution, or RPM 1640 medium,* and 10% bovine fetal serum containing 10 μg penicillin and 100 μg streptomycin. Following incubation in 5% $CO_2$ humidified air atmosphere at 37°C, nonadherent cells are removed by further washing. Adherent cells are gently collected and resuspended by gentle suction into Pasteur pipettes and cells counted with a hemocytometer and phase microscopy. Eosin or 1% trypan blue dye† exclusion can be used to assess cell viability. In studies of cellular function it is important that there is no blood contamination.[2] In addition, local anesthesia contaminating the lavage fluid could potentially alter the cellular function. For that reason some researchers feel that it is important that these cells be collected under general anesthesia, while others have felt that an adequate sample can be collected in the standing sedated horse. For concentration of the BAL supernatant for subsequent analysis of protein a positive pressure filtration system‡ has been used.[8]

The use of different stains for identifying different cell types is important and should not be overlooked. Differential cell counts may be affected by the stain used. Significant overestimation of alveolar macrophages has been reported when using Wright's stain cytocentrifuged preparations compared to the same preparations stained with nonspecific esterase.[5] The latter is more accurate for macrophages.

*Microbiology Associate, Walkeisodle, MD.
†Grand Island Biologic Co., Grand Island, NY.
‡PM 10 Amicon, Danvers, MA.

## BAL Results

Because of the variation of techniques which have been described earlier the total cell and differential cell counts reported from normal horses have varied (Table 4–1). However, when approximately the same volumes of fluid (between 200 and 500 ml) were used the total cell count and differential cell counts were similar in normal horses. From our experience the total cell counts should be less than 500 cells/μl with most horses having approximately 300 cells/μl. The majority of the cells are macrophages or lymphocytes (approximately 40 to 45% of each) (Fig. 4–1). Epithelial cells that are decapitated by trauma of processing or degeneration can be "lymphocyte look alikes" and erroneously classified.[13] The remaining cells include neutrophils which are usually less than 5%, mast cells, epithelial cells, and eosinophils. Additional information on BAL results are available for normal foals, ponies with COPD, transport stressed horses, and horses with various types of lung pathology.[2–9,14,15] On comparing one 300 ml lavage and three 100 ml lavages the percentage of BAL fluid recovered and the absolute cell count of macrophages in the BAL fluid are only slightly less in the former (Sweeney, C.R., unpublished data, 1989). No differences in other cell components are seen. When comparing the total cell count and absolute cell counts of macrophages, lymphocytes and neutrophils in a small volume lavage (50 ml) versus a large volume lavage (300 ml) there is a greater concentration of neutrophils in the small volume lavage (Sweeney, C.R., unpublished data, 1989). Though the absolute cell counts of macrophages and lymphocytes are significantly lower in the small volume the percentage of these cells obtained does not significantly differ between the two volumes. These changes reflect the fact that the small volume is more of a bronchial lavage than a true bronchoalveolar lavage. Similar findings are reported in man, and in human asthmatics, use of a small volume showed cy-

**TABLE 4–1. *Differential Cellular Characteristics of Lavages of the Respiratory Tract (mean % ± SD or SE)***

| # Horses | Vol (ml) | Epithelial Cells | Macrophages | Lymphocytes | PMN | Eosinophils | Mast Cells | Reference |
|---|---|---|---|---|---|---|---|---|
| Bronchoalveolar lavage | | | | | | | | |
| 10 (VE) | 60 | 14.3 ± 13.4 (SD) | 70.3 ± 15.2 | 7.6 ± 3.9 | 6.2 ± 5.0 | 1.0 ± 1.4 | 0.6 ± 1.4 | 3 |
| (NS) | (NS) | 2.3 ± 1.4 (SE) | 48.5 ± 2.5 | 35.3 ± 2.5 | 6.2 ± 2.4 | 2.5 ± 0.9 | 5.2 ± 0.8 | 9 |
| 3 foals (×5) | 1200/2 lungs | 0 | 55–90 | 4.2–30.1 | 1.5–18.3 | 0–0.2 | 0–2.5 | 5 |
| 1 | (NS) | 9.0 ± 5.6 (SD) | 37.9 ± 11.2 | 20.1 ± 5.3 | 22.7 ± 7.3 | 3.9 ± 2.5 | 3.1 ± 2.5 | 15 |
| 10 | 300 | 3.5 ± 0.7 (SE) | 45 ± 2.8 | 43 ± 2.7 | 8.9 ± 1.2 | <1 | 1.2 ± 0.3 | 8 |
| 9 | 50 | — | 54.3 ± 16.4 (SD) | 28.8 ± 16.2 | 14.4 ± 10.1 | 0.4 ± 1.0 | 2.0 ± 1.1 | 17 |
| 9 | 1 × 300 | — | 52.4 ± 9.3 (SD) | 38.3 ± 10.5 | 5.4 ± 3.2 | 0.2 ± 0.3 | 3.6 ± 2.2 | 17 |
| 6 | 1 × 300 | — | 44.7 ± 9.4 (SD) | 46.5 ± 11.4 | 2.4 ± 1.9 | 1.6 ± 3.6 | 4.8 ± 3.4 | 17 |
| 6 | 3 × 100 | — | 59.2 ± 7.4 (SD) | 33.0 ± 8.1 | 1.2 ± 1.2 | 0.2 ± 0.4 | 6.5 ± 2.1 | 17 |
| 9 | 180–500 | 0.9 ± 0.59 (SE) | 31 ± 6.3 | 60 ± 5.9 | 4.7 ± 1.61 | 1.2 ± 0.43 | 2.7 ± 0.71 | 18 |
| Tracheobronchial or transtracheal aspirate | | | | | | | | |
| 42 (VE) | 30 | 49.1 ± 11.5 (SD) | 43.0 ± 10.7 | 2.2 ± 2.4 | 4.6 ± 4.9 | 0.7 ± 0.4 | 0.1 ± 0.2 | 3 |
| 10 (VE) | 20 | 34 ± 6.6 (SE) | 24 ± 4.0 | 8.2 ± 1.9 | 32.0 ± 8.9 | <1 | — | 8 |
| 15 (TT) | 30 | 19.8 ± 6.1 (SD) | 65 ± 13.7 | 7.4 ± 3.8 | 6.4 ± 5.5 | 1.2 ± 1.4 | 0.2 ± 0.4 | 3 |
| Bronchial lavage | | | | | | | | |
| 42 (VE) | 30 | 32.5 ± 10.9 (SD) | 55.5 ± 12.9 | 3.4 ± 2.6 | 8.4 ± 5.9 | 0 | 0.1 ± 0.3 | 3 |
| PM Tracheobronchial lavage | | | | | | | | |
| 92 | (NS) | 2.3 ± 2.6 (SD)<br>10.7 ± 5.8 (AC) | 34.0 ± 18.0 | 4.9 ± 3.1 | 39.0 ± 21.0 | 3.5 ± 2.0 | 1.6 ± 1.9 | 6 |
| Nasal lavage | | | | | | | | |
| 42 | 30 | 80.9 ± 12.7 (SD)<br>14.4 ± 11.9 (SQ) | 2.3 ± 2.0 | 1.5 ± 1.4 | 0.9 ± 0.8 | 0 | 0 | 3 |

NS = Not specified
VE = Via endoscope
T = Tracheal
PM = Postmortem
TT = Transtracheal
AC = Alveolar cell
SQ = Squamous cell

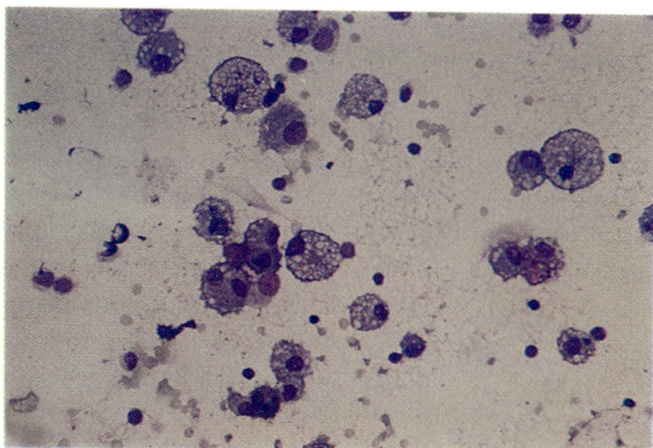

**FIG. 4–1.** Extremely foamy macrophages in an equine BAL. Wright Giemsa ×400.

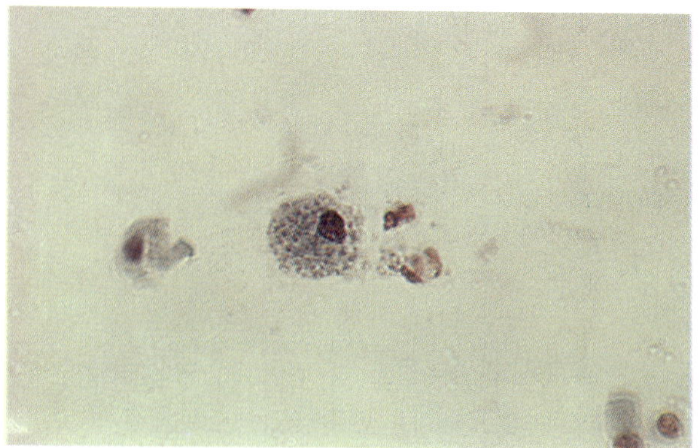

**FIG. 4–2.** Multiple histoplasma organisms in and beside a large macrophage in a bronchial washing from an Arabian foal. Necropsy tissue diagnosis of disseminated histoplasmosis was confirmed by microbiology cultures of lung and kidney. ×315 Sano Trichrome. (Courtesy Dr. J. Roszel.)

tologic changes that would have been missed had only a larger volume been infused.[16] We have not found that there is any difference in the BAL fluid composition recovered from the right and left lung of the same horses (Sweeney, C.R., unpublished data, 1989).

There are age related increases in the total number of cells and macrophages recovered in foals. In a study in 3 foals between 2 to 63 days of age, repeated lavages showed the proportion of macrophages declined (from >80% to 55 to 82%) and the percent of lymphocytes rose from approximately 5% to 13 to 30%.[5] In individual foals the percentage of cells, particularly neutrophils, varied. The percentage of alveolar macrophages was higher than what had been reported in mature horses where mean percentage is reported to range from 30 to 60 (Table 4–1). Percentage of neutrophils in normal foals ranged from 1.5 to 18%. In normal mature horses or ponies the number of neutrophils can vary with environment; one experiment exposing normal and "heavy" ponies to a barn showed normal ponies had an 8-fold increase in neutrophils and the ponies with COPD had a significantly higher percentage increase.[4]

Changes in the eosinophil numbers or mast cells have been inconsistent and difficult to interpret.[3,8,15] Siderophages were found more frequently in BAL than in transtracheal washes from the same horses.[8]

The assumption that BAL reflects the whole lung or lungs is inaccurate. The BAL reflects only the changes in the epithelial lining fluid in that lung segment lavaged. Unless the pulmonary disease or condition is diffuse, (Figs. 4–2 and 4–3) a BAL sample may "miss" the affected area and lavage a normal area of the lung. This has been our experience in performing BALs in horses with moderate to severe pneumonia. In all cases it was our objective to lavage the affected area and the BALs were obtained with a guided fiberoptic endoscope. Despite this attempt, in 50% of the horses, total cell count, differential cell count, and cytologic examination of the BAL were similar to that of a normal horse indicating normal lung was lavaged (Sweeney, C.R., unpublished data, 1988). In the remaining horses there was a significant increase in

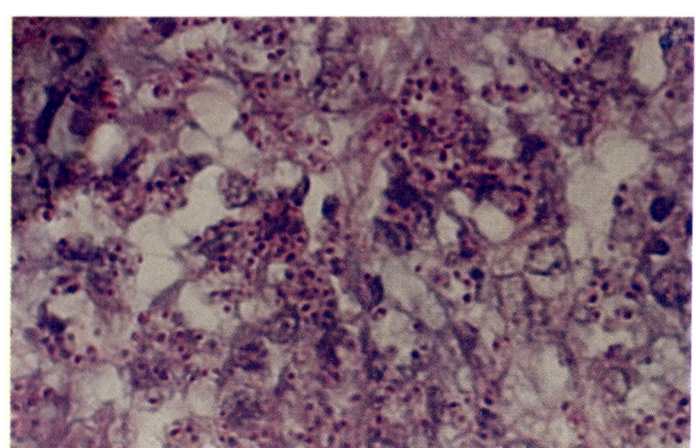

**FIG. 4–3.** Necropsy lung tissue of granuloma with many intra- and extracellular histoplasma organisms. Same case as Figure 4–2. ×260 Periodic acid Schiff/hematoxylin. (Courtesy Dr. J. Roszel.)

total cell counts ranging between 500 to 5000 cells/μl. In horses in which the cell count was abnormal the percent of neutrophils was also greatly elevated from 10 to 91% of the cells obtained. There were some horses in which the total cell count was within the normal range, but there was a significant increase in the percent of neutrophils. Recovery rate of BAL fluid in horses with pneumonia was approximately 60% of the infused 300 ml (Sweeney, C.R., unpublished data, 1989). At this time we still feel that a transtracheal aspirate is a better indicator of the "whole lung" in patients with nondiffuse lung disease. While BAL may accurately diagnose pneumonia, it has an equal chance of missing the affected area.

In human beings postretrieval handling is recognized as affecting results and even when samples have been collected by experienced people using standardized technique, one multicenter study found 30% of 1588 BAL to be unsatisfactory because of a paucity of pulmonary alveolar macrophages, an excess number of epithelial cells, mucopurulent exudate, degenerated cells and laboratory artifact either alone or in combination.[13] Airway disease and bleeding can contaminate the sample. It is likely that as the technique becomes more widespread in equine medicine, sample evaluation will become more sophisticated and more critical and guidelines for the technique, sample processing and interpretation will evolve.

## References


1. Hunninghake GW, Gadek JE, Kawanami O, et al. Inflammatory and immune processes in the human lung in health and disease: Evaluation by bronchoalveolar lavage. Am J Pathol, *97*:149, 1979.
2. Dyer RM, Liggitt HD, Leid RW. Isolation and partial characterization of equine alveolar macrophages. Am J Vet Res, *44*:2379, 1983.
3. Mair TS, Stokes CR, Bourne FJ. Cellular content of secretions obtained by lavage from different levels of the equine respiratory tract. Equine Vet J, *19*:458, 1987.
4. Derksen FJ, Scott JS, Slocombe RF, et al. Bronchoalveolar Lavage in Ponies with Recurrent Airway Obstruction (Heaves). Am Rev Respir Dis, *132*:1066, 1985.
5. Zink MC, Johnson JA. Cellular constituents of clinically normal foal bronchoalveolar lavage fluid during postnatal maturation. Am J Vet Res, *45*:893, 1984.
6. Larson VL, Busch RH. Equine tracheobronchial lavage: Comparison of lavage cytologic and pulmonary histopathologic findings. Am J Vet Res, *46*:144, 1985.
7. Anderson NV, DeBowes RM, Nyrop KA, et al. Mononuclear phagocytes of transport-stressed horses with viral respiratory tract infection. Am J Vet Res, *46*:2272, 1985.
8. Derksen FJ, Brown CM, Sonea I, et al. Comparison of transtracheal aspirate and bronchoalveolar lavage cytology in 50 horses with chronic lung disease. Equine Vet J, *21*:23, 1989.
9. Viel L. Structural-functional correlations of the lung in horses with small airway disease. Ph.D. Thesis. University of Guelph, Guelph, Canada, 1983.
10. Crystal RG, Reynolds HY, Kalica AR. Bronchoalveolar Lavage: The report of an international conference. Chest, *89*:122, 1986.
11. Brain JD, Frank NR. Alveolar macrophage adhesion: Wash electrolyte composition and free cell yields. J Appl Physiol, *34*:75, 1973.
12. Lam S, LeRiche JC, Kijek K. Effect of filtration and concentration on the composition of bronchoalveolar lavage fluid. Chest, *87*:740, 1985.
13. Chamberlain DW, Braude AC, Rebuk AS. A critical evaluation of bronchoalveolar lavage. Acta Cytologica, *31*:599, 1987.
14. Yamashiro S, Viel L, Bast T, et al. The morphological study of airways and cells recovered by bronchoalveolar lavage in a horse with chronic obstructive pulmonary disease (COPD). Anat Rec, *211*:219A, 1985.
15. Yamashiro S, Viel L, Bast T, et al. Mast Cells in Bronchoalveolar Lavage of a Horse with Obstructive Small Airway Disease. Anatomia, Histologia, Embryologia, Bd. 15, Reports of the World Association of Veterinary Anatomists, 1986.
16. Lam S, LeRiche JC, Kijek K, et al. Effect of Bronchial Lavage Volume on Cellular and Protein Recovery. Chest, *88*:856, 1985.
17. Sweeney CR, Rossier Y, Ziemer EL, et al. Bronchoalveolar lavage in the horse: Effect of lavage fluid volume and site. Personal communication, 1989.
18. Traub-Dargatz JL, McKinon AO, Bryninckx WJ, et al. Effect of transportation stress on bronchoalveolar lavage fluid analysis in female horses. Am J Vet Res, *49*:1026, 1988.

CHAPTER 5

# THORACOCENTESIS, PLEUROSCOPIC EXAMINATION, AND LUNG BIOPSY

*JILL BEECH*

## Thoracocentesis

This procedure is indicated when physical, ultrasonographic, or radiographic examination suggests the presence of pleural effusion and/or pleural neoplasia. The latter is rare in horses, but mesotheliomas, lymphosarcoma, and metastatic gastric squamous cell carcinomas have been diagnosed from pleural fluid cytology. Usually pleural effusions are secondary to pneumonia or pulmonary abscessation. Chylothorax is rare but has been diagnosed by thoracocentesis.

### *Technique*

Aseptic technique is important. One should perform the procedure as ventrally as possible into the pleural space while avoiding the heart. Even minor contact with the heart can cause fatal arrhythmias. Massive amounts of fluid or masses that displace the heart can increase the chance of pericardial or cardiac contact. When ultrasonography is available its use is often helpful in locating the best site for thoracic puncture. Not only does it enable visualization and thus avoidance of the heart, it also allows placement in areas likely to yield the greatest volume of fluid, and/or placement into localized pockets of fluid.

If only small volumes of fluid are suspected a 12 to 14 gauge noncutting end cannula can be used; 6 cm (2½ inch) length teat cannulas work well. If larger volumes exist and drainage is required, a larger bore catheter should be placed. Argyle catheters used for thoracic drainage in human beings work well and come in various sizes. They have an indwelling trocar over which the catheter can be pushed into the pleural cavity and the trocar then removed. Both trocar and catheter can be resterilized and re-used multiple times. Unless the fluid is viscid or contains clumps of fibrin, the smaller bore catheters suffice. The flanged outer end of the catheter requires either fitting an adapter for suction or relying on gravity flow alone; even when the latter is used one should have a method for rapidly occluding the catheter should fluid cease to flow. Other tubes and trocars may also be used.

The usual site for thoracic puncture is between the seventh and eighth ribs. A large area of skin should be aseptically prepared so that several areas may be punctured if necessary and contamination of the clinician's hands, the cannula, and the tubing is unlikely. When larger indwelling tubes are placed and require subcutaneous tunneling an even larger area must be prepared.

The site of puncture is anesthetized with sufficient local anesthetic (usually approximately 8 ml) to extend down to and include the parietal pleura. The site should be in front of a rib to avoid the intercostal nerves and blood vessels that lie along its caudal aspect. A small stab incision just large enough to allow introduction of the selected cannula or catheter is made through the skin and the cannula is then pushed through the soft tissue and into the pleural space; the latter is usually recognized by a palpable decrease in resistance. If one is not sure about the presence of fluid, it is important to have the cannula's hub sealed so that no air is aspirated. Also, when a cannula with a pointed closed end is used and the apertures are along the side of the cannula, it is important to advance the cannula sufficiently so that the aperture and not just the cannula end lies within the pleural space. If no fluid is obtained, one can try repositioning the cannula end within the same entry site, instilling a small volume of sterile fluid such as phosphate buffered saline solution (PBSS) and then aspirating, or it may be necessary to remove the cannula and place it elsewhere. Whenever any fluid is instilled, it should approximate body temperature. Always ensure the cannula is long enough for the horse's size. Most mature horses' thoracic walls are 3 to 6 cm (1½ to 2½ in.) thick. Fluid can be placed in ethanol for fixation or collected in EDTA tubes for prompt processing. Aseptically obtained samples can be submitted for culture and sensitivity. When chylothorax is suspected, fluid should be submitted for triglyceride and cholesterol analysis. If thoracocentesis is performed bilaterally fluid from both sides should be examined and cultured. If no fluid is obtained, yet one suspects neoplasia of the pleural cavity, it may be helpful to lavage the pleural space with several hundred ml of warmed pH adjusted PBSS and then aspirate and analyze the fluid. It does not adversely affect the patient if only a small portion of the volume that was instilled is recovered.

When fluid can no longer be obtained the teat cannula can be removed without the necessity of a skin suture. When larger bore tubes are used, skin sutures will be necessary; frequently a "purse string" suture is placed and tightened as the tube is removed. Localized cellulitis is not uncommon when septic fluid is obtained and it requires symptomatic treatment.

## Analysis of Pleural Fluid

Normal horses have either minimal (2 to 8 ml) or no retrievable fluid. Their fluid is clear pale straw yellow and odorless. However, one study on 18 clinically normal horses reported some had hazy fluid.[1] Red tinged coloration can occur secondary to bleeding from the puncture site but this usually clears as more fluid is withdrawn. In normal horses total cell counts have usually been reported to be less than 4,000/mm³ and total protein is usually less than 2 to 3 g/dl. Although a range in cell count of 800 to 12,100 mm³ and total protein range of 0.2 to 4.7 g/dl have been reported in clinically normal horses only a small fraction of these horses was necropsied to be sure there was no pleural abnormality.[1]

When the neutrophils are degenerate and exceed 10,000/mm³, septic disease is likely even though only small volumes of fluid are retrieved. Cell counts can be deceptively low as one may sample only the top layers of fluid; ventral sediment and fibrin may contain large numbers of cells. Cell counts can vary between the beginning and end of a collection. It has been shown that cell counts and total protein content of pleural fluid are not accurate indices for prognostication.[2] If the sample is relatively acellular, it should be centrifuged and smears made from the mixed sediment for cytologic evaluation.

Color and odor of the fluid should be recorded. A foul odor suggests necrosis and possible anaerobic infection. However, although a foul odor suggests the presence of anaerobes, absence of an odor does not eliminate their existence. Nonodorous fluid should never be interpreted as meaning no anaerobes are present. Septic pleural fluid is cloudy, usually yellow, sometimes beige tinted or bloody, and may contain fibrin clots. If the aspirate is mostly blood, one must consider trauma, neoplasia, or an abscess that has eroded a major vessel. Serosanguinous fluid has been seen with neoplasia. Cloudy white, pale pink opaque or opalescent fluid suggests chylothorax which may be idio-

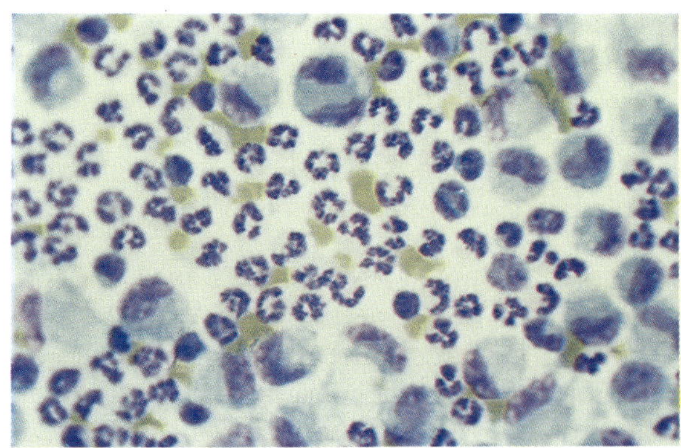

**FIG. 5–1.** Chronic active pleuritis with a predominance of nonseptic neutrophils, scattered large macrophages, some with vacuolated cytoplasm, and few lymphocytes. Wright-Giemsa stain. (Courtesy of Dr. E. Ziemer.)

pathic or occur secondary to lymphatic duct rupture; the fluid will not clear with centrifugation but will clear when ether is added.

When septic effusion exists, total protein and total cell counts are usually high. The predominant cell is the neutrophil and degenerate changes are common. Macrophages may be very active (Fig. 5–1). Reactive mesothelial cells are not uncommon and may be difficult to differentiate from neoplastic cells as there is no clearly defined demarcation between benign and neoplastic mesothelial cells. Even when neutrophils are the predominant cell type a careful cytologic evaluation should always be made to ascertain if any exfoliated neoplastic cells are present. Ulceration and tumor necrosis can cause exudation of large numbers of neutrophils. Many thoracic neoplasms do not exfoliate neoplastic cells or the numbers are so low that they may be obscured by other cells. For example, one mare with metastasis of gastric squamous cell carcinoma to the pleural cavity had approximately 20,000 nucleated cells/mm$^3$ in her pleural fluid and most were neutrophils; it was only by careful searching that a few abnormal clusters of cells were identified and the diagnosis was made (Fig. 5–2). Pleural or pulmonary hemangiosarcomas may cause hemothorax, yet one may aspirate only blood with no evidence of neoplastic cells.

In normal pleural fluid lymphocyte counts are less than 675/mm$^3$ with a reported mean of 211/mm$^3$.[1] If a preponderance of lymphocytes is found or there are unusual or immature forms, variation in cell sizes, increased numbers of nucleoli in nuclei, pleomorphism and increased mitotic figures, lymphosarcoma should be suspected (Figs. 5–3 and 5–4). Unlike effusions associated with other neoplasms, those due to lymphosarcoma may occur in young horses. When there are increased numbers of lymphocytes but morphology is normal, one should check the pleural fluid's triglyceride concentration to determine if it is a chylous effusion.

If many mesothelial cells are seen in a large volume of fluid, one should strongly suspect neoplasia. Diffuse mesotheliomas have been diagnosed. Pleomorphism, multinucleation of cells often arranged in polyps or forming spheres or attached in series by cytoplasmic

**FIG. 5–2.** Large bizarre vacuolated cell in the center with a heavy protein background. Fluid from a horse with pleuritis and effusion secondary to metastasis of a gastric squamous cell carcinoma. Sano Trichrome stain.

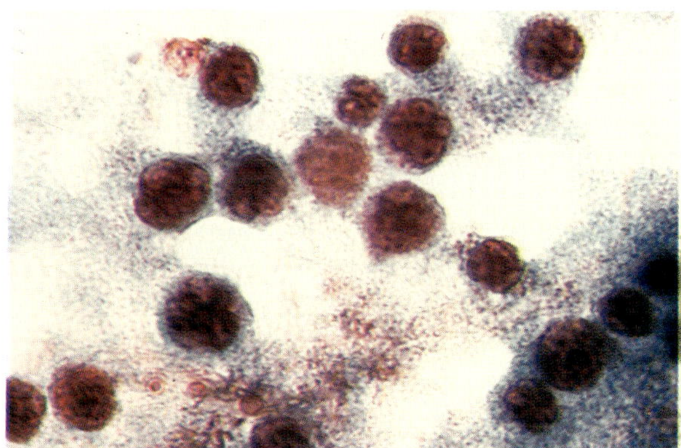

**FIG. 5–3.** Abnormal lymphocytes in pleural fluid from a horse with lymphosarcoma. Sano Trichrome stain.

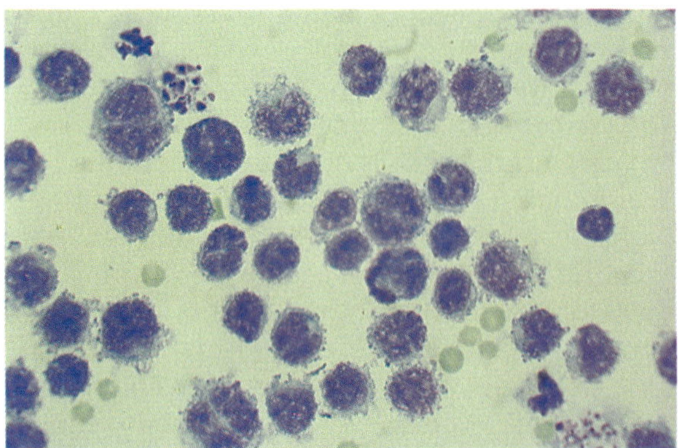

**FIG. 5–4.** Pleural fluid (from a cow with lymphosarcoma) showing predominantly abnormal lymphocytes with great variation in cell size and development, increased numbers of nuclei, mitosis, and karryorhexis. Wright-Giemsa stain. (Courtesy of Dr. E. Ziemer.)

bridges, was seen in one mare.[3] Vacuolation was common, although this can be seen with many inflammatory processes. The large vacuoles remained unstained following PAS staining.[3] If any adenomatous type cells are seen in pleural fluid, PAS staining is advised as the large glycoprotein containing vacuoles of adenocarcinoma cells will stain positive for PAS. As glycogen granules which are common in normal cells will also stain with PAS, it is often helpful to treat suspicious PAS positive cells with malt diastase. This enzyme digests glycogen but not glycoprotein and restaining the cells following diastase treatment differentiates between glycoprotein and glycogen.[3] Tartaric acid inhibition of glucuronidase staining has also been used to differentiate carcinomas with a high level of specificity and sensitivity from macrophages, mesothelial cells, and lymphoma cells.[4] Beta glucuronidase is the lysosomal and microsomal enzyme in mammalian cells and a higher activity exists in cancer cells. Tartaric acid added to the incubation medium does not inhibit this staining of cancer cells but inhibits it in other cells.[4,5] Occasionally, inclusions compatible with herpes virus infection have been seen in mesothelial cells (Fig. 5–5).

Carcinomas may exfoliate single abnormal cells or clusters and sheets of cells. There may be vacuolization or basophilia of the cytoplasm, variation in nuclear size, coarse nuclear chromatin, large bizarre nucleoli, anisocytosis, anisokaryosis and mitotic figures. Presence of nonviable keratinized epithelial cells with no evidence of less mature or bizarre forms should not be interpreted as indicating malignancy as the former cells are probably contaminants exfoliated from the skin.

When a chylous effusion is found, one should measure pleural fluid triglyceride and compare it with serum concentration; an elevation in the former indicates chylothorax. Pseudochylous effusion can occur with chronic inflammation and cellular degeneration and is characterized by a high pleural fluid cholesterol.

I do not advocate determining pleural fluid pH or glucose as they are unlikely to provide additional helpful information.

## Pleuroscopic Examination

When one suspects neoplasia of the visceral or parietal pleura but is unable to confirm it by cytologic examination of pleural effusion or biopsy of masses that may be evident on ultrasonographic examination, direct visual examination may be helpful and also allow visually guided biopsy of any masses. The procedure has allowed definitive diagnosis of intrathoracic masses which would not other-

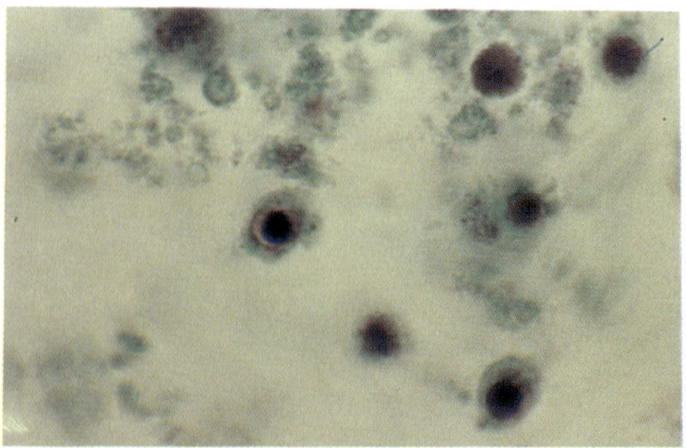

**FIG. 5–5.** Pleural sediment smear from a horse with recent signs of a respiratory problem. There are two mesothelial cells (center and lower right) with a background of precipitation protein. Cell in center has a halo around a large intranuclear inclusion compatible with a herpetic infection. ×400 Sano Trichrome. (Courtesy of Dr. J. Roszel.)

wise have been possible. In one mare, multiple small friable red masses were seen and could be biopsied, resulting in a diagnosis of hemangiosarcoma. In another mare, a large perioesophageal mass seen on radiographs could be seen by pleuroscopy and uterine biopsy forceps introduced through a separate stab incision could be visually guided to obtain a sample of the mass; squamous cell carcinoma was diagnosed.[6] Familiarity with the technique and knowledge of landmarks are needed. Also, the technique as presently performed, allows examination of only the dorsal and middle parts of the thorax; examination of the ventral far cranial and pericardial areas is not possible.[7,8] Both the rigid laparoscope[1] and flexible fiberoptic endoscope have been used; the former is superior as it provides the better visual field because it is designed for examination of a body cavity.

An area over the caudodorsal lung field is aseptically prepared and local anesthesia infiltrated down to and including the parietal pleura at the site of entry. The tenth intercostal space is frequently used. Unless the horse is already sedate, tranquilization or sedation should be used. A stab incision is made through the skin, a "purse string" suture placed, and blunt instruments and an index finger used to enter the pleural cavity, avoiding the caudal aspect of the ribs. The sterilized rigid laparoscope* is passed into the pleural cavity and the "purse string" suture pulled snugly around it. It can then be advanced at an angle to allow examination of the parietal pleura. The lung will collapse due to iatrogenic pneumothorax, producing a large space for examination. Following examination, the endoscope can be withdrawn and a tube inserted for aspirating the air from the thoracic cavity, thus allowing reinflation of the lung. When the laparoscope or endoscope has a suction unit, this can be turned on prior to removing the instrument and lung inflation can be observed. The "purse string" suture is tightened as the instrument is removed. Alternatively, the endoscope can be removed and the site sutured and a separate small puncture site in the same sterilized dorsal area made for aspiration of the air. As this procedure has the potential for introducing sepsis, strict asepsis is necessary and broad spectrum antimicrobial drugs should be instituted prior to and for several days following the procedure. The transient pneumothorax should not pose a significant hazard provided that the opposite lung has adequate function and the former is relieved following the procedure. Local antibacterial ointment and an adhesive elastic bandage are sometimes used.

*Wolf-Lumina 130° rigid fiber laparoscope. Rich Wolf Med Instruments Corp., Rosemont, IL.

## Percutaneous Lung or Pleural Biopsy

The technique for parenchymal biopsy has been published.[9] Indications for a percutaneous lung biopsy would be the presence of diffuse interstitial or miliary nodular lung disease of unknown origin, or focal masses of unknown origin visualized by radiography or ultrasonography. Unless the disease process is diffuse or the area to be biopsied has been selected based on radiographic or ultrasonographic localization of a lesion, the likelihood of obtaining a diagnosis is slim. The danger of lacerating vessels must be weighed against the potential advantages of the procedure. As long as the biopsy is relatively superficial within the lung, vessel damage is unlikely. In a group of 20 horses in which biopsies were obtained from the caudodorsal lung field no significant complications occurred. Two horses had transient hemoptysis, a common occurrence in humans following lung biopsy.[9]

A Tru-Cut(TM) biopsy needle* is easy to use and enables one to obtain a small core of tissue. Several biopsies could be obtained from the same horse. The horse is sedated if necessary, a preselected area is aseptically prepared, and the biopsy site is anesthetized down to and including the parietal pleura. A small stab incision is made in the skin at a site not directly over the expected entry point into the pleural cavity and the biopsy needle pushed through the soft tissue, avoiding the vessels and nerves running along the caudal

*Baxter Health Care Corp., Rocky River, Ohio.

rib margin. A decrease in pressure can be felt when the pleural cavity is entered. The needle is then thrust into the lung parenchyma, and the cutting part of the needle and main sleeve manipulated to cut off a section of lung within the lumen. The biopsy needle can then be removed and the sample placed in appropriate fixative or impression smears made prior to fixation. The skin can be sutured. Provided that the skin opening is not directly over the entry site into the thorax and no airway of significant size was cut no problems with pneumothorax are likely. The horse should be carefully observed for the next few hours to ascertain if any epistaxis or change in respiratory function occurs.

The tissue can be fixed in 10% formalin for routine histologic examination, in Michelle's fixative if immunofluorescent studies are anticipated, or fixed for special purposes according to one's clinical suspicion. A sample can also be submitted for culture if one suspects an infectious agent. If tuberculosis is suspected, all people handling the material should be cautioned.

If a fungal infection is suspected, the laboratory should be advised so that appropriate media can be selected. Where pneumoconiosis is a possibility, x-ray diffraction analysis may be useful.

## References

1. Wagner AE, Bennet DG. Analysis of equine thoracic fluid. Vet Clin Pathol, 11:13, 1983.
2. Raphel CF, Beech J. Pleuritis secondary to pneumonia or lung abscessation in 90 horses. J Am Vet Med Assoc, *181*:808, 1982.
3. Kramer JW, Nickels FA, Bell T. Cytology of Diffuse Mesothelioma in the Thorax of a Horse. Equine Vet J, *8*:81, 1976.
4. Apibal S, Sestapruks P, Bunyaratvej A, et al. Use of tartaric acid resistance of B. glucuronidase for the characterization of cancer cells in pleural effusions. Acta Cytol, *31*:6119, 1987.
5. Hayhoe FGJ, Quaglino D. Haematological Cytochemistry. London, Churchill Livingstone, 1980, p 211.
6. Ford TS, Vaala WE, Sweeney CR, et al. Pleuroscopic diagnosis of gastroesophageal squamous cell carcinoma in a horse. J Am Vet Med Assoc, *12*:1556, 1987.
7. Mansmann RA, Strother SB. Pleuroscopy in horses. Mod Vet Pract, *66*:9, 1985.
8. Mackey VS, Wheat JD. Endoscopic examination of the equine thorax. Equine Vet J, *17*:140, 1985.
9. Raphel CF, Gunson DE. Percutaneous lung biopsy in the horse. Cornell Vet, *71*:439, 1981.

# CHAPTER 6

# ULTRASONOGRAPHIC EVALUATION

*VIRGINIA B. REEF*

Widespread availability of portable ultrasound machines in equine practice has made ultrasonography a useful diagnostic tool for the evaluation of horses with respiratory tract diseases.[1-6] A thorough knowledge of the principles of diagnostic ultrasound is necessary to perform and interpret a thoracic sonogram.[7-10]

## Principles of Diagnostic Ultrasound

Ultrasound is sound which has a frequency above the normal hearing range of the human ear (i.e., greater than 20,000 hertz).[7,9] Medical diagnostic ultrasound commonly employs frequencies from 1.9 to 10 megahertz (MHz). The ultrasound beam is produced by the electrically induced deformation of one or more piezo-electric crystals housed within a transducer. Application of the transducer to the skin using a coupling gel allows the ultrasound waves to propagate through the soft tissues.[7,10] The ultrasound beam is reflected back to the transducer at interfaces between tissues of different acoustic impedance.[7,9] Acoustic impedance is the density of the tissue multiplied by the velocity at which sound travels through that tissue. The larger the difference between the acoustic impedance of two adjacent tissues, the greater the amount of ultrasound that will be reflected back from this interface to the transducer.[7,9] The reflected ultrasound waves are received by the transducer, deforming the piezo-electric crystal, producing an electric current.[7,9] This electrical signal is then processed through a scan converter to produce an image. The ultrasound beam is reflected, refracted, scattered, and absorbed as it passes through soft tissue.[7,9] To produce the best quality image, the ultrasound beam must be perpendicular to the structure being imaged, maximizing the amount of reflected ultrasound. As a result of sound wave attenuation, the highest amplitude echoes will be reflected from tissue interfaces closest to the transducer.[7,9] Thus using time gain compensation (TGC), the amplitude of the returning echoes near the skin surface are suppressed, while those from more distant tissue interfaces are enhanced.[7,9]

Selection of the appropriate transducer frequency is essential to obtain a good quality image. Higher frequency transducers emit ultrasound with shorter wavelengths. This improves the resolution of the soft tissue structures imaged, but results in decreased penetration of the ultrasound wave through the soft tissue.[7,9,10] In contrast, lower frequency transducers produce ultrasound waves which are longer and can penetrate deeper into the soft tissue; but the resolution of the image is less, especially for structures close to the skin surface. Therefore, a thorough knowledge of the anatomy of the tissues to be imaged (i.e., location and depth from the skin surface) is required to select the transducer frequency which will produce the best image.[10] In general, the highest frequency transducer which will penetrate the tissues of interest to the depth desired should be selected.

There are two tissues, bone and air, which are major deterrents to the transmission of ultrasound waves; this is due to their high and low acoustic impedances, respectively, compared to soft tissue and results in nearly complete reflection of the ultrasound waves with no further transmission of the ultrasound beam to deeper structures.[7] An acoustic shadow will be produced when the ultrasound beam strikes bone or mineralization, as the ultrasound waves are reflected by the latter but transmitted through the soft tissue structures on either side.[7,8] The bone appears as a hyperechoic (white) structure from maximal echo reflection, with an anechoic (black) shadow due to lack of echoes returning from the tissue deep to the bone or calcification. Thus the ultrasound beam must be directed between the ribs in the intercostal spaces for adequate visualization of structures within the thorax. Structures normally containing air will also cause complete reflection of the ultrasound beam with artifacts caused by the sound waves reverberating between the highly reflective surface and the transducer.[8]

## Patient Preparation

Excellent contact between the transducer and patient is essential to obtain a diagnostic quality image.[7,9] The skin surface must be clean, as dirt, dander, and other structures attached to the skin will cause scattering of the ultrasound beam before it can be transmitted to the underlying soft tissues. Severe scattering of the ultrasound beam will result in a poor quality image or none at all. As hair traps air at the skin surface, reflecting ultrasound waves before they can penetrate the skin, the area of interest should be clipped to obtain the best possible image. An acoustic coupling gel is then applied to the transducer and the skin surface, eliminating an air-transducer interface at the skin surface and optimizing contact between the transducer and the skin surface.

## Transducer Selection

The depth of the structure under examination relative to the skin surface is the most important consideration in transducer selection.[10] The pleural surface of the horse usually is located 5 cm or less from the skin surface,[3] although this varies with the age, size, and conformation of the horse, and the portion of the thorax under investigation. A 5.0 MHz transducer can usually penetrate to a depth of 10 to 15 cm from the skin surface with optimal image quality usually in the 5 to 10 cm range, depending upon the focal zone of the transducer. Large amounts of fluid in the pleural cavity may result in successful imaging of deeper structures 15 to 20 cm from the skin surface, as little attenuation of the beam occurs in certain fluids, particularly transudates. A 3.0 or 3.5 MHz transducer will also produce an acceptable image of intrathoracic structures, and may be needed to adequately penetrate and "image" the lung and pleural cavity in horses with severe pleural effusions and lung consolidation. In these horses, optimal imaging of the parietal pleural surface will still be obtained with a 5.0 MHz transducer.[3] The amount of subcutaneous fat present in the horse will also affect transducer selection, as a few centimeters of fat can decrease the power of the ultrasound beam by half.[9] Thus a fat horse will require the use of a lower frequency transducer to obtain adequate penetration but there will be some resultant loss in image quality.

## Linear Scanner Versus Sector Scanner

Linear and sector scanners are the two types of diagnostic ultrasound machines currently available to the private practitioner.[10] Both types can be used successfully to image the lung and pleural cavity in the horse.[10] The sector scanners are mechanical, producing a sector image by mechanically oscillating one piezo-electric crystal or rotating several piezo-electric crystals simultaneously.[9] As the transducers normally house 1 to 3 crystals, the head of the transducer is usually small and the beam is in line with the long axis of the transducer. Some companies do make sector scanner transducers containing an offset head, with the beam perpendicular to the long axis of the transducer, enabling the ultrasonographer to have better access to those areas with limited exposure. The sector transducers are much easier to use than the linear scanner for the horse's thorax.[3-10] Because the ribs cause acoustic shadows and reflect all the ultrasound waves back to the transducer, the scanning surfaces are limited to the intercostal spaces. In the horse these are narrow and curved; therefore, a transducer with a small head and an in line beam will have the maximal contact surface and transducer mobility, enabling the ultrasonographer to keep the beam perpendicular to the structures being imaged. The image quality of the sector scanner is also inherently better than that of the linear scanner, due the focusing properties of a single crystal, versus the multiple crystals present in the linear scanner.[9,10] Another advantage of the sector scanners is that a variety of depth settings may be selected for the examination independent of the transducer frequency selected. Therefore, in situations (i.e., pleural effusion), where the ultrasound beam can penetrate deeper than what is normally imaged with the selected transducer frequency, the depth setting can be changed to include these images. Also, the maximal depth settings on many of the portable sector scanners are greater than those on the linear scanners.

The linear scanners are electronic scanners which produce a rectangular image.[9] They are composed of multiple piezo-electric crystals in a row which emit an ultrasound beam perpendicular to the long axis of the transducer. These transducers are usually long and thin, making them ideal for transrectal pregnancy examination of the mare,[10] but their limited contact surface when used in the intercostal spaces makes examination of the equine thorax more difficult. The 5.0 MHz transducer is usually the optimal frequency for this examination. With most linear scanners the depth of field for a 5.0 MHz transducer is usually fixed at 10 to 12 cm, requiring a change to a lower frequency transducer (3.0 MHz), if more depth is needed (15–20 cm).[10] This change will result in a corresponding loss of image resolution. Also, it is difficult to follow the recommendation of scanning abnormalities in two different planes if a linear transducer is being used.[3] Linear scanners are less expensive, however, and thus the decision between a linear or sector scanner should be based upon the range of scanning needed and the suitability of the equipment for each practice's needs.

## The Normal Equine Thorax

The landmarks for the normal equine lung field are the 17th intercostal space (ICS) at the level of the tuber coxae, the 15th ICS at the level of the tuber ischii, the 13th ICS at mid thorax, the 11th ICS at the point of the shoulder and the 9th ICS to the point of the elbow. These landmarks can be used as a guide to locate the underlying lung field, although this will vary somewhat with the stage and depth of respiration (Figs. 6–1 to 6–3).[2] The cardiac window is the area where the heart lies immediately adjacent to the parietal pleura without any overlying lung.[3] The right cardiac window is located in the 4th ICS below the level of the point of the shoulder (Fig. 6–2) and the larger left one is located from the 3rd to 5th ICS below the level of the point of the shoulder. The diaphragm can be visualized from the caudal surface of the heart between the thorax and abdomen back to the 16th or 17th ICS and is imaged as parallel echogenic fascial planes on either side of its hypoechoic musculature ventral to the lung and somewhat parallel to the body wall (Fig. 6–3).[3] The liver is normally imaged ventral to the diaphragm on the right side (Fig. 6–3) unless liver atrophy is present, in which case the large colon will be visualized.[2,3] The liver appears as a triangular organ of intermediate echogenicity with numerous vessels branching throughout the hepatic parenchyma. For comparison the spleen is more echogenic,

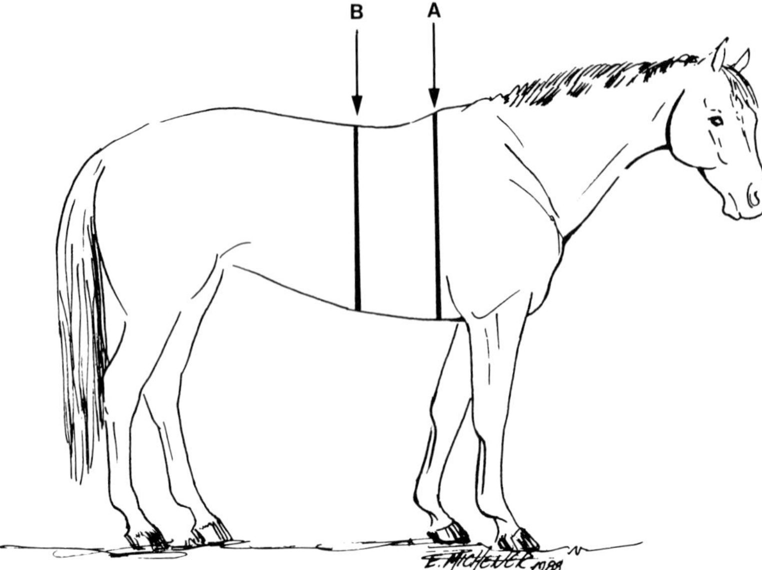


**FIG. 6–1.** Diagram of a horse from the right side. A. Location of cross section shown in Figure 6–2 (area of right cardiac window). B. Location of cross section shown in Figure 6–3 (midthoracic region).

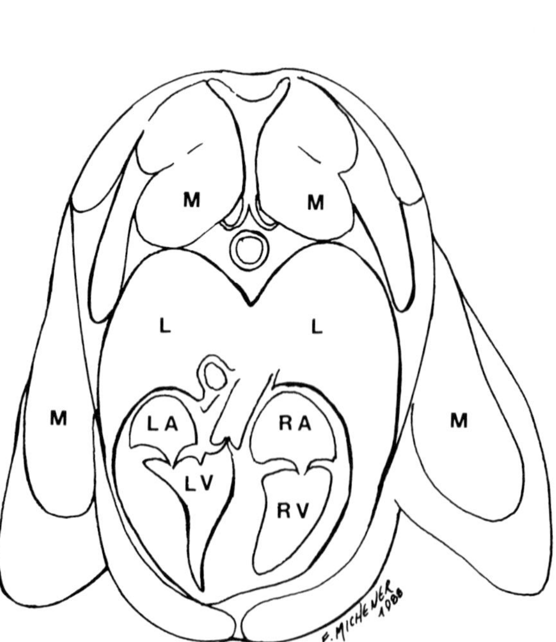


**FIG. 6–2.** Diagram of a cross section of a horse taken at A in Figure 6–1 at the level of the right cardiac window. M—muscle; L—lung; LA—left atrium; LV—left ventricle; RA—right atrium; RV—right ventricle.

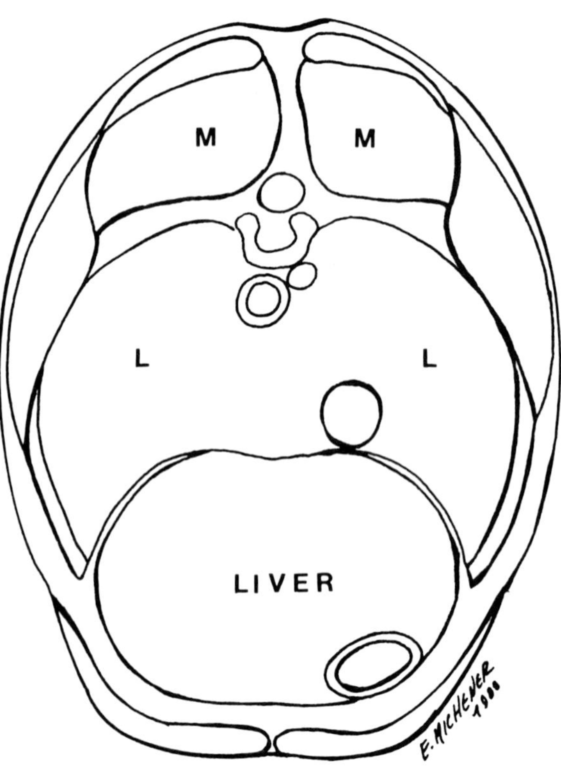


**FIG. 6–3.** Diagram of a cross section of a horse taken at B in Figure 6–1 in the midthoracic region. M—muscle; L—lung.

while the kidney is more sonolucent. The large colon appears as a curvilinear hyperechoic (gas-filled) echo immediately ventral to the liver (or the diaphragm in horses with liver atrophy).[2,3] The liver will also be imaged on the left side immediately ventral to the diaphragm and caudal to the heart for 2 to 3 ICS. The spleen may then be imaged as a more echogenic organ medial to the liver extending caudally from the 7th ICS to the region of the paralumbar fossa.[2,3] High amplitude echoes from the gas filled stomach may be seen in the 10th ICS medial to the spleen.[2,3]

The lung is imaged as a high amplitude echo deep to the intercostal muscles and parietal pleura (Fig. 6–4A, B).[2,3] Concentric reverberation artifacts are produced from the normal visceral pleural surface and appear as multiple equidistant echoes caused by complete reflection of the ultrasound beam from the large, flat, smooth surface of the lung and reverberation of the sound between the lung and the transducer.[2,3] Due to the large difference between the acoustic impedance of air and soft tissue, normal air filled lung does not allow penetration of the ultrasound waves to deeper structures. The normal parietal pleural surface is imaged as a thin white line lateral to the lung surface and medial to the intercostal muscles (Fig. 6–4A, B).[2] Watching the scan in real time (as it is actually happening), one sees the lung sliding past the parietal pleural surface of the thoracic wall with inspiration and expiration.[3,5] In the normal horse it can also be seen to move across the diaphragm and over the heart base with respiration.[3,5] A small amount of pleural fluid can often be imaged in normal horses as an anechoic space separating the parietal pleural surface from the lung in the ventralmost portion of the thorax.[3] In one survey at the racetrack, 85% of horses had visible fluid in the right hemithorax, varying in height from less than 1 to 3.5 cm in the ventralmost portion.[3] Many of these horses also had a small amount of fluid imaged in the left hemithorax. This amount of fluid is normal, and functions to lubricate the pleural surfaces.[3]

Both sides of the thorax should be scanned as unilateral disease may be present. Although the majority of horses with pleural disease have the most severe disease process in the right hemithorax, the left may be equally involved or, on occasion, may be the most severely affected.[3] The thorax is usually scanned initially from the dorsal to the ventral aspect, parallel with the ribs and intercostal spaces and then scanned perpendicular to the long axis of the ribs in a cranial to caudal direction if any abnormalities are noted.

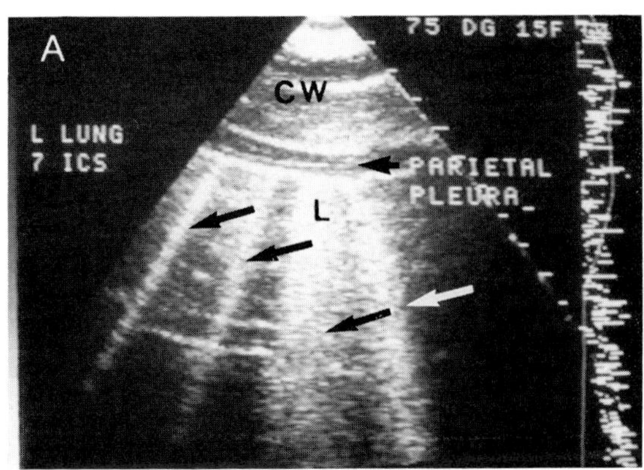


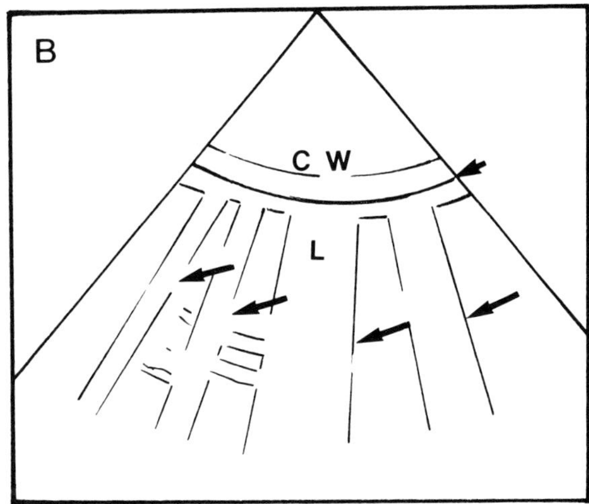


**FIG. 6–4.** Sonogram of the left side of the thorax from a 2-year-old Thoroughbred colt taken at the 7th intercostal space. The right side of the scan is dorsal and the left side is ventral. A. The long arrows point to the reverberation artifacts created from a normally aerated lung periphery. The short black arrow points to the parietal pleura. L—lung; CW—chest wall. B. Diagram of sonogram 6–4A. The long arrows (black and white) point to the reverberation artifacts. The short black arrow points to the parietal pleura. L—lung; CW—chest wall.

## Abnormal Equine Thorax

Selection of horses for ultrasonographic examination of the thorax should be based, in large part, on results of auscultation and percussion. Examination should be thorough and performed in a quiet area; it is important to ensure depth of breathing is adequate for assessment. The detection of normal lung sounds throughout the thorax at rest and with deep breathing indicates normal aeration of the periphery of the lung and a decreased likelihood of detecting any abnormalities of the pleura or pulmonary parenchyma. The auscultation of areas of dullness, large airway sounds, pleural friction rubs, and crackles are indicative of pleural and/or pulmonary disease, close to or involving the visceral pleural surface of the lung. Although abnormalities are occasionally found on ultrasonographic examination of the lung or pleura of horses in the absence of any auscultable changes, the majority of horses with ultrasonographic lesions have abnormal lung sounds.

A line of ventral dullness detected on thoracic auscultation and percussion usually indicates a pleural fluid line. Pleural fluid is easily detected ultrasonographically as an anechoic space between the parietal pleural echo, the diaphragm, and the lung (Fig. 6–5A, B).[1,3–6] With the accumulation of pleural fluid and the dorsal displacement of the ventral lung border, a larger portion of the diaphragm and underlying abdominal viscera can be successfully imaged.[1,3] The type and amount of pleural fluid and opacities and the extent of the underlying pulmonary pathologic condition can be characterized if the periphery of the lung is affected.[1,3–6]

The pleural fluid may be clear and anechoic (Fig. 6–5A, B) or a composite fluid with fibrin (Fig. 6–6A, B), loculations (Fig. 6–7A, B), adhesions (Fig. 6–8A, B) or gas echoes (Fig. 6–9A, B).[1–6] Clear, anechoic fluid has little or no cellular debris, is usually a transudate or modified transudate, and can be imaged in horses with congestive heart failure, pericarditis, and nonfibrinous pleuropneumonia.[1,3,6,11] The pericardiodiaphragmatic ligament, a normal pleural reflection, can be imaged from each side of the thorax as a continuous membrane stretching from the diaphragm to the pericardium (Fig. 6–10A, B) in all horses with pleural fluid. It can be differentiated from fibrin by its ultrasonographic appearance as it usually appears more echogenic than fibrin, is a thicker membrane,

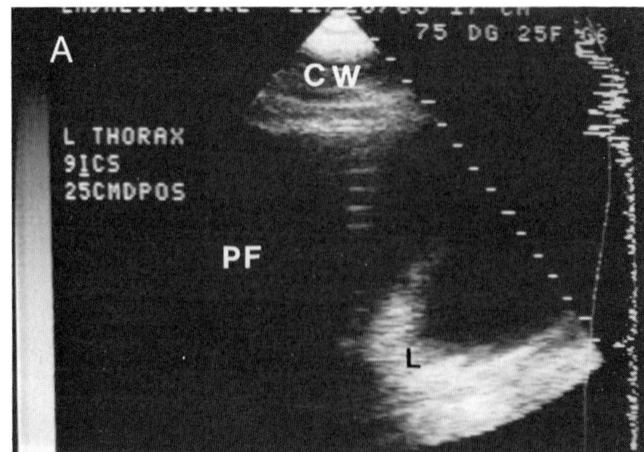


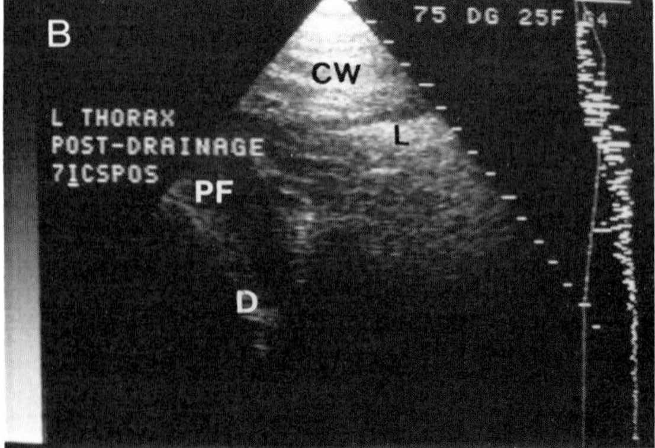


**FIG. 6–5.** Sonograms of the left side of the thorax from a yearling Standardbred filly with pleuritis. A. Sonogram of the left 9th intercostal space taken at a level 25 cm dorsal to the point of the shoulder. The right side of the scan is dorsal and the left side is ventral. A large anechoic (black) pleural effusion (PF = pleural fluid) is imaged surrounding the lung (L), which is compressed cranioventrally by the surrounding fluid. CW—chest wall. B. Sonogram taken level with the point of the shoulder from the same horse immediately after thoracocentesis. Notice the marked decrease in the amount of pleural fluid (PF) in the ventralmost portion of the thorax next to the diaphragm (D) and the re-expansion of the lung (L) with the fluid removed. The aerated (normal) lung is now against the parietal pleural surface at the chest wall (CW).

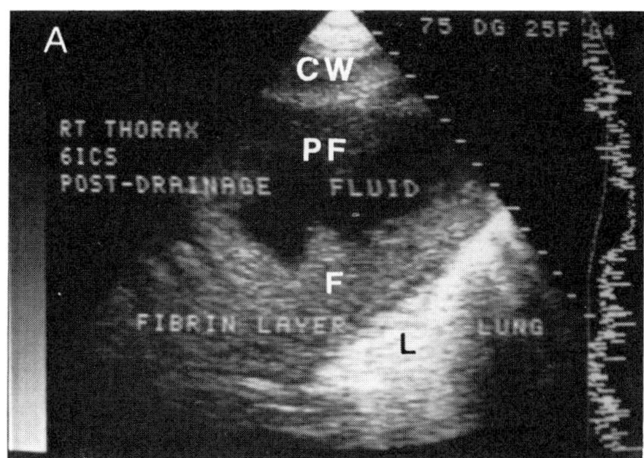


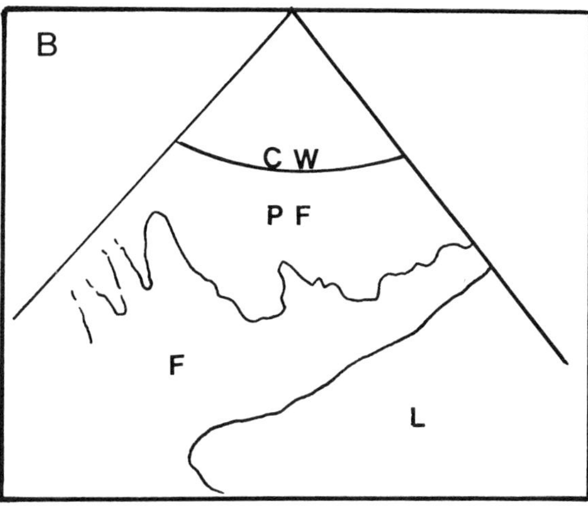


**FIG. 6–6.** Sonogram of the right side of the thorax from a 3-year-old Thoroughbred gelding with pleuropneumonia taken at the 6th intercostal space after drainage of pleural fluid. A. A small amount of pleural fluid (PF) is seen next to the chest wall (CW). Notice the large fibrin (F) layer on the visceral pleural surface of the lung (L). The right side of the sonogram is dorsal and the left side is ventral. B. Diagram of sonogram 6–6A. CW—chest wall; PF—pleural fluid; F—fibrin; L—lung.

floats, and can be imaged continuously from the diaphragm to the pericardium. This ligament was visualized consistently in a group of experimental horses whose thoraxes were infused with sterile saline, as well as in horses with pleuropneumonia, and it can be easily misdiagnosed as fibrin if a careful evaluation is not performed.[6] Fibrin has a filmy, filamentous ultrasonographic appearance and is attached to the parietal and/or visceral pleural surfaces, usually loosely, and may be present in layers (Fig. 6–6A, B) or as strands floating in the fluid, moving with respiration and the heartbeat (Figs. 6–7A, B and 6–8A, B).[3,6] Loculations are common in horses with fibrinous pleuritis and may be infrequent or extensive and multiple. (Figs. 6–7A, B and 6–8A, B).[3,6] The more extensive and organized the loculations, the more difficult successful drainage of the pleural fluid becomes.[3,5] The prognosis for horses with this type of fluid has been reported to be poorer than if a clear anechoic

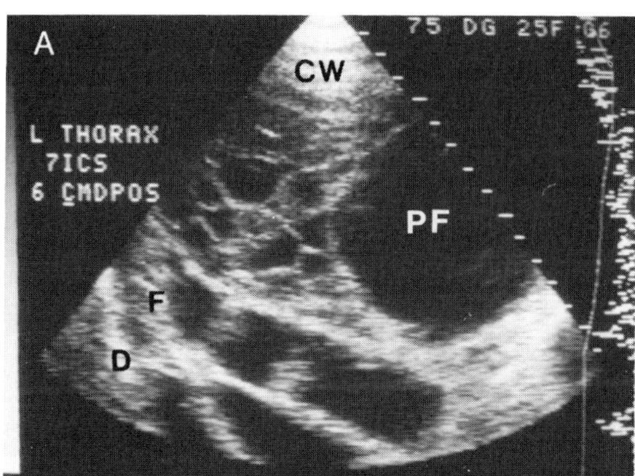


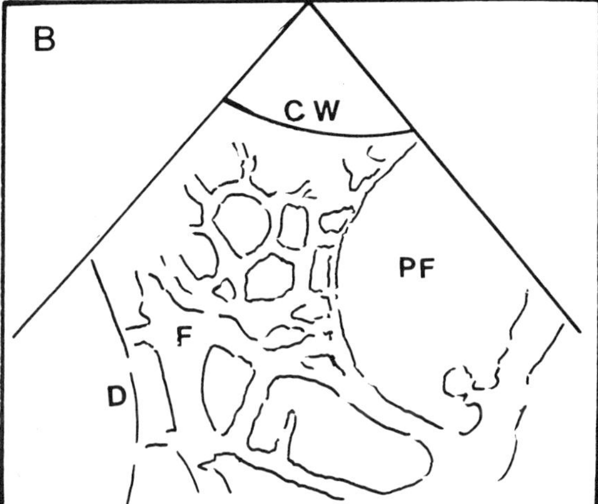


**FIG. 6–7.** Sonogram of the left side of the thorax from a 3-year-old Standardbred filly with pleuropneumonia taken at the 7th intercostal space at a level 6 cm dorsal to the point of the shoulder. A. Notice the extensive fibrinous (F) loculations of pleural fluid (PF) in the ventral thorax extending from the diaphragm (D) to the chest wall (CW). No lung is visible at this level. B. Diagram of sonogram 6–7A. CW—chest wall; F—fibrin; PF—pleural fluid; D—diaphragm.

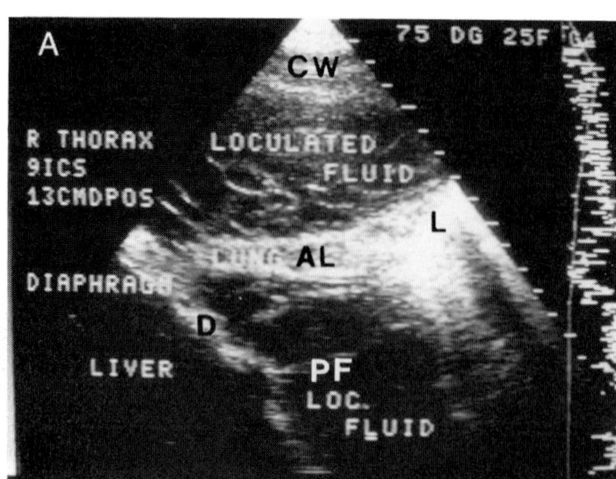


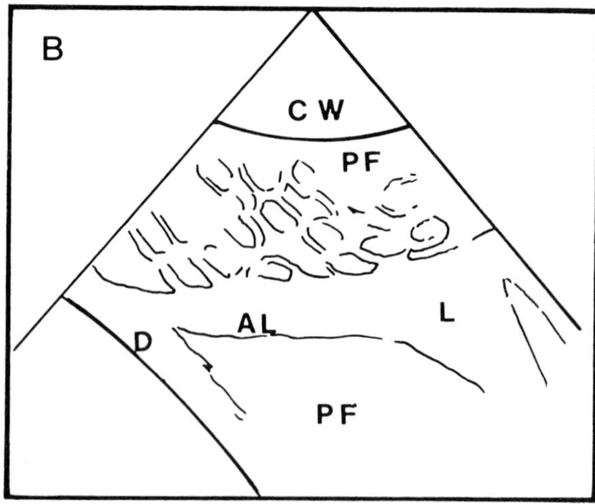


**FIG. 6–8.** Sonogram of the right side of the thorax from a 5-year-old Standardbred stallion with pleuropneumonia taken at the 9th intercostal space 13 cm dorsal to the point of the shoulder. A. Notice the adhesion of the atelectatic lung (AL) to the diaphragm (D) in the ventral portion of the thorax to the left of the sonogram. Normally aerated lung with its characteristic reverberation artifacts can be seen in the dorsal side of the sonogram (to the right). Loculated pleural fluid (PF) is seen both superficial and deep to the adhesion. The atelectic lung is compressed by the surrounding fluid. CW—chest wall. B. Diagram of sonogram 6–8A. CW—chest wall; AL—atelectic lung; L—lung; D—diaphragm; PF—pleural fluid.

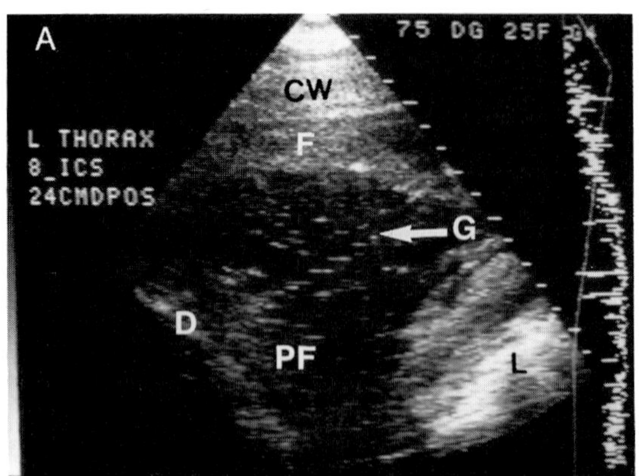


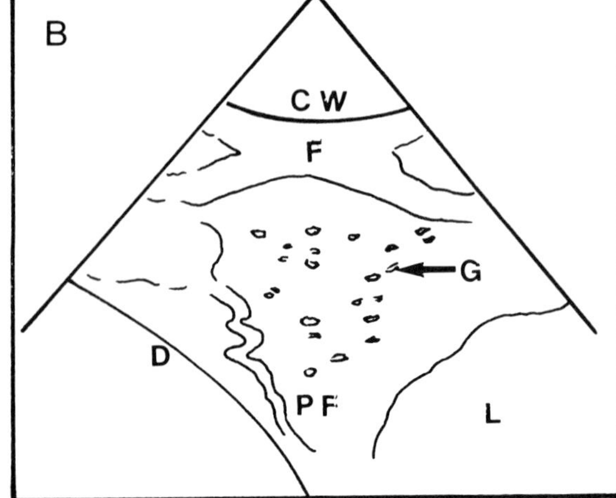


**FIG. 6–9.** Sonogram of the left side of the thorax from a 5-year-old Standardbred gelding with anaerobic pleuropneumonia taken at the 8th intercostal space at a level 24 cm dorsal to the point of the shoulder. A. Notice the layer of fibrin (F) along the parietal pleural surface of the chest wall (CW) and the multiple small hyperechoic (white) free gas (G) echoes (arrow) mixing in the pleural fluid (PF). The diaphragm (D) and ventral part of the thorax are to the left of the sonogram and the lung (L) and more dorsal part of the thorax are to the right of the sonogram. B. Diagram of sonogram 6–9A. CW—chest wall; F—fibrin; D—diaphragm; PF—pleural fluid; L—lung; G—free gas echoes.

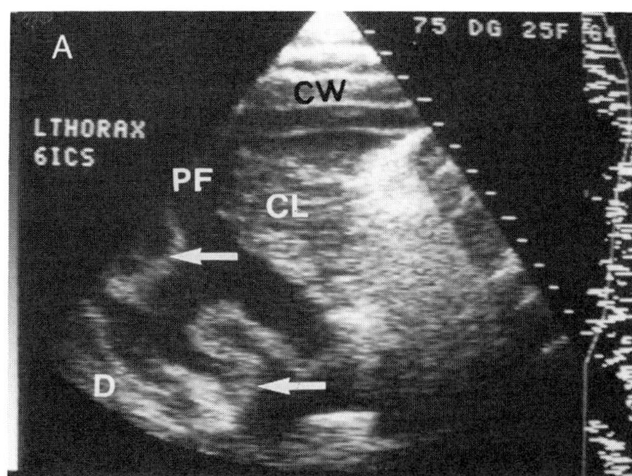


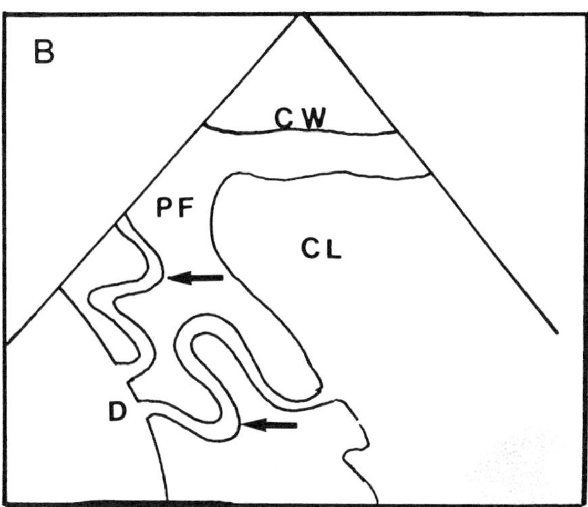


**FIG. 6–10.** Sonogram of the left side of the thorax from a 5-year-old Thoroughbred gelding with pleuropneumonia taken at the 6th intercostal space level with the point of the shoulder. Dorsal is to the right of the sonogram and ventral is to the left. A. Notice the consolidated sonolucent lung (CL) and anechoic pleural fluid (PF). The arrows point to the pericardiodiaphragmatic ligament along the diaphragm (D). CW—chest wall. B. Diagram of sonogram 6–10A. CW—chest wall; PF—pleural fluid; D—diaphragm; CL—consolidated lung. Arrows point to the pericardiodiaphragmatic ligament.

fluid was present, as a longer treatment and recovery time is usually necessary.[3] Many of these horses also have severe underlying pulmonary pathologic conditions with a concomitant poorer survival rate or less successful return to performance.[3] Adhesions may be imaged as echogenic, firm attachments between the visceral and parietal pleural surfaces (Fig. 6–8A, B). When these adhesions between the lung and the parietal pleural surfaces are mature and fibrous they may result in distortion of the diaphragm with exhalation. Adhesions of the lung to the parietal pleural surface of the thoracic wall or diaphragm can also be detected by the lack of independent movement between these surfaces.[3] Slow shallow respiration results in little motion of the lung relative to these structures and if normal movement of the lung against the thoracic wall or across the diaphragm is not seen in the resting horse, the ultrasonographic evaluation should be performed with the horse breathing deeply to differentiate whether it is normal or has pleural adhesions.

Gas echoes are bright hyperechoic floating structures visualized within the pleural fluid which have been associated with the production of free gas in horses with anaerobic pleuropneumonia (Figs. 6–9A, B; 6–11A, B).[4] The gas echoes are often seen swirling in the pleural fluid (Fig. 6–9A, B) or are trapped in fibrinous loculations (Fig. 6–11A, B) in horses with fibrinous pleuropneumonia. Their number usually increases in the more dorsal portions of the pleural fluid. There is a significant association between the recovery of anaerobic organisms from cultures of the pleural fluid or transtracheal aspirates and the presence of gas echoes in horses with anaerobic pleuropneumonia.[4] Several of the horses in which gas echoes were detected, in addition to the anaerobic infection also had bronchopleural fistulas or pulmonary-pleural abscesses communicating with bronchi.[4] No association has been found between the diagnostic or therapeutic use of thoracocentesis and the subsequent appearance of gas echoes.[4]

Pneumothorax can be diagnosed ultrasonographically with or without pleural effusion.[3] The area of contact between the dorsalmost aspect of the lung and the more dorsal air accumulation can be identified. The lung with its characteristic artifact can be imaged moving against the parietal pleural surface of the thoracic wall, while the dorsal pneumothorax is imaged as a non-moving gas artifact. In horses with large volumes of pleural effusion diagnosis is even easier, as a gas (pneumothorax)–fluid (pleural effusion)

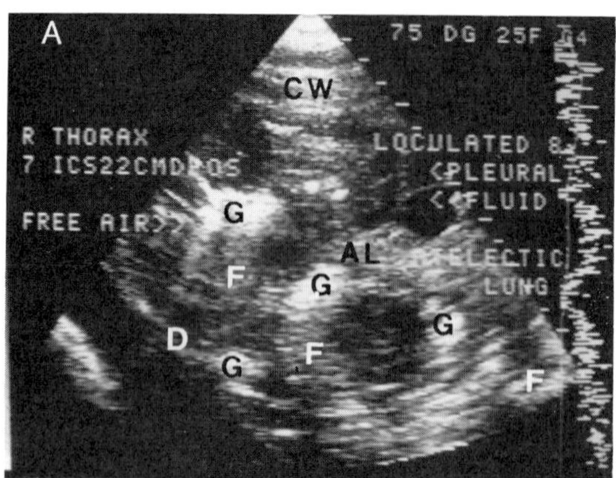


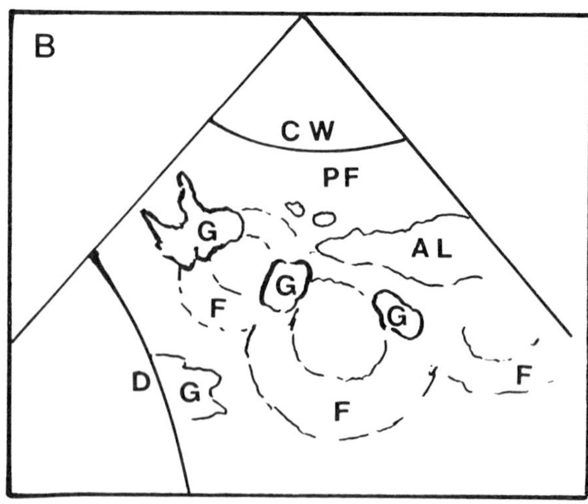


**FIG. 6–11.** Sonogram of the right side of the thorax from a 6-year-old Thoroughbred mare with anaerobic pleuropneumonia taken in the 7th intercostal space at a level 22 cm dorsal to the point of the shoulder. The right side of the sonogram is dorsal and the left side is ventral. A. Notice the multiple hyperechoic gas (G) echoes trapped within the fibrinous (F), loculated pleural fluid ventral to the compressed atelectic lung (AL). D—diaphragm; CW—chest wall. B. Diagram of sonogram 6–11A. CW—chest wall; G—gas; AL—atelectatic lung; F—fibrin; D—diaphragm.

interface can be imaged against the parietal pleural surface, while the visceral pleural surface of the lung is imaged deeper in the thoracic cavity, floating in the fluid (Fig. 6–12A,B).

Careful evaluation of the underlying lung is essential in horses with pleural effusion to determine the presence and severity of pulmonary involvement. Differentiation between compression atelectasis, consolidation, abscess and necrosis can be made ultrasonographically if the periphery of the lung is involved, and it usually is.[3,5,6] With compression atelectasis and collapse of the ventral-most portion of normal lung by the surrounding fluid, the compressed ventral margin of

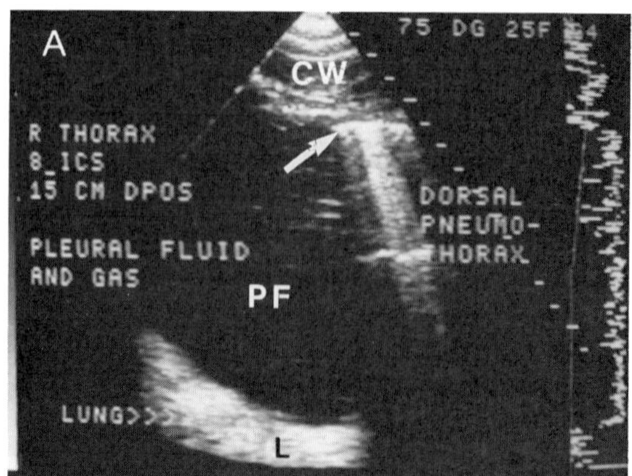


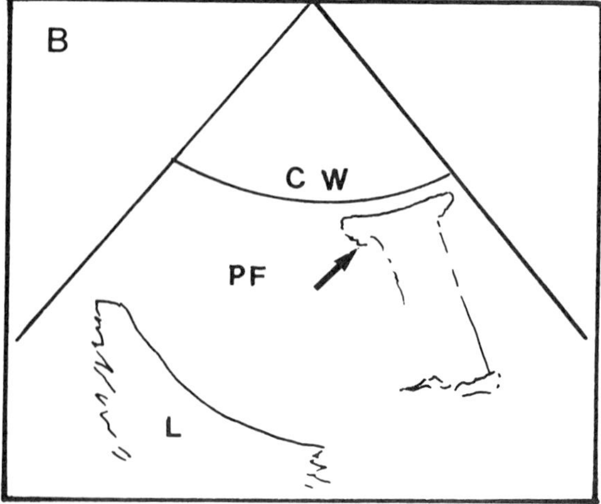


**FIG. 6–12.** Sonogram of the right side of the thorax from a 2-year-old Thoroughbred gelding with anaerobic pleuropneumonia and a dorsal pneumothorax taken at the 10th intercostal space at a level 15 cm dorsal to the point of the shoulder. The right side of the sonogram is dorsal and the left side is ventral. A. The arrow points to the dorsal pneumothorax (hyperechoic gas echoes) at the gas-pleural fluid (PF) interface. The lung (L) is seen deep to the gas-fluid interface floating in the pleural fluid. CW—chest wall. B. Diagram of the sonogram from 6–12A. CW—chest wall; PF—pleural fluid; L—lung.

the lung is seen floating in the pleural fluid.[3,6] In horses with small pleural effusions and normal lungs the ventral portion of the lung will still appear echogenic, with the characteristic gas artifacts. With greater pleural effusions, the ventralmost tip of the lung appears compressed and is more sonolucent due to lack of aeration (Fig. 6–5A). The more dorsal lung is normally aerated and has the characteristic gas artifacts. A similar ultrasonographic appearance has been seen in horses with normal lungs in which a pleural effusion was created experimentally[6] and is also the typical appearance in horses with congestive heart failure, pericarditis, and pleuritis without pulmonary disease.

Consolidation of the pulmonary parenchyma results in several ultrasonographic appearances depending upon the severity of the disease process. In its mildest form small areas of dimpling or irregularities are seen in the otherwise smooth visceral pleural surface.[3] Small portions of consolidated lung are seen as sonolucent areas with radiating artifacts interrupting an otherwise normal visceral pleural surface (Fig. 6–13). This ultrasonographic image may be seen in horses with acute pneumonia, intraparenchymal hemorrhage, or a clinically resolved pleuropneumonia which was originally much more severe.

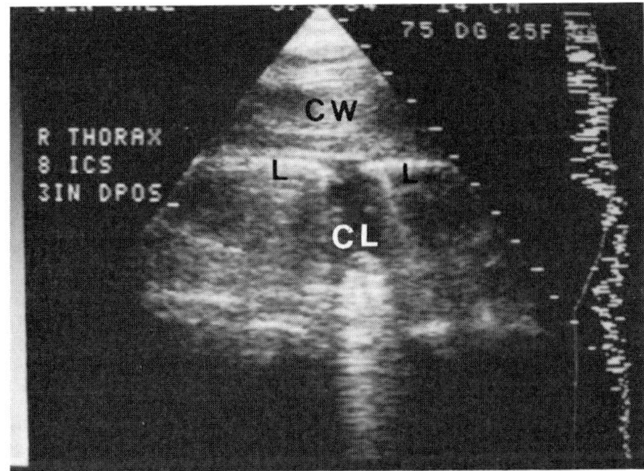


**FIG. 6–13.** Sonogram of the right side of the thorax from a 6-year-old Thoroughbred gelding with pneumonia taken from the 8th intercostal space at a level 3 inches dorsal to the point of the shoulder. There is a small area of sonolucent lung consistent with an area of consolidated lung (CL). Notice the normally aerated lung (L). CW—chest wall.

Larger areas of sonolucent lung correspond to more severe consolidation and pneumonia (Figs. 6–10A, B; 6–14A, B; 6–15; 6–16A, B; 6–17A, B). In these horses the areas of affected lung are wedge shaped and are not compressed by the surrounding fluid (Figs. 6–10A, B; 6–14A, B; 6–15). The normal anatomy of the lung is still visible and appears intact. Often large air echoes can be imaged within the sonolucent lung, consistent with air in the larger airways only, surrounded by nonaerated consolidated lung (Fig. 6–14A, B). With more severe pneumonia the entire portion of the affected lung is uniformly sonolucent and the entire bronchial anatomy can be visualized branching throughout the lung (Fig. 6–17A, B).[3] The lung ultrasonographically resembles liver, consistent with the hepatization seen with severe pneumonia. The most severe consolidation is usually seen in the ventral portion of the lung in the 5th to 7th ICS. Most horses with pleuropneumonia have bilateral lung consolidation although the right side may be the more severely affected.[3,6] Unilateral lung consolidation is less common but when it occurs is more likely to affect the right lung.[6] Other areas of the lung may also be affected, reinforcing the need for careful auscultation of the entire thorax and subsequent ultrasonographic evaluation of any dull areas (Case 1).

The pulmonary parenchyma appears sonolucent and the normal anatomic structures can no longer be visualized when there is parenchymal necrosis. These portions of necrotic lung do not move normally with respiration; instead they appear gelatinous as the lung moves, consistent with collapsing necrotic tissue. A follow-up examination 1 or 2 days later often reveals an area of cavitation where the necrotic tissue previously was visualized. These horses may develop a bronchopleural fistula in this area (Fig. 6–18A, B). Often this coincides with the development of gas echoes in the pleural fluid, suggesting the presence of an anaerobic infection.[4] A dorsal pneumothorax may also result from this cavitation of necrotic lung and the resultant bronchopleural fistula. The prognosis for survival of these horses is poor (less than 50%) and

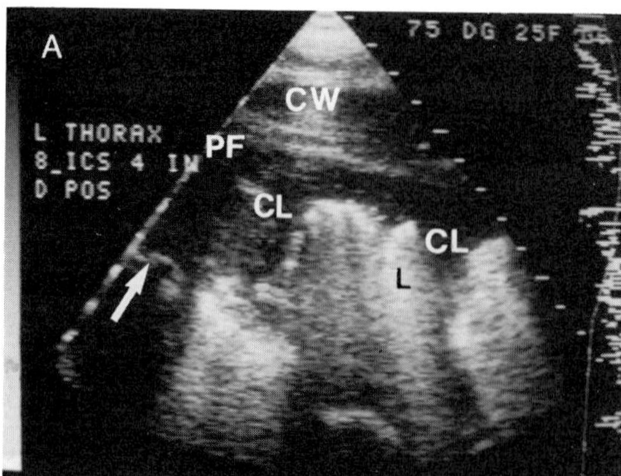


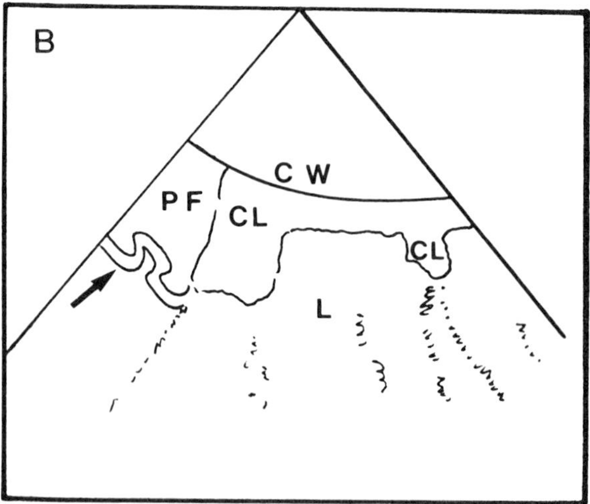


**FIG. 6–14.** Sonogram of the left side of the thorax from a 5-year-old Thoroughbred filly taken from the 8th intercostal space at a level 4 inches dorsal to the point of the shoulder. A. Notice the sonolucent consolidated lung (CL) against the chest wall (CW) in the more dorsal portion of the thorax (the middle and right side of the sonogram). In the more ventral portion of the thorax to the left of the sonogram is some anechoic pleural fluid (PF) and the pericardial diaphragmatic ligament (arrow). B. Diagram of sonogram 6–14A. CW—chest wall; CL—consolidated lung; L—lung; Arrow points to the pericardial diaphragmatic ligament; PF—pleural fluid.

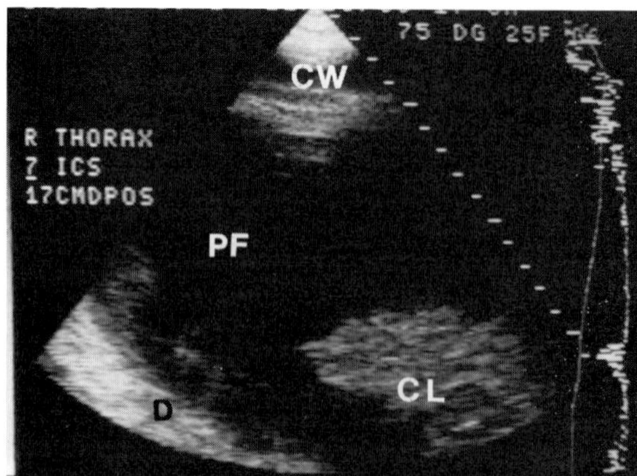


**FIG. 6–15.** Sonogram of the right side of the thorax from a 1-year-old Standardbred filly with pleuropneumonia taken from the 7th intercostal space at a level 17 cm dorsal to the point of the shoulder. The consolidated lung (CL) is floating in the pleural fluid (PF) in the more dorsal portion of the thorax with the diaphragm (D) in the ventral thorax. CW—chest wall.

for return to performance, grave.[4] Prolonged broad spectrum antimicrobial therapy (6 months or longer) may be necessary and the pulmonary disease is usually so extensive that owners frequently elect to breed and not compete these horses.

Abscesses are sonolucent areas within the lung which are usually well circumscribed and lack normal pulmonary anatomic structures.[3,6] They may be encapsulated if they are chronic (Fig. 6–19A, B) or may appear as sonolucent cavities, some of which may contain echogenic debris, if they are of recent origin (Fig. 6–20A, B).[3,6] They may be single or multiple. Those deep within the pulmonary parenchyma will not be imaged ultrasonographically if there is no disease of the more superficial lung. In these horses, if a deep pulmonary abscess is suspected yet thoracic auscultation is normal, thoracic radiographs should be obtained. In most horses and foals, however, the periphery of the lung is affected, enabling the ultrasonographer to successfully image the abscess. Gas caps may be visualized in the abscess and are recognized by the characteristic gas artifact imaged in their dorsal portions (Fig. 6–19A, B).[3] These gas caps may be associated with the presence of a gas forming organism, usually an anaer-

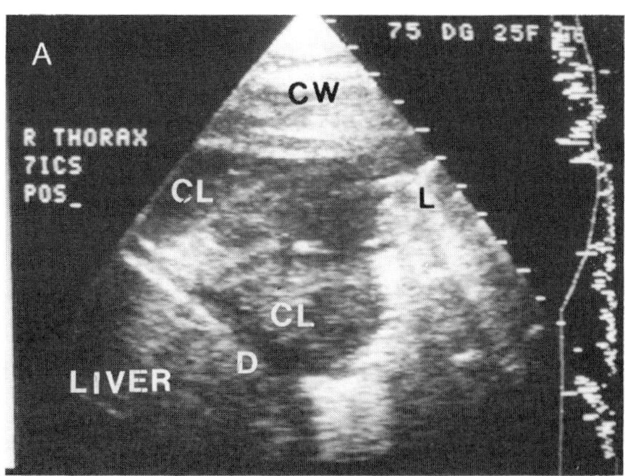


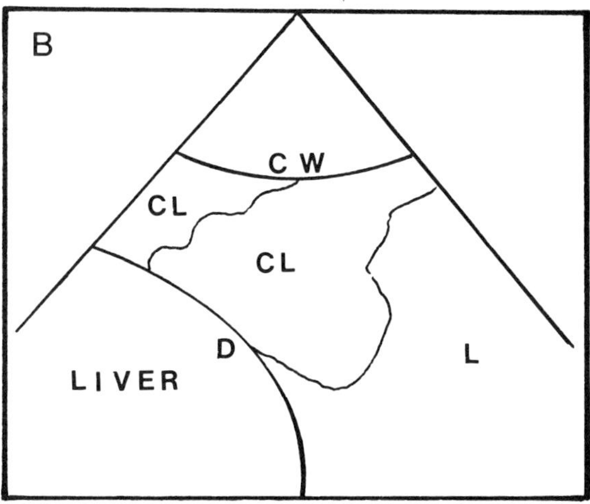


**FIG. 6–16.** Sonogram of the right side of the thorax from a 6-year-old Thoroughbred gelding with pneumonia taken from the 7th intercostal space level with the point of the shoulder. The right side of the sonogram is dorsal and the left side is ventral. A. Notice the large areas of sonolucent consolidated lung (CL) in the ventral portion of the thorax against the diaphragm (D) and chest wall (CW). The more dorsal lung (L) is more normally aerated at the periphery. B. Diagram of sonogram 6–16A. CW—chest wall; CL—consolidated lung; L—aerated lung; D—diaphragm.

obe, or with a bronchial communication between the lung and the abscess.[4] Horses with severe pleuropneumonia will often "wall off" an abscess in the pleural cavity. In these horses the dorsal wall of the abscess is the ventral lung, the lateral wall is the parietal pleural surface of the thoracic wall, the medial wall is either lung or mediastinum, and the ventral wall is the diaphragm (Case 2). Percutaneous drainage of these abscesses can be performed successfully with ultrasonographic guidance.

Evaluation of the thorax for other types of masses, either pleural or pulmonary, in horses with suspected neoplasia is another application of diagnostic ultrasound.[3,5] Pleural masses are much easier to find in horses with a pleural effusion, as the fluid separates

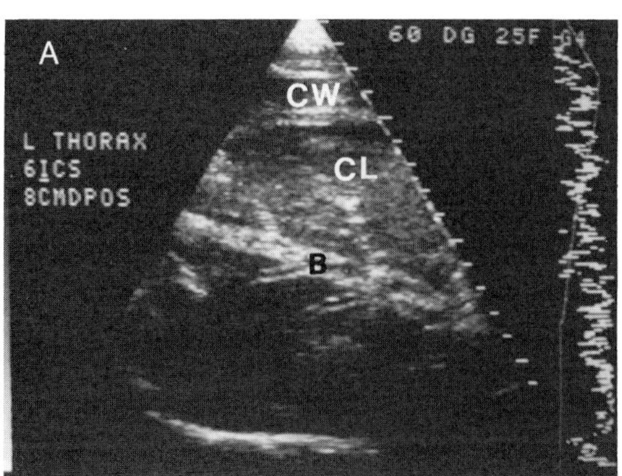


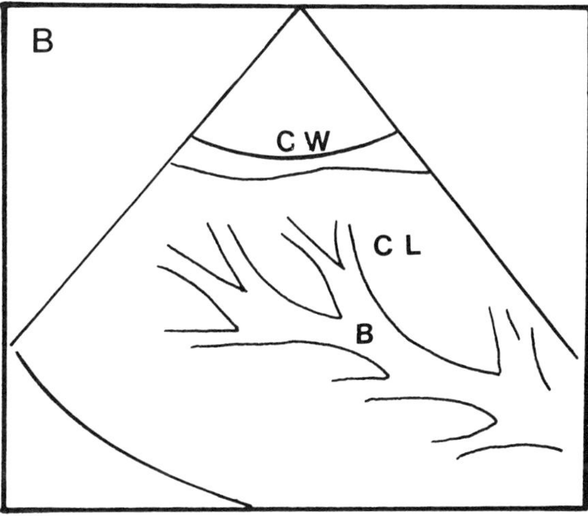


**FIG. 6–17.** Sonogram of the left side of the thorax from a 4-year-old Thoroughbred gelding with pneumonia taken from the 6th intercostal space at a level 8 cm dorsal to the point of the shoulder. The right side of the sonogram is dorsal and the left side is ventral. A. The entire pulmonary parenchyma imaged is highly sonolucent, enabling the bronchial tree (B) to be visualized throughout the consolidated lung (CL). CW—chest wall. B. Diagram of sonogram 6–17A. CW—chest wall; CL—consolidated lung; B—bronchus.

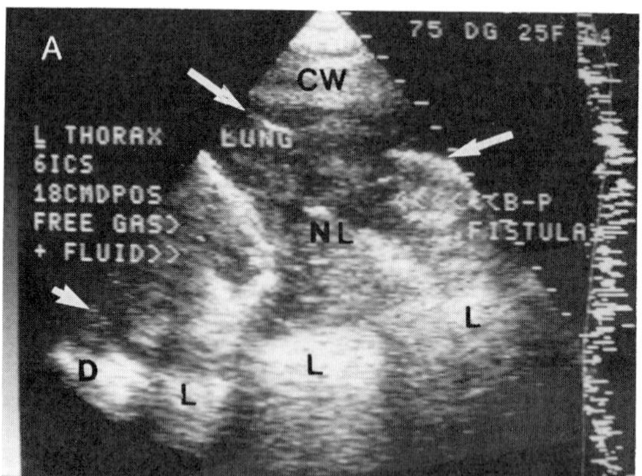


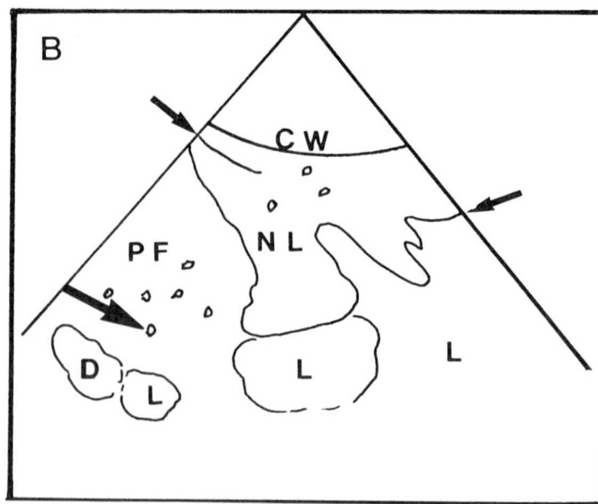


**FIG. 6–18.** Sonogram of the left side of the thorax from a 2-year-old Thoroughbred colt with a necrotizing anaerobic pleuropneumonia and development of a bronchopleural fistula, taken from the 6th intercostal space at a level 18 cm dorsal to the point of the shoulder. The right side of the thorax is dorsal and the left side is ventral. A. The long arrows point to the visceral pleural surface of the lung with a central sonolucent discontinuity in the area of necrotic lung (NL) and a bronchopleural fistula. The hyperechoic areas represent areas of aerated lung (L). The shorter arrow points to free gas echoes in the pleural fluid. D—diaphragm. B. Diagram of sonogram 6–18A. CW—chest wall; NL—necrotic lung; L—lung; D—diaphragm; PF—pleural fluid. The two long arrows point to the visceral pleural surface of the lung, while the larger arrow points to the free gas echoes in the pleural fluid.

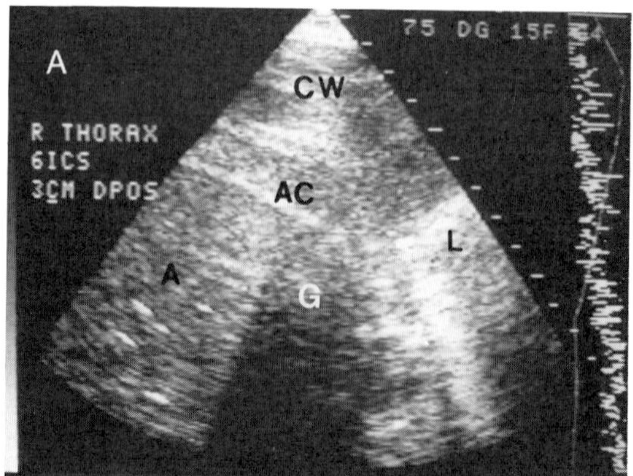


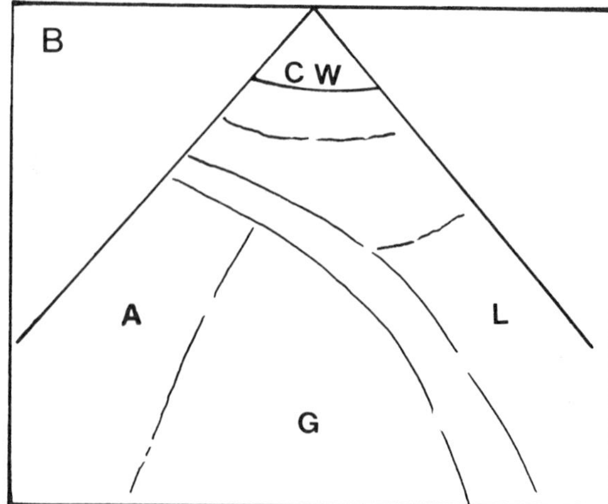


**FIG. 6–19.** Sonogram of the right side of the thorax from a 5-year-old Thoroughbred mare with a pulmonary abscess taken at the 6th intercostal space at a level 3 cm dorsal to the point of the shoulder. A. The normal portion of the lung (L) is dorsal. The abscess (A) is ventral. The abscess (A) is surrounded by a thick capsule (AC) and a dorsal gas (G) cap is present in the abscess associated with a communicating bronchus. CW—chest wall. B. Diagram of sonogram 6–19A. CW—chest wall; L—lung; AC—abscess capsule; A—abscess; G—gas.

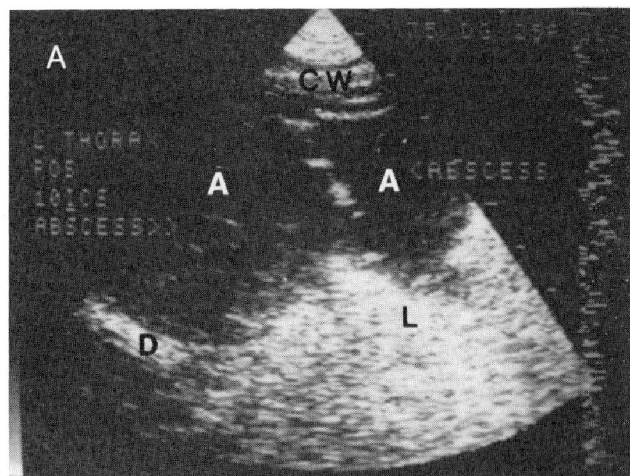


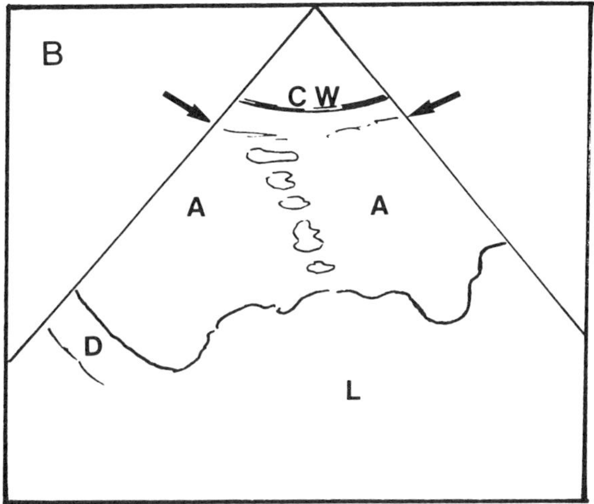


**FIG. 6–20.** Sonogram of a 3-month-old foal with pulmonary abscess caused by Rhodococcus equi, taken from the left 10th intercostal space level with the point of the shoulder. The right side of the sonogram is dorsal and the left is ventral. A. The abscesses (A) are anechoic to sonolucent areas in the periphery of the lung just dorsal to the diaphragm (D). The remaining lung (L) appears relatively normal in this sonogram. CW—chest wall. B. Diagram of sonogram 6–20A. CW—chest wall, A—abscess, L—lung; D—diaphragm.

the parietal and visceral pleural surfaces allowing improved visualization. Neoplasms are relatively rare in horses but lymphosarcoma, one of the more common ones, often involves the mediastinum and thus both the cranial and caudal mediastinum should be evaluated ultrasonographically when possible. The caudal mediastinal region can be visualized only in horses with pleural effusion as the area is normally covered by aerated lung. Limited visualization of the mediastinal region immediately cranial to the heart is possible in most horses from the right 3rd ICS. Masses may occasionally be imaged free in the pleural fluid in horses with lymphosarcoma (Fig. 6–21). If the periphery of the lung is affected ultrasonographic visualization and guided biopsy of masses is possible. A thoracocentesis should be performed and submitted for cytologic evaluation, as exfoliation of neoplastic cells into the thoracic fluid can be diagnostic.

Diaphragmatic hernias may be imaged ultrasonographically by visualizing abdominal viscera in the thorax without the diaphragm separating them from the thoracic viscera (Fig. 6–22A, B). The lung with its characteristic reverberation artifacts can usually be seen in the dorsalmost portion of the thorax moving with respiration. Immediately ventral

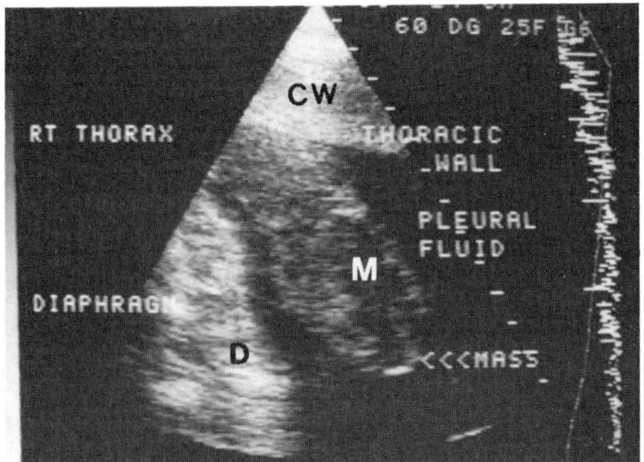


**FIG. 6–21.** Sonogram of a 17-year-old crossbred gelding taken from the right 6th intercostal space below the point of the shoulder. The right side of the sonogram is dorsal and the left side is ventral. Notice the mass (M) with uniform echogenicity in the ventral portion of the thorax between the diaphragm (D) and chest wall (CW) surrounded by pleural fluid (PF). This uniform soft tissue mass is consistent with a neoplasm such as lymphosarcoma, which was diagnosed in this horse.

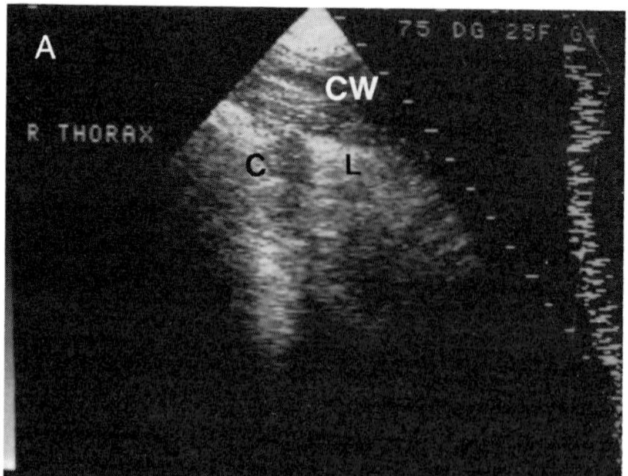


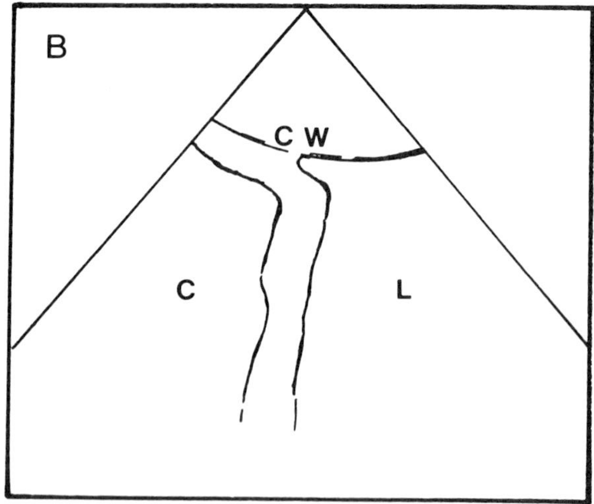


**FIG. 6–22.** Sonogram of a 15-year-old Thoroughbred gelding with a diaphragmatic hernia taken from the right mid-thoracic region. The right side of the sonogram is dorsal and the left side of the sonogram is ventral. A. The cranioventralmost portion of the lung (L) is dorsal and immediately adjacent to the colon (C) and chest wall (CW). No echoes from the diaphragm could be found in this region between the thoracic and abdominal viscera. B. Diagram of sonogram 6–22A. CW—chest wall; C—colon; L—aerated lung.

to this will be the echoes from the abdominal viscera, which often are gas filled, especially if the large colon is in the hernia. Distended portions of fluid filled small intestine may also be imaged and the degree of distention of the small bowel, the wall thickness and the motility of the portion of the intestine indicate the amount of compromise to that portion of the intestine. It is not usually possible to visualize the entire hernial ring as echoes from gas in the bowel prohibit penetration of the ultrasound to the deeper areas. Small diaphragmatic hernias, those which do not involve the portions of the diaphragm nearest the thoracic wall, or those resulting in herniation of abdominal viscera deep to normally aerated lung, will not be seen ultrasonographically. Thoracic radiography is indicated in all horses suspected of having a diaphragmatic hernia. Ultrasonography can provide a diagnosis in some horses when radiographic facilities are not readily available.

## Comparison of Thoracic Radiography and Ultrasonography

There are numerous limitations to obtaining high quality thoracic radiographs from the adult horse.[12,13] First, only lateral thoracic films can be obtained and usually four overlapping areas are radiographed to evaluate the majority of the equine thorax. Thus, characterization of any abnormalities in two mutually perpendicular planes is not possible. Localization of a lesion to one side of the thorax is often difficult, although the use of both right and left lateral radiographs may resolve this. High output radiograph generators are required with high mAs and kVp to overcome the limitations imposed by the size and respiratory motion in the adult horse. This equipment is not portable and is expensive, limiting its use in large animal practice. Recent advances in high speed film and intensifying screens have enabled some decrease in the maximum mAs required; however, radiography is still usually confined to a referral hospital or university setting. The health hazard of continued exposure to x rays is also a consideration.

There are also limitations to obtaining a high quality thoracic sonogram from a horse. Although some images can be obtained from horses with sleek short hair coats and copious amounts of coupling gel, clipping the hair coat in the area under investigation is necessary for optimal image quality. Images can only be obtained through the intercostal spaces as the ribs are excellent reflectors of ultrasound. Air is a near perfect reflector of ultrasound and thus it is impossible to image abnormal areas that are deep to areas which are normally aerated. Two mutually perpendicular views can be obtained with the sector scanner transducers due to the small size of the head, while only one view (dorsal-ventral) can be obtained with the longer linear transducers. The correct transducer frequency, usually 5.0 MHz, must be selected for optimal image quality, but a lower frequency transducer (3.0 or 3.5 MHz) may be needed if extensive pleural or pulmonary disease is present.

The major advantage of thoracic radiography compared to ultrasonography is in the detection of interstitial changes, lesions located deep in the pulmonary parenchyma in an otherwise normal lung field, and in the detection and characterization of diaphragmatic hernias. Thoracic radiography is also superior to ultrasonography in diagnosing pulmonary edema and pneumothorax. Therefore, thoracic radiography is the diagnostic technique of choice in horses which are normal on auscultation, but in whom thoracic disease is suspected. Ultrasonography will not provide any additional information about the pulmonary parenchyma if the periphery of the lung is normally aerated.

Ultrasonography is useful in characterizing pleural and peripheral pulmonary disease.[1,3–6] Abnormal thoracic auscultation except that of airway disease is a good indication that ultrasonography will provide diagnostic information. The ultrasound equipment is portable, readily available to many private practitioners, relatively inexpensive when compared to the equipment needed for thoracic radiography, and can be used to evaluate other areas. Although some practice is necessary to become proficient in its use, the technique is readily mastered with time, patience, and repeated scanning of abnormal animals.

The biggest advantage of ultrasonography in horses with pleuropneumonia is the ability to characterize the fluid and to evaluate the severity of the underlying pulmonary disease.[6] The presence of adhesions, pleural thickening, pulmonary necrosis and compression atelectasis can also only be detected ultrasonographically.[6] The detection and further characterization of the above abnormalities will improve the clinician's ability to assess the severity of the underlying pleural and pulmonary disease and form a more accurate prognosis. For example, the detection of free gas echoes within the pleural fluid indicates a poor prognosis as it is significantly associated with the presence of an anaerobic infection.[4] Survival rates are also poorer in horses with severe fibrinous pleuritis. Treatment and recovery time will also be longer, and thus more costly, in horses with severe fibrinous pleuritis and loculations when compared to horses with a non-fibrinous pleuritis. The horse's ability to return to its previous performance level may be affected if numerous adhesions exist between the parietal and visceral pleural surfaces.[3] Horses with compression atelectasis and a nonfibrinous pleuritis have an excellent prognosis for survival and return to performance. The detection of areas of consolidation, pulmonary necrosis, or abscesses all increase the probable treatment and recovery time and the prognosis for survival decreases as they become more extensive. Although consolidation is detected radiographically in most horses with pleural effusion, ultrasonography is more sensitive and can detect smaller areas of pneumonia.[6] The side of the lung affected can be readily determined and both sides of the thorax accurately compared, unlike with radiography.

Pleural effusions, especially small volumes, are also more frequently detected ultrasonographically than radiographically.[6] The sonogram can also readily distinguish the side or sides of the thorax with pleural effusion and can be used semi-quantitatively to assess the amount of pleural fluid present.[6] In horses with pleuropneumonia with small effusions (surrounding the cranioventral tip of the lung only) less than 1 L of fluid was recovered per side in the majority.[6] One to 5 L was recovered per side in the majority of horses with moderate pleural effusions (the fluid line extending up to the level of the point of the shoulder).[6] In horses with severe effusions (pleural fluid line above the point of the shoulder) fluid volumes in excess of 5 to 10 L can be recovered depending upon the level of the fluid line. The severity of the underlying pulmonary disease also influences the volume of fluid recovered as horses with compression atelectasis will have more fluid recovered than horses with severe consolidation, if the fluid levels are the same, because the consolidated lung occupies more space. Ultrasonography can be used as a guide to sample or drain the area with the largest fluid accumulation or the least loculation.[3,5]

In conclusion, ultrasonography is a valuable diagnostic aid in the evaluation of the pleura, lung, and mediastinum, especially in horses with pleural effusion. Careful auscultation can be an effective tool for selecting horses in which diagnostic ultrasound will provide additional information. Progressive scanning of horses with pleuropneumonia, pneumonia, or pulmonary abscessation to assess response to treatment and need for drainage is also an important application.

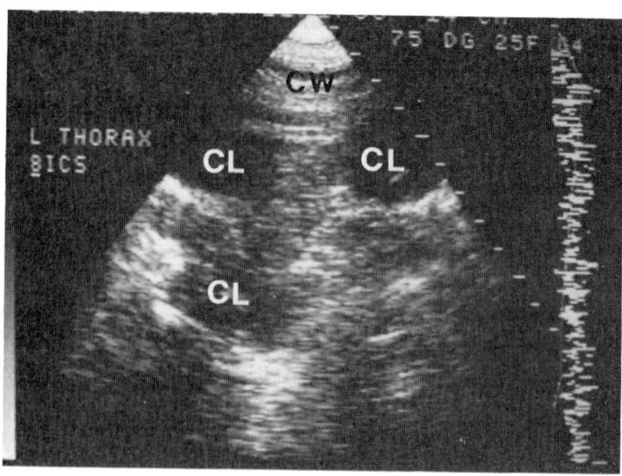


**FIG. 6–23.** A sonogram of the left side of the thorax from a 2-year-old Standardbred filly with pneumonia. The left side of the scan is ventral and the right side dorsal. The large areas of sonolucent lung are areas of consolidation (CL = consolidated lung) in the mid portion of the left lung field imaged in the 8th intercostal space. CW—chest wall.

## Case Studies

### *Case One*

A 2-year-old Standardbred filly was referred to our hospital with a history of fever, coughing, and epistaxis. She had been shipped from Kentucky 6 days earlier and had raced successfully 2 days prior to presentation. The filly had cooled out normally after the race and showed no clinical signs until the morning of presentation.

Initial physical examination revealed the filly to have a temperature of 38.7°C (101.6°F), a pulse of 72 beats per minute, and a respiratory rate of 50 breaths per minute. There was dried blood at both nostrils. Auscultation revealed increased harshness and wheezes in both lung fields. A friction rub was ausculted over the left mid thorax. A transtracheal aspirate revealed a chronic active suppurative septic pneumonia with intra and extracellular Gram negative rods. A culture of the aspirate grew Pasteurella species.

Thoracic radiographs were performed revealing a large radiopaque area in the central caudal lung fields. This area was well circumscribed and consistent with an area of consolidation or an abscess. A sonogram revealed large sonolucent (fluid filled) areas in the mid caudal portion of the left lung (Fig. 6–23) consistent with consolidation and pneumonia or intraparenchymal hemorrhage.

Broad spectrum antimicrobial therapy (intravenous potassium penicillin and gentocin) was started. Two weeks later, therapy was changed to oral trimethoprim sulfa. The filly responded to the broad spectrum antimicrobial therapy and several months later, returned to racing although performance was decreased compared to that prior to pneumonia.

### *Case Two*

A 6-year-old Thoroughbred mare was referred to our hospital with a 4 day history of fever not responsive to antimicrobials beginning 2 days after racing. She had intermittent epistaxis and the lungs sounded dull cranioventrally. Pleuropneumonia was suspected.

At presentation the mare had a temperature of 39.1°C (102.4°F), a pulse of 60 beats/minute, and a respiratory rate of 24 breaths/minute. No lung sounds were auscultable over the right ventral thorax. A sonogram of the left side of the thorax revealed a loculated pleural

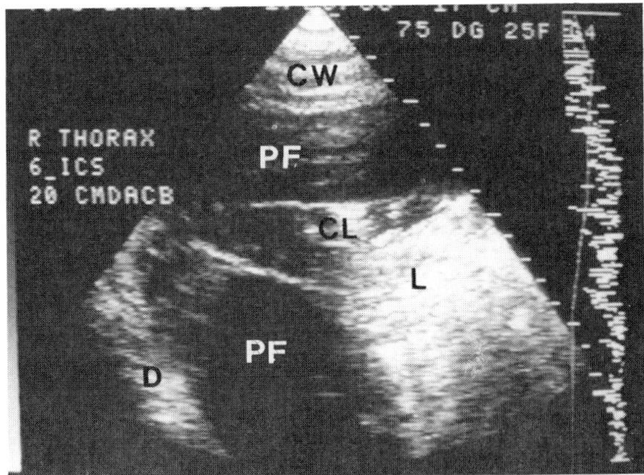


**FIG. 6–24.** A sonogram of the right side of the thorax from a 6-year-old Thoroughbred mare with pleuropneumonia. The left side of the sonogram is ventral and the right side dorsal. There is a large ventral area of consolidation (CL) surrounded by pleural fluid (PF) in the 6th intercostal spaces. The normal lung (L) is dorsal. CW—chest wall; D—diaphragm.

effusion and compression atelectasis of the lung. A sonogram of the right side of the thorax revealed large areas of hypoechoic lung (Fig. 6–24) compatible with consolidation and pneumonia and a loculated pleural effusion. Transtracheal and pleural fluid aspirates revealed an acute suppurative septic pleuropneumonia, and β-hemolytic streptococci were isolated from the cultures of all three samples. Anaerobes were suspected due to the foul odor of the pleural fluid taken from the right hemithorax and Clostridium sp. were isolated from the anaerobic culture.

The mare was treated with intravenous potassium penicillin, gentocin, and oral metronidazole. Nonsteroidal anti-inflammatory drugs were administered as needed. Drainage of the pleural fluid was performed periodically when indicated from clinical and ultrasonographic examination.

The left side of the thorax responded rapidly to the broad spectrum antimicrobial therapy and drainage. Within 1 week, the lung sounds and ultrasonographic examination of the left side of the thorax were near normal. The consolidated right lung became more gelatinous and necrotic and an abscess gradually formed in the ventral thorax. The dorsal border of the abscess was the lung, the ventral border was the diaphragm, the lateral border was the chest wall, and the medial border was the caudal mediastinum. A bronchopleural fistula was suspected due to the prior severe necrosis and liquifaction of the right ventral lung.

Antimicrobial drugs were changed to oral trimethoprim-sulfa and metronidazole after 3 weeks and the mare was discharged on therapy 1 week later. She was returned to the

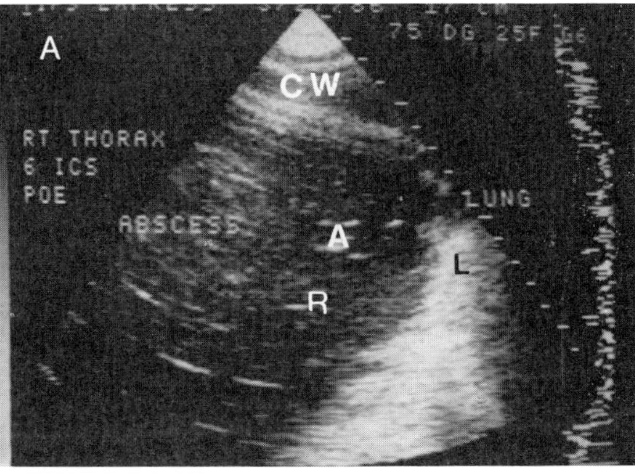


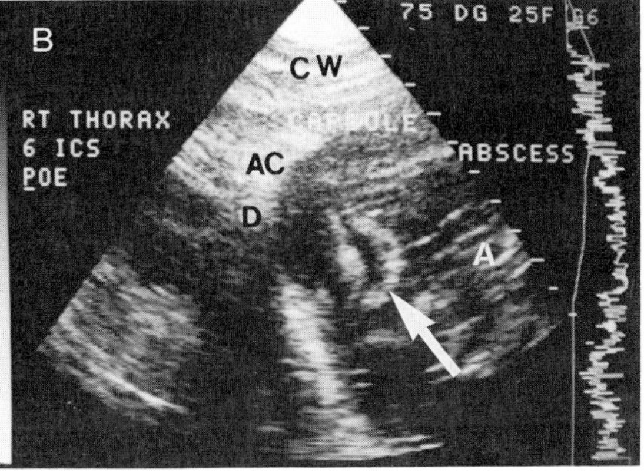


**FIG. 6–25.** Sonogram from the right side of the thorax of the same mare as in Figure 24 taken at the 6th intercostal space 2 months later. A large pleuropulmonary abscess is present in the right ventral thorax. A. Sonogram of the dorsal border of the abscess (A) which is the ventral most portion of the lung (L). CW—chest wall. B. Sonogram of the ventral portion of the abscess (A) formed by the diaphragm (D). The pericardiodiaphragmatic ligament (arrow) is visualized within the abscess. CW—chest wall; AC—abscess capsule.

hospital 1 month later because of persistent fever. The sonogram revealed a 25 cm diameter abscess in the right ventral thorax (Fig. 6–25A, B). This abscess was drained transthoracically several times and a culture and sensitivity were repeated. Beta hemolytic streptococcus, enterococcus, and multiple anaerobes were isolated. Broad spectrum antimicrobial therapy and drainage were continued for the next 4 months but the large abscess and bronchopleural fistula persisted.

Surgical exploration and drainage were performed under general anesthesia 6 months after the initial presentation. Several liters of thick foul smelling exudate were drained, the abscess was debrided and the patent bronchus sutured. The horse experienced severe respiratory distress after surgery and was euthanatized. Postmortem examination revealed an acute inflammatory infiltrate throughout the left lung, compatible with aspiration of the purulent material from the abscess in the right hemithorax.

## References

1. Rantanen NW, Gage ML, Paradis MR. Ultrasonography as a diagnostic aid in pleural effusion of horses. Vet Radiol, *22*:211, 1981.
2. Rantanen NW. Ultrasound appearance of normal lung borders and adjacent viscera in the horse. Vet Radiol, *22*:217, 1981.
3. Rantanen NW. Disease of the thorax. Vet Clin North Am [Equine Pract], *2*:49, 1986.
4. Reimer J, Reef VB, Spencer PA. Ultrasonography as a diagnostic aid in horses with anaerobic bacterial pleuropneumonia and/or pulmonary abscessation: 27 cases (1984–1986). J Am Vet Med Assoc, *194*:278, 1989.
5. Byars TD, Halley J. Uses of ultrasound in equine internal medicine. Vet Clin North Am [Equine Pract], *2*:253, 1986.
6. Reef VB, Boy MG, Reid CF, et al. Evaluation of horses and cattle with thoracic disease: Comparison between ultrasonography and radiography: 56 cases (1984–1985). J Am Vet Med Assoc, in press.
7. Rantanen NW, Ewing RL. Principles of ultrasound application in animals. Vet Radiol, *22*:196, 1981.
8. Park RD, Nyland TG, Lattimer JC, et al. B-Mode grayscale ultrasound: imaging artifacts and principles. Vet Radiol, *22*:204, 1981.
9. Powers RL. Ultrasound science for the veterinarian. Vet Clin North Am [Equine Pract], *2*:3, 1986.
10. Rantanen NW. General considerations for ultrasound examinations. Vet Clin North Am [Equine Pract], *2*:29, 1986.
11. Rantanen NW. Diseases of the heart. Vet Clin North Am [Equine Pract], *2*:33, 1986.
12. Farrow CS. Radiography of the equine thorax: Anatomy and technic. Vet Radiol, *22*:62, 1981.
13. Farrow CS. Equine thoracic radiology. J Am Vet Med Assoc, *179*:776, 1981.

## CHAPTER 7

# RADIOGRAPHIC EXAMINATION AND INTERPRETATION

*CHARLES S. FARROW*

In a medical discussion of the equine respiratory tract, it is possible to present the relevant material in a variety of ways, depending largely on the viewpoint of the writer. From a radiologic perspective, an anatomic approach appears most appropriate; however, no existing scheme is entirely suitable since most still retain human discriptors, e.g. upper and lower airways. I have therefore chosen to avoid the temptation of an anatomic subclassification for the pragmatic simplicity of a traditional nose to alveolus presentation. Since published radiologic observations on pulmonary diseases in the horse are still at a premium, I have relied heavily on my own experience, spanning the better part of the last 2 decades.

## Radiographic Methods, Protocols, and Techniques

It is axiomatic that the analysis and subsequent interpretation of any radiograph are potentially only as good as the completeness and quality of the obtained image. This is even more true of low contrast/low density regional anatomy as exemplified by the respiratory tract. The following comments describe common radiographic errors and how they may be avoided. Examination protocols and techniques follow at the end of each section.*

### *Nasal Cavity*

The combination of multiple air-filled chambers and extremely thin bones, dictates the use of less penetrating radiation when radiographing the nasal cavity. For the purpose of orientation it is best to image the entire head in lateral view, choosing a film size compatible with the size of the horse. A similar field size, but made in the dorsoventral position, is also useful. Limited field or spot views are best made once a specific abnormality is identified. Oblique views are of value in assessing dorsolateral lesions of the nasal bones and maxilla, especially when combined with a lead skin marker indicating the location of a related swelling, lump, depression, or draining sinus on the surface of the face.

***Views.*** Lateral, dorsoventral (if possible), right and left lateral 30° obliques.

***Technique.*** 70 kVp/12 mAs

### *Paranasal Cavity*

Unlike many lesions affecting the nasal cavity which lie in a relatively central position, a paranasal pathologic condition, especially in-

*Most radiographic images shown in this chapter were produced with a high output x ray generator (Picker GX 1500), a focused, linear-type grid with 8:1 ratio, 103 lines/in., and a rare earth imaging system consisting of DuPont, Quanta III intensifying screens and Cronex 7 x-ray film. Focal-film distance was 48 in.

volving the maxillary sinuses, is often eccentrically positioned so that it may be superimposed upon the normal opposite sinus when projected laterally. This problem may be partially overcome by obliquing the x-ray beam to profile the affected side away from the nonaffected side. Because of the variation in oblique views it is best to make a comparable view of the opposite side. This will greatly speed the process of deciding what is diseased and what is merely different (based on the reader's lack of familiarity with the particular view).

***Views.*** Right and left lateral 30° obliques (one of the affected side and one of the opposite side for comparison).

***Technique.*** 70 kVp/12 mAs

## Pharynx

Pharyngeal radiography is often marred by overexposure, resulting in poor structural definition. Use of a hot light alleviates the problem, but does not eliminate it. The use of soft tissue technique, as opposed to the more penetrating skull settings, typically provides the best definition of the pharyngeal soft tissues. The x-ray beam should be centered on the throat region (just rostral and slightly above the mandibular angle) to achieve a distortion-free anatomic perspective. Care should be taken to position the head naturally, avoiding extension or flexion which often distorts the pharynx, and may in this respect lead to a false diagnosis. A 14 × 17 in. film provides ample context in which to view related pathologic conditions.

***View.*** Lateral

***Technique.*** 80 kVp/12 mAs

## Guttural Pouches

The guttural pouches of the horse may be imaged in a manner similar to that previously described for the pharynx. As with the pharynx, it is critical to avoid extremes of head position which may mimic disease. Although lateral oblique views have been advocated by some as a means to establish lesion laterality, I have found such projections to be of little use. An extended ventrodorsal view is beneficial in differentiating unilateral from bilateral involvement, but requires general anesthesia in most cases.

***View.*** Lateral

***Technique.*** 80 kVp/12 mAs

## Larynx

The larynx is best viewed as a composite image along with the pharynx and guttural pouches, and is optimally assessed using a relatively light technique. It is important to keep the horse's head parallel to the cassette to avoid distortion of the soft palate and epiglottis. Like other structures in the throat, the appearance of the larynx may be altered by head position. Respiration may occasionally influence laryngeal size.

***View.*** Lateral

***Technique.*** 80 kVp/12 mAs

## Trachea

The cervical trachea requires at least two 14 × 17, or 7 × 17-inch films to be imaged completely in an adult horse. The exposures are made with the horse in the standing position, right side to the cassette. With the exception of proximal obstructive lesions, there is little difference in the relative appearance of inspiratory and expiratory radiographs. The intrathoracic trachea and the part of the trachea passing through the thoracic inlet may be imaged using thoracic techniques.

***View.*** Lateral (one proximal and one distal)

***Technique.*** 70 kVp/12 mAs

## Bronchi

The larger airways (principal, secondary, and tertiary bronchi) are outstanding in most thoracic radiographs, particularly over the heart base. When normal bronchi are viewed end-on, their walls may appear thickened. Tangentially oriented airways often appear asymmetric with abnormally opaque lumens. All of these normal variations are accentuated by a light technique.

*View.* Lateral thorax (dorsocaudal aspect of lung provides optimal survey)

*Technique.* 80 kVp/40 mAs

## *Lung*

The thorax of a young foal may be completely imaged using a single 14 × 17-in. x-ray film; larger foals require 2 or 3 films. By comparison, 4 films of this size are needed to completely visualize the thorax of an adult horse. A similar degree of difference exists in the radiographic techniques (kVp, mA, and exposure time) required to produce thoracic radiographs of a foal as compared to an adult horse.[1,2]

Generally, the lighter the exposure, the more dense the appearance of the lung. This is particularly true in large animals including the horse, in which normal background lung density is greater than in the dog, the species which is most often used in teaching thoracic radiology in veterinary colleges. Bearing in mind that the lateral thoracic projection in a horse portrays a meter or more of thoracic width in less than a millimeter of film thickness, it is no wonder that equine lung films are frequently misdiagnosed as having abnormal interstitial density.

*Views.* Newborn foal (single lateral); intermediate sized foals (2 to 3 overlapping laterals); adult horse (4 overlapping laterals).

*Techniques.* Adult horse: dorsocaudal field—80 kVp/40 mAs; dorsocranial field—95 kVp/40 mAs; dorsoventral field—80 kVp/50 mAs; cranioventral field—110 kVp/80 mAs. 400- to 500-lb foals: reduce exposure by 50%. Newborn foal: reduce exposure by 75%.

# Abnormal Radiographic Appearance

## *Radiographic Signs*

Radiographic signs are the abnormalities identified on one or more of the films in a particular radiographic examination. These signs, or radiographic indicators of disease, may be of a general nature, for example an increase or decrease in lung density, or alternatively may be relatively specific such as the characteristic airway dilation seen in bronchiectasis. Rarely are radiographic lesions etiospecific, although some by virtue of their physical attributes or distribution may by inference be related to a particular pathological process such as pneumonia, abscess, or tumor. Some radiographic signs such as air or fluid in the pleural space are more indirect in nature, serving primarily to direct the viewer's attention to those organs which may be associated with such findings. Sometimes it is what is not seen that constitutes the major radiographic observation—for example, an enlarged, fluid-filled guttural pouch resulting in a loss of its normal gas content. Other signs are employed in a more interpretive manner such as a cavitary lung lesion, or a displaced soft palate. Occasionally, radiographic abnormalities are described in terms of what they resemble such as "coin" lesions (typically medium-sized, spherically shaped localized opacities) in the lung. The meaning of such lesions, however, is variable, especially among different species of animals. For example: in the young horse "coin lesions" usually reflect abscess, often the result of Rhodococcus (Corynebacterium) pneumonia; while in the dog such lesions usually indicate metastasis or, less commonly, mycosis.

## *Nasal Cavity*

### Orofacial Deformity

Facial deformity accompanied by a corresponding change in the mandible is usually congenital. When comparable abnormalities are not found in the mandible, trauma in addition to congenital deformity should be considered. Irrespective of etiology, the effect of most such deformities is to impede air flow through the rostral part of the upper airways, often resulting in noisy breathing. In my experience, the most common deformity is a lateral deviation of the rostral soft tissues, accompanied by a similar deformity of the upper and lower jaws. Prognathism or brachygnathism may also be present (Fig. 7–1).

## Facial Deformity

Facial deformity, unassociated with a mandibular pathologic condition, may be congenital or traumatic, usually the former. Lateral deviation of the premaxilla typically produces dental malocclusion, mandibular overbite, and septal displacement. Obstruction of the rostral air passages is common.[3]

## Septal Deviation

Deviation of the nasal septum unassociated with orofacial deformity is commonly caused by a contiguous mass, prior trauma, or embryologic error (Fig. 7–2). As with other forms of upper airway obstruction, this condition is characterized by abnormal breathing sounds. A dorsoventral view is required for detection; a lateral view is noncontributory. Symmetric positioning is mandatory, usually requiring tranquilization, sedation, or general anesthesia. Congenital septal deviation may occasionally be seen associated with other anomalies such as cleft soft palate and epiglottic hypoplasia/entrapment.[4]

## Hemorrhage

Free nasal hemorrhage is difficult to identify radiographically, even in large volume. Nasal bleeding often does no more than cause a subtle increase in background nasal cavity density which is difficult to differentiate from normal variation in radiographic technique. Alternatively, contained or trapped hemorrhage, for example an ethmoid hematoma, may be inferred on the basis of increased density in the ethmoturbinate or a mass effect. Hemorrhage per se cannot be differentiated from other fluids.

## Fracture

Facial fractures in the horse may occur following blunt trauma; for example being kicked by another horse, running into a post, striking the inside of a horse trailer during an accident, or being hit by a twitch handle. Fractures of the face may show soft tissue swelling, displacement, and sinus hemorrhage.[5]

Displaced facial fractures lying in the plane of the x-ray beam and disrupting the contour of the nasal bones are best seen in lateral view. Fractures which are at less favorable angles to the x-ray beam, undisplaced, and do not disrupt the nasal margin, are much harder to detect. When fracture fragments are displaced inwardly, the term depression fracture is used.[6] Such injuries often obstruct the dorsal nasal passages, both mechanically and secondary to hemorrhage. Resulting obstruction may be temporary or permanent depending

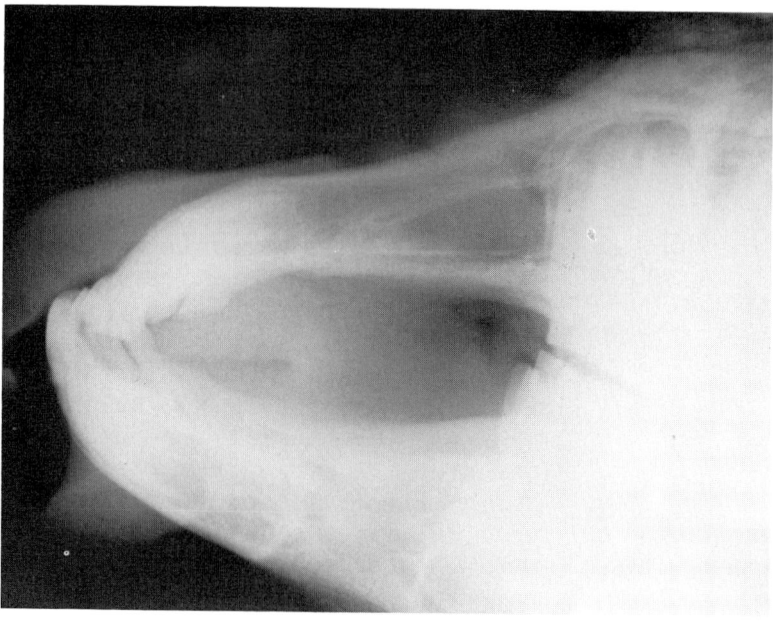

**FIG. 7–1.** Orofacial deformity. Lateral view of rostral aspect of the face shows mandibular prognathism. The apparent obliquity of the incisors is the result of lateral deviation of the associated jaws causing obstruction of the related airways.

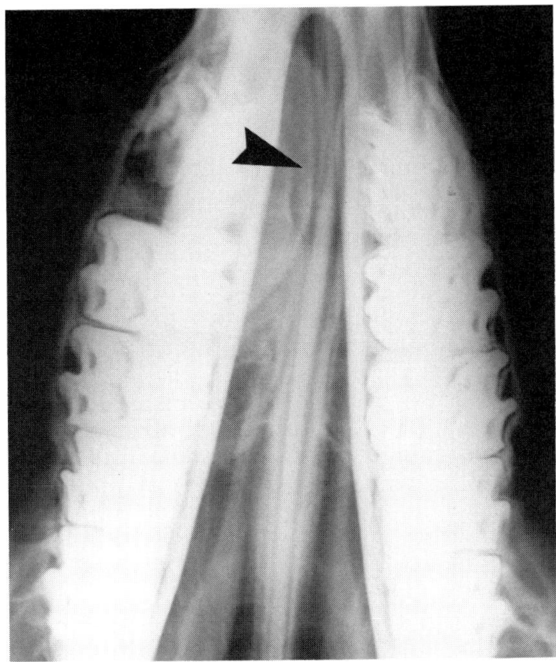

FIG. 7–2. Dental abscess. Ventrodorsal view of face shows rostrally located mass occluding the right side of the nasal cavity and displacing the nasal septum to the left (arrow). An infected tooth was removed previously.

on the extent of the original injury, the method of repair (if any), and the manner of healing. Complications associated with facial fracture include: delayed union, nonunion, osteomyelitis, sequestration, oronasal fistula, and draining sinus formation.

## Gunshot

Facial gunshot wounds may cause external and internal fractures, dental injury, nasal and paranasal bleeding, injury to the nasolacrimal duct, nerve damage, and infection.[7] Determining the probable course of the bullet from its entrance/exit holes and radiographically visible fragments is useful in assessing related soft tissue injury which is otherwise unapparent.

## Infection

Nasal cavity infection is typically diagnosed by clinical, not radiologic means due to the nonspecificity of most infections. As with nasal hemorrhage, much free mucus and pus may go undetected. Structural alteration to the turbinates must be extensive before becoming visible. Alterations in tissue density are difficult to differentiate from variations in radiographic technique.

## Mass Lesions

***Abscess.*** Most medium to large abscesses located in the rostral two thirds of the nasal cavity are readily detectable; small abscesses and larger masses in the caudal third are more difficult to see. Primary or secondary infection of the adjacent paranasal sinuses is often difficult to establish without a ventrodorsal view.

***Granuloma.*** Granulomatous masses may arise within the nasal cavity as a result of fungal infection, particularly Coccidioides spp. These lesions are most often seen as large, spherical masses in the caudal aspect of the nasal cavity.[8]

***Neoplasia.*** Tumors of the nasal cavity are rare; when present they may take the form of isolated mass lesions, or alternatively, appear as relatively vague changes in form or density. Foals, juveniles, and adults may be affected.[9,10] A congenital ethmoid carcinoma has been reported.[11] Tumor-like lesions such as cysts are more common, frequently displacing the nasal septum and contralateral concha and causing obstruction. As with nasal cavity abscesses, a ventrodorsal view is invaluable in assessing the full extent of the injury.

***Neoplastic-like Lesions.*** Intranasal cysts tend to occur in younger horses and are generally believed to be congenital. Some consider such masses a form of benign tumor. These lesions usually appear as large, spherical, discretely walled, fluid-filled masses within the nasal cavity or paranasal sinuses (Fig. 7–3). Facial deformity, septal and/or turbinate deviation, and nasal discharge may result.[12]

***Hematoma.*** Progressive ethmoid hematoma is a slowly enlarging mass originating in an ethmoturbinate bone. Extension into adjacent tissues and spaces is common; distortion and destruction may result. Typically, the lesion appears as a spherical or oval soft tissue mass in the caudal aspect of the nasal cavity as viewed laterally. The normal ethmoid shadow may be hidden or altered accordingly (Fig. 7–4).[4]

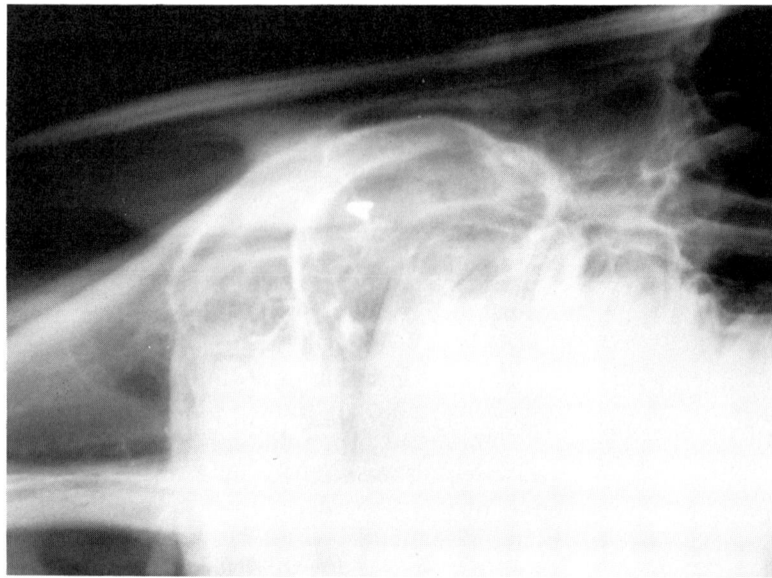

FIG. 7–3. Nasal cyst. Lateral view of central part of the nasal cavity shows a large, discretely walled, compartmentalized mass (arrow). Centrally located lead skin marker (A) indicates point of maximal facial swelling.

*Miscellaneous.* Nasal polyps occur in young horses, appearing as one or more variably sized, soft tissue masses within the nasal cavity.[8] As with other nasal cavity masses, polyps obstruct air flow through the involved part of the nasal passages. The cause of most polyps is unknown, although chronic inflammation is suspected.[13,14]

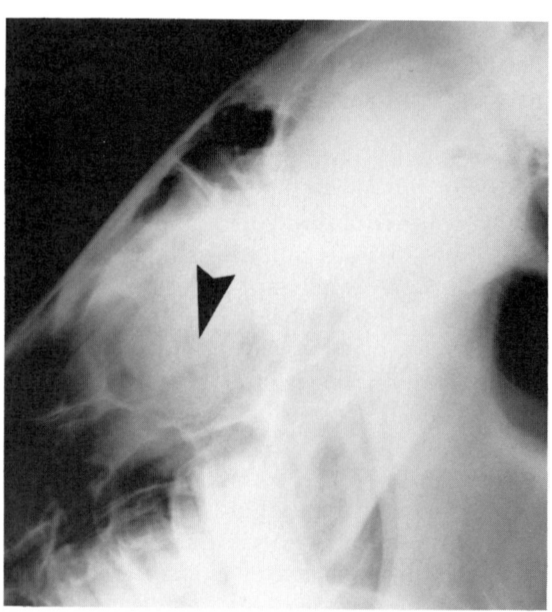

FIG. 7–4. Progressive ethmoid hematoma. Lateral view of the caudal aspect of the nasal cavity shows an ill-defined opacity partially obscuring the ethmoid turbinate bone and adjacent frontal sinus (arrow).

Inspissated pus secondary to chronic sinusitis may be radiographically identified in the ventral conchal sinus above the third to fifth maxillary cheek teeth.[15]

## *Paranasal Sinuses*

### Fluid Line

The presence of a fluid line within a facial sinus is one of the radiographic hallmarks of paranasal sinus disease. Showing as sharply demarcated regions of high contrast (black on top, white on the bottom), fluid lines lie typically in the sagittal plane of the skull within the fields of the paranasal sinuses. Produced by a combination of fluid and air juxtaposed within a confined space, the radiographic appearance of fluid lines is highly labile, often changing greatly or even disappearing with different head positions and beam angles. For this reason it is important to use comparable head positions when reevaluating fluid lines in progressive radiographs. The most common causes of fluid lines are trauma and infection. Chronic sinus obstruction may also produce a fluid line by preventing drainage of naturally produced secretions.

### Trauma

Paranasal fractures often produce sinus hemorrhage. Large volume bleeding may result in complete sinus opacification, while smaller hemorrhages are more apt to generate fluid lines. Persistence of a fluid line beyond a few days following facial injury is unusual, as most hemorrhages are absorbed or drain into the adjacent nasal passages. Recurrence of a traumatically-induced fluid line following earlier resolution may indicate a secondary infection, especially in the context of a related compound fracture of the involved sinus.

## Infection

Sinus infections can be primary or secondary, with the latter usually resulting from an adjacent dental infection. Extension of a dental infection, particularly of the fourth maxillary cheek tooth, into the associated paranasal sinus may cause empyema.[4] Penetrating wounds, especially by nails, often result in a similar outcome. Nasal cavity infection may extend into the paranasal sinuses; and conversely, a sinus infection may infect the nasal cavity. Theoretically, sinus obstruction may also lead to secondary infection by creating an environment conducive to bacterial growth. Radiographically, paranasal sinus infection is most often characterized by varying degrees of sinus opacification or a fluid line.[16] Expansion of the involved sinus cavity is common in chronic cases (Fig. 7–5). Longstanding sinus infections may eventually breach the bone and drain through a surface sinus.

## Cyst

Radiographically, cysts of the paranasal sinuses most often result in generalized opacification. Chronic sinus infection may be characterized by thickening of the sinus wall and expansion of the sinus cavity. Inward growth of the cyst can lead to opacification of the adjacent half of the nasal cavity, and deviation of the nasal septum to the contralateral side.[17]

## Neoplasia

Sinus tumors are uncommon. A recent review of equine facial disorders indicated that neoplasms were twice as likely to develop in the paranasal sinuses compared with the nasal cavity.[9] Of 16 tumors identified, one-half were malignant; carcinomas predominated. A second report on equine facial disease showed facial tumors in the horse to be even less frequent.[10]

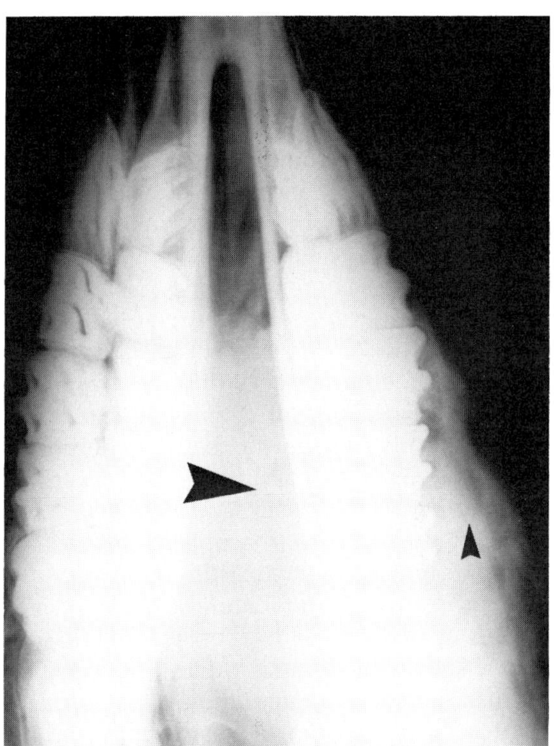

**FIG. 7–5.** Paranasal sinus abscess. Ventrodorsal view of nasal cavity shows a large centrally located mass obliterating the nasal passages on the left (large arrow), expanding and opacifying the associated maxillary sinus (small arrow) and displacing the adjacent nasal septum.

Radiographically, paranasal sinus tumors may show one or more of the following features: sinus opacity, fluid line, expansion and/or destruction of the sinus wall. Extension of the tumor to the nasal cavity may produce secondary septal deviation as well as conchal deformity or destruction, depending on the nature of the tumor.[8,9]

# *Pharynx*

The pharynx, as viewed in a lateral radiographic projection, consists of a large, roughly rectangular, air-filled chamber that is subdivided into three regions: the nasopharynx, which constitutes the major part of the cavity; the laryngopharynx (the area immediately dorsal to the arytenoepiglottic folds), and the oropharynx (the area ventral to the caudal aspect of the soft palate, which is typically not visualized radiographically because of insufficient contrast).

Dorsally, the pharynx is bounded by the paired guttural pouches, readily identifiable by their large gas content. The larynx forms the caudal pharyngeal margin as well as a portion of the ventral border. The soft palate completes the remainder of the ventral pharynx. The rostral aspect of the pharynx is radiographically nonspecific, being a composite image of multiple contiguous and overlapping structures or cavities.

Roentgen signs of pharyngeal disease include decreased gas content, alterations in size or contour, and changes in the size, shape, or position of the soft palate. Reduction in pharyngeal gas content is usually of an extrinsic nature, stemming from disease-induced enlargement of surrounding structures, such as the guttural pouches and retropharyngeal lymph nodes. These lymph nodes often produce a distinctive convexity in the caudoventral margin of one or both guttural pouches.[18]

Normal pharyngeal/laryngeal dimensions have been determined radiographically against which questionable cases may be compared.[19]

## Congenital Malformation

Hypoplasia of the soft palate may produce upper airway obstruction and interfere with laryngeal closure during swallowing; the latter in turn may lead to inhalation pneumonia.[18,20] Congenital pharyngeal cysts may do likewise.

## Obstruction

***Intrinsic.*** Intrinsic pharyngeal obstruction may be caused by acute or chronic inflammation. Necrotizing pharyngitis and follicular pharyngitis may both substantially reduce the size of the laryngeal field as evaluated in a lateral radiograph. Depending on location within the pharyngeal cavity, a pharyngeal cyst, abscess, granuloma, tumor, or localized adenopathy may obstruct the upper airway.

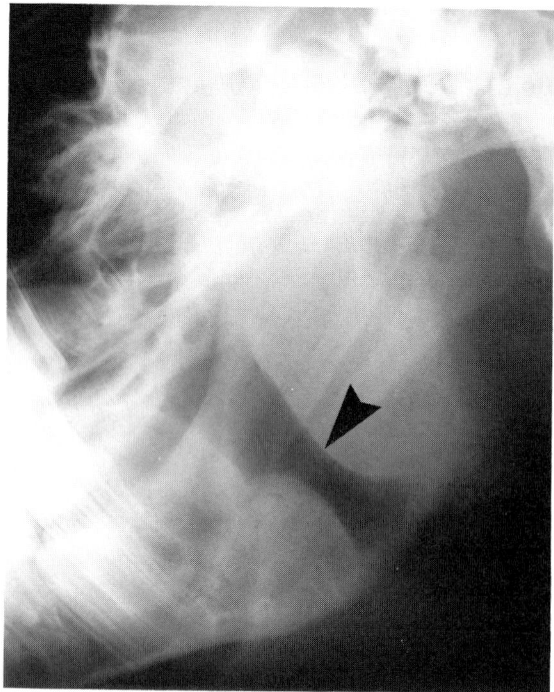

**FIG. 7–6.** External pharyngeal compression. Lateral view of pharynx shows marked dorsal pharyngeal compression (arrow) secondary to guttural pouch abscess and regional adenopathy.

***Extrinsic.*** Guttural pouch empyema, tympany, and retropharyngeal lymph node abscess are the most common sources of pharyngeal compression (Fig. 7–6).[21]

## Trauma

Pharyngeal injury may be the result of internal or external trauma, usually of the penetrating variety, with the former occasionally being iatrogenic.

## Dorsal Displacement of the Soft Palate

Dorsal displacement of the soft palate may be associated with organic or functional disorders of the larynx or pharynx. Occasionally, normal horses may have dorsal palatal displacement; however, this is usually an intermittent finding. When present radiographically, dorsal displacement should be considered abnormal until proven otherwise. Possible laryngeal etiologies include epiglottic hypoplasia, persistent epiglottic frenulum, epiglottic cicatrix, and epiglottic entrapment by diseased or malformed arytenoepiglottic folds. Pharyngeal causes of dorsal palatal displacement may include palatal hypoplasia, palatal myositis, ninth and tenth cranial nerve deficits, and pharyngitis, and secondary causes include disorders of the guttural pouches and parapharyngeal structures.[17] Persistent dorsal displacement of the soft palate may also be associated with epiglottic shortening or other types of laryngeal pathology (Fig. 7–7).[22,23]

## Guttural Pouches

The guttural pouches—large, thin-walled, air-filled extensions of the pharynx—are radiographically outstanding. Unfortunately, their superimposition and close relative proximity afford minimal opportunity for radiographic separation in all but the ventrodorsal view. This view, optimally obtained with the head fully extended, requires the use of general anesthesia. Accordingly, in many centers and in most practices, assessment is usually based on a lateral projection only.

The roentgen signs of guttural pouch disease include increased air content, decreased air content, a fluid level, deformity, intraluminal mass, extraluminal gas or fluid level, and pharyngeal compression and laryngotracheal displacement.[17]

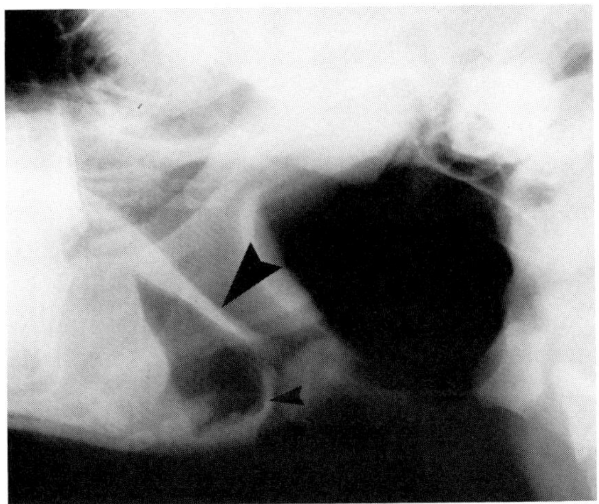

**FIG. 7–7.** Displaced soft palate. Lateral view of pharynx shows proximally displaced soft palate (large arrow), and hypoplastic epiglottis (small arrow).

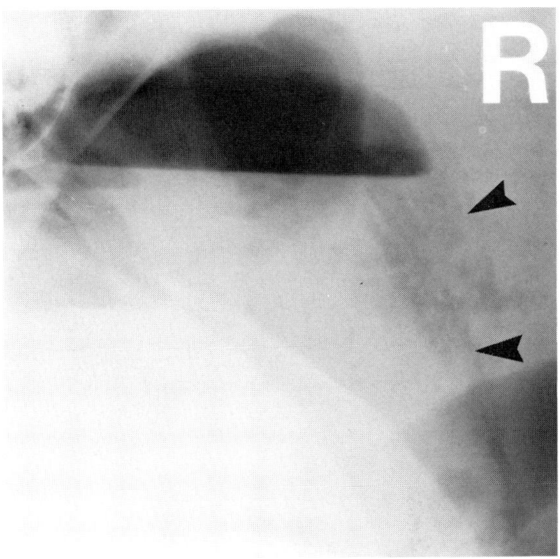


**FIG. 7–8.** Guttural pouch empyema. Lateral view of guttural pouches shows large fluid line proximally, with adjacent mixed gas/fluid accumulations (arrows).

### Congenital Malformation

Presumably due to dysplasia of its pharyngeal communication, the guttural pouch may become distended with air, often bilaterally. This condition is termed tympany, and is most common in foals and young horses. The degree of associated swelling is often so great that it compresses the pharynx and displaces the larynx and proximal trachea ventrally. This relocation may severely retard breathing.[17]

### Infection

Guttural pouch infections may assume a wide variety of radiographic appearances. These range from little or no detectable change in early or internally draining infections to total opacification or a distinct fluid line in advanced disease (Fig. 7–8). Infections may erode the wall of the affected pouch and drain to the regional soft tissues, producing swelling, extraluminal gas, and abscess.[17] Tympany may occur due to inflammation of the mucosal flap of the nasopharyngeal orifice which then acts as a one-way valve potentially trapping gas and secretions. Infections also occasionally may lead to the formation of a fistula between the affected guttural

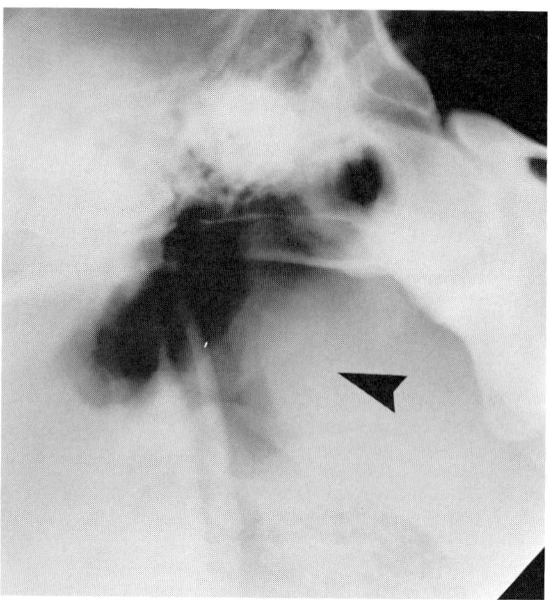

FIG. 7–9. Retropharyngeal adenopathy. Lateral view of guttural pouches shows severe compression of their caudoventral aspects secondary to contiguous abscessation (arrow).

pouch and adjacent pharynx.[24] Rarely guttural pouch infections may produce concurrent facial and vestibulocochlear disease. Contiguous infection or adenopathy frequently compresses the pouches (Fig. 7–9).

## Hemorrhage

Guttural pouch bleeding is most often the result of head trauma or mycotic infections which erode the wall of the internal carotid artery. Hemorrhage may also occur following a necrotizing bacterial infection, foreign body penetration, gunshot, and facial injury. Radiographically, guttural pouch hemorrhage is typified by varying degrees of opacification or a fluid line. Blood clots in the form of intraluminal masses may occasionally be identified provided there is sufficient background contrast.[18]

# *Larynx*

In terms of what may be specifically identified in a radiographic image, the larynx consists of the epiglottis, aryepiglottic folds, corniculate process of the arytenoid cartilage, lateral ventricles, and body of the larynx. Architectural or spatial alterations to these structures constitute the basis for the roentgen signs of laryngeal disease.

These signs include abnormal epiglottic position relative to the soft palate; epiglottic thickening, distortion, or marginal irregularity; decreased epiglottic size (includes length if measurable); displaced, deformed, indistinct arytenoepiglottic folds or corniculate processes; and laryngeal mineralization.*

Normal pharyngeal/laryngeal dimensions have been determined radiographically against which questionable examinations may be compared.[19]

## Congenital Malformation

Epiglottic hypoplasia or shortening may be a solitary anomaly or combined with other laryngeal or pharyngeal malformations. Structural epiglottic abnormalities often result in epiglottic as well as palatal dysfunction. Epiglottic cysts may have a similar affect. A single case of laryngeal web has been reported as a source of mild respiratory distress in a 10-day-old foal.[25]

## Cysts

Laryngeal cysts, at least those detected radiologically, most commonly involve the ventral aspect of the epiglottis. Such cysts may be either congenital or acquired subsequent to inflammation and blockage of related mucus glands.

## Infection

Unless pharyngeal volume is reduced or the shape of the pharyngeal cavity altered, for example secondary to swelling, granulation, necrosis or scarring, pharyngitis, epiglottitis and laryngitis are likely to be radiographically undetectable. The aftermath of some of these conditions, however, such as an epiglottic abscess, cyst or granuloma, may be identified at a later time. Chronic chondritis, naturally occurring or following laryngeal surgery, may cause visible laryngeal de-

*It should be noted that mineralization of the equine larynx may occur naturally and be unrelated to a past or present pathologic condition.

formity, and may produce calcification in one or more of the laryngeal cartilages.[26] Perilaryngeal abscessation may develop subsequent to pharyngeal infection.[27]

### Neoplasia

Laryngeal neoplasia is rare, at least in regard to its radiographic recognition. Lesions affecting the epiglottis usually develop ventrally, resulting in both deformity and dorsal displacement.

### Trauma

Laryngeal trauma is occasionally seen in horses, usually following a deep laceration or penetrating wound. In addition to whatever structural damage may occur, deep and superficial emphysema often develop, typically from laryngeal air leakage. The escaping air may migrate along the deep fascial planes of the neck into the mediastinum, producing a pneumomediastinum, or conversely can extend proximally to the head region.

## *Trachea*

The normal equine cervical trachea may be imaged sufficiently to detect the following structures: the caudal aspect of the larynx, the tracheal lumen, the inner tracheal surface (mucosa), the tracheal rings, and the annular ligaments (by inference the space between tracheal rings). The absence or alteration of these normally visible shadows forms the basis for a diagnosis of tracheal disease.

The caliber of the equine trachea normally changes little with differences in lung inflation, although it may change slightly. However, with dyspnea the tracheal lumen may enlarge considerably, returning to normal once breathing again becomes normal. Localized tracheal narrowing is usually the result of trauma or infection, and occasionally tumor. Regional reduction in the tracheal lumen may be an illusion stemming from the superimposition of an adjacent organ or mass. Rarely, a peritracheal mass may produce compression. A contiguous mass, for example a retropharyngeal abscess, or alternatively, a mass affect such as a dilated esophagus, may cause tracheal displacement and various degrees of compression.

Roentgen signs of tracheal disease include extraluminal gas (usually linear but sometimes focal), mediastinal gas (secondary to tracheal leakage), decreased definition or absence of normally visible tracheal soft tissues; luminal alteration; and deformity, deviation, or displacement. The cervical trachea is an uncommon site of a primary, radiographically discernable pathologic condition. More frequent are the mass related, secondary effects caused by contiguous structures such as the guttural pouch and esophagus; these effects are primarily dislocating, but may also produce localized or regional compression.

### Congenital Malformation

Congenital malformations of the equine trachea are rare. In the scabbard anomaly the trachea is compressed laterally, producing a reduction in cross-sectional area and a commensurate decrease in air flow.[28] Tracheal hypoplasia is usually associated with a uniform reduction in tracheal caliber, often substantially less than the vertical diameter of the larynx. I have not encountered tracheal collapse in the horse or foal.

### Trauma

Blunt neck injury may cause tracheal fracture or avulsion at the laryngotracheal junction, while penetrating wounds may lacerate or puncture the tracheal wall. In any case, extraluminal gas is the best radiographic indicator of such injury. Escaped tracheal gas, assuming more than a small volume transient loss, typically migrates distally, ultimately producing a pneumomediastinum, and with larger volumes, subcutaneous emphysema.[18,29]

### Infection

Tracheitis, even when associated with a large volume of exudate, is difficult and in most cases impossible to recognize radiographically.[18]

### Neoplasia

Tumors of the equine trachea are rare. When present, they typically originate from the tracheal wall and grow inwardly, thereby reducing air flow secondary to a reduction in luminal, cross sectional area (Fig. 7–10).

### Iatrogenic

The trachea may be injured by the injudicious use of an endotracheal tube or the inadvertent introduction of substances intended for the stomach. Diagnostic transtracheal aspiration often produces deep cervical and mediastinal emphysema (Fig. 7–11),[30] which is rarely of clinical importance.

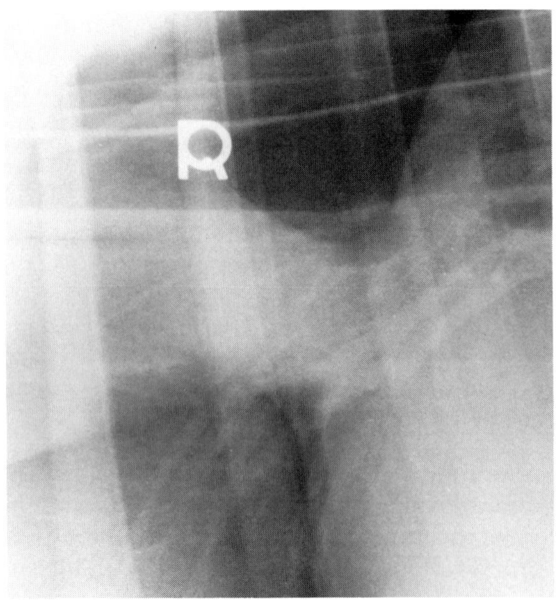

**FIG. 7–11.** Pneumomediastinum. Lateral view of midcranial part of thorax shows mediastinal air outlining the trachea 1 hour after a tracheal wash.

## *Conducting Airways*

The conducting airways in the horse include the principal bronchi, subsidiary bronchi, and proximal and terminal bronchioles. Respiratory bronchioles are rare and poorly developed in this species. Conducting airway disease may involve the endobronchial, bronchial, or peribronchial tissues, as well as any combination of these tissues. In the horse, it is not possible to distinguish between these levels of involvement radiographically.

Often the roentgen signs of airway disease are absent or barely detectable.[1] When present, the major radiographic indicators of conducting airway disease are increased bronchial visibility, size, and number; the former often described as line or ring shadows depending on whether the affected airways are viewed laterally or end-on. Dilated airways may result from functional or mechanical obstruction (chronic obstructive lung disease), structural weakening (bronchiectasis), or normal compensatory mechanisms (increased ventilatory demand). The number of identifiable, medium-sized airways is primarily a function of bronchial size. As the bronchial tree becomes better inflated, smaller airways, normally invisible, become radiographically detectable by virtue of their increased diameter. Smaller airways may also become pathologically enlarged, similarly resulting in improved detectability.[32] It has not been established if older horses develop increased bronchial density as a result of advancing age, although some speculate that this occurs.

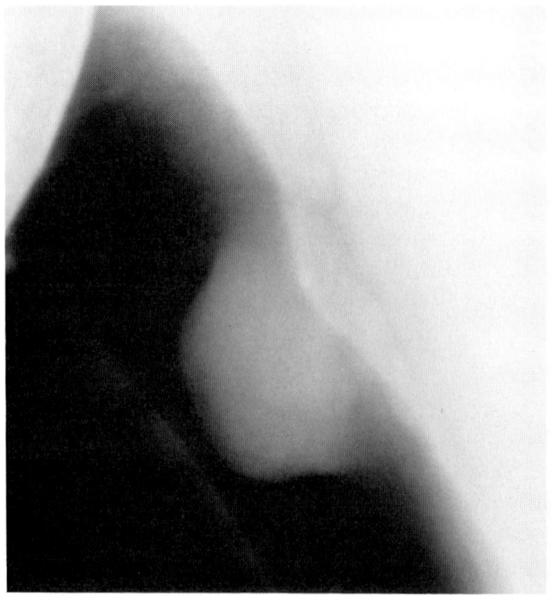

**FIG. 7–10.** Tracheal tumor. Lateral, close-up view of the proximal trachea shows a large, broadly based luminal mass.

### Bronchitis

Bronchitis is typically associated with a normal radiograph.[31] The belief held by many veterinarians that bronchitis can be radiographically diagnosed with confidence is false.[32] Thin horses, because of reduced perithoracic soft tissues, allow better radiographic visualization of the conducting airways. This improved bronchial clarity may be mistaken for bronchitis.

### Chronic Bronchitis

Only the most severe and long-standing cases of bronchitis may be expected to show radiographic signs such as ring and line shadows representing end-on and profile views of large and medium sized bronchi respectively (Fig. 7–12).[4]

### Bronchiolitis

Bronchiolitis cannot be recognized radiographically as a primary condition of middle or distal airways. When bronchiolitis does result in a radiographic abnormality, it is most apt to take the form of a nonspecific interstitial pattern, often without accompanying ring or line shadows.[4] A slight, generalized dilation of the bronchial tree may be present.

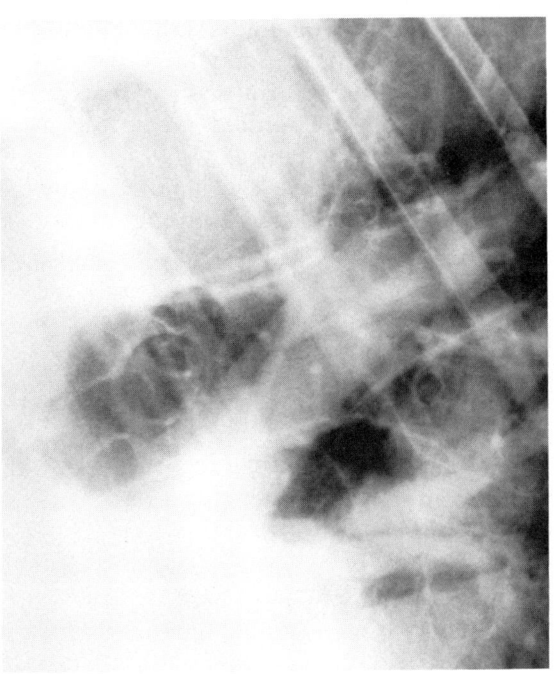

**FIG. 7–12.** Severe, chronic bronchitis. Lateral, close-up view of central thorax shows numerous line and ring shadows representing thickened bronchial walls.

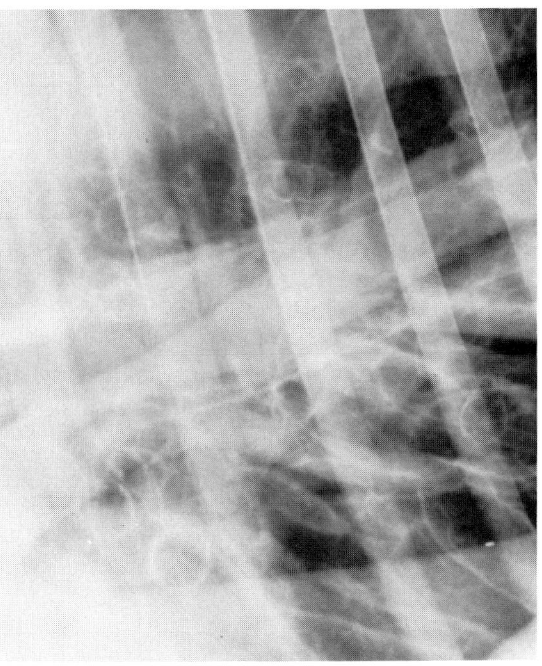

**FIG. 7–13.** Bronchiectasis. Lateral, close up view of central thorax shows thickened, cylindrically dilated bronchial walls.

### Bronchiectasis

Bronchiectasis is an irreversible dilation of the pulmonary airways, in horses believed to stem from chronic obstructive lung disease. Based on the radiographic appearance of the affected airways, bronchiectasis has been classified into three types: cylindrical, varicose, and saccular—the first being the most common in the horse (Fig. 7–13). Conducting airways may become temporarily dilated secondary to local, regional, or diffuse luminal obstruction or upper airway obstruction, and to compensate for anemia, blood loss, or shock.[31]

## *Pulmonary Vasculature*

Radiographically identifiable vascular disease in adult horses is limited to an evaluation of individual size and the overall number of vessels. In foals in which a ventrodorsal view may be made, it is possible to compare the right pulmonary vasculature to the left, possibly then inferring a thrombus in the absence of a vessel present in one half of the lung but not the other. Generally though, the pulmonary vasculature of the horse is assessed for size and number. In suspected congenital heart disease, the appearance of the pulmonary vessels may establish the presence of an intracardiac shunt. For example, an atrial or ventricular septal defect would typically shunt blood from the left to the right side of the heart, thereby increasing the size and number of visible lung vessels (Fig. 7–14). Conversely, a tetralogy of Fallot would result in a right to left shunt, in turn decreasing the size and number of pulmonary vessels.[33]

The vascular bed of the equine lung also enlarges with most types of inflammatory lung disease, depending in large part on the degree of associated inflammation. This increase in blood supply may be termed pulmonary hyperemia.

## Lung

Before describing the radiographic pathologic condition of the equine lung, it is necessary to mention pattern recognition technique, a diagnostic scheme developed and refined by physician radiologists for the purpose of diagnosing the nature and causes of diffuse human lung disease. This method was later adopted by Suter and applied with some modifications to the dog and cat. Largely based on these earlier efforts, a similar approach has been used in the horse. The pattern approach to diffuse lung disease is as follows. Abnormal lung densities are relegated to one of four subanatomic components of the lung: the interstitium, alveoli, bronchi or vasculature.

The interstitial pattern is typically characterized by a mild overall increase in lung density causing the pulmonary vasculature to appear indistinct or blurred. This loss of vascular detail results from a reduction in contrast between the pulmonary vessels and the surrounding lung secondary to interstitial fluid or cellular accumulations. Interstitial patterns may be further described as structured or nonstructured, depending on whether or not the abnormal interstitial density is composed of discrete, repetitive shadows, for example small nodules or lines.

The alveolar pattern (also termed air space pattern or terminal air space pattern) is best illustrated by a moderate to marked increase in lung density and the presence of air bronchograms—branching black bands representing air-filled bronchi or bronchioles surrounding by consolidated lung.

Since much of what may ultimately accumulate in the alveoli originates in the pulmonary vasculature, and must first traverse the interstitium, it is understandable that abnormal lung densities may be found in both the interstitium and alveoli concurrently. Such patterns are termed mixed, acknowledging their dual nature.

The bronchiolar pattern is indicated by line and ring shadows representing end-on or profile views of thickened bronchial walls. Al-

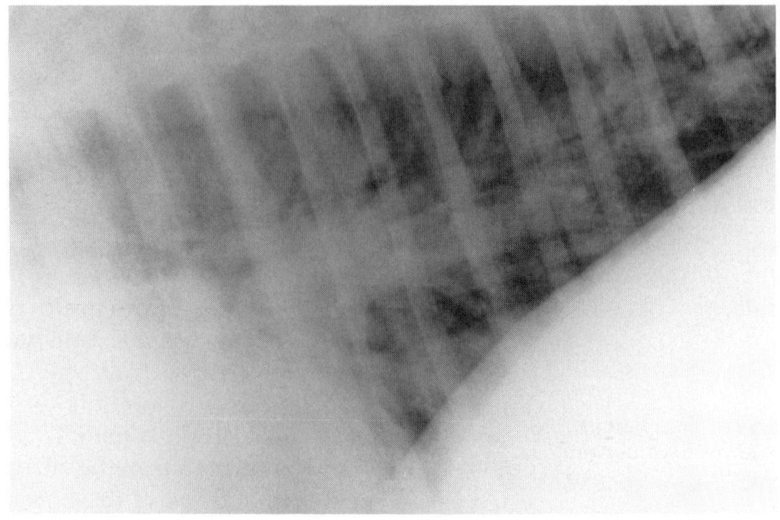

**FIG. 7–14.** Ventricular septal defect. Lateral view of foal's thorax shows generalized cardiomegaly with pulmonary overcirculation.

ternatively, line and ring densities may be produced by peribronchial disease, with or without associated bronchial involvement. Bronchial dilation may also indicate an airway disorder, although it must be clearly established that the observed dilation is not merely a transitory finding associated with increased ventilatory effort.

The vascular pattern is best demonstrated by alterations in the individual size, and number of pulmonary blood vessels. From such findings one may infer abnormalities in the cardiovascular or pulmonary systems (Fig. 7–15). When more than one area is involved, that which is most affected is chosen. If two areas are equally affected, terms are combined, or the more general term mixed is used, for example, interstitial pattern, bronchovascular pattern, mixed pattern. Knowing which structural part of the lung is involved, one may devise a list of differential diagnoses which are typified by such a lesion pattern. It is claimed by proponents of this technique that it is superior to the more traditional etiologic approach in which one must rely on having seen or read of the disease previously as well as being able to recall its radiographic particulars. In my view both methods have

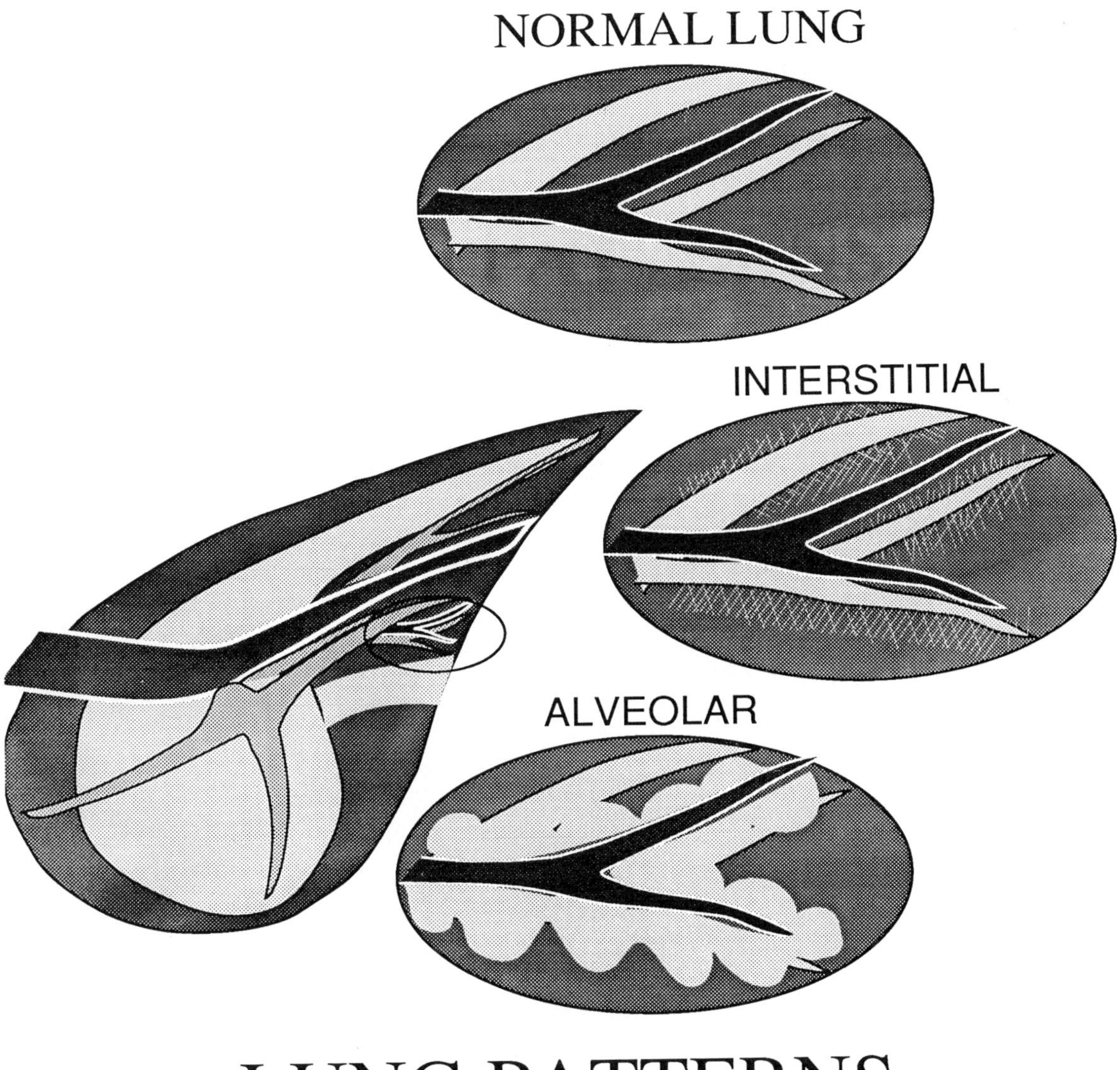


**FIG. 7–15.** Patterns of lung disease. See text for explanation.

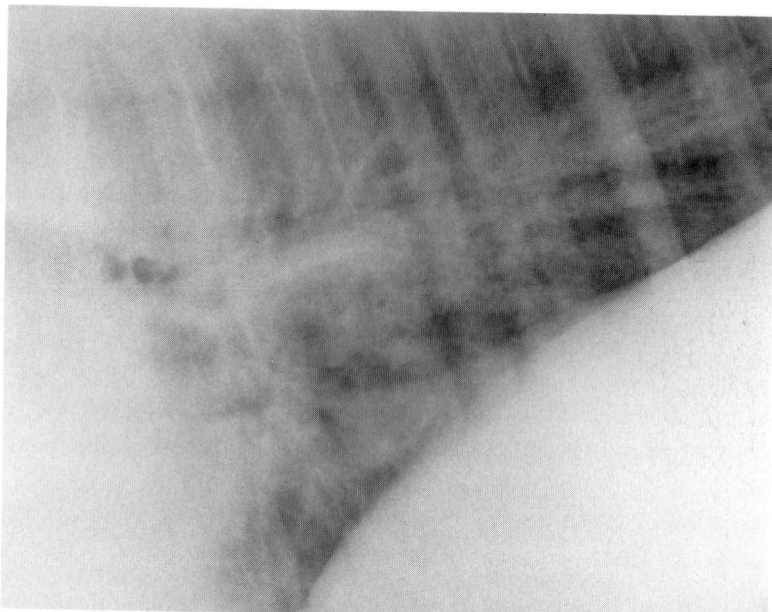

**FIG. 7–16.** Pneumonia. Lateral view of caudodorsal lung shows increased background lung density which reduces vascular contrast, and therefore detail.

virtue: an etiologic approach for commonly encountered entities such as bacterial pneumonia, pleuritis and abscess, and pattern recognition for atypical or unfamiliar conditions patterns such as fungal pneumonia, heart disease, or neoplasia.

## Pneumonia

***Bacterial.*** Bacterial pneumonia in the horse is highly variable, ranging in radiographic appearance from a barely detectable increase in background lung density to overt consolidation (Figs. 7–16 to 7–19); most, but not all pneumonias are unstructured (lack a repetitive lesion pattern), and few are etiologically specific. In cases of suspected bacterial pneumonia, when structured lung patterns are present, fungal pneumonia, diffuse abscesses, and metastasis also require diagnostic consideration (Fig. 7–20). Distribution may be localized, regional or diffuse, unilateral or bilateral.[30–32] Many bacterial pneumonias are first seen in the central lung field partially superimposed over the caudal part of the heart as patchy consolidation (Figs. 7–21 and

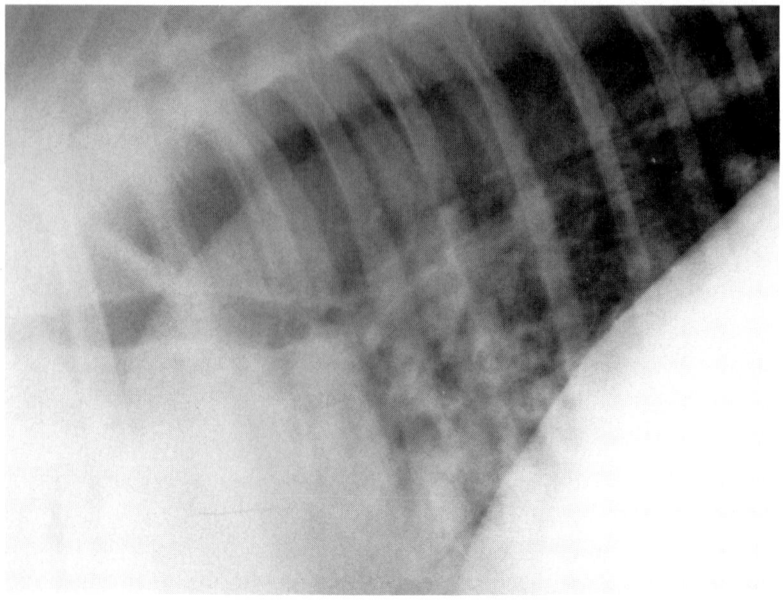

**FIG. 7–17.** Pneumonia. Lateral view of thorax shows patchy lung consolidation obscuring the dorsocaudal aspect of the heart.

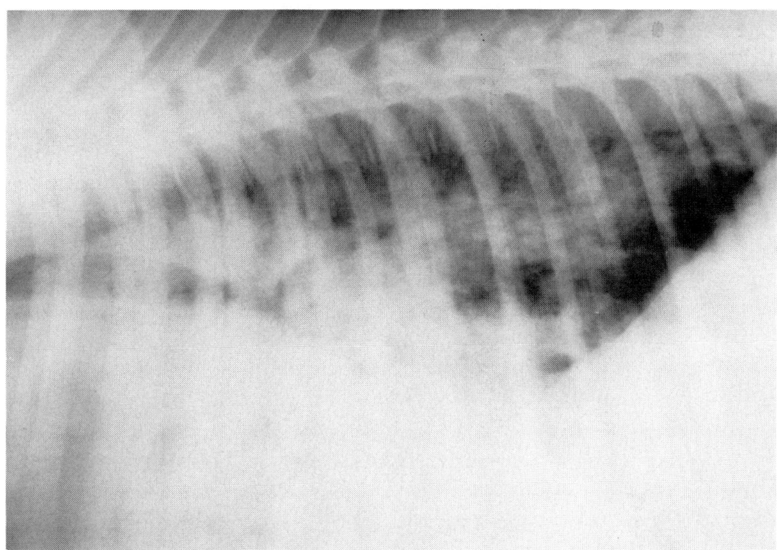

**FIG. 7–18.** Pneumonia. Lateral view of thorax shows near total consolidation of the ventral two thirds of the lung.

7–22).[34] Solid or cavitated lung abscesses may result.[35] Extension to the pleural space may occur, producing a pleuropneumonia. Dyspnea resulting from pneumonia rarely produces hyperinflation, but may result in esophageal air accumulation which must not be mistaken for a gas-capped abscess (Fig. 7–23). Immunodeficient (CID) Arabian foals frequently develop pneumonia (Fig. 7–24).

***Fungal.*** Fungal (mycotic) pneumonias, more than other diffuse lung diseases in the horse, typically produce structured lung patterns, usually discrete nodules or circular masses. Most occur in the warmer southwestern part of the United States. Aspergillosis superinfections have been described, occasionally associated with a mycetoma.[4]

***Viral.*** Viral pneumonias, equine herpesvirus for example, often do not produce a sufficiently large increase in lung density to be reliably or consistently detected on a radiograph. Usually it is not until a concurrent or secondary bacterial pneumonia has developed that the radiograph becomes convincingly abnormal.[31]

***Inhalation.*** The inhalation of liquid or particulate matter into the tracheobronchial tree is termed aspiration pneumonia. There are

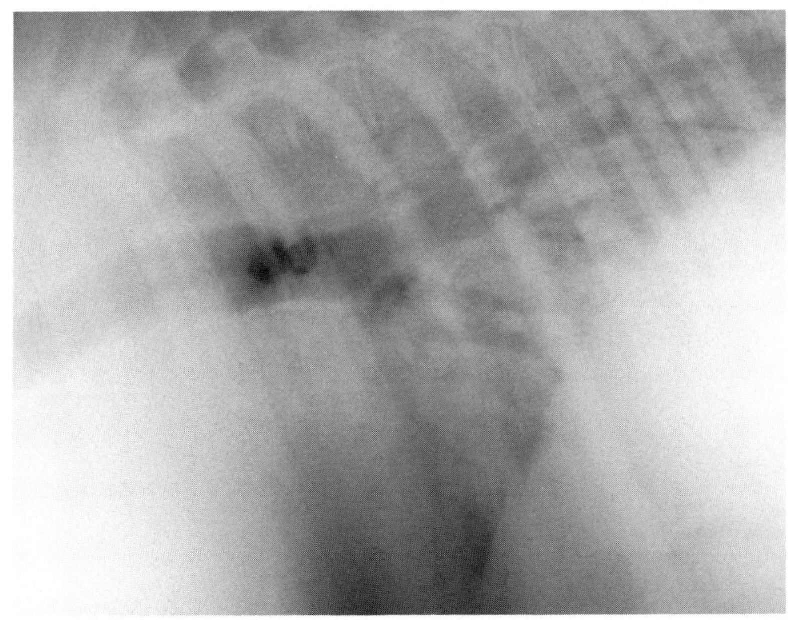

**FIG. 7–19.** Pneumonia. Lateral view of thorax shows consolidation of the majority of the lung field.

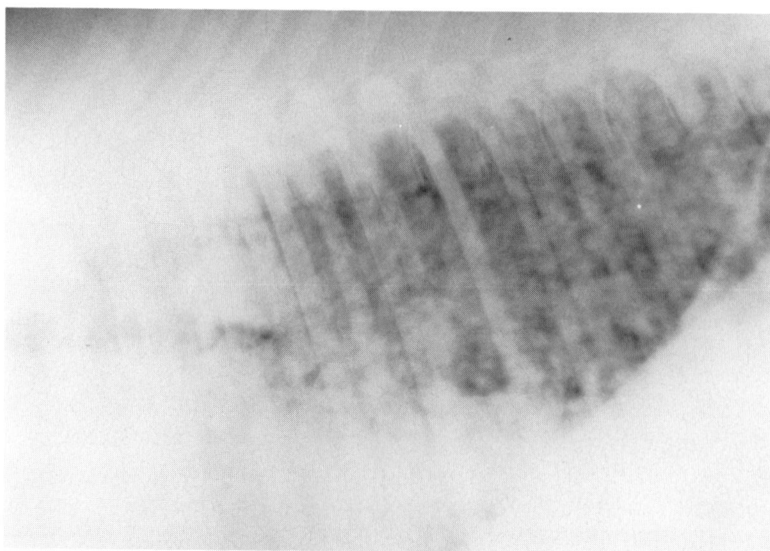

**FIG. 7–20.** Pneumonia. Lateral view of thorax shows diffuse lung nodules which coalesce ventrally.

two forms, acute and chronic. The acute form results from the inhalation of foreign material over a short span causing an acute onset of clinical signs. The aspirate may be either a solid or liquid. Aspiration of solid particulate matter results primarily in bronchial obstruction. Aspiration of liquid material, particularly low pH gastric contents, commonly produces dyspnea, cyanosis, and occasionally shock. The chronic form results from repeated episodes of aspiration producing chronic pneumonia or granulomatous disease. It is most common in foals or horses with swallowing disorders or long-standing esophageal obstruction. Chronic aspiration of oil base medicaments may result in lipid pneumonia.

The radiographic findings in aspiration pneumonia vary according to the nature and volume of the aspirate. The initial radiographic appearance will change depending on treatment, complicating infections, and the duration of the disease process. Typically, on the early radiographs the lung is affected by a combination of peribronchial and parenchymal disease. The bronchial shadows are usually ringlike in character when viewed end-on or resemble train tracks when seen in profile. They appear clearest dorsocaudal to the heart base. The parenchymal shadows are patchy, somewhat fluffy densities liberally distributed throughout the lung. Later these densities may coalesce and become more vis-

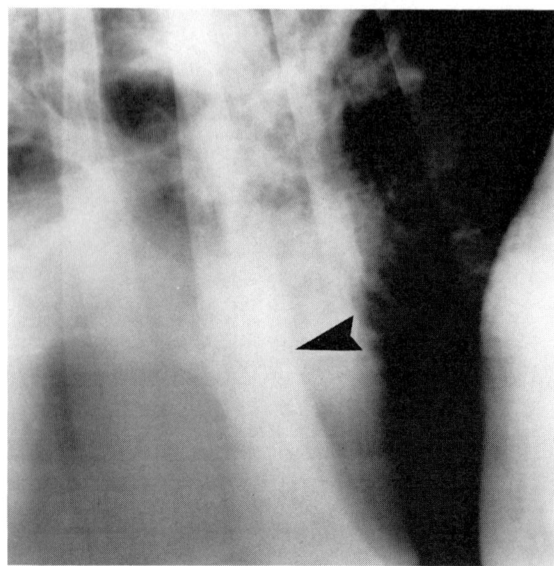

**FIG. 7–21.** Focal pneumonia. Lateral view of central thorax shows vertically oriented consolidation forming a cardiopulmonary silhouette sign (arrow). Deliberate overexposure was used to better define the lesion, causing the adjacent normal lung to be "burned out."

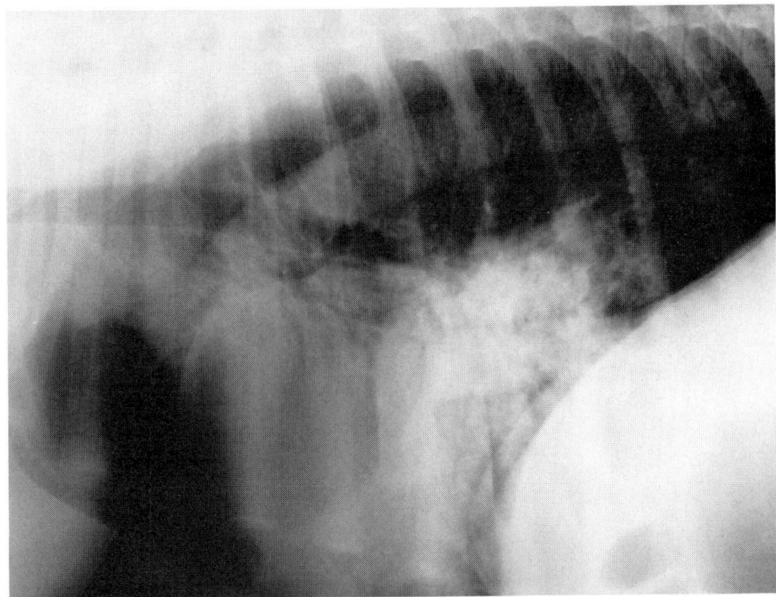

**FIG. 7–22.** Focal pneumonia. Lateral view of thorax shows horizontally oriented consolidation superimposed on caudal heart base.

ible. This usually indicates consolidation and/or abscesses. In either case, these radiographic findings represent a worsening of the animal's condition.[36]

***Immune Related.*** Immunologic lung disease (allergic, hypersensitivity pneumonia) can seldom be diagnosed solely on the basis of radiographic appearances. A diagnosis of immune mediated lung disease is at best suggested radiographically if probable cause exists historically and alternative radiographic diagnoses have been ruled out (Fig. 7–25).[3]

***Parasitic.*** Parasitic pneumonias lack a typical appearance, appearing variably as interstitial, alveolar or mixed patterns. Some parasitic pneumonias are associated with a normal radiograph.[4]

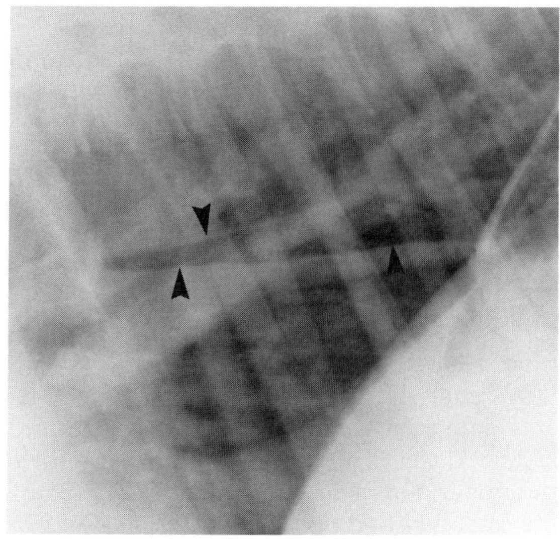

**FIG. 7–23.** Esophageal gas. Lateral view of caudodorsal lung field shows air in the esophagus (arrows). Since no evidence of esophageal or lung disease was found, the described finding was considered incidental.

## Pleuropneumonia

Pleuropneumonia is the concurrent infection of the lung and pleural cavity. Its appearance varies according to the amount of pleural fluid, which if present in large volume obscures the lung, and therefore the observer's ability to establish lung involvement. Pleural fluid in small volume is difficult to detect radiographically as it is often hidden by the heart and proximal part of the forelimbs. Sonography is useful in this regard. Theoretically, infection may extend from the lung to the pleural space, or alternatively, from the pleural space to the lung. In some cases, lung inflation may become restricted secondary to surface fibrin deposition, although this can be difficult to differentiate from the effects of pleural fluid alone. Again, ultrasound is useful in this situation.

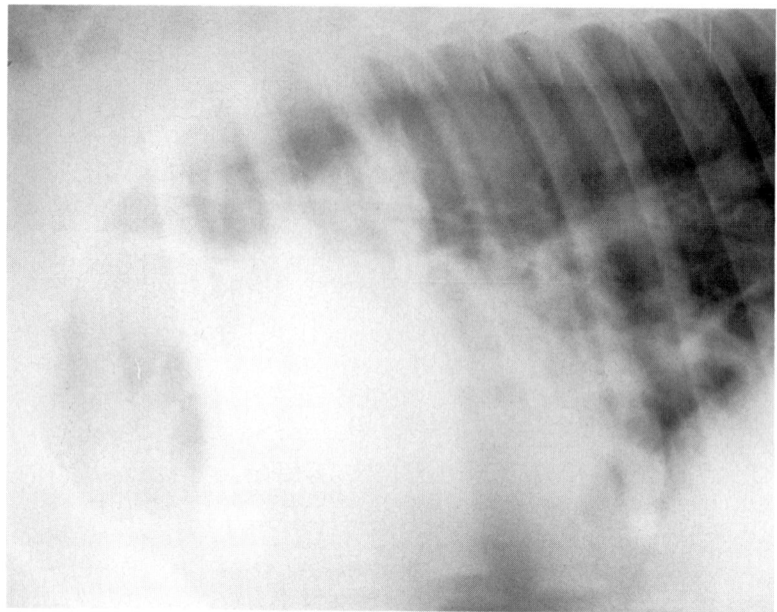

**FIG. 7–24.** Pneumonia. Lateral view of thorax shows patchy consolidation over much of the ventral half of the thorax in a foal suffering from combined immunodeficiency (CID).

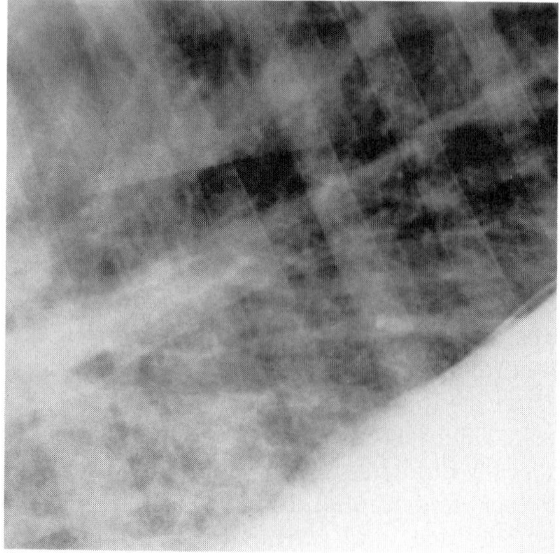

**FIG. 7–25.** Immune-mediated lung disease. Lateral view of thorax shows a coarse interstitial lung pattern. The ventral two thirds of the lung show relatively greater density than the upper third. This is likely a result of a combination of factors, including the relative thinness of the region, resulting in greater penetration and therefore a darker image; greater involvement of one half of the lung than of the other; or a relative difference in pulmonary ventilation. Regional interstitial emphysema is also a possibility.

## Pleuritis

Equine pleural diseases often result in the production of an excessive volume of pleural fluid. Pleuritis may be primary without known cause, or secondary to a wide variety of conditions including bacterial or fungal pneumonia, pulmonary abscessation, granuloma, and tumor.[37] Pleural fissure lines are rarely visible because of minimal lobation in the horse's lung. Fluid lines will also be undetectable radiographically, unless there is accompanying air in the pleural space. Combined, fluid in the dependent portion of the pleural cavity and air above it will result in a distinctive air-fluid interface or fluid line. This finding should prompt the observer to seek the source of the air.

## Abscess

Abscesses, like pneumonia, are polymorphic. Lesions may vary in appearance from large, well-defined solid masses, to multiple, small ill-defined nodules (Figs. 7–26 and 7–27). Coalescent abscesses may resemble pulmonary consolidation (Fig. 7–28). Some are cavitated and contain fluid (Figs. 7–29 to 7–31). Visibility is first a function of size, and less so of location. Dorsocaudal lesions are most easily seen due to enhanced lesion contrast provided by the lung, while cranioventral masses are often obscured by regional soft tissue. Alternate side radiography may assist

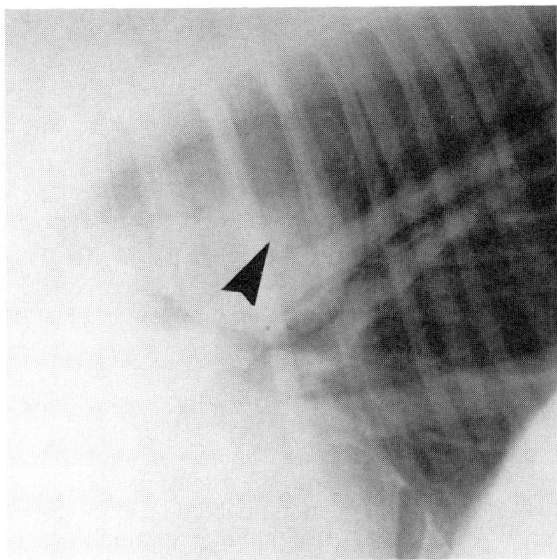

**FIG. 7–26.** Pulmonary abscess. Lateral view of thorax shows a solitary lung abscess over the heart base (arrow).

in establishing whether a lesion is in the right or left hemithorax.

## Infectious Cavitary Lesions

Cavitary lesions in the horse are most often of infectious origin. They are typically created when a lung abscess or area of consolidation communicates with an airway sufficiently large to allow air to enter the abscess cavity and produce a fluid line, thus establishing the cavitary nature of the lesion. Cavitary lesions that are completely filled with fluid are radiographically indistinguishable from solid masses.[35] Occasionally, abscesses may drain completely into a communicating airway, revealing a predominantly air-filled lesion (Fig. 7–31). Fungal balls, or pulmonary mycetomas are also usually air-filled, but differ from a communicating abscess by being compartmentalized (Figs. 7–31 to 7–33).

## Pulmonary Edema

***Cardiogenic.*** Pulmonary edema arising from cardiac causes may produce, depending on its severity, an increase in the size and number of pulmonary vessels, an increase in background lung density which may diminish vascular clarity, and varying amounts of pulmonary consolidation as a result of edema replacing air in the terminal air spaces. It is this last radiographic sign, pulmonary edema, which constitutes the basis for a radiographic diagnosis of congestive heart failure. Pleural fluid, ascites, or subcutaneous edema may also develop depending on the nature of the heart disorder. Cardiomegaly is difficult to establish in the adult horse due to the inability to include the entire thorax on one radiograph. The multiple films required for evaluation of the thorax lead to a radiographically segmented appearance, which makes accurate film evaluation of heart size

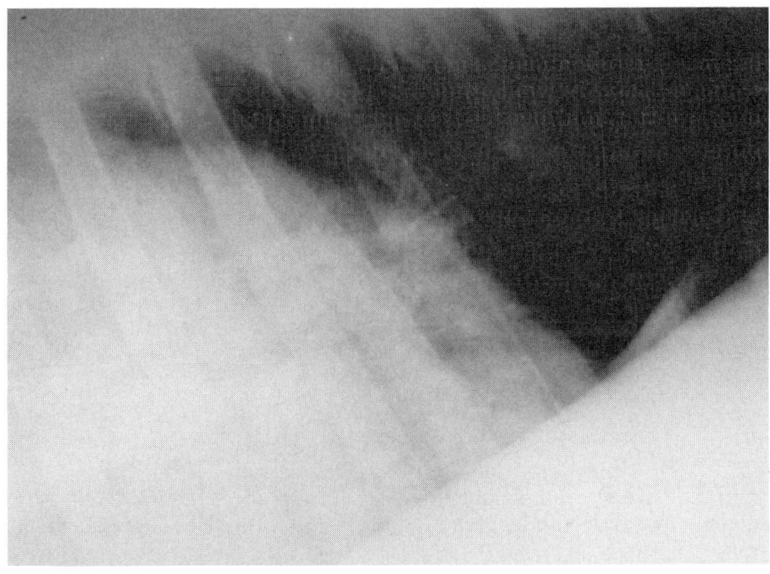

**FIG. 7–27.** Pulmonary abscess. Lateral view of thorax shows the caudal half of a large pulmonary abscess in the dorsal aspect of the lung.

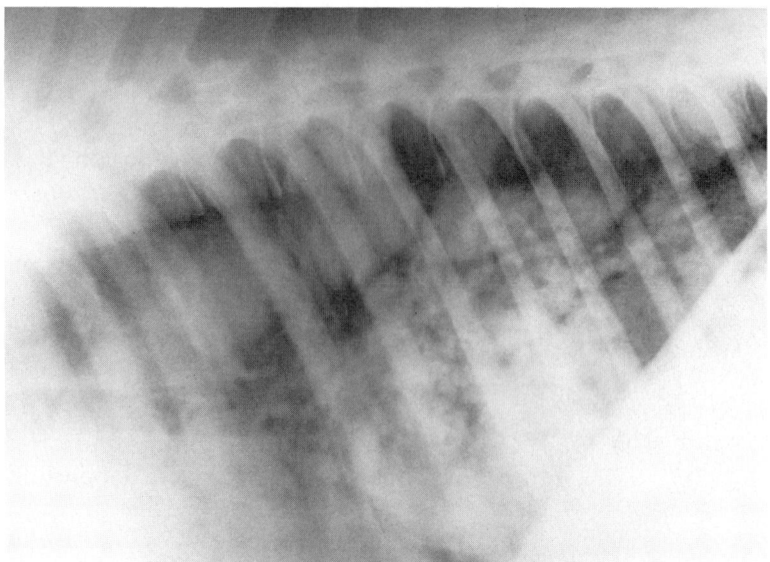

**FIG. 7–28.** Pulmonary abscess. Lateral view of thorax shows coalescence of multiple, variably sized abscesses resembling pulmonary consolidation.

difficult.[31] Moderate or severe heart enlargement is far easier to identify in foals, in which the entire heart may be seen as a single image, and in the context of the surrounding lung and related structures. Congestive heart failure in foals may be due to either congenital or acquired heart disease, usually the former, while in adult horses failure is more likely to stem from acquired cardiovascular disease.[38]

***Noncardiogenic.*** Noncardiac edema may be produced by a variety of direct and indirect mechanisms including: head trauma, heat stroke, strangulation, electrocution, smoke inhalation, near-drowning, certain poisons, some bacterial pneumonias, and often following the inhalation of esophageal or stomach contents. Fluid overload, especially in young foals or anesthetized adult horses, is one of the more common causes of pulmonary edema.

## Chronic Obstructive Lung Disease

Pulmonary emphysema, as in man, is now included in the broader functional category of chronic obstructive lung disease (COLD).[39,40]

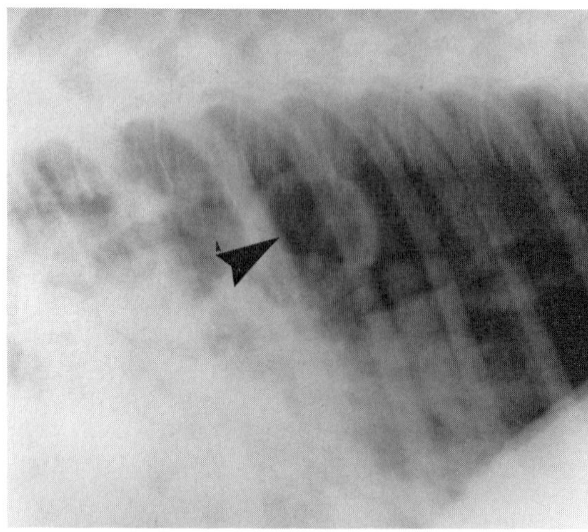

**FIG. 7–29.** Infectious cavitation. Lateral view of thorax shows a small, solitary cavitary lung lesion (arrow) overlying widespread ventral consolidation.

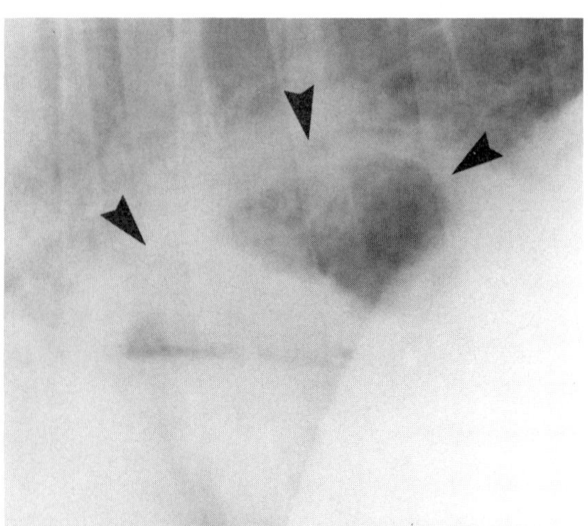

**FIG. 7–30.** Infectious cavitation. Lateral view of thorax shows a medium-sized, rough-walled, partially fluid-filled, cavitary lesion (arrows).

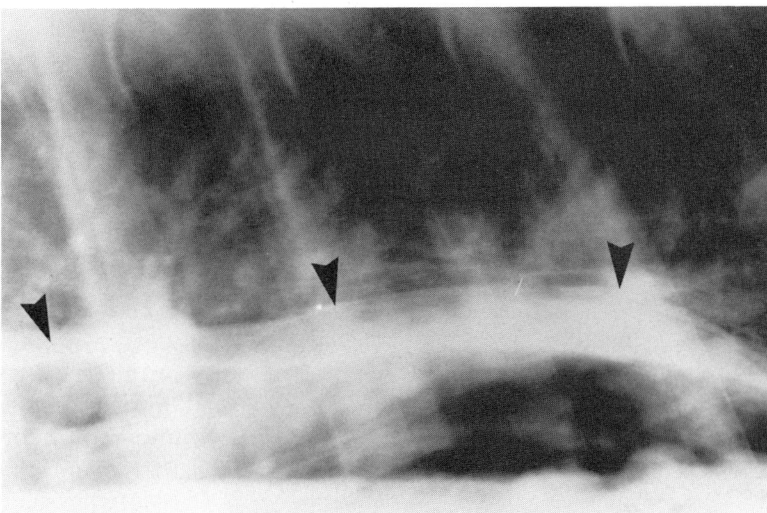

**FIG. 7–31.** Infectious cavitation. Lateral view of thorax shows the dorsal aspect of a massive, smooth-walled, partially fluid-filled, cavitary lesion (arrows).

Some workers contend that emphysema is rarely a primary disorder as once generally believed, but instead develops as a further progression of advanced obstructive lung disease.[40]

Radiographically, COLD is often undetectable; in advanced cases of emphysema, the diagnosis may be inferentially made on the basis of three coexistent radiographic signs: pulmonary hyperinflation, hyperlucency, and diminished vascular size and number.[31]

## Pulmonary Contusions

Pulmonary contusions in the horse typically occur following severe, blunt thoracic trauma, for example, being hit by a car or secondary to a trailer wreck (Fig. 7–34). Penetrating thoracic wounds are more apt to produce localized or regional hemorrhage, while all but the most serious falls cause neither. The usual radiographic picture is that of pulmonary consolidation, ranging from patchy areas of increased lung density to total re-

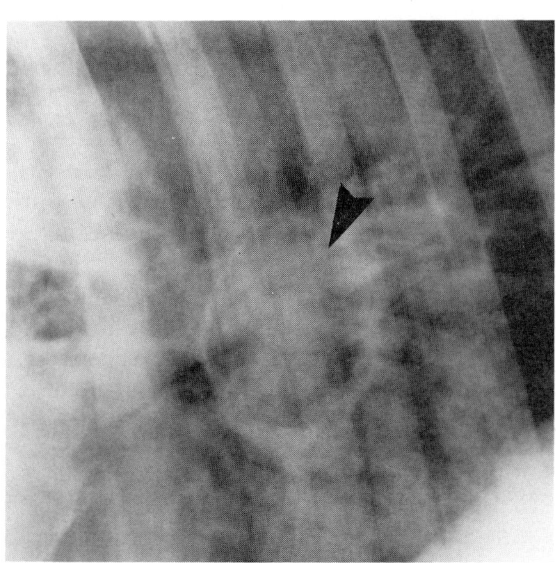

**FIG. 7–32.** Infectious cavitation. Lateral view of thorax shows a solitary cavitary lesion caudal to the carina (arrow).

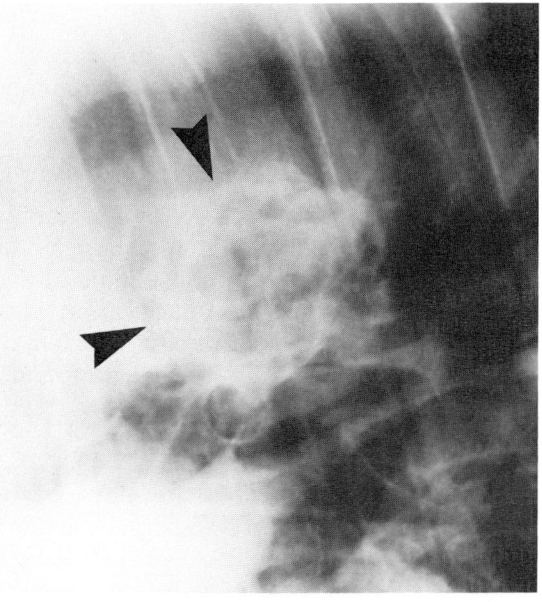

**FIG. 7–33.** Infectious cavitation. Lateral view of thorax shows a solitary compartmentalized, cavitary lesion proximal to the carina (arrows).

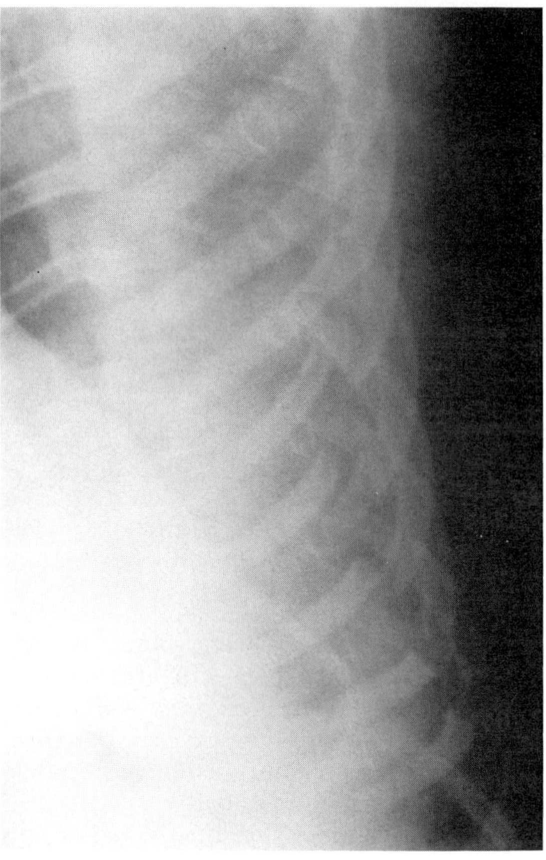

**FIG. 7–34.** Chest wall trauma. Ventrodorsal oblique view of thorax shows multiple rib fractures, pulmonary contusions, and a small pneumothorax.

gional opacification. As in other commonly radiographed domestic animals, contusions usually begin to resolve within 24 hours, with the lung often being clear in a week. Pneumonia rarely ever develops secondary to pulmonary contusions, although resorbing blood frequently causes severely consolidated lung to change from complete opacification to a mottled density after a day or two, which may be mistaken for a complicating pneumonia.

## Traumatic Cavitary Lesion

Traumatic bullae or pneumatoceles are rare in the horse, and like pulmonary contusions are usually the aftermath of severe thoracic injury. They may also occur in foals as secondary complications of mechanical ventilation. As in pet animals and people, most resolve spontaneously within a week. I have not seen such lesions subsequently lead to pneumothorax, although theoretically it is a possibility. Like other cavitary lung lesions, traumatic bullae are radiographically characterized by an oval appearance, a discrete wall, and a fluid line.[32]

## Penetrating Chest Wound

Penetrating thoracic foreign bodies, particularly wooden stakes, carry the potential for multiple internal injuries including pneumothorax, hemothorax, pulmonary hemorrhage and/or pulmonary contusion, traumatic cavitation, and pneumomediastinum (Fig. 7–35). Related infections may include abscess, pneumonia, and pleuritis. Draining sinus tracts may develop, and occasionally fistulas form (Fig. 7–36).[1,41]

## Pneumothorax

Pneumothorax represents the abnormal accumulation of air or gas within the pleural space (between the visceral and parietal pleura). In the horse, pneumothorax most often develops during chest drainage, secondary to a penetrating chest wound, or as a complication of pneumonia or an abscess (Fig. 7–37). Limited in the adult horse to a lateral view, the radiographic diagnosis of pneumothorax is typically made on the basis of one or more visible pleural surfaces in the dorsal aspect of the caudal lung field.[32] Occasionally, a spontaneous pneumothorax (cause undetermined) will develop following a period of great distress such as a barn fire, often accompanied by a pneumomediastinum (Fig. 7–38). It is my belief that pneumothorax occurs in this context as a result of alveolar rupture with retrograde movement of air into the mediastinum and subsequently the pleural space. Pneumothorax has been described following near drowning, possibly due to the same mechanism.[43]

## Hemothorax

Most commonly the result of thoracic wall or lung injury, a medium or large volume hemothorax appears radiographically like any other pleural fluid accumulation—a ventral region of near total opacity obscuring the as-

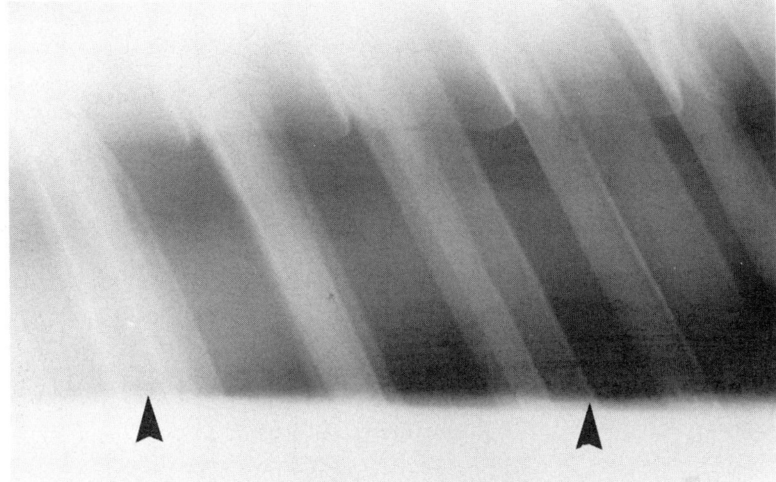

**FIG. 7–35.** Hydropneumothorax. Lateral close-up view of mid-dorsal thorax shows a fluid line (arrows) and an absence of lung markings following a penetrating chest wound. The cylindrical opacity dorsal to the fluid level is the aorta.

sociated parts of the heart and lung. There is no fluid line, but rather a fluid zone: a less discrete opacity lacking the contrast of a fluid line, and formed by the submerged portion of the lung, surrounding fluid, and chest wall.

## Exercise Induced Hemorrhage

The cause or causes of exercise related lung bleeding in race horses is unknown. Radiographically, the lesion is fairly characteristic, usually appearing as a relatively discrete opacity in the dorsal aspect of the caudal lung field (Fig. 7–39). Occasionally the lesion is cavitated and contains a fluid line.[42]

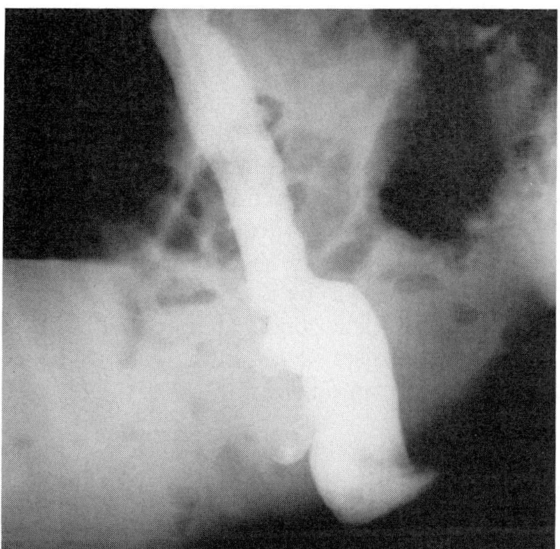

**FIG. 7–36.** Thoracoabdominal sinus tract. Sinogram: lateral view of abdomen shows a large sinus tract coursing diagonally through subcutaneous tissues of the lateral abdominal wall. The draining sinus into which the catheter was placed was located on the dorsolateral aspect of the thoracic wall.

## Smoke Inhalation

My experience with smoke inhalation in horses has been similar to that which I have previously described in dogs.[43,44]

Related injury results from a combination of factors including oxygen deprivation, car-

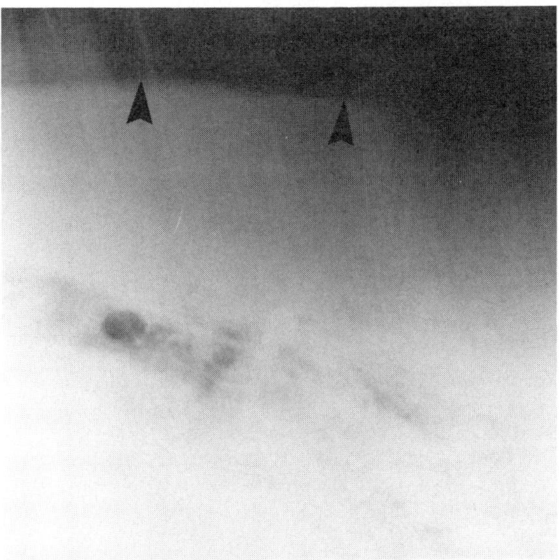

**FIG. 7–37.** Infectious pneumothorax. Lateral, close-up view of thorax shows a dorsal pneumothorax outlining consolidated lung (arrows indicate lung margin).

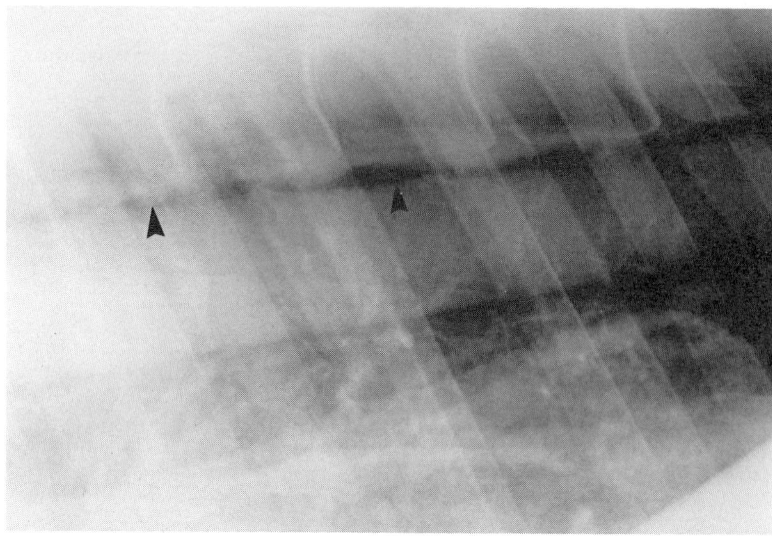

**FIG. 7–38.** Spontaneous pneumothorax. Lateral, close-up view of caudodorsal thorax shows air outlining the aorta (arrows). The dorsal margin of the partially collapsed lung is clearly visible.

bon monoxide poisoning, heat, and mechanical-chemical irritation. Additionally, toxic gases other than smoke may be produced by the combustion process and are also inhaled, producing additional injury. Pneumonia and adult respiratory distress syndrome often develop subsequently. Fatalities may occur as a direct result of the inhalation injury or secondary to its complications. Associated burns worsen the prognosis.

Radiographically, great variability exists, ranging from normal to interstitial or alveolar lung patterns. Diffuse peribronchial densities are most common, followed by mixed (alveolar-interstitial) patterns (Fig. 7–40). The appearance of the lung may change markedly

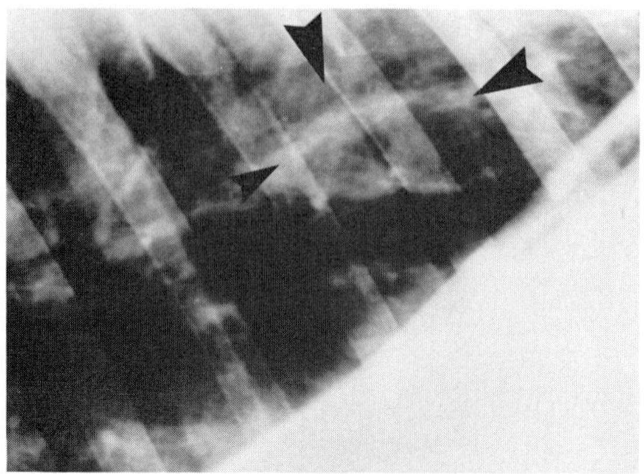

**FIG. 7–39.** Exercise-induced pulmonary hemorrhage. Lateral, close-up view of caudodorsal thorax shows an oval, partially cavitated lung opacity (arrows).

within 72 hours following the fire, depending on the nature and extent of the inhalation injury, and the effectiveness of treatment.

## Near Drowning

Veterinary reports on near drowning deal almost entirely with the dog.[45,46] Typical early radiographic observations consist of consolidation in the dorsocaudal aspect of the lung, or alternatively, diffuse interstitial lung density. Later films may show resolution of earlier lung densities signifying effective treatment and likely recovery. Spreading of existing lung densities or transition to an alveolar or mixed pattern suggests treatment ineffectiveness, complicating pneumonia or adult respiratory distress syndrome (ARDS). A recently described case of near drowning in a horse, but not seen by the referral center until the next day, described patchy consolidation in the caudal part of the lung, and pneumothorax/pneumomediastinum.[47]

## Strangulation

Strangulation occasionally occurs in horses. The pathogenesis is imperfectly understood, but strangulation generally is believed to be caused by the following sequence of events: circumferential pressure on the neck; occlusion of the regional venous blood supply, leading to cerebral anoxia and ultimately unconsciousness; involuntary relaxation of the neck muscles; upper airway obstruction; ar-

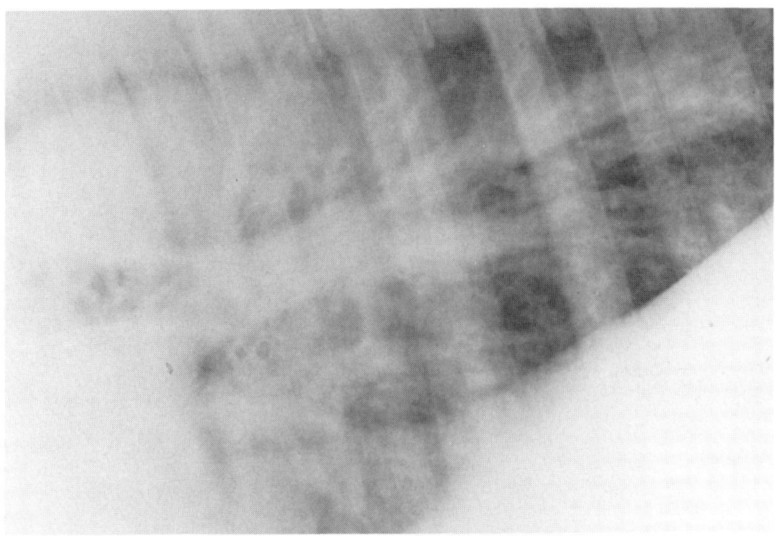

**FIG. 7–40.** Smoke inhalation. Lateral view of mid and central thorax shows increased lung density (mixed pattern).

terial blockage; and brain death. Surviving animals may develop pulmonary edema and inhalation pneumonia may also occur.

Radiographically, the lung is often normal. When pulmonary edema is present, appearances vary according to the amount and distribution of the edema. When inhalation has occurred, its distribution often reflects the animal's position at the time it inhaled the vomitus. For example, if the horse were on its back, the dorsal part of the lung would be most apt to be affected.

## Tumors

Both primary and secondary lung tumors are uncommon in the horse, with the latter being seen with relatively greater frequency. Mediastinal tumors are also rare in horses as compared with pet animals.

## Miscellaneous

***Respiratory Distress Syndrome.*** A foal born without pulmonary surfactant is unable to maintain alveolar inflation; predictably, this critical chemical deficiency results in uneven inflation, atelectasis, hypoxia, and often death. Radiographic appearances vary widely depending on the degree of volume loss (Fig. 7–41).

***Pulmonary Eosinophilia with Pulmonary Infiltrates (PIE).*** PIE, a form of immuno-

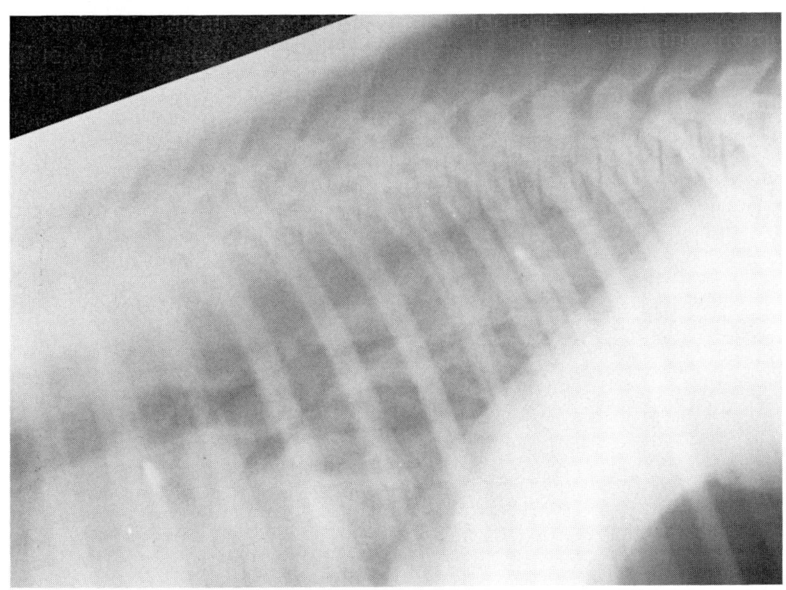

**FIG. 7–41.** Neonatal respiratory distress syndrome. Lateral view of thorax shows a generalized increase in lung density resulting from atelectasis secondary to surfactant deficiency. The foal died approximately 55 hours following premature birth. Histologically, the lung had extensive hyaline membrane formation in the terminal air spaces with no evidence of pneumonia or aspiration.

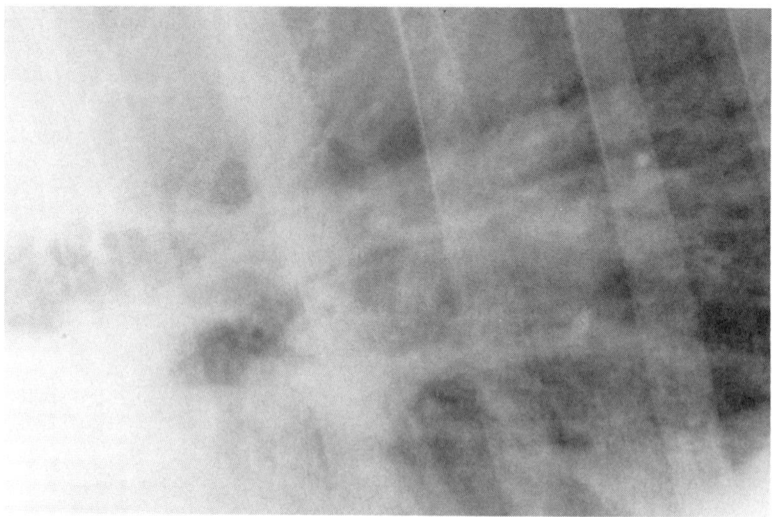

**FIG. 7–42.** Pulmonary infiltrates with eosinophilia (PIE). Lateral close-up view of caudal thorax shows a generalized increase in lung density which reduces vascular clarity.

pneumonia first described in man, apparently has a counterpart(s) in domestic animals. Unlike in the dog, however, the lung is most apt to assume a generalized increase in background density, as opposed to regional, symmetric consolidation (Fig. 7–42).

## Extrapulmonary Disorders Which May Affect the Lung

***Diaphragmatic Hernia.*** Unlike in pet animals in which two projections are customarily made, a diagnosis of diaphragmatic hernia in the horse is usually made from a lateral view only; consequently it is often impossible to establish the laterality of the lesion. However, even with this limitation a diagnosis may be possible based on loss of a discrete diaphragmatic interface, and abnormal lung density (opacity or lucency), depending on the nature of the herniated viscera (Fig. 7–43).

***Transdiaphragmatic Abscess.*** Occasionally liver abscesses may extend into and eventually through the diaphragm, ultimately involving the lung. The extent of the resulting pulmonary diseases depends on whether the infection is locally confined to a small area of the lung, or disseminates widely into the pleural cavity with ensuing pyothorax (Fig. 7–44).

***Pulmonary Compression Secondary To A Large Volume of Abdominal Fluid.*** Ascites or peritonitis associated with a large volume of abdominal fluid causes cranial displacement of the diaphragm, which in turn may create compression atelectasis of the caudal part of

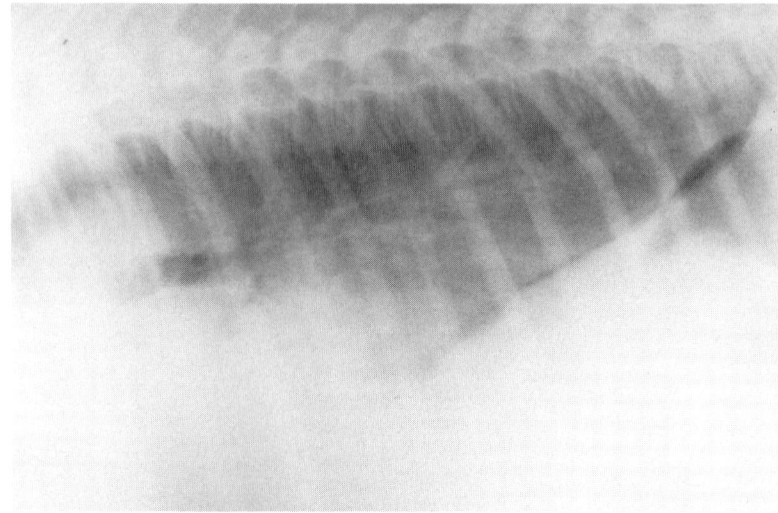

**FIG. 7–43.** Diaphragmatic hernia. Lateral view of thorax shows increased density in the ventral half of the thorax with associated loss of the diaphragmatic interface. The apparent increased lung density is caused by compression atelectasis.

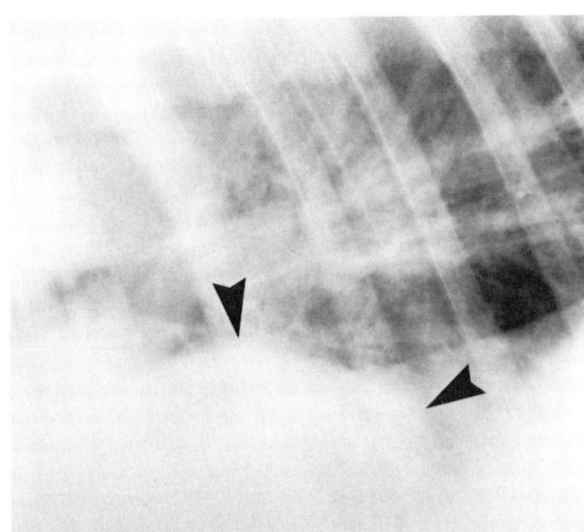

**FIG. 7–44.** Transabdominal abscess. Lateral view of central thorax shows an ill-defined mass superimposed on the caudal vena cava (arrows), and loss of lung detail ventrally secondary to pleural fluid and atelectasis.

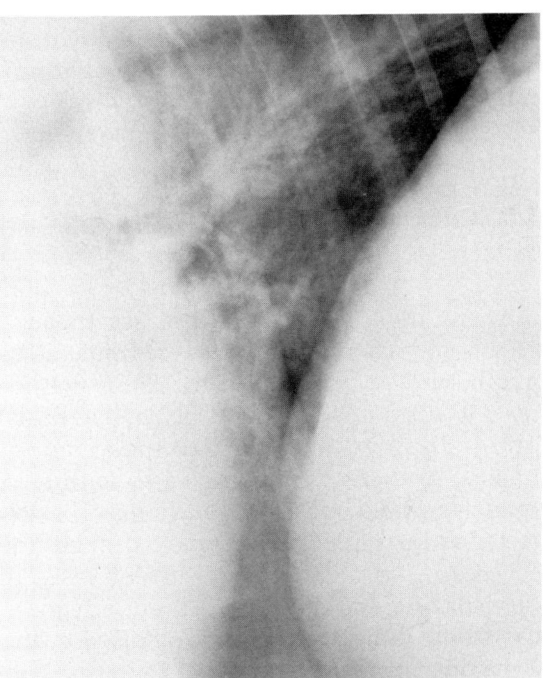

**FIG. 7–45.** Lung compression secondary to ascites. Lateral view of the caudoventral aspect of the thorax shows a regional increase in lung density, associated vascular crowding, and cranial displacement of the diaphragm.

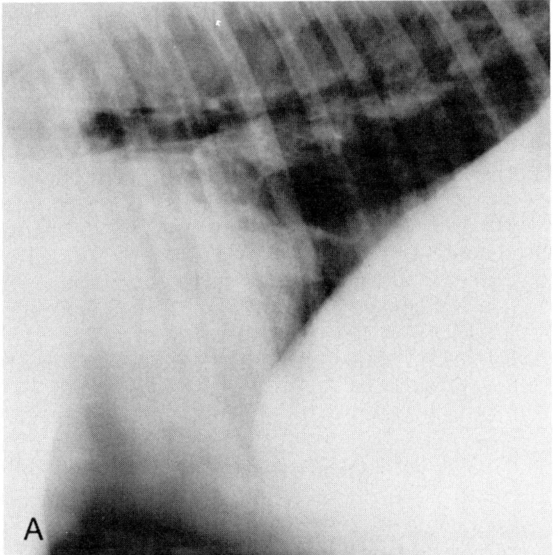


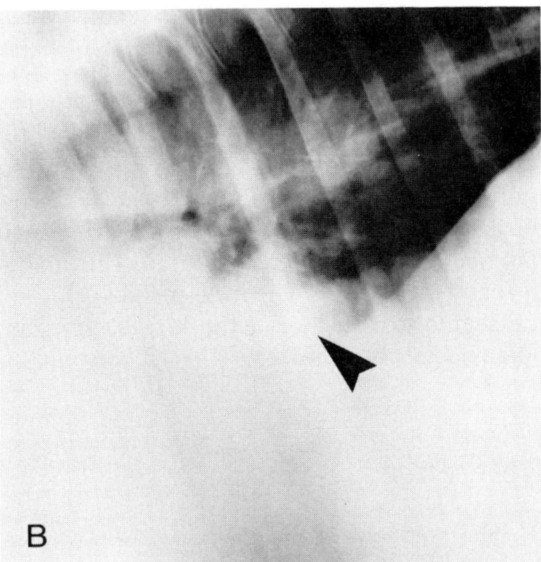


**FIG. 7–46.** A. Pneumonia, initial examination. Lateral view of thorax shows normal lung in foal suspected of having pneumonia. B. Pneumonia, 2-week progress examination. Lateral view of thorax shows consolidation forming a positive silhouette sign with the caudal aspect of the heart (arrow).

the lung. This volume loss combined with related vascular crowding may resemble pulmonary consolidation (Fig. 7–45).

## Diseases With A Normal Radiograph

There are a number of diseases that are commonly associated with a normal radiograph, and in this respect the latter may be used to support a tentative clinical diagnosis. These disorders include uncomplicated sinusitis; laryngitis (excluding cases with multiple lymphoid masses, which may be detected radiographically); tracheitis; all but the severest forms of bronchitis; most cases of bronchiolitis and alveolitis; all but advanced cases of chronic obstructive lung disease; and a majority of cases of early and intermediate duration allergic lung disease. Parasitic and viral pneumonia create a generalized but subtle increase in background lung density which is difficult to distinguish from technical variation. Even bacterial pneumonia may be difficult to detect initially, especially in foals. Where uncertainty exists, repeat the examination in a week or two, and compare with the original examination (Fig. 7–46A, B). Chronic conditions tend to change slowly, and are unlikely to show change, even with effective treatment, much before 1 or 2 months. Cardiac disease may also escape radiographic detection, either because the heart has not become sufficiently large, especially in foals, or because it is indiscernible due to the segmented nature of the image typically obtained in adult horses.

## References

1. Farrow CS. Equine thoracic radiology. J Am Vet Med Assoc *179*:776, 1981.
2. Farrow CS. Radiography of the equine thorax: anatomy and technique. Vet Radiol *22*:62, 1981.
3. Valdez H, McMullan WC, Hobson HP, et al. Surgical correction of deviated nasal septum and premaxilla in a colt. J Am Vet Med Assoc, *173*:1001, 1978.
4. Haynes PF, Qualls CW. Cleft soft palate, nasal septal deviation, and epiglottic entrapment in a Thoroughbred filly. J Am Vet Med Assoc, *179*:677, 1981.
5. Stickle R. The equine skull. In: Thrall DE, ed. Textbook of Veterinary Diagnostic Radiology. Philadelphia, WB Saunders Co, 1986, p 57.
6. Turner AS. Surgical management of depression fractures of the equine skull. Vet Surg, *8*:29, 1979.
7. Farrow CS, Munger W. Gunshot wounds of the equine head. WCVM Bulletin, *8*:2, 1980.
8. Hodgin EC, Conaway DH, Ortenburger AI. Recurrence of obstructive nasal coccidioidal granuloma in a horse. J Am Vet Med Assoc, *184*:339, 1984.
9. Boulton CH. Equine nasal cavity and paranasal sinus disease: a review of 85 cases. Equine Vet Sci, *5*:268, 1985.
10. Gibbs C, Lane JG. Radiographic examination of the facial, nasal and paranasal sinus regions of the horse. II. Radiological findings. Equine Vet J, *19*:474, 1987.
11. Acland HM, Orsini JA, Elkins S, et al. Congenital ethmoid carcinoma in a foal. J Am Vet Med Assoc, *184*:979, 1984.
12. Lattimer JC. Equine nasal passages, sinuses, and guttural pouches. In: Thrall DE, ed. Textbook of Veterinary Diagnostic Radiology. Philadelphia, WB Saunders Co, 1986, pp 64–68.
13. Leyland A, Baker JR. Lesions of the nasal and paranasal sinuses of the horse causing dyspnea. Br Vet J, *131*:339, 1975.
14. Moulton JE. Tumors of the respiratory system. In: Moulton JE, ed. Tumors in Domestic Animals. Berkeley and Los Angeles: University of California Press, 1961, pp 115–124.
15. Schumacher J, Honnas C, Smith B. Paranasal sinusitis complicated by inspissated exudate in the ventral conchal sinus. Vet Surg, *16*:373, 1987.
16. Boles C. Abnormalities of the upper respiratory tract. Vet Clin North Am [Lg An Pract], *1*:89, 1979.
17. Lane JG, Longstaffe JA, Gibbs C. Equine paranasal sinus cysts: A report of 15 cases. Equine Vet J, *19*:537, 1987.
18. Farrow CS. The larynx, pharynx, and trachea. In: Thrall DE, ed. Textbook of Veterinary Diagnostic Radiology. Philadelphia, WB Saunders Co, 1986, pp 318–338.
19. Linford RL, O'Brien TR, Wheat JD, et al. Radiographic assessment of epiglottic length and pharyngeal and laryngeal diameters in the Thoroughbred. Am J Vet Res, *44*:1660, 1983.
20. Bertone JJ, Traub-Dargatz JL, Trotter GW. Bilateral hypoplasia of the soft palate and aryepiglottic entrapment in a horse. J Am Vet Med Assoc, *188*:727, 1986.
21. Sweeney CR, Benson CE, Whitlock RH, et al. Streptococcus equi infection in horses—part II. Comp Cont Ed, *9*:845, 1987.
22. Haynes PF. Persistent dorsal displacement of the soft palate associated with epiglottic shortening in two horses. J Am Vet Med Assoc, *179*:677, 1981.
23. Koch DB, Tate LP. Pharyngeal cysts in horses. J Am Vet Med Assoc, *173*:860, 1978.
24. Jacobs KA, Fretz PB. Fistula between the guttural pouches and the dorsal pharyngeal recess as a sequela to guttural pouch mycosis in the horse. Can Vet J, *23*:117, 1982.

25. Lees MJ, Joann CL, Barber SM, et al. A congenital laryngeal web in a Quarterhorse filly. Equine Vet J, *19*:561, 1987.
26. Haynes PF, Snider TG, McClure JR, et al. Chronic chondritis of the equine arytenoid cartilage. J Am Vet Med Assoc, *177*:1135, 1980.
27. Farrow CS, Barber SM. Perilaryngeal abscess—What is your diagnosis? J Am Vet Med Assoc, *179*:830, 1981.
28. Carrig CB, Groenendyk, Seawright AA. Dorsoventral flattening of the trachea in a horse and its attempted surgical correction: a case report. J Am Vet Rad Soc, *14*:32, 1973.
29. Caron JP, Townsend HGG. Tracheal perforation and widespread subcutaneous emphysema in a horse. Can Vet J, *25*:339, 1984.
30. Farrow CS. Pneumomediastinum in the horse: a complication of transtracheal aspiration. Vet Radiol, *17*:192, 1976.
31. Farrow CS. Radiographic aspects of inflammatory lung disease in the horse. Vet Radiol, *22*:107, 1981.
32. Farrow CS. Inflammatory lung disease in the horse: A radiologic perspective. Presented at the annual meeting of the AVMA, St. Louis, 1981.
33. Farrow CS. The lung. In: Thrall DE, ed. Textbook of Veterinary Diagnostic Radiology. Philadelphia, WB Saunders Co, 1986, pp 339–355.
34. Kangstrom L.E. The radiological diagnosis of equine pneumonia. Vet Radiol, *9*:80, 1968.
35. Silverman S, Poulos PW, Suter PF. Cavitary pulmonary lesions in animals. J Am Vet Radiol Soc, *17*:134, 1976.
36. Farrow CS. Exercise in diagnostic radiology: inhalation pneumonia in a horse. Can Vet J, *23*:340, 1982.
37. Smith BP. Diseases of the pleura. Vet Clin North Am [Lg An Pract], *1*:197, 1979.
38. Reef VB. Cardiovascular disease in the equine neonate. Vet Clin N Am: Equine Pract, *1*:117, 1985.
39. Beech J. Diseases of the lung. Vet Clin North Am [Lg An Pract], *1*:149, 1979.
40. Breeze RG. Heaves. Vet Clin North Am [Lg An Pract], *1*:219, 1979.
41. Farrow CS. Sinography in the horse. In: Proceedings of the 32nd annual convention of the AAEP, 1986, pp 505–521.
42. Pascoe JR, O'Brien, Wheat JD, et al. Radiographic aspects of exercise-induced pulmonary hemorrhage in racing horses. Vet Radiol, *24*:85, 1983.
43. Farrow CS. Inhalation injury. In: Kirk RW, ed. Current Vet Therapy VIII. Philadelphia, WB Saunders Co, 1983, pp 173–179.
44. Farrow CS. Smoke Inhalation. In: Emergency Radiology in Small Animal Practice. Toronto, BC Decker, 1988, pp 78–79.
45. Farrow CS. Near drowning. In: Kirk RW, ed. Current Veterinary Therapy VIII. Philadelphia, WB Saunders Co, 1985, pp 167–173.
46. Farrow CS. Near drowning. In: Emergency Radiology in Small Animal Practice. Toronto, BC Decker, 1988, pp 80–81.
47. Humber KA. Near drowning in a gelding. J Am Vet Med Assoc, *192*:377, 1988.

# CHAPTER 8

# XERORADIOGRAPHIC EXAMINATION

*PAUL G. ORSINI*

Xeroradiography* is a radiographic process which has greater resolution for soft tissue structures when compared to standard radiography. It is most useful when contrast differences between various tissues of a subject are small but sharply defined. In human medicine, xeroradiography has received most attention in mammography where it is essential to differentiate small nodular masses and cysts from surrounding blood vessels, ducts, adipose tissue, and skin. In veterinary medicine xeroradiography can be helpful in evaluating small bony lesions, such as hairline fractures and osteolytic changes. When evaluating the upper respiratory tract in the horse, it has been used to demonstrate normal variations in the radiographic anatomy of the region and also in the diagnosis of certain disease conditions such as arytenoid chondrosis.

## Xeroradiography

In xeroradiography, the detecting medium is a thin layer of selenium which acts as a photoconductor. It is a two-stage process in which the selenium surface is first given a uniform surface charge and is then enclosed in a plastic cassette. This is then exposed to the radiation penetrating through the irradiated subject. The original uniform charge is partly dissipated by the radiation exposure and the residual charge pattern forms a "latent image" of the radiation which has passed through the subject. The second step in the process is to develop and thereby make visible this image by exposing the selenium layer to an aerosol of electrically charged colored powder particles (toner) which adhere to the surface primarily in the regions of high field strength and therefore clearly delineate gradients in the charge density. This development process gives a positive or negative image of the subject depending on the charge given to the powder. The image is then preserved by transferring it to paper.

*Xerox 126 Conditioner and Processor, Xerox Corporation, Pasadena, CA.

## *Technique*

When evaluating the upper respiratory tract of the horse, lateral xeroradiographs are the most beneficial projection as the dorsoventral projection is usually of little value because of the superimposition of the skull and cervical vertebrae on the larynx. Oblique projections can be useful in delineating unilateral lesions. The head can be held in different positions depending on what is to be evaluated. Initial survey films should be taken with the head and neck in the normal resting position. A thin rope halter should be used to restrain the horse so that an unobstructed exposure can be obtained. The charged cassette is held against the left side of the neck so that the exposed picture will be routinely oriented with the rostral aspect of the animal to the left. The cassette is held perpendicular to the central x-ray beam centered on the palpable rostral aspect of the larynx. The focal film distance should be 90 cm with an exposure technique of 50 mAs at 95 kV in most average sized horses.

## Anatomy

Xeroradiography has been of paramount importance in describing the normal radiographic anatomy of the equine pharynx, larynx, and associated structures.[1] Because of its high soft tissue resolution, one can identify the majority of pharyngeal and laryngeal structures with one exposure. As can be seen from Figures 8–1 and 8–2, the lateral xeroradiograph allows visualization of a number of structures including the soft palate, aryepiglottic folds, palatopharyngeal arch, corniculate process of the arytenoid cartilages, laryngeal ventricles, vocal folds, and cricoid cartilage.

Although some individuals consider mineralization of the laryngeal cartilages abnormal, it has been determined that in the horse, as in man and the dog, mineralization of certain laryngeal cartilages is a normal process.[1–4] The body of the thyroid cartilage appears mineralized independent of age (Figs. 8–1 and 8–2). The laminae of the thyroid cartilage are the second most common areas of mineralization in the horse's larynx. One study showed mineralization of this region in 74 of 80 (93%) normal horses ranging in age from 4 days to 24 years (mean age of 6.0 years).[1] This mineralization (determined to be calcification) appears xeroradiographically as a diffuse lacy pattern (Fig. 8–1). The lamina has two centers of mineralization, one in the caudal aspect of the mid-lamina, the other in the caudal cornu (Figs. 8–1 and 8–3). With advancing age these two centers become confluent (Fig. 8–4). Since the caudal cornu is the caudalmost aspect of the thyroid cartilage and

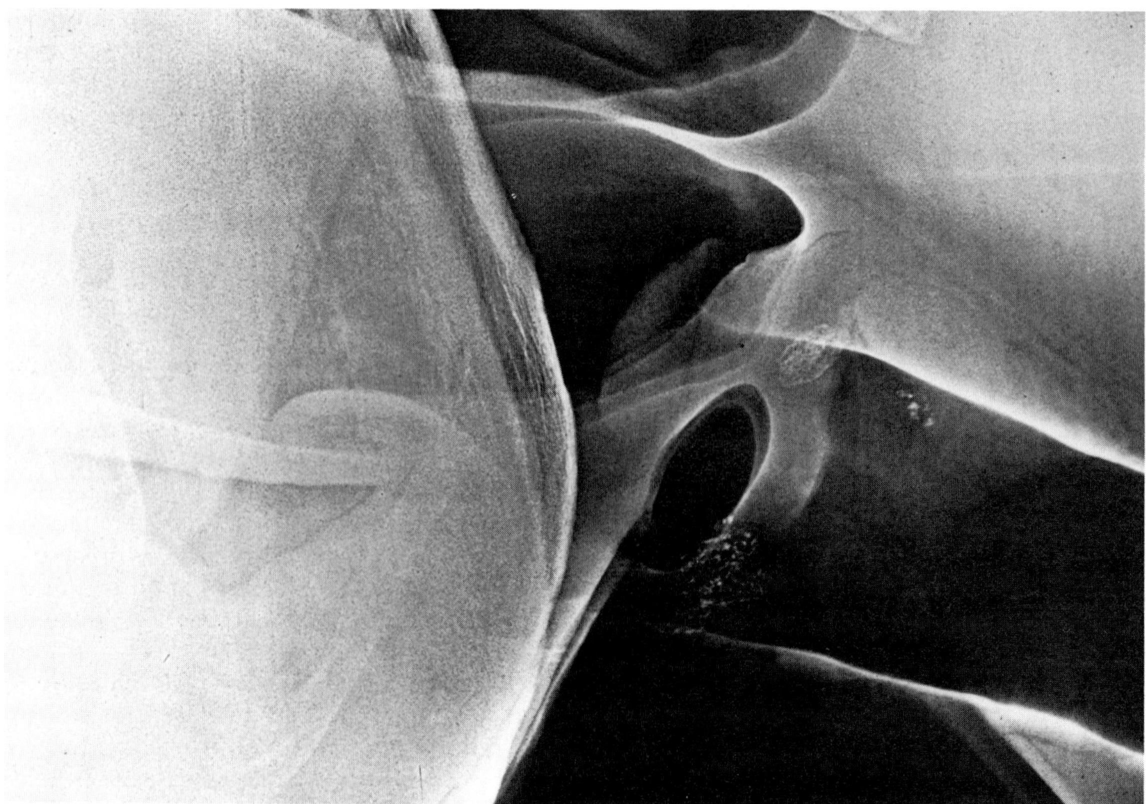

**FIG. 8–1.** Lateral xeroradiograph of the laryngeal region of a normal 7-year-old Thoroughbred.

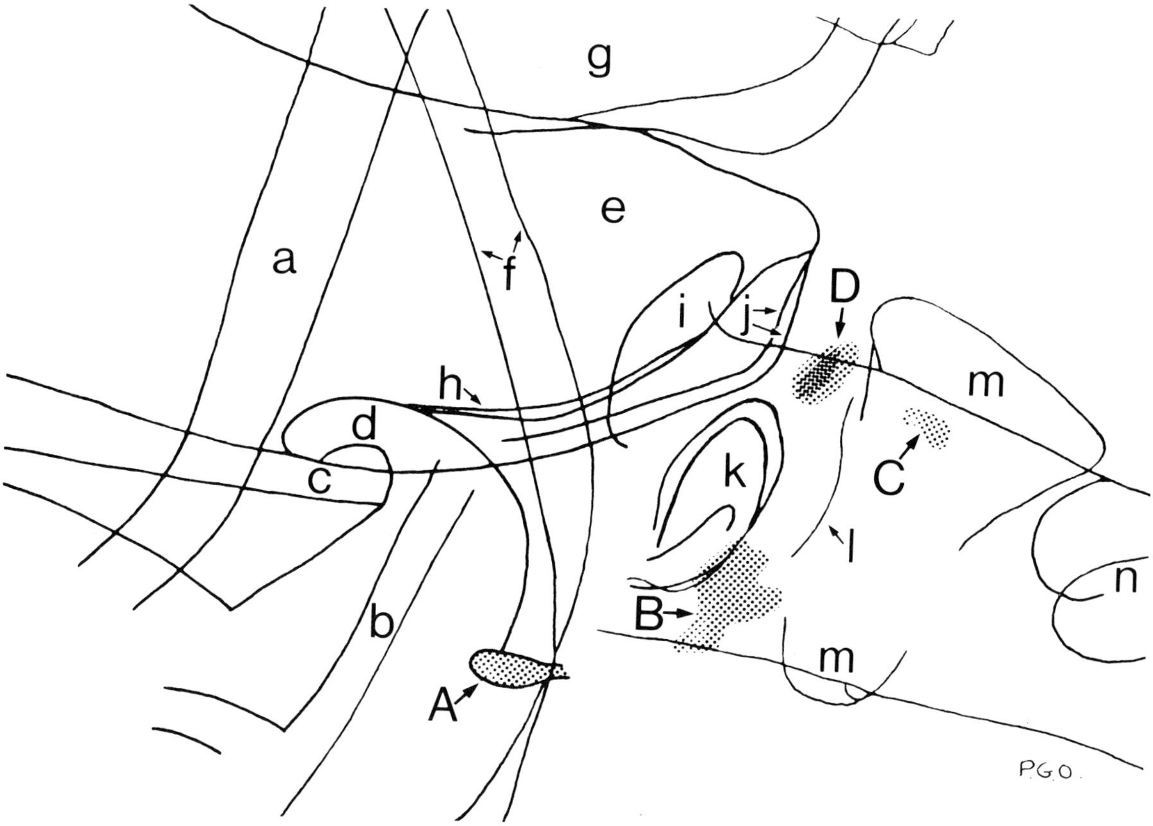

**FIG. 8–2.** Diagram of Figure 8–1. A. Body of thyroid cartilage. B. Calcification of thyroid laminae. C. Calcification of thyroid caudal cornua. D. Calcification of muscular processes of arytenoid cartilages. a. Stylohyoid bones. b. Thyrohyoid bones. c. Soft palate. d. Epiglottis. e. Nasopharynx. f. Rami of mandibles. g. Guttural pouches. h. Aryepiglottic folds. i. Corniculate cartilages. j. Palatopharyngeal arch. k. Lateral laryngeal saccules. l. Vocal process of arytenoid cartilage. m. Cricoid cartilage. n. Thyroid glands.

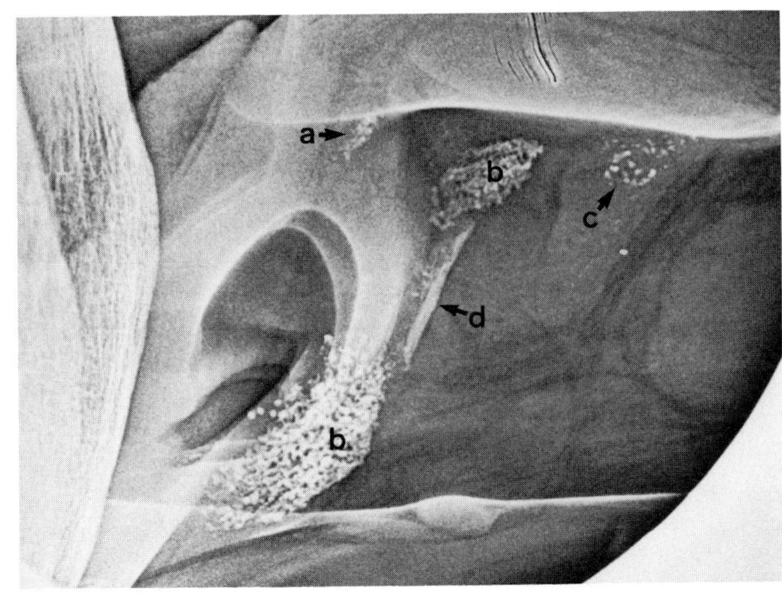


**FIG. 8–3.** Lateral xeroradiograph of the laryngeal region of a normal 14-year-old Thoroughbred showing calcification of the muscular processes of the arytenoid (a), thyroid (b), and cricoid (c) cartilages. Note the dense caudal border of the thyroid laminae (d).

thus the part that articulates with the cricoid cartilage, this area can be used as a radiographic landmark for the cricothyroid articulation. In older horses, the mineralization in the thyroid laminae has a denser and more linear appearance which corresponds to the caudal border of the cartilage (Figs. 8–3 and 8–4).

The muscular process is the only part of the arytenoid cartilage to mineralize in the normal horse and is the next most common area to show this change. It has been shown to undergo mineralization in 64% of the study group mentioned previously.[1] The core of mineralization appears as a discrete elliptical density dorsal to the laryngeal ventricles and just cranial to the cricoid cartilage. The average size and shape of this density can be seen in Figure 8–1. Located just caudal to the muscular process is the area of the arytenoid cartilage that articulates with the cricoid cartilage and therefore this can be used for a radiographic landmark to identify the cricoarytenoid articulation. Both the thyroid laminae and arytenoid cartilage mineralization have been shown to increase with age.[1]

The cricoid cartilage shows mineralization in only a small percentage of normal horses.[1] This mineralization is restricted to the caudal aspect of the lamina and dorsal arch region of the cartilage (Figs. 8–3 and 8–4). Unlike in the thyroid and arytenoid cartilages, there has been no correlation shown between degree of mineralization of the cricoid cartilage and increasing age.[1]

The epiglottic cartilage shows no tendency to mineralize, unlike in the dog in which it often undergoes mineralization. The cuneiform cartilage (cuneiform process of the epiglottis) and corniculate cartilage (corniculate process of the arytenoid cartilage) also show no tendency towards mineralization in the normal horse.[1]

When evaluating the cervical region, one has to remember that the cartilaginous tracheal rings undergo normal mineralization (Fig. 8–5). This finding is more common in the aged horse but has been seen in horses as young as 3 years of age.

In the lateral laryngeal xeroradiograph the two lateral laryngeal ventricles are easily visualized superimposed on each other in the center of the thyroid lamina region (Fig. 8–1). They normally have an elliptical shape with a dorsoventral long axis. They are usually symmetric in shape, one being slightly bigger than the other due to magnification of the ventricle farthest from the cassette (i.e., right ventricle). The size of the ventricles can vary depending on the stage of respiration at the time of exposure.

## Clinical Applications

Standard radiography is usually adequate as an adjunct to physical examination and endoscopy for the diagnosis of most upper airway disorders. Xeroradiography in most of

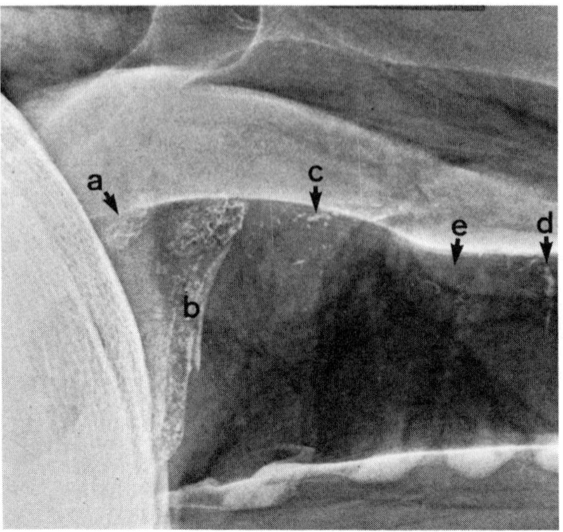


**FIG. 8–4.** Lateral xeroradiograph of the laryngeal region of a normal 24-year-old Thoroughbred showing calcification of the muscular processes of the arytenoid cartilages (a), thyroid (b), and cricoid (c) cartilages, as well as the tracheal rings (d). The thyroid glands (e) are also well delineated.

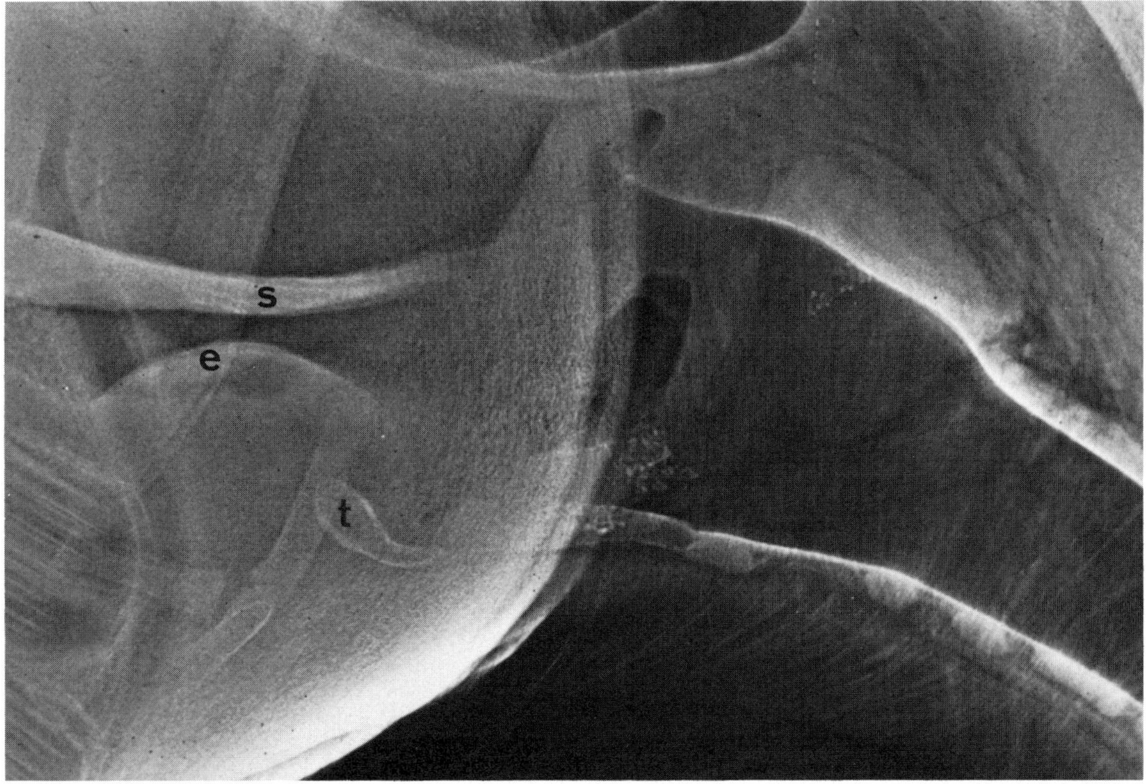


**FIG. 8–5.** Lateral xeroradiograph of the laryngeal region of a horse with persistent dorsal displacement of the soft palate (DDSP). Soft palate (s), hypoplastic epiglottis (e), body of the thyroid cartilage (t).

these cases gives a clearer, more easily discernable picture, but whether this is worth the added radiation exposure is up to the discretion of the clinician and radiologist. Examples of dorsal displacement of the soft palate (DDSP) and epiglottic entrapment (EE) are demonstrated in Figures 8–5 and 8–6. As described in the previous chapter, measurement of epiglottic length can be useful in the determination of the etiology of both these problems.[5] Although this measurement can be obtained from a standard radiograph, the xeroradiograph can facilitate it. Since DDSP and EE can occur simultaneously, in a case of persistent DDSP, the xeroradiograph can be helpful in determining whether the epiglottis is entrapped as the latter cannot be evaluated endoscopically in such cases. Pharyngeal and laryngeal masses such as subepiglottic cysts and abscesses as well as retropharyngeal

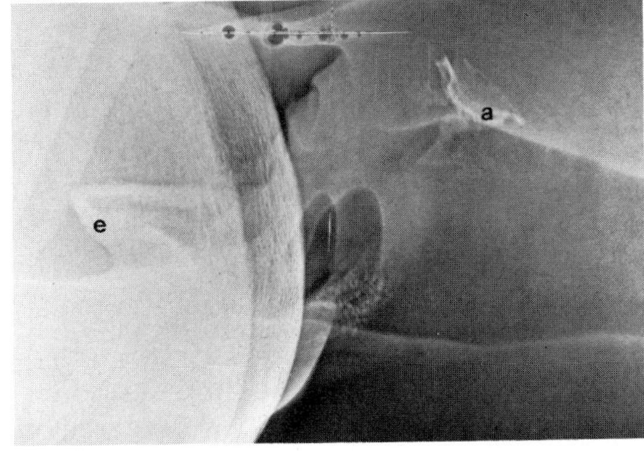


**FIG. 8–6.** Lateral xeroradiograph of the laryngeal region of a horse with an entrapped epiglottis as well as arytenoid chondrosis. Entrapped epiglottis (e), abnormal calcification of arytenoid cartilage (a).

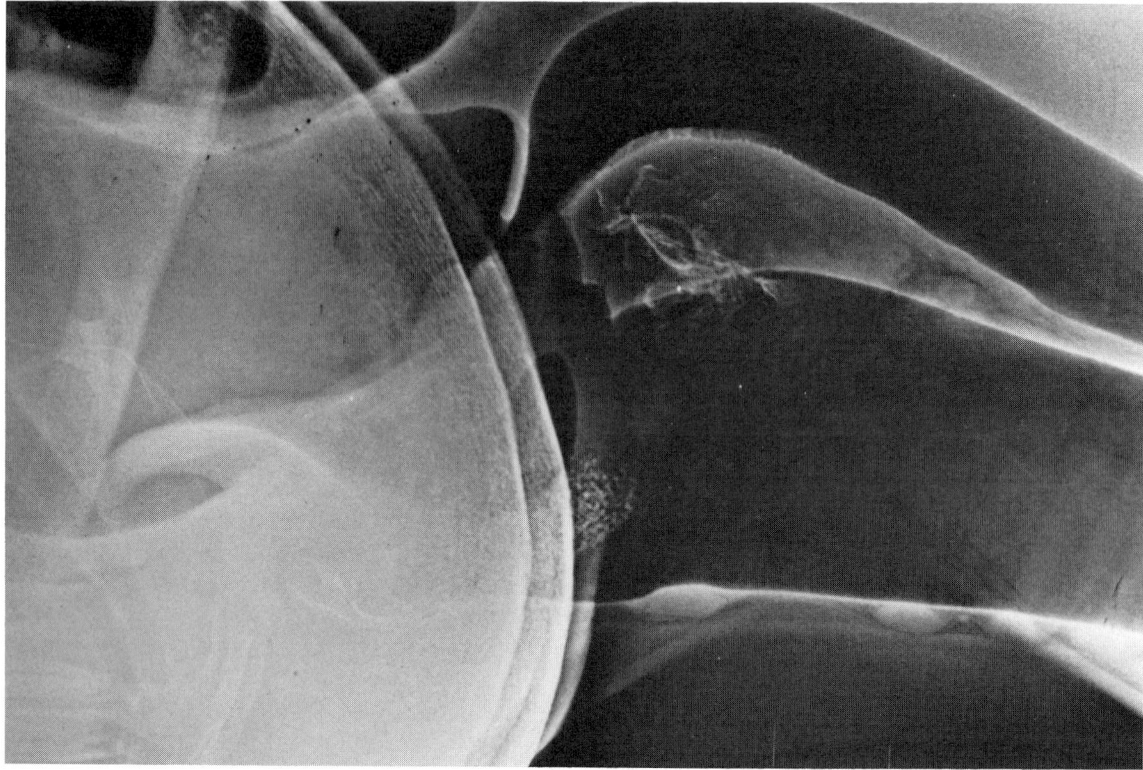

**FIG. 8–7.** Lateral xeroradiograph of the laryngeal region of a 3-year-old Standardbred with arytenoid chondrosis demonstrating the stellate configuration of calcification in the area of the dorsocaudal region of the arytenoid cartilage. Note the outline of only one laryngeal saccule. Note also the air distention of the esophagus due to sedation.

lymphadenopathy or an abscess can be more readily observed with the use of xeroradiography.

The most valuable use for the xeroradiographic evaluation of the upper respiratory tract of the horse is in the diagnosis of the early stages of arytenoid chondrosis. As has already been discussed in other chapters, arytenoid chondrosis is usually diagnosed by history, physical examination, and a thorough endoscopic examination. Diagnosis may be difficult in less severe cases and, in some instances, is confused with laryngeal hemiplegia. When evaluating for arytenoid chondrosis, the horse's head and neck should be in the extended position for the best xeroradiographic evaluation of the laryngeal cartilages. Abnormal radiographic findings in horses with arytenoid chondrosis are (in order of most common occurrence):

1. enlargement and overall increased density of the arytenoid cartilage region (Figs. 8–7 and 8–8)
2. abnormal amount and pattern of mineralization (dystrophic calcification) in the region of the arytenoid cartilage (Figs. 8–7 and 8–8)
3. abnormal contour of the corniculate processes of the arytenoid cartilage (Figs. 8–7 and 8–8)
4. soft tissue masses within the larynx, often obliterating part or all of the laryngeal ventricles (Fig. 8–8)

It is important that the radiographic demonstration of normal, age-related mineralization not be confused with the abnormal changes associated with arytenoid chondrosis.

## Conclusion

Xeroradiography is by no means essential for the diagnosis of most upper respiratory disorders. Its greater soft tissue resolution makes it helpful in a relatively small number

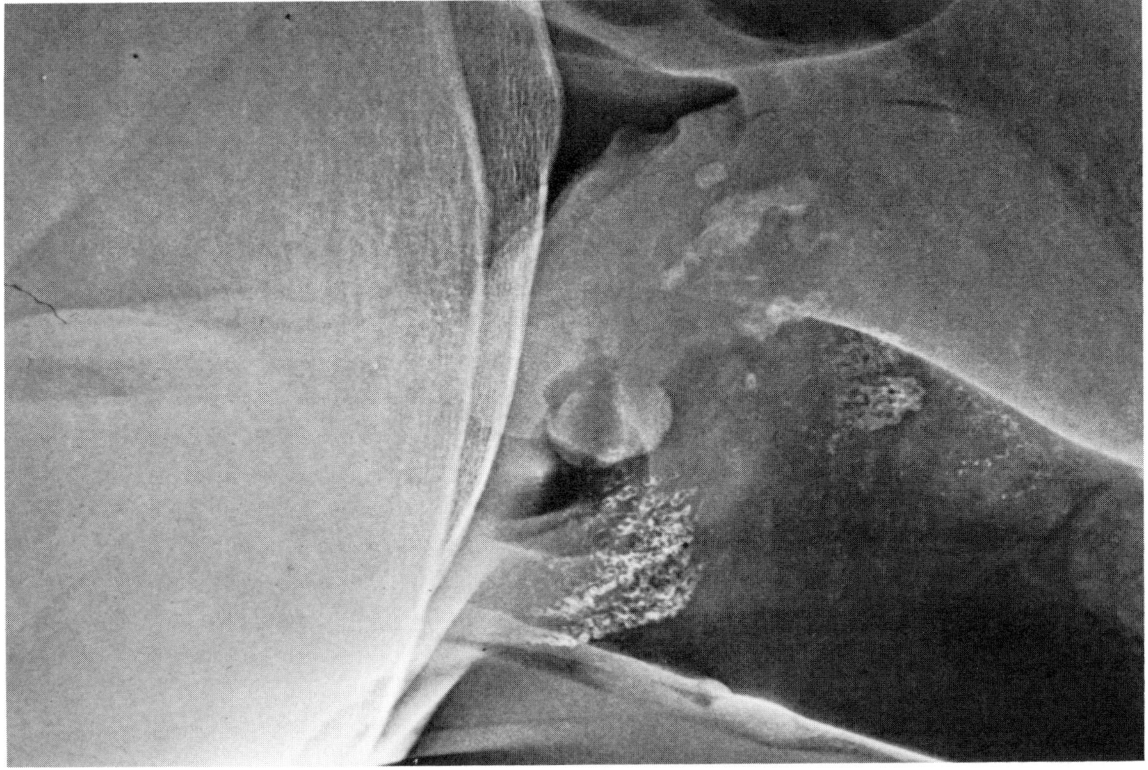

**FIG. 8–8.** Lateral xeroradiograph of the laryngeal region of a 5-year-old Thoroughbred with arytenoid chondrosis. Note the increased density of the arytenoid region with the abnormal calcification, the abnormal contour of the corniculate cartilages, and the soft tissue mass obliterating the laryngeal saccules.

of cases but that does not detract from its importance. It has been beneficial in describing the normal radiographic anatomy of the area and therefore has allowed a more thorough and thoughtful evaluation of standard radiographs of the region.

## References

1. Orsini PG, Raker CW, Reid CF, et al. Xeroradiographic evaluation of the equine larynx. Am J Vet Res, *50*:845, 1989.
2. Getty R. Sisson and Grossman's The Anatomy of the Domestic Animals. 5th ed. Philadelphia, WB Saunders Co, 1975.
3. O'Brien JA, Harvey CE, Tucker JA. The larynx of the dog: Its normal radiographic anatomy. J Am Radiol Soc, *10*:38, 1969.
4. Hately W, Evison G, Samuel E. The pattern of ossification in the laryngeal cartilages: A radiographic study. Br J Radiol, *38*:585, 1965.
5. Linford RL, O'Brien TR, Wheat JD, et al. Radiographic assessment of epiglottic length and pharyngeal and laryngeal diameters in the Thoroughbred. Am J Vet Res, *44*:1660, 1983.

# CHAPTER 9

# SCINTIGRAPHIC IMAGING OF LUNG DISEASE

*MICHAEL W. O'CALLAGHAN*

Nuclear medicine imaging (scintigraphy) provides a means of displaying or mapping a variety of lung functions. Compared to other lung function tests, scintigraphy has the advantage of displaying, in image form, regional variations of the parameter under study, instead of providing only a global measurement for the lung as a whole.

Until recently, evaluation of pulmonary conditions in horses has relied heavily on thoracic radiography. In spite of the satisfactory image resolution of modern rare earth screen/film combinations, many equine lung conditions are recognized radiographically only when accompanied by gross changes in lung architecture and lung tissue mass. Thus pleural effusion, bronchopneumonia, cardiac-induced pulmonary edema, and lung abscesses demonstrate well recognized radiographic patterns. However, many conditions implicated in poor performance such as bronchiolitis, COPD (chronic obstructive pulmonary disease), EIPH (exercise-induced pulmonary hemorrhage), and intralobular emphysema only occasionally produce distinctive patterns, even when severe. The major drawback of thoracic radiography, however, is the absence of direct information on lung functions such as air exchange, blood flow, ventilation/perfusion matching, solute exchange, and mucociliary clearance.

The value of scintigraphy lies in providing this functional information as a complement to radiographic examination and other lung function tests. Potentially, a wide variety of parameters can be imaged depending on the isotopes or the carrier medium chosen for the particular examination. Currently, in human medicine, scans of pulmonary ventilation and perfusion are the most commonly performed, using a wide variety of isotopes and administration methods. Other parameters under investigation for their clinical relevance are the clearance of aerosolized solutes (potentially sensitive indicators of subclinical interstitial disease and respiratory distress syndrome) and mucociliary clearance rates (reflecting clearance of particulate matter from the airways and hence integrity of the mucociliary elevator). Cell labeling techniques are also being investigated for their ability to demonstrate accumulations of specific white cell populations. At present only ventilation/perfusion scans are employed on a wide scale, most other procedures being limited to research applications or clinical trials.

The first scintigraphic examinations on horses were performed to demonstrate pulmonary arterial perfusion and ventilation in equine lung disease.[1] Most reports on ventilation/perfusion imaging relate to experimental studies.[2–5] The rate of solute clearance from the lung using DTPA (diaminetriaminepenta acetate) aerosol has been determined for normal horses[4] and a limited number of clinical cases studied using the technique. Mucociliary clearance rates have also been investigated in horses, mainly using nuclear probes placed over the trachea.[6] Preliminary investigations of camera images have been carried out in a few institutions.

## Scintigraphic Technique

Scintigraphy is performed by first administering to the patient a gamma emitting radioisotope either by itself or attached to a carrier substance. The passage or accumulation of the isotope, or the label to which it is attached, is then recorded by a gamma camera placed over the organ of interest. Alternatively, a gamma counter or probe can be used to record the accumulated gamma photon emission rate at different points over the thorax. Probes are suitable only for recording count rates or generating time function curves, but not an image. With a gamma camera a planar image of the area subtended by the face of the camera is displayed, demonstrating regional variation in count rates (scintigraphy). When linked to a dedicated computer system, the recorded data can be subjected to a wide range of image manipulation methods and analysis.

To produce satisfactory images of the horse's lung, radionuclides are limited to those with gamma energies in the range of 100 to 500 kev. For practical reasons and safety, only isotopes with relatively short half-lives are suitable (i.e., less than 3 to 5 days). The ideal energy for equine lung imaging lies between approximately 140 to 200 kev. Higher energies require heavy collimation and result in "shinethrough" from the opposite lung, while lower energy photons are heavily absorbed (attenuated) in the chest wall. Attenuation of emerging photons also occurs in the lung tissue, an effect which increases with distance from the thoracic wall. Scintigraphic images of the lung are therefore heavily weighted in favor of counts arising in the superficial layers of the lung. This effect is greatest for isotopes with the lowest energies.

Radioisotopes administered to the patient emit radiation in all directions. Therefore, in order to determine the planar origin of each

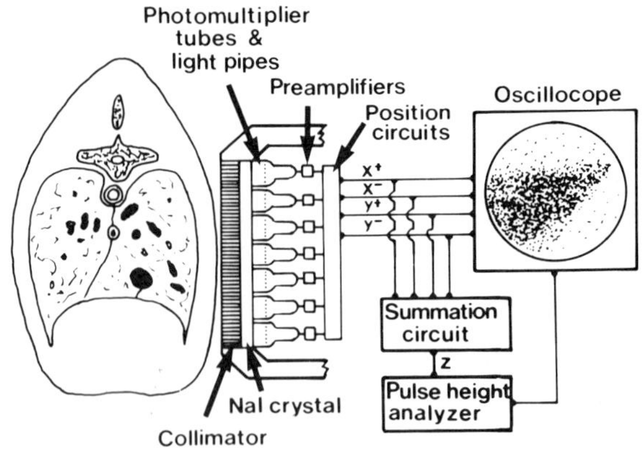


**FIG. 9–1.** Essential components of a gamma camera and recording system. Photons of gamma energy originating from the radioactive material in the horse's lung (left) penetrate the collimator causing the sodium iodide crystal to flow at each point of strike. The light generated by each strike is recorded simultaneously at each photomultiplier tube, the strongest signal arising from the tube immediately over the strike. The amplified signals generated by the strike are then summed electrically to provide X+, X−, Y+ and Y− coordinates. These determine the physical position of the strike on the camera face. Provided the summed strength of these signals falls within a preset energy window, determined by the pulse height analyzer, a Z pulse is generated resulting in projection of a single point of light on the oscilloscope at the calculated x,y position. The x,y, and z signals can also be transmitted to a multiformat camera or computer.

scintillation, the camera is fitted with a collimator which allows only photons traveling at a particular orientation to the camera face to enter the camera. Most collimators are designed to allow parallel, converging, diverging, or selectively angled photons to reach the camera face. Photons penetrating the collimator strike the face of a large, flat crystal (usually made of sodium iodide) which fluoresces at the point of each photon strike. Behind the crystal is an array of photomultiplier tubes (typically 37 or 91 tubes in a large-field-of-view system) each responding to the glow by generating an electrical pulse (Fig. 9–1). The amplified signal from each photomultiplier tube is fed into a discriminator which first rejects counts from photons not in the correct preset energy range (photopeak and window). By analyzing the strength of the signal from each tube the exact spatial origin of the incident photon is determined.

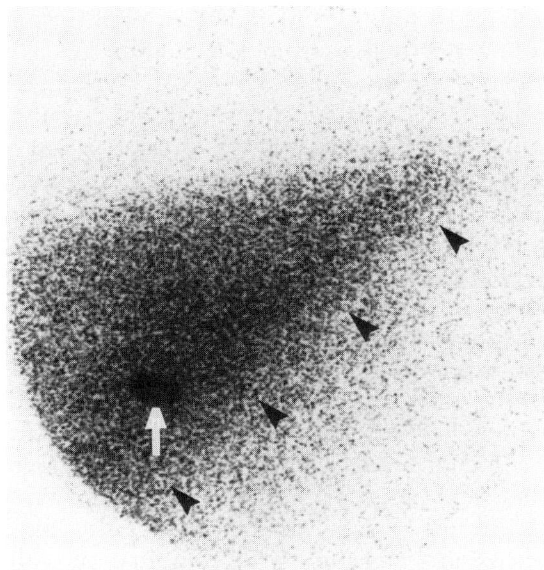

**FIG. 9–2.** Ventilation image of the caudal left lung of a normal horse generated with $^{99m}$Technetium-DTPA aerosol. The image is composed of numerous small dots generated in a multiformat camera. The lower diagonal border (arrowheads) represents the diaphragmatic margin. A darker focal area (arrow) represents activity from a radioactive marker placed on the skin as a reference point.

The resulting signal is then transformed into x,y coordinates and a point is displayed on an oscilloscope or transmitted to photographic film for subjective analysis (Fig. 9–2). The same digitized x,y signal can be recorded on a dedicated computer system for later analysis under program control. Numerous computer systems are available for nuclear medicine applications. Unfortunately, most software provided for lung function analysis is suitable only for human studies. Therefore if analysis beyond subjective evaluation of the raw images is required, it is necessary for end users to develop their own software.

## Ventilation/Perfusion Imaging

### *Ventilation Imaging*

Scintigraphic images taken to demonstrate ventilation function in man are obtained using a variety of radionuclides.[7] Many studies employ the poorly soluble, noble gas, $^{133}$Xenon, which has an energy of 80 kev and a half life of 5.2 days. The relatively long half-life allows a variety of diagnostic maneuvers in the cooperative patient. For clinical imaging three sequential steps are routinely followed: a single breath image, an image at equilibrium after rebreathing, followed by sequential washout images. With a single "breath and hold," which can be performed in human beings but not in horses, the image obtained reflects ventilatory flow or regional distribution of tidal volume. Washin or washout studies highlight areas of the lung with restricted ventilation and air trapping, conditions in which aeration of affected lung is achieved by collateral supply. For washin or washout the patient breathes the xenon over several minutes. Images are recorded at regular intervals, either during inhalation until equilibrium is reached, or from equilibrium until most of the gas has been eliminated. In both cases areas of slow or restricted exchange (increased time constants) are either slow to reach equilibrium during washin or demonstrate delayed washout of the radioactive gas. Images recorded at equilibrium display information effectively representing lung volume, i.e., counts are proportional to the volume of air contained in the lung, some of which may not have been exchanged with the tidal volume, but reached diseased areas by collateral flow. Unfortunately, the low 80 kev gamma energy of $^{133}$Xenon is inadequate for horses, resulting in severe attenuation of the emerging photons in the thoracic wall and unsatisfactory images.

$^{81m}$Krypton, another of the noble gases, has also been used in man and the horse. It is almost ideal for ventilation flow mapping with a 13-second half-life and a gamma energy of 190 kev. Because of its extremely short half-life, activity recorded from the lungs is derived predominantly from gas contained in inspired air. Images are thus heavily weighted in favor of ventilatory flow. Unfortunately, $^{81m}$Krypton is generated from a parent isotope, $^{81}$Rhubidium, which has a half-life of only 4.7 hours, thereby reducing its ready availability and making it impractical for most clinical situations. The techniques required for satisfactory delivery are also exacting, making it suitable only for research purposes. Several other radioactive gases have been employed for pulmonary ventilation studies but have major disadvantages: $^{15}$Oxygen and $^{13}$Nitrogen (short half-lives and require an on-site cyclotron), $^{127}$Xenon (long half-life—34.6 days), and $^{85m}$Krypton (cyclotron produced).

Various attempts have been made to use radioactive aerosols for ventilation imaging since 1965,[8,9] however, until recently the technical difficulty of producing a uniform aerosol with droplet sizes less than 2 μm has limited the use of this technique. When the median aerodynamic diameter of aerosol droplets is greater than 2 μm there is significant deposition in the trachea and large bronchi. This produces focal artifacts which obscure the pattern of deposition in the lung. Recent improvements in nebulizer design and reliable production of aerosols between 0.5 to 1.5 μm has resulted in rapid and widespread acceptance of aerosols for lung scanning.[10] While aerosols may lack the flexibility of $^{133}$Xenon and the precision of $^{81m}$Krypton, they have the advantage of allowing the use of $^{99m}$Technetium, the most widely used and easily managed radionuclide for scintigraphy. Other nuclides such as $^{111}$Indium have also been employed in human medicine. Owing to its high energy $^{111}$Indium is useful only for frontal views in man and impractical in horses because of shine through from the opposite lung. Recently a new solid particle aerosol called "Technegas" has been developed, produced by heating $^{99m}$Technetium in a carbon crucible under an argon atmosphere.[11] Tiny particles of carbon measuring approximately 0.005 μm each containing a single atom of technetium are released. Such fine particles behave more like gases, but with the advantage of remaining in the alveoli for long periods without reabsorption.

## Perfusion Imaging

Perfusion studies in man and other species are generally performed using $^{99m}$Technetium-MAA (macro-aggregated albumin) injected intravenously.[12] This agent remains the main method of demonstrating pulmonary perfusion deficits. $^{99m}$Tc-MAA is prepared from a lyophilized preparation reconstituted with $^{99m}$Technetium in the form of the pertechnetate, eluted from a generator or obtained as a unit dose. MAA particles range from 10 to 60 μm, most of which are trapped in the alveolar vascular bed on first passage through the lung after intravenous injection. Deficits in distribution therefore reflect reduced pulmonary flow to the affected area. Pulmonary perfusion can also be measured using $^{81m}$Krypton delivered intravenously in a saline perfusion. Most of the poorly soluble gas diffuses into the alveoli on first pass through the lung vasculature. Owing to the extremely short half-life, activity recorded in the image reflects pulmonary arterial flow. This method is technically difficult and limited to use in experimental studies. In man, perfusion scans alone or in combination with ventilation scans are particularly valuable in the diagnosis of pulmonary embolism. Deficits are also readily identified in conditions such as COPD, cystic fibrosis, lung abscesses, and pneumonia.

## *Ventilation/Perfusion Balance*

Evaluation of separate ventilation and perfusion images is of limited value since efficiency of the lung depends on matching of these two functions. Ventilation/perfusion matching can be assessed in a variety of ways varying from subjective viewbox comparisons of the separate images to complex computer controlled analyses derived from pixel-by-pixel estimates of ventilation/perfusion match. In the horse, a number of experimental studies using $^{81m}$Krypton have been employed to investigate ventilation/perfusion balance in the conscious standing and anesthetized state.[2,3] For these studies $^{81m}$Krypton was employed for both the ventilation and perfusion images. Delivery of the gas for both ventilation and perfusion studies requires exacting technique, considerable patient cooperation and carries significant exposure risk despite the short half-life of the isotope. Amis et al (1984)[2] demonstrated that adult standing horses have a gravity dependent gradient of ventilation and perfusion per unit alveolar volume, with lowest values dorsally and greatest values ventrally (0.5 to 1.4 in arbitrary units). In contrast to man and the dog, in the horse well-balanced ventilation/perfusion ratios were detected at each vertical level in the lung, concluded by these authors to be a natural adaptation of the horse to high exercise demand and the need for optimal lung efficiency. In anesthetized horses ventilation/perfusion ratios in the nondependent lung were shown to be significantly higher than the lowermost lung, so that severe mismatch occurred.[3] These findings support physiologic measurements of global lung function determined on anesthetized horses, but also demonstrated the side involved and the relative extent of mismatch.

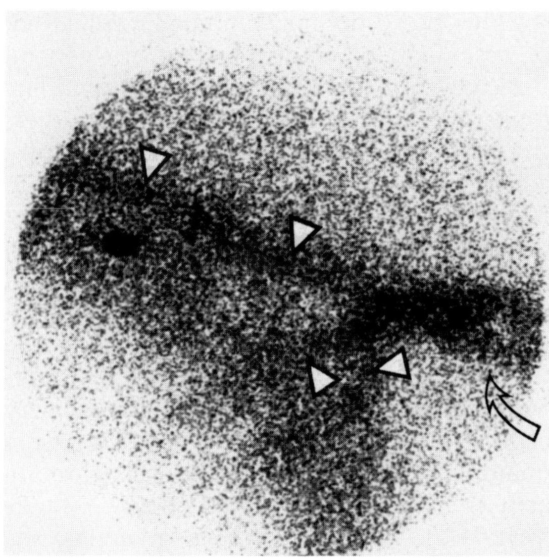

**FIG. 9–3.** Increased turbulence has caused aberrant deposition of radioaerosol in the trachea (arrow) and larger airways (arrowheads) of a horse with severe chronic obstructive pulmonary disease. Aerosol droplet size (0.3 to 1.0 μ) was the same as that employed for the normal horse in Figure 9–2. A radioactive skin marker is evident ventral to the caudal mainstem bronchus.

## *Equine Studies*

Only limited numbers of equine clinical cases have been reported.[1] Perfusion deficits are seen in the caudodorsal angles of the lung field in horses with EIPH, with and without evidence of radiographic lesions.[5] Large perfusion deficits as a result of intrathoracic masses detected on first pass flow studies have also been reported.[13]

For more complete analysis of lung function, ventilation imaging is required to complement perfusion studies, particularly as balanced ventilation/perfusion is critical to optimal lung function. Currently the aerosol of choice for ventilation studies in horses is DTPA, a chelating agent easily attached to $^{99m}$Technetium from freeze dried preparations. For delivery to the lungs a specially adapted nebulizer is required. Aerosol droplets must have a median aerodynamic diameter in the range of 0.3 to 1.5 μm with a narrow geometric standard deviation to avoid upper airway deposition and ensure delivery to the alveoli and terminal bronchioles. Aerosol deposition in the lungs occurs as a result of either inertial impaction or sedimentation. Larger particles are more often deposited by impaction as a result of their inertia, an effect enhanced by turbulence at bends and branches in the airways or by partial airway obstruction. Smaller particles are carried on the decreasing air currents until their settling velocity exceeds air flow velocity resulting in sedimentation. For droplets in the range of 0.3 to 1.5 μm, most have been shown to reach the alveoli.[14] Aerosols with droplets only slightly above this range (2 to 10 μm) deposit mainly in the upper airways by inertial impaction, particularly at the carina and upper airway branching points. In the presence of partial airway obstruction such as in cases of COPD, even particles in an acceptable range for normal animals accumulate in the upper airways and trachea (Fig. 9–3).

For delivery to the horse the aerosol from the nebulizer(s) must be discharged into a breathing circuit which allows only filtered exhaust air to enter the room. The mask system for delivery to the horse must also have a tight seal around the horse's nose to avoid contamination of the room air. Various systems have been devised for delivery of aerosols to human patients and have also been developed for horses.[4] Aerosol can be generated by a venturi or other style of nebulizer or an ultrasonic system, provided mean aerodynamic droplet diameter is between 0.3 to 1.5 μm. Compressed air or a pump capable of supplying air to two or more nebulizers at 15 L/min is necessary for a Venturi system.

Clinic protocols for combined ventilation/perfusion studies vary; however, the general principles are the same. Since the same isotope, $^{99m}$technetium, is used for both studies, the only way to separate ventilation-derived activity from activity delivered during perfusion is to use a considerably greater amount (5 to 6×) of radioactivity for the second procedure. In published protocols the ventilation study is performed first with delivery of approximately 3 mCi of $^{99m}$Tc-DTPA aerosol to the airways, followed by 15 to 20 mCi of $^{99m}$Tc-MAA for the perfusion image.[5] This delivery sequence also avoids having to deliver large quantities of aerosol; higher doses of radioactivity are more easily handled as injectable $^{99m}$Tc-MAA. In practice after attaching the horse to the mask and ventilation circuit, $^{99m}$Tc-DTPA made up to 20 mCi/ml is delivered as an aerosol from two nebulizers over 4 minutes. Immediately following delivery, four images each of 1 minute's duration are acquired, two from each side—cranial and caudal. Most views average 100 to 150K counts/field. Immediately 15 to 20 mCi of $^{99m}$Tc-MAA is injected intravenously through a preplaced catheter. Four 30-second images are then recorded, averaging 800 to 1000K/per field. Whole images are recorded on a microdot imager and on the computer system as a series of 2.5 second dynamic frames. The frames recorded on the computer are then reframed into full images under operator control. Any frames with obvious movement are excluded and the final image scaled up by the average of the frame total (Fig. 9–4). Alternatively, acquisition can be in list mode, a sequential method of recording counts and timing data which allows for more flexible reframing later. The disadvantage of this method is the computer space required.

Even with a large-field-of-view gamma camera a single lateral view of an adult horse's lung cannot be obtained. It is therefore necessary to record cranial and caudal images of the lung and merge them under computer control if a single image suitable for numeric analysis is required.[5] To assist in merging, a reference point common to the two lung halves is needed—a radioactive Cobalt or Americium marker placed on the skin is suitable (Fig. 9–5). The marker is then employed to

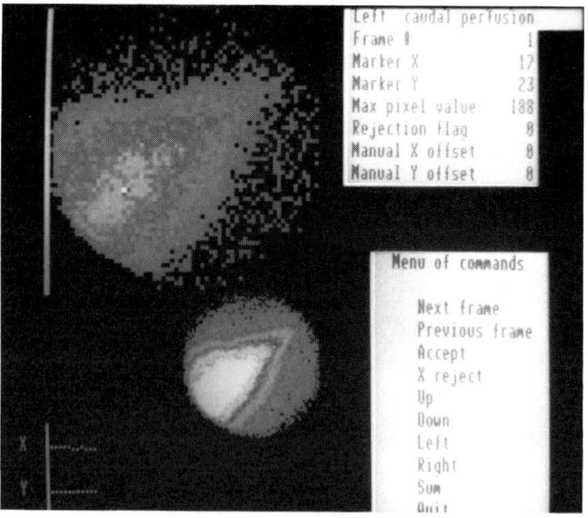


**FIG. 9–4.** Screen display for operator-controlled summation of 2.5 second image frames to form a composite image. This method of image handling allows rejection of frames with movement artifact. The image at top left is a single 2.5 second frame from a perfusion study of the left caudal lung. On the lower left a histogram of the x and y movement of a radioactive marker on the body surface is displayed for the 12 recorded frames. The summed image of the 12 frames appears in the middle of the screen. Relevant image related data and instructions to the operator are displayed in the boxes on the right of the screen.

overlay the ventilation and perfusion images for assessment of regional $\dot{V}/\dot{Q}$ matching analysis. Other mathematical methods of aligning images such as summed least squares pixel count differences are also possible.

In order to compare ventilation and perfusion images acquired in the above described protocol the ventilation component incorporated in the raw perfusion image must first be removed by subtracting a mask of the ventilation image. The ventilation image is then scaled up to the perfusion image, either using the maximum count in the frame as a reference or by calculating the mean count in each frame and scaling the ventilation frame mean up to the perfusion mean. Both methods have their advantages and disadvantages.

Numerous methods for displaying the resulting ventilation and perfusion images are possible. For convenience it is helpful to include in the same display, an image of the ventilation/perfusion ratios obtained by dividing the ventilation image by the perfusion image. A frequency histogram scaled be-

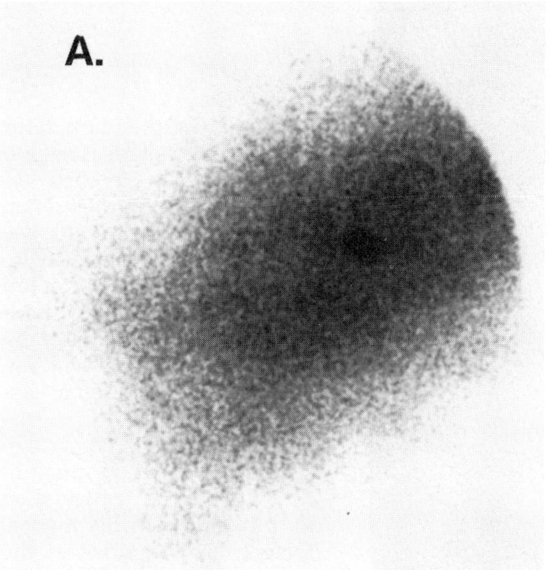


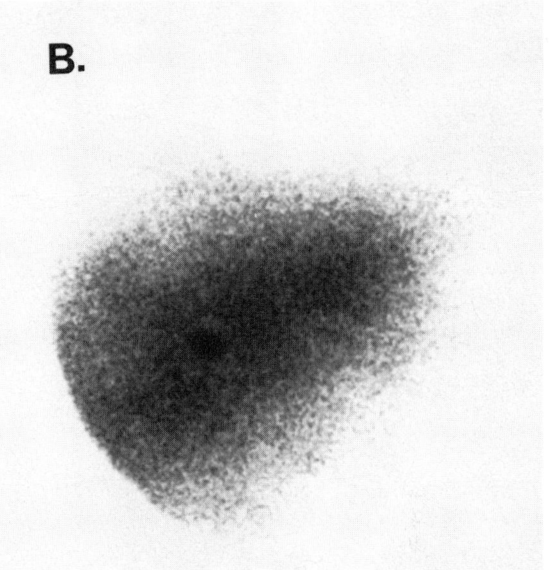


**FIG. 9–5.** The radioactive skin marker used for merging is shown on the cranial (A) and caudal (B) perfusion images of a horse with moderate COPD. Note the uneven count density over the lung, the irregular diaphragmatic margin and the blunt caudal tip, all characteristic findings on both ventilation and perfusion images of COPD cases.

tween arbitrary limits of 1:4 to 4:1 also assists the reader in assessing the case (Fig. 9–6). Other scales have been incorporated into our software in order to highlight minor or major differences.

## *Clinical Case Evaluation*

As there are few reports on scintigraphic evaluation of lung disease in horses, preliminary results from the Tufts University New England Veterinary Clinic are presented to demonstrate the value of scintigraphy in these conditions. Our clinical case evaluations include approximately 100 horses referred for assessment of:

1. Exercise induced pulmonary hemorrhage (EIPH)
2. Chronic obstructive pulmonary disease (COPD) or "heaves"
3. Poor performance thought to be of cardiopulmonary origin
4. Pre-training and pre-racing evaluation of young horses
5. Miscellaneous cases, some with radiographically obvious lung diseases such as pleuritis, interstitial infiltrate or abscesses.

### EIPH

The pattern of ventilation and perfusion in a limited number of horses with EIPH and radiographic signs of the disease has been described as a caudodorsal deficit in perfusion resulting in a high $\dot{V}/\dot{Q}$ ratio in the same area.[5] In a number of cases with more recent histories of bleeding and no overt radiographic signs similar dorsocaudal distributions of perfusion deficits have been observed with similar high $\dot{V}/\dot{Q}$ ratios. In most of these the perfusion (and in the worst cases ventilation) deficits were more confined to the dorsocaudal margin than in a previously reported study.[5] A prominent horizontal gradation from dorsal to ventral was also noted (Fig. 9–7).

### COPD

COPD cases have displayed three distinctively different patterns. In the majority of cases patchy distributions of increased and decreased counts were evident throughout the lung on both ventilation and perfusion

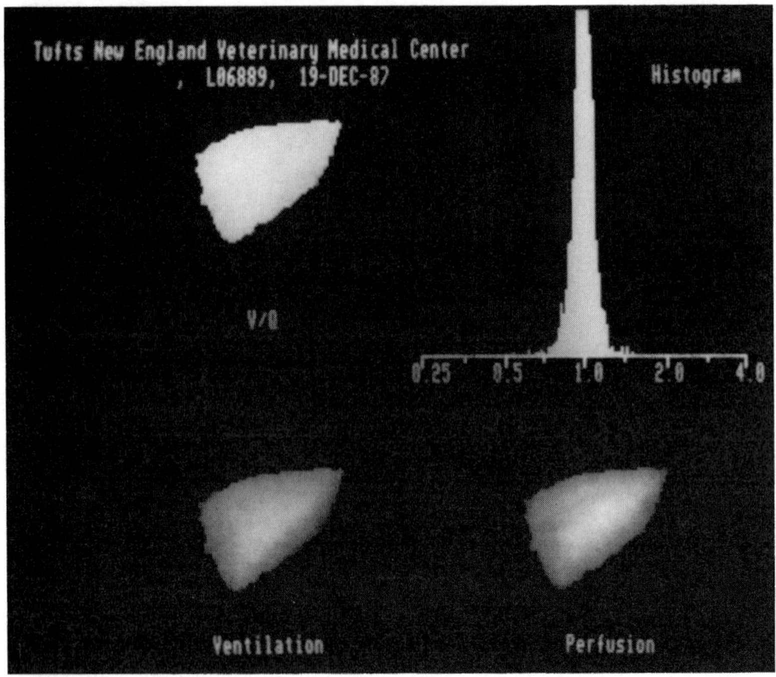


**FIG. 9–6.** Display format for final merged images. The two lower images were each obtained by merging the cranial and caudal images using the radioactive marker as a common reference. The upper left image was derived by dividing the ventilation image by the perfusion image to obtain an image of the regional distribution of $\dot{V}/\dot{Q}$ ratios. A histogram of the frequency distribution of the $\dot{V}/\dot{Q}$ ratios in the $\dot{V}/\dot{Q}$ image is displayed on the top right. In this normal horse count densities in the images were evenly distributed and the $\dot{V}/\dot{Q}$ ratios were tightly centered around 1 in the histogram.

images (Fig. 9–8). This distribution was also patchy on the $\dot{V}/\dot{Q}$ image suggesting that the deficits were not evenly matched throughout the lung. The most prominent deficits, and those recognized most easily in the milder cases, were in the costophrenic angle along the caudoventral diaphragmatic margin, an area of the lung not visible on routine radiographs. In many of these cases tracheal deposition was also noted reflecting increased airway turbulence and impaction deposition (Fig. 9–9). This pattern of ventilation and perfusion is similar to that reported for human COPD cases. A second but much less frequent pattern was a severe unmatched ventilation deficit in the mid dorsal area of the lung (Fig. 9–10). The remainder of the lung was evenly perfused and ventilated; however, there was some tracheal deposition, severe in one case. The third pattern noted in a small number of cases was similar to that in cases with confirmed EIPH. In these cases, however, ventilation and perfusion were both fairly equally impaired with better balance of the $\dot{V}/\dot{Q}$ ratios in the dorsocaudal lung. We have interpreted this to be evidence of small airway disease or bronchiolitis confined to the dorsocaudal lung. From this preliminary information there appear to be several different mechanisms (and possibly different etiologies?) contributing to cases with the clinical COPD syndrome. Further study of these cases is required, particularly correlation between the ventilation/perfusion images and the extent and nature of the pathologic lesions.

## Poor Performance

More than half of the poor performance cases demonstrated a pattern of ventilation and perfusion similar to cases of EIPH. One case also demonstrated a cranioventral cutoff of ventilation and perfusion plus a high $\dot{V}/\dot{Q}$ ratio in the dorsocaudal lungfield typical of the pattern in EIPH. Radiographic examination in this case revealed pleuritis. Another case displayed a mid dorsal area of severely reduced perfusion. Radiographs of this horse showed a hyperlucent dorsocaudal lung with reduced pulmonary vasculature in the area ventral to the aorta, suggesting emphysema. No obvious deficits were detected in the remaining cases. Further analysis of these cases is continuing.

## Pretraining and Preracing Evaluations

In young horses prior to training most showed an even pattern of ventilation and

A.

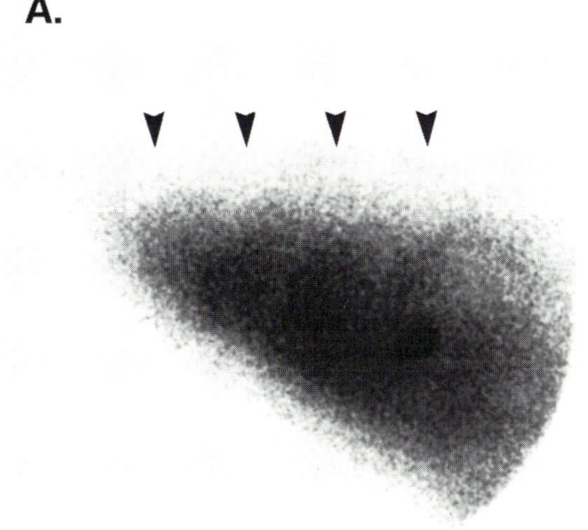

B.

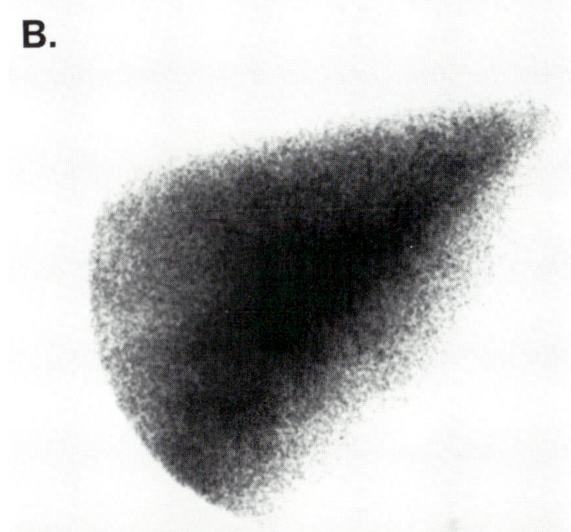

C.

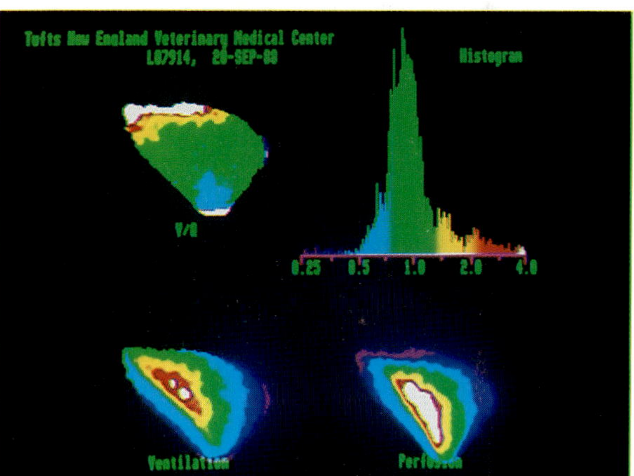


**FIG. 9–7.** A. Perfusion scan of the right lung in a horse with a history of chronic EIPH. Note the somewhat horizontal deficit along the dorsocaudal surface of the lung (arrowheads) and the low count density at the apex. A horizontal gradation of count densities is noted beneath the deficit (the horse's head is to the right). B. Perfusion scan of the left lung in a normal horse for comparison. Note the sharp caudal angle to the lung and the even count densities dorsally. C. Ventilation, perfusion, and $\dot{V}/\dot{Q}$ images in a horse with EIPH demonstrating a dorsocaudal perfusion deficit and corresponding high $\dot{V}/\dot{Q}$ ratios in the same area.

perfusion, a balanced $\dot{V}/\dot{Q}$ ratio and sharp acute angles to the dorsocaudal tip of the lung (Fig. 9–11). A small number showed slightly patchy ventilation. Sequential scans were performed in one horse and this pattern was repeatedly found. In all cases this improved once horses were in training. The significance of this finding is uncertain, but could indicate immature lungs in which aeration only improved with training stress. Horses in the trained, prerace group, with few exceptions, demonstrated even distribution of ventilation, perfusion and $\dot{V}/\dot{Q}$ ratios. Two horses showed a faint increase in $\dot{V}/\dot{Q}$ ratio along the dorsocaudal margin of the lung. Both subsequently bled from the lungs at their first and second starts respectively. One was scanned several days after the bleeding incident, displaying a pattern similar to that seen in other EIPH cases.

### Miscellaneous Cases

In cases with radiographically obvious lesions ventilation and perfusion deficits generally corresponded to the visible lesions.

## Imaging Other Parameters

In man, the clearance rate of $^{99m}$Tc-DTPA aerosol from the lung, expressed as the clearance half-time is a sensitive index of certain conditions affecting the interstitium such as acute respiratory distress syndrome (ARDS), COPD and cystic fibrosis. In normal humans and horses, clearance follows a monoexponential function with an average half-time of 50 to 60 minutes (Fig. 9–12).[4,15] Under experimental or clinical conditions of accelerated clearance, curve analysis indicates that a biex-

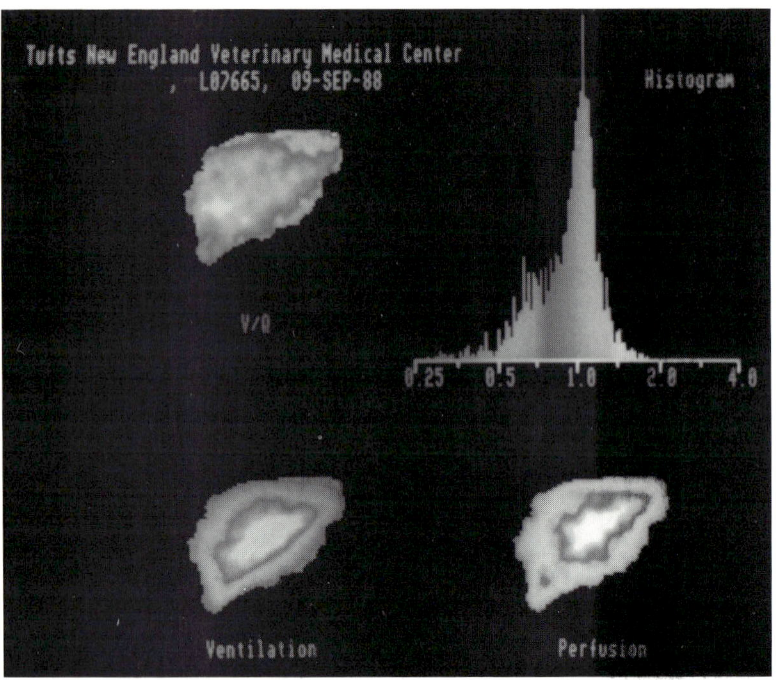


**FIG. 9–8.** Ventilation, perfusion and $\dot{V}/\dot{Q}$ ratio images of a horse with moderately severe COPD, but displaying only mild symptoms at the time of the scan. Note the patchy distribution of counts in all images and the skewed histogram indicating considerable ventilation-perfusion mismatching.

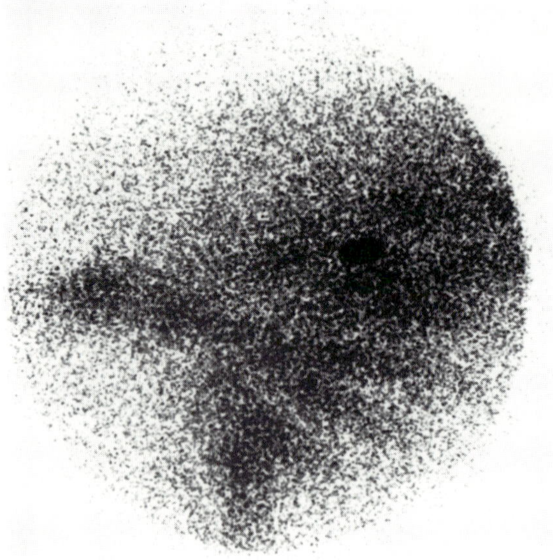

**FIG. 9–9.** Ventilation image of the left cranial lung field of a horse with moderately severe COPD. Patchy distribution of aerosol in this case is accentuated by impaction deposition in the trachea and larger airways. Excessive airway turbulence is considered the main reason for the increased deposition in the upper airways.

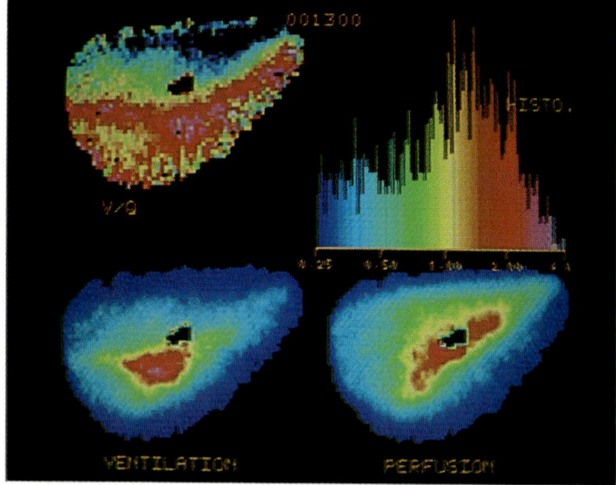


**FIG. 9–10.** Ventilation, perfusion, and $\dot{V}/\dot{Q}$ ratio images of a horse with moderate COPD. The horse had responded well to treatment and had no clinically obvious symptoms at the time of the scan. This pattern of severe ventilatory deficit in the dorsal lung fields has been noted in a small number of horses with COPD. Note also the increased deposition of aerosol in the large airways and the asymmetric distribution of $\dot{V}/\dot{Q}$ ratios on the histogram.

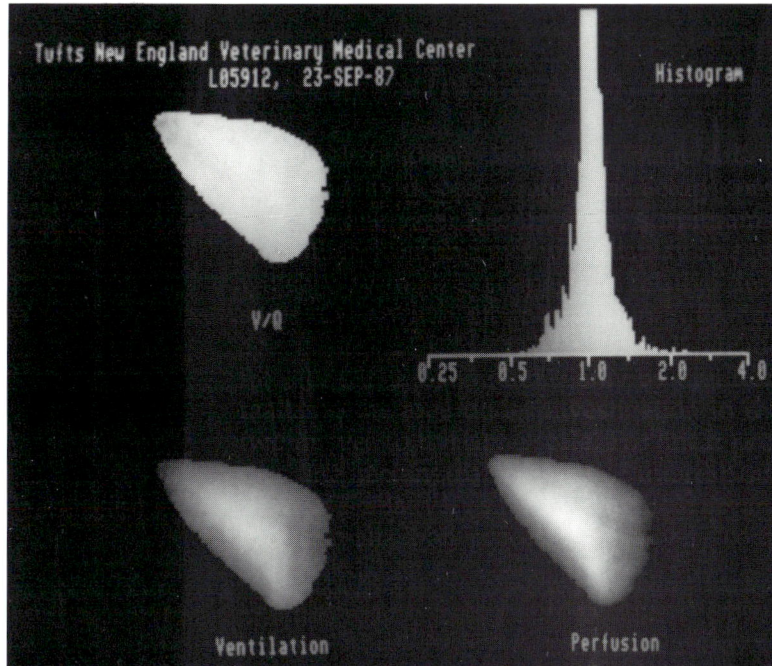


**FIG. 9–11.** Preracing scan on a young horse demonstrating normal ventilation, perfusion, and $\dot{V}/\dot{Q}$ ratio images. Note the even distribution of counts in the images and the narrow histogram of $\dot{V}/\dot{Q}$ ratios centered around 1.

ponential component becomes important in clearance dynamics, the first exponent of which has an extremely short half-time. The clinical relevance of this technique in horses has not been adequately evaluated, but in sheep with pneumonia, clearance dynamics similar to those seen in man have been documented.[16] Further investigation of this technique is needed to determine its clinical potential.

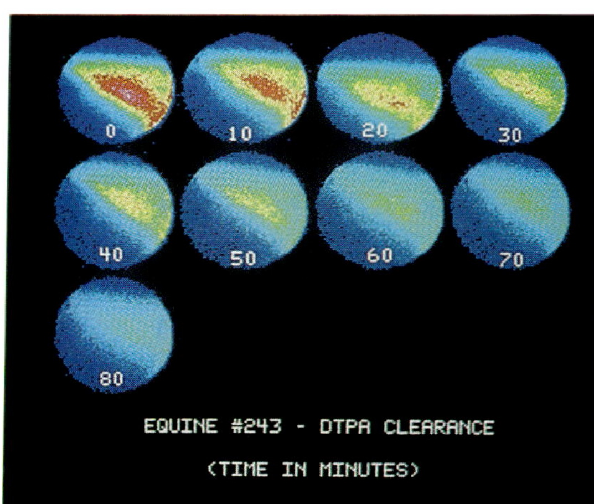


**FIG. 9–12.** Ventilation images of the caudal right lung demonstrating clearance of $^{99m}$Tc-DTPA over time. Images are recorded every 10 minutes. Clearance half-time for normal horses is between 50 and 60 minutes.

Determination of mucociliary clearance is another technique suited to scintigraphy. Experimental studies have employed a variety of methods to analyze clearance of labelled insoluble particles administered as aerosols.[17] Despite promising results from research data, the value of the technique in clinical cases has yet to be proven. In horses preliminary data on tracheal clearance using a probe have been reported.[6]

## Advanced Image Analysis

One of the disadvantages of image data is the difficulty of performing satisfactory comparative analyses. Radiographs, scintigrams, and other scanning methods display images which vary in size, shape, and relative densities. Even when the information in the image is digitized comparisons can be made from one image to another only by first normalizing the area under investigation in the two images to the same scale. For linear profiles and rectangular regions of interest this process is relatively simple. For whole organs the normalization process is relatively com-

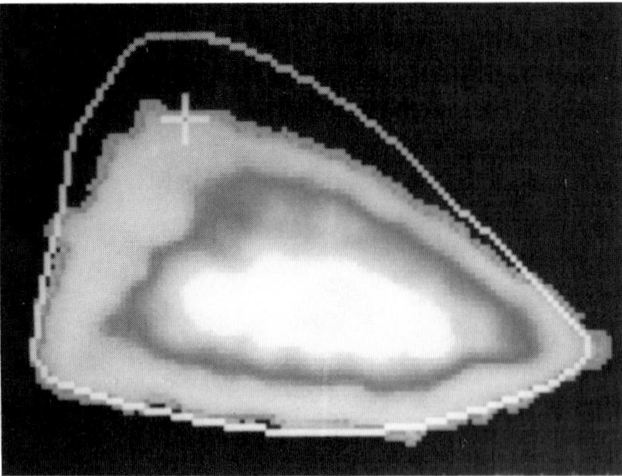

**FIG. 9–13.** Method for normalization of lung images. The image displayed is being fitted into a standard outer contour derived from the average outer lung contour of 12 normal horses. The sample left lung has been rotated clockwise to lie along its diaphragmatic margin and expanded horizontally by bilateral interpolation to fit the length of the contour. A cursor has been placed at the highest point of the rotated lung and will provide the coordinates for vertical interpolation of the image into the reference contour.

plicated. In this laboratory we have recently developed a method for normalizing equine lung images, details of which are to be published elsewhere. Lung images are first rotated to lie on a common diaphragmatic axis then expanded to a common length in a craniocaudal direction. Finally they are expanded vertically into a common outer contour derived from the average of 12 normal outer lung contours (Fig. 9–13). The resulting normalized or standard lung images can then be used for a variety of comparisons. Individual lung images can be compared with a group of horses of a similar type with estimates of the percentage and standard deviation difference (Fig. 9–14) or comparisons can be performed between groups of horses, either as a paired or non-paired Student t-test analyses (Fig. 9–15). Preliminary testing with these analysis methods suggests that they are sensitive to individual or group differences from comparison populations. The potential value of these techniques is in being able to identify early regional lung changes in individuals with suspected lung disease and making comparisons between treatment regimens or the pattern of a particular parameter in various lung conditions. The main advantage of these analyses is the numerical format of the result, expressed in commonly understood and accepted statistical terminology.

## Conclusions

Scintigraphy for equine pulmonary conditions is only beginning to demonstrate its considerable potential. Recent experimental studies confirm its value in determining ventilation and perfusion parameters in a variety of disease states. Extension of these techniques to standardized or normalized images may offer considerable benefits not only for research, but for clinical comparisons and evaluation of individual cases against a population of normals in the same peer group.

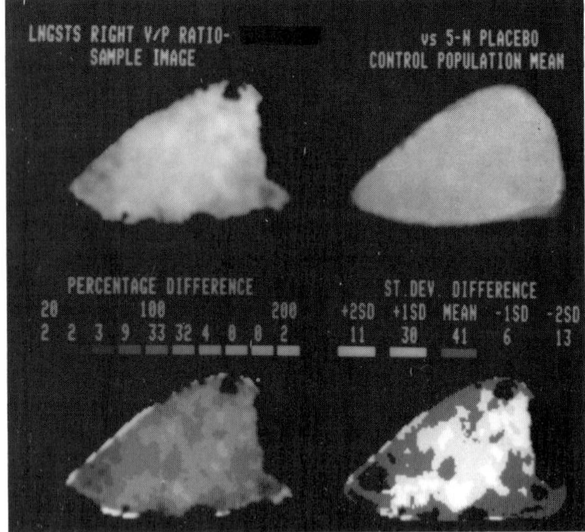


**FIG. 9–14.** Method of comparing an individual against a group of normal matched peers. The sample image from a horse with moderately severe COPD demonstrates patchy irregular distribution compared to the mean image of the normal group. The lower left image shows the degree of difference between the two upper images expressed in percentages, e.g., 33% of the sample lung has $\dot{V}/\dot{Q}$ ratios the same as the control group (100%); 2% of the lung has ratio values only 20% of the normal group. The lower right image displays the same data expressed in standard deviations, e.g., 41% of the sample lung was within 1SD of the group mean, whereas 11% was greater than 2SD above the group mean. (Note: not all colors on the original display are shown on this black and white image.)

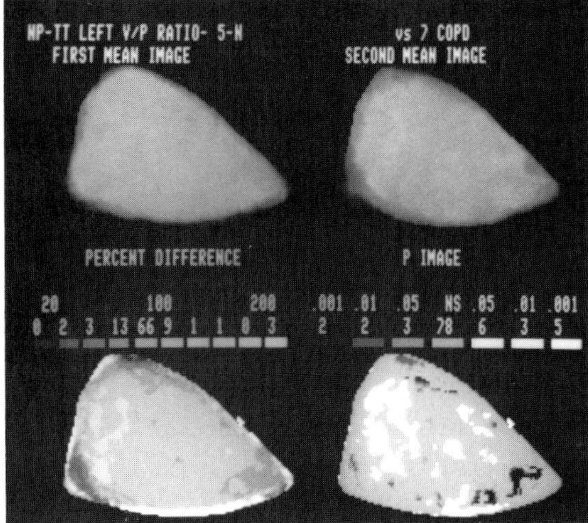


**FIG. 9–15.** Method of comparing different groups of horses. Here a group of 5 normal horses is compared with 7 COPD cases using a non-paired t-test method (the lower right image contains the results of approximately 6500 individual t-tests). The display format is similar to that of Figure 9–14. The P-image displays the regional differences between the two groups of horses expressed in p-values, e.g., 78% of the lung in the two groups was not significantly different for $\dot{V}/\dot{Q}$ ratios, whereas 6% of the lung in the COPD group had $\dot{V}/\dot{Q}$ ratios greater than the normal group at a significance level of 0.05.

Clinical evaluations also indicate that scintigraphy provides information that cannot be obtained by other imaging methods, notably radiography. Until further research and clinical trial data become available the main role of lung scintigraphy will be to complement radiography by providing functional information on the lung not provided by other methods.

## References

1. Devous MD, Theodorakis MC, Hillidge CJ. Scintigraphic evaluation of pulmonary perfusion and ventilation in equine respiratory disease. Proc Am Assoc Equine Pract, *25*:373, 1980.
2. Amis TC, Pascoe JR, Hornof W. Topographic distribution of pulmonary ventilation and perfusion in the horse. Am J Vet Res, *45*:1597, 1984.
3. Hornof WJ, Dunlop CI, Prestage R, et al. Effects of lateral recumbancy on regional lung function in anesthetized horses. Am J Vet Res, *47*:277, 1986.
4. O'Callaghan MW, Hornof WJ, Fisher PE, et al. Ventilation imaging in the horse with $^{99m}$technetium-DTPA radioaerosol. Equine Vet J, *19*:19, 1986.
5. O'Callaghan MW, Hornof WJ, Fisher PE, et al. Exercise-induced pulmonary haemorrhage in the horse: Results of a detailed clinical, postmortem and imaging study. VII. Ventilation/perfusion scintigraphy in horses with EIPH. Equine Vet J, *19*:423, 1987.
6. Boothe DM, Jenkins WL, Hightower DW, et al. Effect of clenbuterol on tracheal mucociliary transport rate (TMTR) in healthy horses (Abstr). ACVIM Proceedings, Washington, DC, 1988.
7. Alderson PO, Line BR. Scintigraphic evaluation of regional pulmonary ventilation. Semin Nucl Med, *10*:218, 1980.
8. Taplin GV, Poe ND. A dual lung scanning technique for evaluation of pulmonary function. Radiology, *84*:365, 1965.
9. Pircher FJ, Temple JR, Kirsch WJ, et al. Distribution of pulmonary ventilation determined by radioisotope scanning. Am J Roentgen, *94*:807, 1965.
10. Alderson PO, Biello DR, Gottschalk A, et al. Tc-99m-DTPA aerosol and radioactive gases compared as adjuncts to perfusion scintigraphy in patients with suspected pulmonary embolism. Radiology, *153*:515, 1984.
11. Burch WM, Sullivan PJ, McLaren CJ. Technegas—A new ventilation agent for lung scanning. Nucl Med Commun, *7*:865, 1986.
12. Newman GE, Sullivan DC, Gottschalk A, et al. Scintigraphic perfusion patterns in patients with diffuse lung disease. Radiology, *143*:227, 1982.
13. Hornof WJ, Koblik PD, O'Brien TR. Use of nuclear scintigraphy to characterize an intrathoracic mass in a foal. J Am Vet Med Assoc, *180*:1319, 1982.
14. Kay J, Coates G, O'Brodovich H. Pulmonary deposition sites of an inhaled radiolabeled submicronic aerosol. Pediatric Res, *20*:1297, 1986.
15. Jones JG, Royston D, Minty BD. Changes in alveolar-capillary barrier function in animals and humans. Am Rev Respir Dis, *127*:S51, 1983.
16. Hornof WJ, O'Callaghan MW, Gunther RA, et al. Lung clearance of $^{99m}$Tc-DTPA aerosol in conscious sheep. Resp Physiol, *72*:375, 1988.
17. Agnew JE, Bateman JRM, Pavia D, et al. A model for assessing bronchial mucus transport. J Nucl Med, *24*:170, 1984.

## CHAPTER 10

# POSTMORTEM EXAMINATION

*JAMES R. ROONEY*

The postmortem examination of the respiratory system has, as its specific purpose, the same significance and justification as the postmortem examination in general. This is, the prosector is moving from the collection and evaluation of clinical signs to the collection and evaluation of anatomic signs. The eventual goal, of course, is as complete an understanding as possible of the natural history of a disease or processes in an animal.

As a student one is taught to carry out the physical examination of a live animal and the postmortem examination of a dead one in a systematic, thorough manner. Clinical experience allows one to develop mental shortcuts, a quick glance enabling the prepared brain to interpret a whole set of physical signs without following an overt step-by-step sequence. Similarly, postmortem experience often allows the practicing pathologist to visualize and interpret an entire organ or system before complete and detailed dissection. The mental habits developed as a clinician or practitioner, however, should not be carried over to the postmortem examination any more than those mental habits developed as a pathologist can be carried over to clinical examinations. The clinician has daily experience with the live animal, and that experience allows rapid and reasonable interpretation and hypothesis formation. That same practitioner, however, does not have daily experience with postmortem work, and it is incumbent upon him to return to student habits of step-by-step, systematic examination. This is particularly true because, often, the postmortem is followed by laboratory and histopathologic examinations. The usefulness and value of those follow-up studies are strictly limited by the quality of the work done at postmortem and the descriptions provided.

The postmortem techniques presented here are based on my book.[1] It is assumed that the animal is positioned on the back, in dorsal recumbency. If the animal is in lateral recumbency, the same basic procedure may be used but with more difficulty. It is further assumed that the evisceration of the abdomen has been completed. Since the inexperienced or part-time prosector may well cut the diaphragm inadvertently during the removal of the abdominal viscera, it is important that the status of the diaphragm be determined as soon as the abdominal cavity has been opened and before evisceration begins. It is to be noted, also, that the ribs have not been and will not be cut away during this procedure. A variant for the foal will be given later in this chapter.

## Diaphragm

### *Hernia, Rupture*

Palpate the entire diaphragm to determine if it is tight or loose on one or both sides. Diaphragmatic hernia is to be located and defined at this time. There may be a smooth-edged defect in the diaphragm, most commonly on the left dorsal quadrant, with or without herniation of abdominal viscera into the pleural cavity. This type would appear to be congenital. Ragged edged tears with hemorrhage in the torn borders are most often seen in the left, middle third of the diaphragm but have been seen in the right half of the diaphragm as well. This type appears to be traumatic in origin although it may not be possible to associate any specific traumatic event.

The most common rupture of the diaphragm occurs near the xiphoid cartilage, ventral midline. This is a postmortem rupture without hemorrhage in the torn diaphragmatic tissue. Postmortem, autolytic changes can, on occasion, give an appearance of hemorrhage in the tissue. This rupture occurs because of gaseous distension of the gut, particularly the large intestine, together with handling of the carcass. I have not seen an intravital rupture of the diaphragm in this area.

## *Pneumothorax*

If the diaphragm is loose on one or both sides without evidence of fluid or exudate as determined by palpation, consideration must be given to pneumothorax. This is the only way to determine if such a condition is present. Before proceeding with the opening of the pleural cavities, a detailed and careful search of the thoracic inlet and thoracic walls should be made for evidence of a penetrating wound, whether accidental (impaling on a post or fence rail) or malicious (gunshot wounds). The wound may not be "gaping." A wound which appears closed at postmortem may well have acted as a valve in the live animal, opening during inspiration, allowing air to enter the pleural cavity, and closing again during expiration (the "sucking chest wound" of military medicine). Fractured ribs, particularly in foals, may lead to pneumothorax (see below). Most often a postmortem "wound," an inadvertent stab or cut by the prosector or assistants, will be found to be the cause. In the presence of pneumothorax and the absence of such wounds, a ruptured emphysematous bleb may eventually be found in the lung. This is, however, rare in the horse.

## Opening Diaphragm; Complete and Incomplete Mediastinum

The diaphragm is now incised on the right side in its middle third. Watch carefully as air enters the right pleural cavity. In the adult horse the right portion of the diaphragm will loosen and the loosening will continue past the midline to the left as the caudal mediastinum is displaced to the left. In most horses the shifting of the mediastinum will stop about halfway with the dorsal half of the left half of the diaphragm remaining tight. In the remaining cases the entire left half of the diaphragm will loosen. This occurs because of fenestrations present in the caudal mediastinum which allow communication between the two pleural cavities. While these fenestrations can be seen with careful subsequent dissection, one cannot be certain of their presence before dissection unless the above observations have been made. It is of interest that such mediastinal shifting and fenestration is not the case in young foals, apparently developing with age and growth and generally being present sometime after about 4 months.

These observations have both clinical and pathologic significance. In the case of pneumothorax, clearly, either one pleural cavity or both may contain air as the result of a single wound, depending upon the presence or absence of fenestrations. In the absence of fenestrations the diaphragm, at postmortem, will be loose not only on the wound "side," but on part of the opposite side as well because of caudal mediastinal shifting.

## Pleuritis, Clinical Signs

Pleuritis is frequent in young, working horses. The disease process begins almost invariably in the right pleural cavity (this will be explained in the section on the lung). In the earlier phases of the disease, the accumulation of fibrinopurulent exudate occurs in the right pleural cavity. Clinical signs, however, may indicate that there is involvement of the left side as well. This is, obviously, to be explained by the shifting of the caudal mediastinum toward the left by the accumulating exudate. The differentiation between unilateral, right side involvement (earlier stage of the disease process) and bilateral (later stage) involvement is to be made by percussion or ultrasonography. A fluid line on the right but not on the left or much lower on the left suggests that the process is still unilateral. With fluid lines at the same height on both sides, there is bilateral disease whether by extension from right to left through fenestrations or through the diseased mediastinum.

## Opening Pleural Cavities

The initial incision in the diaphragm is now carried carefully around to the left, so that the diaphragm drops down. Both phrenic nerves, the caudal vena cava and part of the thoracic aorta are readily visualized. There is normally about 100 ml of clear yellow fluid in each pleural cavity. Fluid should be collected now if desired for eventual cultural or cytologic examination. The diaphragm is now pulled down completely, transecting the nerves and the vena cava and "popping" the aorta out of the aortic hiatus of the diaphragm. Examine the pleural cavity, the lungs and the available portion of the pericardial sac. If the lungs are largely normal and the postmortem takes place within a short time after death, the lungs will collapse as air enters the pleural cavities. Postmortem accumulation of blood and fluids (postmortem "edema") as well as antemortem edema and pneumonia may prevent such collapse.

The massive serofibrinopurulent exudate of pleuritis will have been apparent. Fibrinous adhesions between parietal and visceral pleura are usual in such cases. Thin fibrous adhesions may be found between the visceral and parietal pleura. These should be carefully broken down with attention to possible cause such as healed fractures of ribs. In the absence of such a cause the adhesions may be attributed to pleuritis some time in the past.

## Fractured Ribs, Foals

In young foals, particularly neonates, the ribs should be carefully inspected and palpated. Costochondral fractures are common and generally of no significance. Fractures of the ribs themselves, however, may lacerate the lungs, heart, or intercostal arteries. In the latter two cases there may be significant hemothorax. Such fractures usually affect one or more of the fourth through eighth or ninth ribs, unilaterally or bilaterally. Pneumothorax may be present as a result of laceration of the lung (and be undetected unless the precautions noted above have been taken). I have not seen fractured ribs penetrate the skin, but there are usually hemorrhage and bruising of the tissues of the external thoracic wall. The location of the fractures of the ribs suggests that they occur because of compression of the chest wall by the incompletely extended shoulder and elbow as the foal passes through the pelvic canal of the mare.

## Dissection, Continued

Pericardial fluid should be collected with a syringe and needle at this time if eventual culture or cytology is anticipated as the pericardial sac may be torn during the removal of the thoracic viscera. The left hand is run forward in the right pleural cavity, the cranial mediastinum identified and torn into. The hand is pulled backward and upward, tearing loose the sternal attachment of the pericardial sac, so that the pericardium and heart drop down. In the foal the entire sternum may now be removed by cutting through the costal cartilages on both sides. This is not done with the older animal.

Now the prosector moves to the head and neck. The skin is removed from the ventral surfaces. Incisions are placed just inside the rami of the mandible on each side, and the tongue withdrawn. Pulling firmly caudally on the tongue, transect the palate. Incise deeply just lateral to the larynx on each side and cut forward. With palpation one can locate the angle between the greater and lesser cornua of the hyoid bones and cut easily through the cartilage forming that angle. Strip the tongue, pharynx, larynx, and trachea back to the thoracic inlet. In the foal with sternum removed cut just inside the first rib on each side to sever the vessels and nerves exiting to the foreleg and continue to pull caudally to remove the heart and lungs. In the older horse transect the trachea and esophagus in the middle of the neck. Open the thoracic inlet by a circular cut around the esophagus and trachea, severing the vessels and nerves. Insert the distal cut ends of the esophagus and trachea into the thoracic cavity. Within the thoracic cavity grasp the cut end of the trachea (a small incision between two tracheal rings helps provide a grip) and strip the heart and lungs out of the thoracic cavity. A small amount of additional sharp dissection may be necessary in the thoracic inlet. Unless identified and brought along as the stripping is done, the thoracic aorta may break near its middle. The organs are now placed on a table for examination. Even in the field a table is desirable in order to provide a reasonably comfortable working level.

## Pharynx

The dorsal wall of the pharynx is opened and the pharynx examined. There is an abundance of solitary lymphoid nodules scattered throughout the pharyngeal mucosa. These nodules are prominent in the foal and horse up to about 2 years of age, becoming smaller and less obvious after that time (this is characteristic of lymphoid tissue in general in the horse). Foreign material may be found imbedded in the crypts associated with the nodules with or without purulent exudate. In acute strangles (a rarity at postmortem) there are multiple small abscesses throughout the pharyngeal mucosa. Rhinopneumonitis infection induces reddening and excess mucus production (again, a rarity at postmortem). Gentle pressure on the mucosa often expresses cheesy material from the pharyngeal crypts which should not be mistaken for pus. It is largely keratin and debris and of no pathologic significance.

Elsewhere in this volume pharyngitis is discussed as a clinical entity particularly in young, working horses. Despite the clinical experience there is no pathologic evidence to support either acute or chronic pharyngitis as a usual or common condition in such horses. Even biopsy material from putative cases does not present the accepted criteria for either acute or chronic inflammation. Hyperplasia of the lymphoid nodules is cited, but such hyperplasia has not been quantified and, indeed, even if present, is not sufficient evidence for a diagnosis of acute or chronic pharyngitis.

Redundant pharyngeal mucosa, often encasing the epiglottis, is seen occasionally at postmortem, particularly in Standardbred horses. It is discussed elsewhere in this volume. There are no pathologic changes associated with such redundant mucosa. Partial pharyngeal and/or soft palate paralyses are discussed elsewhere. Those few cases with such a clinical diagnosis presented for postmortem examination have shown no significant lesions, including histologic examination of the relevant nerves. The other respiratory structures of the head will be discussed below.

## Cysts

Cysts may be encountered at virtually any level from the pharynx to the thoracic inlet. They are more often dealt with clinically but may be encountered as incidental findings at postmortem. Most of these cysts appear to be of embryonic origin whether of thyroglossal duct, lymphoepithelial (branchial cleft), parathyroid, or thymus primordium origin. Their presence is obvious, of course, if sufficiently large. If located in the subcutaneous tissues, "dimpling" of the skin may be apparent. Histologic examination often (but not always) permits determination of the probable origin of the cyst unless there is significant secondary infection.

## Larynx and Trachea

The larynx is opened through its dorsal wall after examination and removal of the esophagus. Laryngeal hemiplegia is readily ascertained as atrophy with a gradual change of color of the muscles from red to white. This is easily seen in the dorsal cricoarytenoid muscle, specifically, of course, on the left side. Hypoplasia of the epiglottis is occasionally found. Chondromas of the vocal folds are generally sequelae of "roaring" operations, although not necessarily so. The cartilaginous larynx tends to ossify with age in some horses. This is of no clinical significance.

Lesions of the trachea are uncommon. Tracheal stenosis is usually the result of traumatic lesions. I have not seen a bona fide case of tracheal collapse at postmortem. Fusions of tracheal rings are not uncommon and of no known significance.

## Dissection of Heart and Lungs

Since the examination of the lungs cannot proceed adequately until the heart and its vascular connections with the lungs have been examined, the entire procedure for such examination is included here. The method to be described is superior to the usual "blood-flow" method but is somewhat more difficult to learn.

Separate the aorta from the mediastinum to the base of the heart. Free the esophagus from the mediastinum and strip it cranially. If present, the thymus may be examined before proceeding. Turn the heart and lungs upside down, so that the ventral surfaces of the lungs are uppermost and the trachea to the prosector's left. The left lateral surface of the heart is presented by drawing the apex of the heart toward the prosector.

Slice the pleural connection between the middle (a lobe of the right lung) and left lobes of the lung, continuing the incision to open the pericardial sac. Open the pericardium to the apex of the heart and fold it under the heart. Do not attempt to remove the pericardium at this stage. Open the left atrium at the cranial border and continue the incision caudally to open the right and left pulmonary veins a short distance into the lungs. (The connections of the pulmonary veins and atrium are destroyed before examination in the blood-flow method.) Palpate the left atrioventricular orifice through the atrial incision. With the knife cut through the atrium and orifice to the apex of the heart, close and parallel to the caudal border of the heart, the right longitudinal groove, opening the left ventricle. The ventricle is examined in a preliminary manner at this time.

Without lifting the heart/lungs, spin them around, so that the trachea is directed to the right. Tip the apex of the heart toward the prosector presenting the right side of the heart for examination. Remove the pericardium. Open the right atrium at the cranial border, continuing caudally to open the coronary sinus, caudodorsally to open the caudal vena cava, and craniodorsally to open the cranial vena cava. The right atrioventricular orifice is palpated. With the knife cut through the atrium and orifice to the apex of the heart close and parallel to the same right longitudinal groove. Redirect the knife from the apex parallel and close to the left longitudinal groove toward the origin of the pulmonary artery and cut. Now, tip the apex of the heart away from the prosector. The origin and course of the pulmonary artery are clearly displayed. Cut a distance into the left and right branches of the pulmonary artery.

The vascular connections between heart and lungs have now been examined. Grasp the aorta and heart and, exerting traction, cut between heart and lungs to separate them. Before reorienting the lungs' dorsal surfaces uppermost, carefully examine the rather small middle lobe of the right lung, particularly in cases of pleuritis. In such cases a purulent process (either an abscess, per se, or a more diffuse purulent infiltration) will often be found as the nidus for the pleuritis. If not found here, the nidus is usually in the right apical lobe.

Most cases of pleuritis arise by extension of the purulent process in one of these two sites to the right pleural cavity. Streptococcus zooepidemicus is the usual organism. The purulent exudate associated with S. zooepidemicus infection is more often greyish and of a watery consistency and can be overlooked unless the area is carefully examined. Other causes of pleuritis include surgical interventions, inhalation of foreign materials (stones, hay, straw, rose branches, pieces of plastic), and diaphragmatic hernia. In such unusual cases the nidus is not, of course, in the middle or apical lobes, and different organisms or numbers of organisms may be cultured. Diaphragmatic hernias are not always massive. A portion of small or, more often, large intestine may herniate through and become adherent to a small 3 to 4 cm defect. Unless strangulated, these small herniations cause no further problem. If strangulated, however, leakage of bacteria, particularly Escherichia coli, into the pleural cavity induces severe pleuritis.

Orient the lungs, dorsal surfaces uppermost. Examine and slice the mediastinal lymph nodes and the left and right bronchial lymph nodes. These nodes are prominent in the younger animal but may be, normally, quite small in the older animal. Significant enlargement, hyperemia, or edema of the nodes suggests they be saved for histologic or cultural examination. The nodes may be abscessed, most frequently in Rhodococcus (Corynebacterium) equi infections.

The trachea is opened along the dorsal midline into the major, main stem bronchi with attention to the mucus content and the appearance of the mucosa. Frequently, strings or threads of blood are seen admixed with the mucus on the ventral mucosal surface. It is routine for bleeding to occur in the lungs during the agonal period, and this blood is moved up the trachea in the mucous blanket. Careful subsequent attention and examination will show that most of this bleeding is occurring in the dorsal part of the diaphragmatic lobes of the lungs.

## Edema

Foam may be present in the trachea as a rather stiff, creamy mass often tinged with blood. Such foam indicates that pulmonary edema was an antemortem event, though the event may have been agonal and not primarily related to the cause of the animal's illness or death. As already noted fluid ("edema") accumulates in the lung as a postmortem event, preventing collapse of the lungs and causing the unwary to think that either true edema or pneumonia is present. The absence of foam in the trachea is a clear sign that fluid accumulation in the lung occurred after death.

True or "pure" edema of the lungs (not agonal, postmortem, or accompanying pneumonia) is not common in the horse. It has been seen with severe trauma to the head and with certain anesthetic agents (chloroform, ether, methoxyfluothane). The lungs are usually hyperemic as well as edematous. Edema may occur, as well, in foals receiving heroic parenteral fluid therapy, although some degree of septicemic pulmonary involvement is usually present in such cases, making a distinction difficult.

## Lungs

Color changes are reliable indicators of pulmonary status and lesions in the absence of significant postmortem change. Since the majority of postmortems are not done immediately after death, however, color changes can be deceptive and must be evaluated with care.

Hypostasis, increased redness resulting from accumulation of blood in the down lung, is usual and well-known. Less well-known is the hypostasis of the dorsal portions of both lungs which occurs in horses which have been in dorsal recumbency for surgical procedures. Such dorsal hypostasis may have down-lung hypostasis superimposed, giving an initial impression of bilateral pneumonia.

Autolysis causes rapid color changes, a normal pink lung becoming darker and darker red. Eventually greenish-black discoloration occurs together with accumulations of gas caused by putrefaction. These should not be mistaken for emphysematous bullae. Greenish-black discoloration may also be associated with inhalation pneumonias in the absence of significant autolysis, but such pneumonias are not common in horses. Inhalation is somewhat more common in foals as a result of intubation feeding, but the animal apparently dies before such putrefactive changes occur and/or the appropriate organisms are not present in the feeding mixture.

The evaluation of color change must always be accompanied by the most important technique for examination of the lungs, palpation. The consistency of the lung parenchyma is a reliable indicator of status in all but the most advanced stages of autolysis. The normal, aerated lung has a delicate, spongy, elastic consistency. The hypostatic lung loses the delicate quality, becoming somewhat more densely rubbery in character. Atelectasis requires definition, most frequently in the neonate. Atelectasis does occur in connection with pneumonias in older foals and with pleuritis (in the latter the subpleural parenchyma is routinely atelectatic when a fibrinous "rind" is present on the pleural surface). The atelectatic lung has the denser consistency of the hypostatic lung but with a much less rubbery texture. The consolidated pneumonic lung is characteristically stiff and hard with little or no rubbery or delicately elastic consistency.

These descriptions of lung consistency are but attempts to put into words a tactile experience. It is only by palpation of each and every lung at postmortem that the prosector will gain an ability to assess accurately such changes in consistency in his or her own terms. In any event a description of what is seen and felt should be provided for the use of the histopathologist. As so often stressed, and as often ignored, the condition of the organ should be described before any attempt to arrive at an anatomic diagnosis.

## Pneumonia

Pneumonia as a self-standing clinical and pathologic entity is much less frequent in the horse than in many other species. By far the greatest majority of pulmonary lesions encountered in animals beyond the first 5 to 6 months are not pneumonia. One type which does occur is an acute, hemorrhagic pneumonia most frequently seen in younger, working and traveling animals. Characteristically, the onset is acute with severe respiratory distress either during or in the immediate post-travel period. Without heroic treatment (and, often even then) death is inevitable and rapid. At postmortem there may be serosanguinous pleural fluid or even free blood in the pleural cavities. The lungs are uniformly intensely red with a consistency like that of the hypostatic lung or even that of a hematoma. Free blood oozes freely from the cut surface. S. zooepidemicus has been isolated most frequently but other organisms may be present.

Rarely, so-called "bastard strangles," S. equi infection disseminating from its usual sites of involvement, may affect the lungs. There is multifocal consolidation of the lung with dark, plum-red discoloration. There may be small abscesses or purulent involvement of bronchioles. The focal areas of consolidation are scattered randomly in the lungs, suggestive of an hematogenous origin.

## Focal, Chronic Lesions

In older horses it is not uncommon to find focal, chronic, granulomatous lesions unrelated to the cause of death. These lesions appear to be located randomly in the lung without a specific site predisposition. While fungi (Aspergillus spp.) may be found in some, more often the lesion is of such chronicity that a cause is not apparent. Such focal lesions are frequently located deep in the parenchyma of the lung and are most readily detected by palpation.

## Ox Warble

Tracks of subpleural hemorrhage may occasionally be encountered, particularly in the dorsal part of the lung. These are caused by the migration of the ox warble (Hypoderma bovis) although the warble may have moved on by the time of postmortem examination.

## Heaves

As is now well-known, pulmonary emphysema ("heaves" of horses) is not a primary emphysema but rather a bronchiolitis (acute and/or chronic) which induces functional or, less often, structural emphysema as a secondary phenomenon. If structural emphysema is present, the lungs will be paler than normal, overexpanded and may be bearing rib impressions. In the less severe case the gross postmortem findings may be disappointing despite significant clinical evidence of disease. Careful palpation may reveal irregular, knobby thickenings along the course of the bronchioles. Histologic examination, however, is usually required in order to establish a diagnosis.

## Lungs in Foals

The evaluation of the lungs of foals can present difficult challenges to the prosector. Foals may be born dead or barely viable, expiring within a short period. Those foals born dead may simply have dark red, atelectatic lungs. Many, however, particularly those which have been delayed (dystocia) will have small, scattered areas of aeration, appearing as a pinkish mosaic in the dark red background. Evidence of aeration is more obvious in the thin borders of the lung. There will often be delicate rib impressions on such lungs, suggesting that gasping did pull the lungs against the rib cage without successfully expanding the major mass of the parenchyma. One can, of course, test the aeration status by flotation in water.

The newborn may have become infected with a septicemic organism before, during, or immediately after birth. In such cases there will be general evidence of septicemia in many organs and tissues as well as the lung. The latter will usually be aerated but darker red than normal with a consistency similar to the hypostatic (congested, hyperemic) lung. The microscope will reveal severe congestion with early evidence of inflammatory change (pneumonia). Meconium will almost invariably be seen microscopically in varying amounts. Small amounts are quite normal; however, large amounts suggest gasping while the foal was still in the amniotic sac. Fluid in the lungs may be compressed along alveolar walls, giving the impression of "hyaline membrane disease." There is no hard evidence, however, that hyaline membrane disease as a distinct entity occurs in the foal. In my experience so-called hyaline membrane is most widespread and of greatest severity with influenza infection of the foal lung.

The premature foal, one born 2 weeks or more before the expected foaling date for the mare, presents no specific or pathognomonic lesions of the respiratory system. Any of the conditions discussed above for neonatal lung may apply. Hyaline membranes in the lung are not characteristic of prematurity in foals.

In this same connection, "neonatal maladjustment syndrome" seems to have become a favorite academic veterinary medical diagnosis. From the pathologic standpoint this is incoherent. If such cases come expeditiously to postmortem, without intensive care, the pattern discussed in the previous paragraph is usually found. Other, even more obvious lesions, such as lacerated lungs caused by fractured ribs, or congenital heart defects, may be present. With intensive care preceding the death of the animal, more severe degrees of pneumonia and septicemia are generally found. Neonatal maladjustment may describe the clinical situation in a general way, but it is not an etiologically or pathologically distinct syndrome.

A specific and severe pneumonia accompanies rhinopneumonitis infection of the foal delivered at term. Fetuses aborted before term will usually show significant pleural effusion and interlobular edema of the lungs. The term foal, on the other hand, will have severe interlobular edema accompanied by lobular consolidation, often with effusion of fibrin into the interlobular spaces and onto the pleural surface. Such foals are in respiratory distress when delivered and usually die within 24 hours. (Again, such foals have been presented for postmortem examination with the clinical diagnosis of neonatal maladjustment syndrome.)

Moving on past the immediate neonatal period, lesions of the lung are usually associated with bacterial septicemias, appearing as described above or as frank bacterial pneumonias. In such cases the apical and cardiac portions of the lung are most heavily involved, being firm, consolidated, and dark red. Frank abscesses are uncommon though careful examination may indicate the presence of miliary purulent foci (purulent bronchiolitis). These pneumonic lesions are almost invariably of the character of bronchopneumonia. Fibrinous pneumonia is rare. As already noted, inhalation pneumonia often occurs during this period, associated with nasogastric intubation. It is difficult to distinguish such a pneumonia unless foreign material is seen in the trachea and bronchi and, indeed, bacterial and inhalation pneumonia frequently coincide.

The most frequent pneumonia of the older foal, beyond 1 month of age, is that caused by Rhodococcus equi (Corynebacterium equi) infection.

### Rhodococcus equi pneumonia

***Peracute.*** An apparently normal foal is found dead or dies rapidly after onset of severe respiratory signs. Both lungs are extensively consolidated, firm, dark plum-red with, perhaps, a small amount of mucoid or mucopurulent bronchial exudate. This is the least common form, an overwhelming infection.

***Acute.*** The clinical signs are less fulminating but clearly those of pulmonary involvement. Relatively few animals die during this stage. If they do, there is a diffuse consolidating pneumonia characterized by multiple pinhead to pea-size or larger abscesses scattered at random through the lungs. The abscesses have a cheesy, caseous character.

***Chronic.*** This is the commonest form. After an acute onset, which may even pass unnoticed, the animal shows variably severe respiratory signs, loss of condition, and exercise intolerance. With involvement of the large intestine, variably severe diarrhea is common. After a usually protracted clinical course the animal dies. Multiple large, caseous abscesses are found scattered through the lungs. The chronically ill animal may die suddenly and/or unexpectedly. At autopsy the large abscesses will be seen as well as a diffuse consolidation of the lungs as described for the peracute cases. This appears to be a sudden, miliary dissemination from one or more of the large abscesses.

R. equi infection, as discussed elsewhere in this volume, is an opportunist infection. In that vein it should be noted that solitary R. equi abscesses may be encountered at postmortem of the older, chronically ill or debilitated horse. Such abscesses are usually seen in the lung but may involve the splenic lymph nodes, external iliac lymph nodes, or other unusual sites.

### Viral Infections

Other than rhinopneumonitis, discussed above, there are only two known viral infections of the lung of young foals, neither of which is seen with any significant frequency at postmortem. Adenovirus infection results in a plum-red consolidation, particularly of the more cranial portions of the lung. This virus seems to be the usual "first-in" agent in cases of R. equi pneumonia. In early cases (such as the peracute) the virus may be isolated although it is not usually possible to discern its specific effects with microscopic examination.

Influenza can cause pneumonia of an almost identical gross appearance. The virus can be isolated, and the histologic appearance is characteristic (as already mentioned) in the absence of secondary bacterial infection. The A2 virus is the only strain which has been found in foals at postmortem.

## Epistaxis

While all the relevant pathophysiologic facts are yet to be elucidated about bleeding in working horses, there are certain pathologic facts. In all horses which have come to postmortem with either a recent or chronic history of bleeding, a discrete lesion was invariably found in the caudodorsal part of the diaphragmatic lobe of the lung(s). In the recent case this lesion consists of an area of hemorrhage, often with a greenish tinge, which extends no more than 2 to 3 cm into the parenchyma. The greenish color is caused by hemosiderin present in macrophages. The recurring, chronic case will have, as well, fibrotic thickening around vessels in the area. These appear as whitish or grayish-white bands of scar tissue, most apparent on thin, transilluminated slices of the affected area. It is to be noted that these lesions are located in the same area as the agonal, asphyxial bleeding discussed earlier.

## Upper Respiratory Tract

Examination of the upper respiratory tract under field conditions is difficult. It is usually desirable to examine the head under more controlled conditions. The guttural pouches and much of the respiratory portion of the pharynx can be examined without further dissection. For a more complete examination the head should be sawed on the midsagittal plane. While a band saw is obviously desirable, this can be accomplished by hand. After removing the skin, saw across just behind the incisor teeth. With the ventral surface uppermost saw from rostral to caudal until the head is split. A rather coarse toothed saw is best and should be applied with short strokes which are more effective with tissue than the smooth, long strokes of proper carpentry technique. Further cuts may be required to completely explore the sinuses.

Gross lesions of the turbinates and nasal passages are uncommon. Tumors apparently arising from the mucosa of the ethmoturbinate area occur infrequently and only in older horses. They are to be differentiated from so-called ethmoid hematomas involving the same area in younger, working age horses. Apart from the age difference, confusion may arise because the adenocarcinomas of this area are often quite hemorrhagic in character.

The ethmoid hematoma is a bulging, bluish mass protruding into the nasopharynx. The tough, fibrous capsule of the mass often displays a tracery of white strands (thickened fibrous tissue) and biopsies of these masses usually yield only capsular tissue. The histologic finding of large numbers of hemosiderophages in the capsule strongly suggests ethmoid hematoma. The site of origin and cause or causes of this lesion are not known.

## Guttural Pouch

Empyema of the guttural pouches may be encountered in either acute or chronic form. Such empyema is most commonly a sequela of strangles (S. equi) infection. In the more acute form there is a quantity of creamy, yellowish pus in one or both guttural pouches. In longer standing cases the pus becomes inspissated, presenting as balled-up, cheesy masses. The empyema may be either unilateral or bilateral. In the latter case, particularly with the chronic form, the pharynx may be sufficiently compressed to cause asphyxia and death.

Guttural pouch mycosis affects the dorsal portion of the guttural pouch, almost invariably unilaterally. The greyish-white, tough necrotic mass is surrounded by a reddened rim of guttural pouch mucosa. Such cases may be encountered unexpectedly at postmortem. Most, however, are presented because of fatal hemorrhage following invasion of the internal carotid artery. In such cases there usually will be partially clotted blood in the involved guttural pouch. Aspergillus spp. are usually isolated from such lesions and can be seen microscopically.

Guttural pouch tympanitis remains an etiologic mystery. There are no frank lesions present to indicate the cause. It is my impression, based on the few cases examined, that the pharyngeal orifice is anatomically normal but smaller than average in such cases. There are no relevant histologic findings.

Purulent infection of the sinuses, specifically the maxillary sinus, is most often associated with dental lesions and infections. They are not often seen at postmortem. Sawdust may admix with the normal mucus covering the mucosal surfaces and be mistaken for an acute mucopurulent exudate. Squamous cell carcinoma has been reported but is rare.

## Reference

1. Rooney JR. Autopsy of the Horse. New York, R.E. Krieger Publishing Co, 1976.

## CHAPTER 11

# INFECTIONS CAUSED BY VIRUSES*

*JILL BEECH*

Viral infections are an important cause of acute illness in horses, can predispose them to secondary bacterial pneumonia, and may predispose them later to chronic obstructive pulmonary disease (COPD). They have been implicated as causing follicular lymphoid hyperplasia and contributing to chronic poor performance.[1,2]

At present the most important viruses that cause equine respiratory diseases are: equine Influenza A/equine 2 (H3N8 strain) and equine herpesvirus type 4 or Rhinopneumonitis, previously called equine herpesvirus 1 subtype 2. Although significant earlier, the A/equine 1 (H7N7) strain of influenza has not been an important cause of disease in the USA or Europe for about 10 years.[3,4] The significance of equine herpesvirus type 2 as a respiratory pathogen remains somewhat controversial. Except for causing severe and often fatal respiratory infections in immunocompromised foals, adenovirus's role in contributing to equine respiratory disease has not been clarified. Both rhinoviruses and parainfluenza viruses have been associated with mild respiratory disease in horses but, in general, are not considered important.

## Pathogenesis of Viral Pneumonia

The pathogenesis of viral pneumonia probably has been most extensively studied in mice experimentally infected with influenza, and extrapolations have been made to other species including horses.[5] The amount of virus delivered to the respiratory tract as well as host defenses determine the severity and duration of illness. With uncomplicated viral pneumonia there is loss of airway epithelial cells and influx of neutrophils into the airways, peribronchial mononuclear cell infiltrate, thickening and hyperemia of alveolar septae, exudate with an increase in lymphocytes and neutrophils and edema in alveoli, interstitial infiltration with white blood cells, and capillary thrombosis. The response to viral infections and the recovery depend on complex interactions between antibody, complement, macrophages, lymphocytes, lymphokines, and cell mediated immunity in the host.

Following infection, virus particle reactions with receptors on cell surfaces are important in triggering the cascade of events leading to immune responses and phagocytosis by macrophages and neutrophils, and usually intracellular destruction. The virus proteins present on the surfaces of macrophages and dendritic cells in association with class II major histocompatibility (MHC) antigen and are recognized by delayed hypersensitivity type ($T_d$) and helper ($T_h$) lymphocytes. Major histocompatibility antigen I glycoprotein on infected cell surfaces is also important as it activates cytotoxic T ($T_c$) lymphocytes. Macrophages secrete monokines or lymphokines, including interleukin I and interferon. Interleukin I initiates and amplifies T (lymphocyte) cell dependent immune responses and in-

*I thank and acknowledge D.G. Powell for reviewing the chapter and for his suggestions.

flammation. It acts on the temperature regulating center in the hypothalamus and is the principal mediator of pyrexia. The T lymphocytes are divided into helpers ($T_h$), suppressors ($T_s$), and those which have cytotoxic activity ($T_c$) or are important in delayed hypersensitivity ($T_d$). The $T_d$ lymphocytes secrete various lymphokines that enhance the immune reaction by attracting and activating macrophages and other T cells. The $T_h$ cells secrete helper factors. $T_c$ are important in recovery and offer a degree of heterotypic immunity but it is unclear exactly how they function, although it may be through gamma interferon.[6] The $T_s$ cells recognize viral antigen either as it is presented by the antigen presenting cell or probably by direct binding following processing, and they secrete suppressor factors which regulate the immune response by suppressing other lymphocytes, usually when the latter are no longer needed. The interferons can activate macrophages, $T_c$ lymphocytes and natural killer (NK) cells and inhibit replication. The NK cells are immunologically nonspecific and seem to be important in early defense in killing virus infected cells. They may limit viral spread by lysis of virus infected cells and production of interferon.[5] The $T_c$ and $T_d$ cellular activity usually peaks about 1 week post infection and then declines over several weeks. However, memory $T_d$, $T_c$ and $T_h$ cells may persist for years.

In addition to the activity of the T lymphocytes, beta (β) lymphocytes are important. Beta (β) lymphocytes have specific Ig receptors on their surfaces. Beta cell growth and differentiation are dependent upon growth factor interleukins released by $T_h$ but a "cycle" exists as these cells also act to process viral antigen and present it to T cells. The β lymphocytes differ from T cells in origin, in function and in their surface markers and antigen receptors. The β lymphocytes produce antibodies. The rise in IgM antibodies occurs early in the immune response but is transient and, therefore, elevated specific antibodies are usually diagnostic of recent or ongoing chronic infection. The rise in IgG usually occurs later but persists longer. At least for influenza, the time of rise in virus specific serum IgA varies according to whether infection is primary or secondary. Submucosal lymphoid tissues can be stimulated by overlying antigens to produce antibodies, especially IgA, and antibodies are also produced in lymph nodes, bronchus-associated lymphoid tissue (BALT) and the spleen. IgA is especially important on mucosal surfaces as it can neutralize viruses and decrease or prevent attachment of bacteria to mucosal surfaces, thus acting as an important defense. IgA is most important in the upper respiratory tract, whereas in the lower respiratory tract secretions there is a greater proportion of IgG relative to IgA.[5] The re-exposure of memory B cells to an antigen rapidly activates them within 1 or 2 days to produce specific antibodies, primarily IgG. Although both IgG and IgM are produced in the lung, the former is reported to predominate.[7]

Interferons are important early in infection. In other species several have been characterized; at the time of writing, to my knowledge there are no published studies on horses' interferons. In general there are three types of interferons: alpha (α), beta (β) and gamma (γ). Alpha and beta interferon are produced by most cells following viral infection but gamma interferon ("immune interferon") is produced mostly by $T_c$ cells involved in an immune response. Interferons induced by one virus are effective against most other sensitive viruses. Interferons interfere with intracellular viral replication primarily by inhibiting viral transcription and translation. Gamma interferon induces enzymes which inhibit protein synthesis in virus infected cells, activates $T_c$ lymphocytes, NK cells and macrophages, and enhances expression of both Class I and II major histocompatibility antigens on cell surfaces. These activated cells then produce more interferon. Interferons indirectly enhance the lysis of infected cells by increasing NK cell activity, but at the same time as they enhance the immune response they also have some suppressive activities. Interferons enhance resistance to viral infection in uninfected cells.

The immune response is also enhanced or "complemented" by complement activation which leads to inflammation and destruction of infected cells and virus. Complement activation can occur secondary to the presence of antigen-antibody complex (IgG and IgM complexes primarily) and also via an alternate nonantibody-dependent pathway. Complement opsonizes virus particles, leading to their phagocytosis. A number of different plasma proteins can act as complement components.

Factors affecting clearance of viral particles play a role in response to viral infections. Mucociliary clearance is important in lung defenses, but distal regions of the lungs lack ciliated epithelium and depend on the alveolar macrophages (PAM). During infection PAM action is augmented by the influx of neutrophils, blood monocytes and antibodies. Pre-existing macrophage dysfunction could enhance viral infection. The association of transport and other stresses with predisposition to infectious respiratory disease in horses could be at least partially due to altered macrophage activity, although presently available data leave this unclear.[8-10]

Secondary bacterial pneumonias are common sequelae to viral infections. Viral-bacterial synergy in the lung is probably the culmination of multiple events. In vivo experimental studies in other species have shown that sublethal viral infections do not affect antibacterial defenses during the first few days, but in overwhelming infections intrapulmonary bactericidal activity is depressed on the first day of infection.[11,12] Although mucociliary clearance is important, it has been claimed that its dysfunction is not the major reason for the lowered bactericidal activity of virus infected lungs as biocidal depression has been seen at times when removal of radiotracer labeled bacteria is only minimally decreased.[12] Alveolar macrophage dysfunction is thought to be the major cause of lowered pulmonary defenses. Whether viral infection has a direct suppression on macrophages is controversial.[11-13] At the time of peak macrophage dysfunction many cells contain viral antigen, probably due to ingestion of desquamated epithelial cells which contain viral antigen. Antiviral immune responses will then interact with these macrophages and can alter phagocytic function or destroy the macrophages.[12] Destruction of surfactant producing alveolar Type 2 pneumocytes occurs and may also play a role because surfactant is important in phagocytosis of organisms by alveolar macrophages. A loss of surfactant also leads to atelectasis and thus local hypoxia which impairs macrophage function. Any cell injury increases bacterial adherence and could enhance bacterial colonization; experimental studies in other species have demonstrated that normal upper respiratory tract flora frequently colonize and multiply in virus infected lung.[13] There is evidence for viruses directly suppressing pulmonary alveolar macrophage (PAM) function, peripheral neutrophils (PMN), monocyte and lymphocyte function, indirectly suppressing PAM function and peripheral blood elements and acting via immune mediated mechanisms to depress macrophage function.

Viruses may affect the quantity and quality of mucus secretion and induce inflammatory edema. Influenza viral infections in mice can induce inflammatory edema which may promote bacterial growth and suppress macrophage bactericidal activity.[11] In vitro studies have shown that airway mucus interferes with pulmonary macrophage function and this may further impair pulmonary defenses especially when combined with the decrease in bactericidal activity of macrophages. The exact interactions in virus infected horse lung have not been reported.

## Diagnosis of Viral Infections

Unfortunately, in most situations when there is no obvious epidemic and only small groups of horses or individuals show signs of acute viral respiratory disease, few diagnostic tests are performed and careful records of clinical signs, temperature charts, movement of horses, accurate vaccination histories, and other epidemiologically important data are often lacking. The identity and even the existence of the suspected "virus" remain unknown. Some of the problems leading to failures in diagnosis include lack of adequate surveillance and reporting, inability to collect and process appropriate samples in a timely manner, difficulty in interpreting the results, and the economics involved. To a trainer or owner, delayed serologic identification of the causative virus may be of little interest as it provides no immediate value. The horses either will have recovered or developed complications. For a veterinarian interested in recording and reporting outbreaks of respiratory disease, and particularly when a new respiratory pathogen is suspected, an epidemiologic approach should be instituted.[14]

## Epidemiologic Investigation of Virus Diseases

The aims of an epidemiologist are to define where and when a condition occurs, how much is occurring and who is affected; to search for the primary cause and contributing factors; to suggest a means of control; and lastly, to evaluate the efficacy of control measures.[14]

Signs shown by each case must be carefully tabulated to ascertain if one or more diseases exist. Age, sex, and breed of affected animals, time of onset and pattern of spread, geographic distribution (country or state, county, particular farm(s), show grounds, racetrack(s) or similar areas, buildings, fields, etc.) should be ascertained. Age is important as new virus diseases in a naive population tend to affect all age groups, whereas a virus introduced into a population previously exposed to it will cause disease primarily in young or unvaccinated animals. Use of a map to record location of affected horses can be helpful. On a racetrack, for example, a map of the track and use of dated markers for each case as it occurs would clearly demonstrate the pattern of spread.

When there is a point source of infection the numbers of affected horses rise abruptly and then gradually decline, whereas with contact infection there is a slower more gradual rise in numbers of sick horses and a more rapid decline. A persistent low level of infection leads to a rather constant and low number of diseased animals as seen in endemic infections.[14]

The veterinarian can try to ascertain the incidence or attack rate (number of new cases of disease over a specific period of time) as well as the prevalence rate (total number of cases, both new and old, over a period of time) and morbidity (number of diseased horses/number of horses at risk) and mortality rates (number of deaths/number of horses at risk). To further refine these data, age, sex or breed specific rates can also be calculated.[14] Serology and virus isolation as well as postmortem information are important. If and when a viral agent is isolated, provided its incubation period is known, one can ascertain the time of probable infection by subtracting the incubation period from the date of onset of the disease. It is important to seek help from trained epidemiologists and virologists as well as regulatory veterinarians early in the stages of what potentially could progress to become an epidemic.

## Collection of Samples

Ocular conjunctival, nasal, or fecal swabs can be used for isolation of adenovirus. Nasal and pharyngeal swabs can be used for isolation of the other viruses. The swabs should be obtained from the nasopharyngeal areas by vigorous rubbing of the mucosa. Shedding of the virus depends not only on the individual virus and stage of the disease, but also on the horse's immune status and exposure history. Although viral shedding usually coincides with pyrexia, it may precede onset of clinical signs by several days.[1] Coughing, enlarged submandibular lymph nodes, and nasal discharge may be the first abnormalities noted when temperatures are not routinely monitored and generally they are noticed when shedding has ceased.[1] For EHV-1, if affected horses have been previously infected, viral excretion may be minimal and occur for only 24 to 48 hours, whereas horses infected for the first time will excrete for more than a week. It is, therefore, important to sample in-contact horses even if they show no signs, and it may be most productive to sample younger previously unexposed or more naive horses in the stable.

Samples should be collected in special transport medium which contains antibiotics to prevent bacterial growth and proteins to stabilize the virus. Tissue culture media with fetal calf serum has been used for nonadenoviral agents; normal saline solution may suffice for adenoviruses.[15] Samples should be transported on ice so that the temperature is maintained between 0° and 4°C.[1] If transit time is less than 1 day and the weather is not hot, ice or cold packs (< 4°C) should suffice if they are packed with the sample(s) and sent in a styrofoam container. If the environmental temperature is high and transit time is likely to exceed 1 day, it is best to pack the sample in wet ice with provision to replenish it as needed. Dry ice can be used if replenishing wet ice is not possible. Once in the laboratory, following inoculation, identification may take up to 3 weeks. However, many viruses if present in large numbers will cause cytopathic effects in cell culture or hemagglutinating activity within a few days.[1] Postmortem samples submitted for virus isolation should include normal and affected areas as viable virus is often at the edge of the lesion. Each specimen should be packaged separately in an airtight container to prevent cross contamination between samples and to help prevent virus inactivation.

Nasal or pharyngeal scrapings or pharyngeal biopsies can be obtained for immunofluorescence and for cytology using electron-microscopy (EM) to identify virus particles. Indirect immunofluorescent tests are used to identify EHV 1 and 2 and adenovirus.[1,16] In order to detect viruses successfully by EM, $10^8$/ml particles must be present; ultracentrifugation of samples is frequently necessary to achieve this concentration.[1] Samples for EM examination for virions can be sent to the laboratory under ambient conditions as the test does not rely on infectivity of the virus. However, attempts should be made to avoid bacterial contamination as this can interfere with virus identification.

Serology is probably the most commonly used diagnostic tool, although its use requires that one has tentatively identified the infectious agent(s). It is important to obtain the first sample in the acute stage of the disease as a delay in sampling may obscure a rise in titer. With some exceptions a 4-fold rise in titer of the convalescent serum is generally regarded as diagnostic of infection. Except for equine herpesvirus where maximal virus neutralizing antibodies may not be reached for 4 to 6 weeks post infection, most viruses cause a high rise 2 to 3 weeks post infection.[1] There are numerous antibody tests available and titers vary quantitatively amongst the tests. There also may be interlaboratory variation.

## *Techniques for Identification of Viruses and Antibodies*

Electron microscopy can be used to directly detect virions and the sensitivity is enhanced by using immune serum or specific antibodies in immunoelectron microscopy. It may be used on specimens as well as on cell cultures. Electron microscopy identifies to the family level of virus but immunoelectron microscopy is more specific.

Direct detection of viral antigens utilizes specific prelabeled antibodies applied in situ to tissues, excretions, or secretions. If virions or viral antigens are present, they will interact with the antibody and thus be detected. Immunofluorescence is rapid, relatively simple, specific, and sensitive.[7] The direct immunofluorescent test uses fluorescein labeled antivirus antibody to detect the viral antigen. Indirect immunofluorescence is more sensitive than the direct test and uses fluorescein labeled anti-immunoglobulin specific for the antiviral antibody which detects the viral antigen. Careful detail is needed, however, to avoid false positives. The test can also be used in reverse to detect serum antibodies by taking slides with known viral antigen, flooding them with the test horse's serum and then washing the slide and applying a fluorescein labeled anti-horse antibody to detect whether the horse's serum had antibodies that bound to the viral antigen.[7] Use of immunofluorescence in the presence of herpesviruses can lead to false positive reactions because some herpesvirus-infected cells will nonspecifically bind immunoglobulins, not just those antibodies with herpesvirus specificity.

Radioimmunoassay (RIA) is sensitive and allows detection of low concentrations of viral antigens. Usually the "capture" antivirus antibody or antigen is bound to a solid medium and then direct or indirect radioimmunoassay techniques are applied. In the direct RIA, the "capture" antivirus antibody is exposed to the test sample suspected to contain virus or viral antigen, then washed and a radiolabeled "detector" antiviral antibody is added followed by a further washing. A gamma counter is then used to measure any bound labeled antibody. If there was no antigen in the test sample, no binding will have occurred. Indirect RIA is more commonly used and is similar to the indirect immunofluorescent method except labeling is with a radioisotope, not fluorescein, and the detector antibody must be from a different animal species than that used as the capture antibody. In this technique, after the test sample is added to the capture antibody, the detector antivirus antibody is added but unlike in direct RIA is unlabeled; radiolabeled antiglobulin to this antivirus antibody is then added as the "indicator" antibody.[7] When RIA is used to detect antibody and not antigen, antigen and not antibody is used as the "captor."

Enzyme linked immunoabsorbent assay (ELISA) or enzyme immunoassay (EIA) employs the same principles as RIA and is equally sensitive. For the direct ELISA, the test sample suspected to contain antigen is added to the substrate which contains antivirus antibody and after a reaction time and washing, an enzyme labeled antivirus antibody is added, the contents are rinsed following appropriate reaction time and a substrate for the enzyme is then added. Color change which can be quantitated reflects the amount of enzyme labeled antibody. In a modified ELISA a biotin labeled antibody is added prior to adding enzyme labeled avidin and then substrate; avidin has a high affinity for biotin and increases the assay sensitivity. Viral antibody in a sample can be measured with ELISA if antigen is bound to the plate first.[7] An advantage of ELISA is that it does not require the use of radiolabeled isotopes, unlike RIA.

Of the various serologic procedures used, virus neutralization (VN), ELISA, RIA, hemagglutination inhibition (HAI or HI) and complement fixation (CF) are most common. Plaque reduction neutralization, or serum neutralization tests which are unaffected by extraction procedures or single radial hemolysis (SRH), may relate more closely to protective antibody but the assays are more costly and time consuming. Studies on equine influenza have demonstrated the increased sensitivity of SRH compared to HI.[17] Recently a sensitive radioisotopic antiglobulin binding assay has been developed for influenza; although it does not differentiate between the two subtypes, it is sensitive and rapid, detecting both the early rise in IgG antibodies and their persisting levels.[18]

In the VN assay, test serum dilutions are made in wells to which a standard amount of virus is added. After incubation cells are added and the cytopathic effect is evaluated; the titer of the test serum is the greatest dilution that prevents cytopathic effects. The plaque reduction assay is a version of VN using cell monolayers inoculated with virus and test serum overlaid with agar or methyl cellulose and incubated until plaques develop; the greatest dilution of serum that decreases the number of plaques by at least 50% is the titer.[7]

Hemagglutination (HA) and hemagglutination inhibition (HAI or HI) tests are used to titrate antibodies to viral hemagglutinin, a glycoprotein of the virus particle. Virions of several families have these glycoproteins in their outer coat that bind erythrocytes and cause hemagglutination. If antibody is mixed with virions prior to exposure to erythrocytes the process will be inhibited. The test is sensitive and specific as it measures antibodies that bind to the cell surface protein that is most subject to antigenic change.[7] Titers are expressed as a reciprocal of the dilution of test serum that inhibits hemagglutination. The test is often used as it is rapid and relatively inexpensive but it can be used only for hemagglutinating viruses such as adenoviruses and influenza viruses. When HA is used for detecting the virus and not antibody, it is not a sensitive indicator of the presence of small numbers of virions.[7] Temperature at which the test is performed is important because viruses such as influenza virus contain neuraminidase which can destroy erythrocyte receptors resulting in virus elution. At least for influenza there may be considerable interlaboratory variation in HAI titers and the pattern of antibody change in individual test samples may even vary between laboratories.[19–21] Use of receptor destroying enzymes can affect antibody titers and cause some of the interlaboratory variation.

In the complement fixation test, test serum is heated to inactivate complement, serially diluted and then antigen and guinea pig complement are added and incubated to allow complement to be "fixed." Hemolysin (sheep red blood cells sensitized with rabbit antiserum) is added and after further incubation each dilution is examined for lysis. When complement has been "fixed" by the virus antibody, lysis is prevented; when there is no antibody in the test serum, hemolysis occurs because of the reaction with free complement.[7]

In the single radial hemolysis technique, virus is coupled to sheep erythrocytes and gels prepared with these sensitized erythrocytes and guinea pig complement. Heat treated test sera are added to wells in the gels and hemolysis measured with a calibrating viewer coupled to a digital recorder.[18]

In the radioisotopic antiglobulin binding assay (RABA) microwells are coated with virus antigen to which test serum is added and incubated. The wells are then washed and filled with monospecific antiserum to equine IgG and then incubated with radiolabeled Staphylococcus aureus protein plus a reducing agent. Gamma spectroscopy is then used to detect bound radioactivity and the counts compared with antigen and antibody control wells.[18]

## *Interpretation of Test Results*

Respiratory viruses may cause subclinical infections in horses and serologic evidence of infection may not be clinically significant. The role of viral infections in adversely affecting exercise tolerance or performance may be difficult to document. Also, as previously mentioned, the test method itself can be a major influence on detection of infections. One study in ponies over a 5-year period showed that most EHV-1, picornavirus, adenovirus and rhinovirus 1 and 2 infections were subclinical; however, the authors pointed out that clinical responses in stressed race horses might be different.[21]

Picornaviruses and adenoviruses may be isolated from healthy as well as diseased animals. Adenovirus is rarely isolated from adult horses with signs of respiratory disease and usually causes clinical disease only in those foals which have impaired immune function. For parainfluenza 3 the CF antibody can persist for 4 months post infection, and HAI and VN antibodies may persist for more than a year;[22] presence of antibodies to this virus should not be interpreted as indicating recent infection or respiratory disease.

## Equine Adenovirus

Equine adenovirus is a DNA virus which was first isolated in 1969.[23] It is highly stable and resistant to changes in pH and temperature. Although it has been accepted that there is only one serotype (EAdV-Austral 75 strain) two separate isolates in Australia and New Zealand were found to differ from previous adenovirus isolates, suggesting antigenic diversity as is seen in adenoviruses infecting other species.[24–26] It has a high prevalence of infection in horses and distribution is worldwide.[15,27] Most isolates have been from Arabian foals with combined immunodeficiency disease (CID) but the virus has also been isolated from clinically normal foals of various breeds and from immunocompetent foals with signs of respiratory tract disease. Infection has also been reported in Thoroughbred race horses in training.[27,28] Subclinical infections are not uncommon, at least in unstressed animals. Presence of antibodies may be age related as some studies show 50% of horses less than 1 year of age lack antibodies.[21,29] Forty-one percent of randomly tested horse sera in the USA had significant titers.[15] Serologic studies in Japan in 1978 showed that 44% of racehorses had CF antibody but a study from 1980 to 1986 showed only 24/3102 racehorses seroconverted.[30,31] Both HAI and VN tests are suitable for identification of its presence. Use of CF and immunodiffusion has shown equine adenovirus has group antigens common to other adenoviruses. Although infections are common in horses, except in immunocompromised hosts, adenovirus's contribution as an important respiratory pathogen remains controversial.

## Pathogenesis

Equine adenovirus can infect multiple sites and can be excreted in conjunctival and nasal discharges, urine, and feces. Following cell entry by direct translocation across the plasma membrane the virus core migrates to the nucleus and replicates forming intranuclear inclusion bodies. Virions are released by cell lysis. Shedding following infection has been documented to last up to 68 days.[26]

## Clinical Signs

Clinical signs can be variable and have been described in most detail in foals. The incubation period is 3 to 5 days in experimental infection and 5 to 7 days following natural exposure. Experimental infection in neonatal foals caused polypnea, intermittent fever, mucoid nasal and ocular discharges, deep coughing, inappetence, mild depression, and scleral and conjunctival hyperemia in some. The foals recovered by 7 days post infection although pneumonia and atelectasis were present at necropsy.[32,33]

Lymphocytopenia occurs initially but lymphocyte counts usually increase by the fourth day. Serum antibodies increase by the tenth day at which time cell changes regress and virus is seldom isolated.[32,33] By 21 days after exposure recovery is virtually complete.[32,33] It is likely that age and prior exposure to the virus as well as immune function influence development and variability of clinical signs. Infection can occur even when foals have been passively immunized by colostrally derived serum antibodies.[32,33] Even when clinical signs are mild, necropsy has shown that severe pneumonia can occur.[29] This could be important in predisposing infected foals to other infections.

In the reports of infection in mature horses, signs have been mild and transient. Two horses in Japan had fever and nasal discharge of less than 2 days' duration and one also had soft feces. Nasal swabs for virus isolation yielded only adenovirus and one horse had a significant rise in CF, HAI and SN antibody titers 2 weeks following illness.[27] Post exercise coughing, nasal discharge and submandibular lymphadenopathy and soft feces have been reported.[28]

## Pathology

Necropsy of infected foals having no immunity to the infection reveals conjunctivitis, rhinitis, tracheitis, and pneumonia. Histology reveals acute bronchopneumonia and peribronchiolar interstitial pneumonia with mononuclear cell infiltration. Affected airways have hyperplastic or degenerated and sometimes ulcerated epithelium and necrotic debris and neutrophils in the lumens. Alveoli also are affected with a mononuclear cell response. Intranuclear inclusion bodies may be present in epithelial cells and also have been found in renal tract epithelial cells. Bronchial lymph nodes may be edematous. Duodenal villous atrophy and pancreatitis have been reported.[29,32,33]

## Diagnosis

Diagnosis is based on virus isolation, immunofluorescent techniques, or serology. The virus can be rapidly inactivated by immunocompetent animals, therefore, virus isolation or IF tests from nasal swabs or scrapings should be performed early in the disease. As the virus occasionally can be isolated from the nasal mucosa of healthy mature horses, interpretation of isolates from this group must be cautious. Fluorescent antibody techniques can be used to identify inclusion bodies in cells from conjunctival or nasal mucosa, and nasal mucus can be examined by negative contrast electron microscopy.

Routine hematology is nonspecific and not diagnostically helpful except to indicate if there is an extreme lymphocytopenia. Persistent lymphocyte counts of less than 1000/ml$^3$ in Arabian foals should make one suspect CID and perform additional tests to examine immunoglobulin status.

## Treatment Control and Prophylaxis

Prognosis for recovery is good provided the animal is immunocompetent and does not develop a significant secondary infection. There has been no scientific evidence to date that any purported immunomodulating drug would benefit infected horses and most recover uneventfully. Individual horses should be given good nursing care and stress should be avoided. Secondary infections should be appropriately treated. In neonatal foals, immune status should be evaluated. If inadequate colostrum has been absorbed, plasma (20 to 40 ml/kg body weight) or another source of IgG should be administered intravenously and the foal's plasma IgG levels rechecked. If CID is documented the owners should be advised on the extremely poor prognosis for survival even if the foal recovers from the current infection.

Other than good management and hygiene, maintaining good ventilation and air quality, and isolating sick horses from clinically healthy animals, there are no prophylactic measures.

As the virion can remain infective under a wide variety of conditions (more than 90 days at ambient room temperature) and is continually eliminated in urine, respiratory tract secretions, and feces, widespread infection is possible. Even though virus is usually not recoverable by 10 days post exposure in affected foals, a contaminated environment could provide a source of infection.

## Influenza

Influenza, a disease of high morbidity but relatively low mortality, economically is claimed to be the most important equine respiratory disease. Widespread transport of horses contributes to its dissemination but to date (March 1990) it has not been reported in New Zealand or Australia; it could cause epizootics if introduced into such countries due to the highly susceptible populations. A severe epidemic of influenza type 2 (H3N8) occurred in South Africa in 1986 and was thought to be due to lack of immunity within the horse population.[34] Most outbreaks occur in 2- to 3-year-old horses which are assembled in large groups in an enclosed environment such as a racetrack, training center, or horse show stabling area. In 1 year slightly more than 40% of respiratory disease in this age group was directly associated with influenza and it has been claimed that resistance usually develops by 4 years of age.[35] The stress of transport, crowding, and poor ventilation are conducive to infection. The virus survives better in low humidity air and like all viruses in aerosols its survival is favored by low temperatures. Transmission by aerosol is aided by the explosive coughing of affected horses, the short 1- to 3-day incubation period, and shedding which can persist for up to 8 days. An especially dangerous source of infection is the infected horse showing few signs but shedding virus. Decreased ventilation increases the amount of virus in environmental air samples, further enhancing spread in enclosed housing.[36]

The virus is a myxovirus with affinity for mucopolysaccharides and glycoproteins in mucus. It has three envelope associated proteins: neuraminidase (N or NA), hemagglutinin (H or HA which accounts for about 25% of the viral protein) and matrix protein (M protein).[5] The matrix protein is not important antigenically. The major antigenic surface proteins neuraminidase (N) and hemagglutinin (H or HA) distinguish the two recognized subtypes, H7N7 and H3N8. The hemagglutinin of subtype 1 (H7) is related to some fowl plague virus strains and that of subtype 2 (H3) is related to human and some avian H3 strains.[7] The N7 and N8 neuraminidase antigens differ. Each strain is often named according to its geographic origin and year of isolation. The H3N8 strain most common in the United States is A/equine 2/Miami/1/63; other strains within this subtype include A/equine 2/Ky/81, A/equine 2/Solvalla/79, A/equine 2/Tokyo/71 and A/equine 2/Fontainbleau/79, and A/equine 2/Newmarket/79, A/equine/Tennessee/86, A/equine/Johannesburg/86, A/equine/Joinville/1/78.[3,20,37–40] In the United States, A/equine 1/Prague/1/56 is the most commonly recognized H7N7 strain but this subtype also includes the strain A/equine/Newmarket/1/77. Genetic sequencing for equine 1 influenza has shown a division into two genetic and antigenic groups based on time periods 1956 to 1963 and 1964 to 1977.[41] In 1964 a major drift occurred, thought to be due either to mutation of a variant with resultant infectious advantage or possibly due to the introduction of a highly related virus from another species.[41,42] Considerably more antigenic drift has been reported for A/equine 2 (H3N8) than for A/equine 1 (H7N7). The Solvalla and Ky strains of H3N8 differ considerably from the earlier Tokyo and Miami strains, but the A/equine 2/Newmarket/79 is antigenically very close to A/equine 2/Fontainbleau/79.[21] Hemagglutinins of recent isolates differ antigenically from the prototype Miami/1/63 strain and these studies were the basis for recommending including A/equine/ Fontainbleu/1/79 or A/equine/Ky/81 in the type 2 component of vaccines.[40] These studies also showed that variants cocirculate in the same horse population. Knowledge of antigenic variation becomes important when selecting a vaccine. If the latter does not contain all strains to which vaccinated horses are likely to be exposed and cross protection is inadequate, prophylactic efficacy may be decreased. Despite heterogeneity, strains have been similar to the original reference strain,[3] with homology reported to be >70% according to one study[40] and >90% in another.[5] The equine 2 viruses' limited antigenic change contrasts to the greater variation that has occurred in human strains.[40]

A/equine 2 is generally thought to be more virulent and more pneumotropic than A/ equine 1, yet is less antigenic.[17,39] In contrast, one study at racetracks in Ontario, reported that A/equine 2 strains were less frequently associated with disease and the outbreaks were less explosive and less severe than the A/equine 1 epidemics.[35] It is possible that factors not associated with viral virulence influenced this latter study. There is no cross immunity between the two strains and, therefore, it would be possible to see two outbreaks of influenza within a short time period in the same group of horses. Mechanisms for antigenic variation in influenza virus strains are unknown but could occur by mutation of existing strains, recombination between equine and other mammalian or avian strains, and direct transmission from other animal sources.[42] Birds have been implicated as the source of both A/equine 1 and A/equine 2.[43]

## Pathogenesis

When influenza viruses are inhaled, most deposit in the upper airway but some aerosolized particles may penetrate more deeply. If there has been previous recent infection with the same or a similar strain of influenza, the viruses may be neutralized by local antibodies which bind predominantly to the HA protein. A relationship between secretory antibody and resistance has been demonstrated in ponies.[44] However, it is not clear whether IgA or IgG in nasal secretions is more important; in humans, the latter is thought to be more important.[36] The relative importance of each may depend on the site of virus deposition because, as previously mentioned, there is proportionally more IgG in the lower respiratory tract and more IgA in the upper respiratory tract. Regardless of type, to be protective, the anti HA antibody must be present at the mucosal surface. The time sequence of rises in IgG, IgM and IgA differ and also vary with whether infection is primary or secondary. Although antibodies are important, based on studies in agammaglobulinemic human beings with influenza infection, their presence is not essential for recovery. Also glycoproteins in the mucus may combine with the virions and prevent the latter's attachment to epithelial cells. This protection is lost if there is sufficient viral neuraminidase to destroy the mucus glycoprotein, allowing virus attachments to epithelial cells. The virus attaches via its hemagglutinin to a receptor (N-acetylneuraminic acid) in glycoproteins and glycolipids, undergoes endocytosis, and fuses with the phagolysosome membrane; the nucleocapsid is then released into the host cell cytoplasm. Replication occurs and virions are released into the airway by budding from the cell's plasma membrane. Spread of virus can occur initially with the help of cilia moving the particles along. The virus spreads throughout the respiratory tract within 1 to 3 days, damaging cilia and epithelial cells.[3] Mucociliary clearance is decreased, secretions accumulate in the airways, and underlying tissues become inflamed. Large areas of airway epithelium may be denuded, increasing susceptibility to secondary infections, exposing irritant receptors and enhancing potential penetration by antigens. In human viral respiratory tract infection transient airway hyperreactivity, impaired mucociliary clearance, and pulmonary function changes have been documented.[45,46] Although similar effects are suspected to occur in horses, to my knowledge they have not been documented to date.

## Clinical Signs

Clinical signs are rapid acute onset of fever, often 40 to 41.1°C (104 to 106°F), serous nasal discharge, hyperemic nasal mucosa and conjunctivitis, frequent dry nonproductive explosive coughing, malaise, inappetence, sometimes limb edema, muscle stiffness and reluctance to move. Prior to the fever the pharyngeal lymph nodes may transiently swell. Incoordination, muscle spasms and myoglobinuria also have been seen.[38,47] Previous exposure and local antibody responses influence severity of clinical signs. In a second infection with the same subtype as in the first exposure there is a rapid increase in local IgA and IgG which could obviously affect virus attachment and replication.[48] Naive foals may succumb within 48 hours to acute viral pneumonia.[38] Lung sounds may be harsh but unless secondary infection occurs, there are no sounds of mucus. Endoscopic examination often reveals pharyngitis, laryngitis, and tracheitis for up to a week. If there are no secondary complications improvement is usually seen by 5 to 7 days. However, resolution of the damage to the epithelium of the respiratory tract may take at least 3 weeks and recovering horses should be regarded as abnormally susceptible to other respiratory infections, allergens or irritants during that time period. Persistent airway lesions have been seen as long as 6 weeks post infection (Rooney, J. personal communication, 1988). Severe infections reportedly have caused horses to remain unfit for competition for 50 to 100 days post infection.[49] Cardiomyopathy is a rare complication; affected horses develop fever, depression, tachycardia, and sometimes arrhythmias. In severe cases, valvular insufficiency and congestive heart failure may occur and cardiac isoenzymes CKMB and HBDH have been elevated.

Hematologic findings are nonspecific and variable; however, a sudden lymphopenia usually occurs and may be detected for up to 4 days. It is then usually followed by a monocytosis.[2]

## Diagnosis

Virus isolation and paired serum samples for serology are required for definitive diagnosis. Viremia is rare and brief when it occurs. If there were significant antigenic drift in field strains, antibodies may not be detected by the prototype strains used for serologic testing.[28,50] However, at least to date this has not been a major problem. By 7 days after infection antibodies are detectable by either HAI or VN tests and they peak by the third week and may persist for up to 18 months.[3] CF titers develop later and remain low and, therefore, are not useful. Both SRH and RABA are more sensitive than the HI (HAI) test.[18] It has been suggested that measurements of virus specific IgM (by RABA) may be useful in detecting recent or multiple infections when levels of IgG are already high.[48] The same authors also suggested the SRH test was similarly useful and that RABA for IgG was more sensitive for identifying infections that had happened more than six months previously.[18] Studies with influenza virus H3N8 infections showed levels of virus specific serum IgG as measured by RABA persisted for at least 62 days (at which time ponies were again infected) but IgM rise had decreased 50% by that time.[48] There was an amnestic response with a rise in IgG after a second infection but the secondary rise in IgM was not amnestic and had shown a major decline by 32 days.[47] Levels of circulating IgA rose approximately 10 days after infection and did not show a major decline for at least 62 days and rose again with a secondary infection. However, these levels are not usually measured in diagnostic laboratories. At the present time measurements of locally produced antibody would not appear helpful as there has been a large variation in proportions of locally produced antibody following infection.[48] Occasional horses fail to seroconvert despite documented infection with A/equine 2 and some may take up to 28 days to show a rise in HAI titer.[51,52] Similar unexplained failure to seroconvert is also seen in some people following influenza infection. As mentioned previously, serum antibody titer results may differ among laboratories.

Nasal mucus taken early in infection or

lung tissue is the best material for virus isolation. The virus grows well in embryonated eggs incubated at 35 to 37°C by the amniotic or allantoic route and presence of virus is indicated by detecting HA activity in either the amniotic or allantoic fluid, depending on route of inoculation. Canine kidney cell line and chick embryo fibroblasts are used for cell culture systems. The difficulty of successful isolation is demonstrated by the fact that in one study, despite respiratory illness and seroconversion, positive cultures occurred in only 8 of 212 samples.[35]

## Treatment

Treatment consists of good nursing care and symptomatic therapy, trying to prevent secondary infections and treating them when they occur. It is important to monitor water intake to ensure that it is adequate and the horses are not becoming dehydrated. When fever exceeds 39.7 to 40°C (103.5 to 104°F) or the horse appears depressed or stiff and is anorexic, it is common to administer nonsteroidal anti-inflammatory drugs such as phenylbutazone or flunixin meglumine to enhance the horse's feeling of well being and decrease the fever. Antipyretics such as aminopyrine have a shorter duration of effect. It is important not to use these drugs to mask secondary complications or prolong their use. Careful examination of the respiratory tract should be performed frequently in affected and exposed horses as bacterial pneumonia and pleuritis can be serious and even fatal complications. Injudicious use of phenylbutazone has allowed insidious progression of disease, resulting in severe pneumonia and pleuritis that is difficult to successfully treat. As long as the horse appears relatively bright, even if its temperature is up to 40 to 40.3°C (104 to 104.5°F), I do not advocate use of antipyretics; the temperature should be monitored and the horse's thorax carefully auscultated periodically for any indication of progression of the disease. It is important not to stress affected or exposed horses. Foals should not be weaned. Transport should be avoided, and moving horses over long distances in the face of an outbreak or following exposure is probably contraindicated. In one study of pleuritis, 22 of 90 horses had been transported over 500 miles[53] and some studies have suggested that transport may adversely affect horses' pulmonary macrophages.[8,9] Whether the prompt use of antibiotics is effective as prophylaxis against secondary bacterial infections has not been proven. If the viral infection appears severe or persistent, they are probably helpful.

The use of antiviral drugs has not been studied in horses. In humans, amantidine has been used and interferon has also been used prophylactically. Substances that would modulate the horse's response to viral infection, decrease viral infection, multiplication and shedding, and enhance recovery would obviously be beneficial. Alpha interferon has been suggested for prophylaxis and treatment of respiratory infections. Dimethyl glycine is reported to enhance cellular and humoral immunity to certain stimuli in man[54] but, to my knowledge, this effect has not yet been documented in horses. Propionibacterium acnes* has been claimed to increase the rate and degree of recovery from respiratory infection in horses.[55] However, to date there are no published studies unequivocally proving the efficacy of any immunomodulating substances in equine viral respiratory tract infections.[56]

Horses should be rested for at least 3 weeks following infection and longer if they were severely affected or the duration of illness was prolonged beyond 3 to 7 days. The tendency to return prematurely to training and racing ignores the required healing time of the horse's respiratory tract epithelium and probably predisposes the horse to developing secondary problems such as chronic coughing. Influenza infection has been claimed to predispose infected horses to later develop COPD.[2]

Duration of immunity following infection probably varies among individuals and published information varies. Also, extrapolation from results of experimental infections in unstressed ponies to clinical racetrack conditions may not always be accurate. Despite experimental evidence that infection with H3N8 (A/equine/Newmarket/79) resulted in complete protection for at least 32 weeks and partial

*TM Immunoregulin, Immunovet, Inc.

clinical protection for 62 weeks[18] and observations on a pony herd indicating that immunity persists for at least a year, it has been suggested that infected horses may be susceptible to reinfection within 3 to 4 months following an infection. In a study on four outbreaks of A/equine 2, only those horses which had not been vaccinated within 6 months showed clinical illness.[51] Other surveys showed similar protection.[3,52]

## Control and Prophylaxis

The disease can spread extremely rapidly. As for all airborne infections, transmission can be interrupted by eliminating the sources and infectious particles in air and protecting and decreasing the number of susceptible horses. The virus is shed during the incubation period and horses remain infectious for at least 5 days after onset of clinical signs.[7] As virus may be shed by partially immune animals that show no clinical signs, these animals pose a significant often unrecognized hazard.[18] Duration of virus excretion varies among individuals and with their immunity. A 4-week quarantine period has been suggested. Movement of personnel dealing with diseased or exposed horses should be limited and they should be educated regarding their role in potentially disseminating disease. Stables, transport vehicles, and equipment should be cleaned and disinfected with a viricidal product (such as those containing quaternary ammonium compounds, phenol, formalin, or chlorine).

Vaccination of exposed previously vaccinated horses may afford some protection but is unlikely to protect naive horses in the face of an outbreak. It has been suggested that over 70% of the equine population should be fully vaccinated in order to prevent epidemics.[38] The number of doses and timing of vaccination have been found to be important in protecting against epidemics. Also, pre-vaccination titers affect the amnestic response and the response to A/equine 2 is much lower than to A/equine 1.[1] There may be an attenuated response to vaccination in horses with pre-existing moderate to high levels of antibodies and foals may be more difficult to immunize than adults.[57] Passively acquired colostral antibody may have limited protective effect; in ferrets and mice, protection is limited to the lower respiratory tract.[5] Also, as unexposed foals' HI titers drop quickly following initial vaccination, they may be susceptible to infection a few months after initial immunization.[57] Serum antibody responses to yearly booster vaccinations appear to vary, sometimes exceeding and sometimes being lower than the response to the initial vaccination; when using a killed bivalent vaccine one cannot rely on consistent and rapid "boosting" of antibody titers in individual horses.[1,19] One study in 1- to 4-year-old horses using an aluminum hydroxide adjuvanted formalin inactivated bivalent whole virus vaccine showed the magnitude of increase in antibody titer and rate of titer decline following the second injection of the initial series varied considerably amongst individuals. By 6 months some had no residual HAI titer to either A/equine 1 or A/equine 2.[57] Revaccination of these horses with a third dose 6 months later caused a transient increase in titers which had usually declined considerably within the next 6 months.[57] Again, responses were variable and occasional horses did not develop significant titers.[57] Low serum antibody titers and susceptibility to infection have been reported in some horses despite vaccination every 3 months.[58] Local antibodies (IgG and IgA), as measured in nasopharyngeal washing and transtracheal aspirates, increase following vaccination and may provide some protective benefit.[48]

Inactivated virus vaccines containing A/equine 1 and A/equine 2 are used in the USA and Europe. The killed virus is usually combined with an adjuvant for parenteral administration. Adjuvanted vaccines elicit higher antibody responses than nonadjuvanted aqueous preparations even when their viral antigen content is lower.[17] Not all commercial vaccines elicit the same antibody responses.[58] One of the problems with currently (1989) available vaccines is the lack of standard requirements for potency, purity and efficacy testing. Equine influenza vaccines would benefit from the use of the single radial immunodiffusion (SRD) assay which is reproducible, specific, correlates with clinical efficacy and is used for standardizing human influenza vaccines.[17,59] Already, its application to equine vaccines (three bivalent aqueous and one adjuvanted bivalent equine influenza vaccine) has shown marked variation in HA antigen activity/virus strains per dose.[17]

A vaccine administered by aerosolization might be expected to provide better protection; however, use of live viruses would not be practical as it would render vaccinated horses infectious for a short period of time. Administration would also be more cumbersome. Recently there has been investigation of the use of a live temperature sensitive mutant of Influenza A.[60] Temperature sensitive mutants of human Influenza A viruses have been studied as potentially useful for vaccines in man because they induce systemic and local immune responses without infection of the lower respiratory tract where the temperature is higher. In the equine study, subclinical infections were elicited following vaccination by nebulization of the temperature sensitive mutant, and challenge with wild type H7N2 virus 4 weeks later elicited neither clinical signs nor virus shedding.[60] Further studies are needed to evaluate its efficacy and safety. Because of genetic instability and reversion to virulence of some temperature sensitive mutants there has been interest in cold adaptant mutants for vaccines.[5] An immunostimulating complexes (ISCOMS)-based vaccine for A/equine 2 influenza virus has received some investigation.[48] To date, there is no evidence to demonstrate that other substances administered concurrently enhance a horse's response to vaccination. Use of dimethyl glycine, which was reported to enhance antibody response to pneumococcal vaccination in man, had no significant effect on serum HI antibody response (as measured by two different methods in two different laboratories) to influenza vaccination in horses.[19]

The usual vaccination program involves two primary injections given several weeks apart, usually between 4 to 8 months of age, followed by booster injections. Although manufacturer recommendations are for annual or semi-annual boosters, it has become common practice to revaccinate heavily stressed competing horses every 3 to 4 months. Influenza A/equine 2 infections have occurred in horses that have been reimmunized within the preceding 4 months.[39] Long-term studies using different commercial vaccines showed a rapid decline in antibodies after 3 months; the decline was related more to the initial titer than to the vaccine.[61] The minimal protective antibody level has not been determined unequivocally for either subtype of influenza and some work has failed to correlate protection with these levels. Horses with HI titers equal to or greater than 1:40 were found to have less than 30% probability of developing respiratory disease but having titers exceed 1:80 gave no additional protection.[35] In one study of an outbreak of A/equine 2 influenza, out of 30 unaffected horses that were sampled, none had an HI antibody titer of 1:80, although, statistically, unaffected horses had a higher frequency of low level serum antibodies than affected horses.[52] In another survey, 46 of 54 affected horses had low HI titers (1:10), whereas 38 of 39 unaffected horses had acute HI titers ≥1:20.[51] Similarly, HI titers of ≥1:16 were reported to prevent infection and disease with A/equine 2/Miami/1/63.[57] However, as method of HI testing affects titers, until there is standardized testing, these parameters could be misleading and unhelpful. The disparity of results with HI titers is avoided by use of the SRH test which is reported to be sensitive and reproducible and also correlate with protection.[17,20] Samples which have been negative on HI have frequently had high (protective) SRH titers.[17] Concentrations of nasal antibodies, or antibodies in other respiratory tract secretions which are not routinely measured, may be the best index of protection. As individual horses' antibody responses to the same vaccine are known to be quite variable, duration of immunity is likely to vary among individual horses.[19,57,58] Regardless of whether adequate testing is available, at present there is no economic incentive to measure antibody levels to determine if a horse requires vaccination. Despite controversy over the best vaccination regimen the value of vaccination in protecting horses has been clearly demonstrated. Even if vaccinated horses are affected during an epidemic, the duration and intensity of clinical signs are reduced. It is advisable to time vaccinations so that the greatest immune response occurs at the time of year when risk of disease is greatest.

Although some trainers believe that influenza vaccination adversely affects the horse and its performance, there have been no studies that support this. Few systemic or local reactions appear to have been reported and controversy over possible adverse side effects appears to be more prevalent in the United Kingdom than in the United States.[62] Mild muscular stiffness and training off form for a day or two have been reported.[52] A preliminary survey of adverse reactions to equine vaccinations showed a low percent.[63] One of 171 horses vaccinated for influenza developed a local abscess and 6 of 389 horses receiving vaccines combining influenza and tetanus toxoid developed adverse respiratory reactions.[63] Of the 6 horses, 2 had a history of chronic obstructive pulmonary disease (COPD) and 5 of 6 adverse reactions occurred following use of a vaccine combining a non-adjuvanted influenza vaccine plus adjuvanted tetanus toxoid. It was postulated that a vaccine's adjuvant might stimulate hypersensitivity responses of the lower airways to inhaled allergens, thus precipitating or enhancing signs of COPD as shown by 4 of 6 horses with adverse respiratory reactions.[63] One study on mucociliary clearance in the respiratory tract in vaccinated horses showed no adverse effects.[64] Because of possible adverse side effects it is unwise to administer any vaccinations, regardless of type, close to racing or other strenuous performance.

An unanswered important question is how or where do equine influenza viruses persist between epidemics? Equine influenza A/1 has been recovered from horses showing clinical signs of influenza that are isolated from other horses. Although it has been speculated that the virus may persist in asymptomatic carriers within the horse population, there has been no evidence for persistence of the virus in individual horses in either a masked or inactive form, therefore, persistence in other hosts and direct transmission from animal reservoirs has been suggested. Antibodies to A/1 have been found in wild rats.[65] It has been suggested that the virus could be carried by birds, rodents, or humans.[43]

## Equine Herpesviruses

Three alphaherpesviruses, which are rapidly growing cytolytic viruses, affect horses: equine herpesvirus types 1 and 4, both previously referred to as EHV-1 (subtype 1 and 2); and type 3 (EHV-3).[66] Infections range from subclinical to severe. Types 1 and 4 were previously thought to be the same virus; although antigenically related, they are genetically distinct and their DNAs show less than 20% homology.[7,67–69] EHV-1 causes abortion, perinatal disease and death, and sometimes neurologic deficits; it also may cause respiratory infections. Unlike other strains of herpesviruses, EHV-1 strains can change significantly in a population of horses, over a period of a few years.[68] Type 4 (EHV-4 or EHV-1 subtype 2) causes rhinopneumonitis and has low abortigenic potential. EHV-2, a slow growing beta "cytomegalic" herpesvirus, has been isolated from horses with respiratory disease as well as from normal horses and its role as a pathogen is controversial. EHV-3 causes coital exanthema. EHV-types 1 and 4 are distinct from the two other equine herpesviruses, EHV-2 and EHV-3.

### *Equine Herpesviruses-1 and -4*

Infection with either EHV-1 or EHV-4 can cause respiratory disease but not severe epidemics. Reports on prevalence of the two types vary although each is important. In the United States EHV-4 has been the strain more frequently associated with overt respiratory tract infections. In one survey 86% of 36 outbreaks of respiratory disease were caused by EHV-4.[68] In the United Kingdom, EHV-4 was more prevalent but EHV-1 infections have been increasing.[70] In central Kentucky, serologic surveys showed that approximately 85% of foals contract infections during their first year of life and most infections are with EHV-4.[66] Virus attachment and penetration is rapid. The virions are enveloped by cell membrane pseudopods and a vacuole is formed around the virions. Uncoating occurs in the cytoplasm and nucleocapsids are enveloped by the host cell's nuclear membrane when the latter either buds outwards or invaginates.

Viral replication rapidly commences, and cell culture work has shown a depression of cellular RNA and sometimes DNA synthesis.[71] Herpetiform vesicles may develop in the tracheal and bronchial mucosa.

Transmission may occur by contact, and intranasal, oral, conjunctival, intratracheal, vaginal, or parenteral inoculation. The incubation period may range from 2 to 10 days. Following multiplication within the upper respiratory tract EHV-1 enters lymphatics and capillaries and viremia develops. Viremia is reported not to occur with EHV-4 infections.[72,73] EHV-1 can replicate within mononuclear cells of peripheral blood with up to 25% of circulating monocytes infected.[7,74] A decrease in monocyte phagocytosis and killing results. T and B lymphocytes, monocytes, and plasma can contain virus following experimental infection and isolates of EHV-1 have been made from the buffy coat of naturally infected horses.[75] The virus can persist in nasal secretions for 20 days post infection and in mononuclear cells for 14 days. Although the site of latent infection has not been identified there is substantial evidence for latent infections. Spontaneous shedding following stress and periodic elevations in serum neutralizing antibody titers have been demonstrated in ponies having no contact with other horses for 10 years.[76] Although persistence of EHV-1 in cells or tissues such as the trigeminal ganglion has been suggested, to date attempts to reactivate the virus from these tissues have been unsuccessful.[76,77] Monocytes or lymphocytes could harbor the virus in a noninfective or subviral form that is then triggered to reactivate, and this could explain the delay between events such as abortion and the original onset of viremia.[75,78] A study in ponies showed virus reactivation and isolation from nasal swabs and leukocytes following administration of high doses of steroids; however, the site of latency remained unknown.[79] It has also been suggested that subneutralizing subtype 2 (EHV-4) antibody may predispose horses to severe infection by subtype 1 (EHV-1).[79] Differences in virulence and in the immune status of affected horses may contribute to the variability of clinical signs. Studies have shown that infection and/or repeated antigenic stimulation with EHV-1 can activate mononuclear phagocytes and make them resistant to virus replication on subsequent exposures.[80]

## Clinical Signs

In foals less than 4 months old, silent infections are not uncommon and may be detected only by routine periodic serologic testing. In one study of experimental infection with EHV-4 in 2- to 4-month-old pony foals, a fever developed at 12 hours, persisted for 36 hours and then transiently recurred on day three. A leukopenia developed by 24 hours but the cell count returned to normal by 3 days. As in other studies there was no rise in VN antibodies.[72] Severe respiratory signs have been reported when subtype 1 (EHV-1) virus is inoculated.[81,82] In another study in conventional foals clinical signs occurred only when there was a sudden appearance of Streptococcus zooepidemicus and/or Bordetella bronchiseptica.[83] The classical signs seen in the field due to EHV-4 infection can rarely be experimentally induced and EHV-1 strains seem to grow better in the nasopharynx, be excreted in larger amounts and elicit greater antibody response in experimentally infected horses.[68,84] Nasopharyngeal swabbing of foals with primary infections may yield virus for up to 10 days.[70,85] Diarrhea and limb edema also have been reported in foals.[85]

In weanlings between 4 to 8 months of age signs may be severe. At this stage passive immunity has waned and these relatively immunologically naive foals are frequently being stressed by weaning and other management changes. The role of stress in clinical disease has been suggested by studies on the abortigenic properties of EHV-1 infection; in one study on 8 mares, all 4 that were transported long distances before and after infection aborted, whereas, only ¼ unstressed mares aborted.[86] Weanling foals become febrile and develop a serous nasal discharge. Hematologic findings are nonspecific although both neutropenia and lymphopenia occur.[87] Secondary bacterial infections are common and the nasal discharge then becomes purulent and the foal may develop a frequent productive cough. The duration of fever varies but usually abates within a week unless there is secondary infection; as the latter is common, fevers and chronic respiratory tract infection often persist unless the animals are treated. Pharyngeal lymphoid hyperplasia is common. A study in 8- to 12-month-old ponies showed that challenge infection with EHV-4 usually caused submandibular lymphadenopathy, fevers, and nasal discharge; however, concurrent B. hemolytic streptococcal infections may also have contributed to the signs.[70] Foals may have repeated infections during their first year of life. Following recovery reinfection may occur within 2 months but usually does not cause clinical signs of respiratory tract disease.

The importance of EHV-1 as a respiratory pathogen in adult horses remains undefined. The virus has rarely been isolated from normal animals.[28,76] Serologic testing in many countries has revealed infection is widespread. A study in Thoroughbreds in training in England showed that EHV-1 infections existed with or without other viruses in about 45% of the outbreaks of respiratory disease. However, many infections were subclinical.[3] In the USA up to 33% of upper respiratory tract infections have been blamed on EHV (subtype unspecified).[74] Inoculation of mature pony mares with EHV-4 (EHV-1 subtype 2) caused a transient (12 to 24 hour) fever and sometimes leukopenia but no clinical signs.[72] Following EHV-1 (or subtype 1) infection, fevers for up to 6 days, nasal and ocular discharge, and less frequently coughing, have been seen in infected 2-year-old ponies, and pregnant mares had mild fevers and nasal discharge and sometimes aborted.[88] However, signs of respiratory tract disease are not consistently seen in pregnant mares. Depending on the stage of gestation at which a pregnant mare is infected with EHV-1, abortion may occur 3 weeks to 4 months later.

Its role as a cause of follicular lymphoid hyperplasia in young adult horses and the role the latter plays in poor performance remain to be defined. Increases in VN antibodies to EHV-1 sometimes have been associated with or closely followed poor performance or mild signs of respiratory disease.[28] Horses that do show signs of EHV-1 infection often have enlarged submandibular lymph nodes and a fever. One survey reported increased amounts of tracheal "mucopus" in a year when there was serologic evidence of EHV-1 infection.[89] Unlike horses with influenza that cough even at rest, those with herpes infection reportedly tend to cough only after exercise.[28]

Abortion due to EHV-1 infection may occur in mares in their last trimester of pregnancy following an incubation period that may last from 9 days to (rarely) several months. Abortion is subsequent to the transplacental passage of virus via infected leukocytes in mares that have previously been infected; because of previous exposure these mares rarely show signs of respiratory disease. Cell associated viremia occurs in these mares despite high levels of circulating VN antibodies.[90] Mares with repeated exposure to EHV-1 become more at risk of abortion or neurologic disease as their last exposure becomes more remote from the current infection.[66] As most epizootics of respiratory infections in young horses are caused by EHV-4 infection, not the abortigenic strain EHV-1, it has been suggested that latently infected carrier horses in which stress reactivates infection and causes virus shedding are the source of infection for most mares.[68] Although recrudescence of a latent infection within a mare could result in abortion, most cases occur subsequent to reinfection via the mare's respiratory tract.[66]

Most mares show few or no signs of impending abortion and recover uneventfully. Provided no dystocia or secondary complications occurred, future reproductive capacity is unimpaired. The fetus is usually born dead.

Neonates infected in utero with EHV-1 but born alive usually die shortly after birth with extensive lesions in the lungs, liver, lymphoreticular tissues, and sometimes adrenal glands. Secondary bacterial infections are also likely.

Occasionally neurologic disease occurs following EHV-1 (but not EHV-4) infection.[66,92–95] It frequently affects several horses in a group, can occur in either sex and may also affect foals, although usually less severely than mature horses. Mortality and morbidity rates have been highly variable; the former being as high as 40%[68] and the latter as high as 90%.[91] Signs have been reported to occur following respiratory disease or abortions or may be the only clinical evidence of infection. The incubation period is usually 6 to 9 days[66,92,93] but signs of ataxia have been seen as early as 1 day following onset of fever.[91] Several horses may be affected over a few weeks but quiescent periods have been reported between new cases.[91] Clinical signs are highly variable but usually do not progress after the first 2 to 3 days. The rate and extent of recovery vary considerably, with some animals completely recovering rapidly, others only partially recovering and others requiring euthanasia.

## Diagnosis

Diagnosis is based on virus isolation, serologic conversion or necropsy and histology. Equine derived cell lines or primary equine cell cultures are required for successful isolation of EHV-4 but EHV-1 may be isolated in either equine cell lines or rabbit kidney.[66] Virus may be recovered from the nasopharynx for up to 12 days following infection in young horses infected for the first time and for shorter periods in horses undergoing subclinical respiratory infection as a result of previous exposure and some resulting immunity.[68,90] Virus is most successfully isolated from horses with respiratory disease by swabbing the nasopharyngeal area with a 2 × 2 inch gauze sponge during the febrile period and immediately transporting this swab in cold transport medium.[68] Citrated blood may also serve as a source for virus isolation. Outbreaks of respiratory disease caused by the two subtypes usually cannot be differentiated by clinical signs. In horses with neurologic signs the cerebrospinal fluid may be xanthochromic with an elevated protein but normal cell count. Peak VN antibody titers occur between 2 and 6 weeks post infection, making association of titer rise with clinical disease somewhat difficult.[84] Indirect immunofluorescent staining of cells from the nasal mucosa is the simplest way to diagnose EHV-1 and -4.

Pathologic findings are often diagnostic. With EHV-1 infection aborted fetuses may have pleural and peritoneal effusion, pulmonary edema, and miliary white foci on the liver surface. Histologically, there is focal necrosis of the liver and necrosis of lymph nodes, thymus, and bronchiolar and alveolar epithelium. If foals are born alive, they are usually "floppy" and weak and die with acute pneumonia or pleuritis; necropsy findings are similar to those described for the fetus. Gross postmortem lesions of rhinopneumonitis include hyperemia, vesicles or ulcers or necrosis of the epithelium of the respiratory tract and miliary plum-red foci in the lungs.[68,96] Microscopically these epithelial lesions show inflammation, necrosis and intranuclear inclusions, and the lung lesions are characterized by infiltration of the terminal bronchioles with neutrophils, peribronchial and perivascular mononuclear cell infiltration and serofibrinous exudate in the alveoli. Pharyngeal lymphoid follicles are hyperplastic and necrotic and contain intranuclear inclusions.[68,96] Horses with the neurologic form of EHV-1 may have grossly obvious small focal hemorrhages in the meninges and neural parenchyma or frequently no gross lesions. Microscopically lesions in the central nervous system vary in severity but all are characterized by vasculitis of small blood vessels, perivascular hemorrhage and cuffing with neutrophils and mononuclear cells and adjacent areas of malacia.[68,95] In aborted fetuses or neonates tissues preferred for virus isolation are lung, liver, spleen, and thymus. Attempts to isolate EHV-1 from confirmed cases of EHV-1 paresis have often been unsuccessful.[68]

For confirmation of EHV-1 infection in individual horses, use of a single serologic test has been claimed to be unreliable due to antigenic variation of virus strains, variability of individual horse's immune responses and variability in the different antibody responses. Virus neutralization (VN), complement fixation (CF) and immunofluorescence (IF) techniques have been advised.[1] The IF technique is the most sensitive and is also ideal for rapid screening.[97] The CF test is more sensitive than VN but CF antibody titers decrease more rapidly than VN titers following infection; a 4-fold decline in CF titer indicates infection within the previous 10 weeks. As clinical infection does not always stimulate a 4-fold rise in VN titers, the latter is not suitable as the only test for an individual horse. However, as the (VN) test is highly reproducible, it is suitable for surveys.[1] In individual horses with neurologic disease due to EHV-1, VN antibody in the CSF is corroborative evidence for diagnosis.[92]

## Treatment and Control

There is no specific therapy and patient care should be directed at good nursing and minimizing and/or treating secondary infections. The same general comments made regarding influenza apply, except for adult horses with subclinical infections where rest may not be needed. However, it has been suggested that if EHV-1 is immunosuppressive as herpesvirus infections are in other species, then infected horses may be predisposed to other infections.[98] A decrease in monocyte function but not neutrophil function has been documented with EHV-1 infection.[74] Horses with the neurologic syndrome may require special care. Those with atonic bladders will need to be catheterized; manual removal of manure from the rectum may be needed if the horse is unable to defecate; recumbent horses require deep bedding, frequent turning, protective bandaging, and sometimes slinging. Sedation may be needed in some.

Infected horses including those with latent infections can shed large amounts of virus from the respiratory tract thus contaminating the environment. Aborted infected fetuses and the placenta and fluids also are sources of infection. Horses with recognized infections should be isolated and it is advisable to prevent movement of horses until 3 weeks following recovery of the last clinical case (be it the neurologic or respiratory form).[68] When it is not possible to adhere to this 3-week period, housing should be disinfected with a viricidal substance, all contaminated materials should be disposed of and horses should be vaccinated. Handlers should wear disposable gloves and change clothes and footwear if caring for infected horses. Preferably, infected horses should be handled by separate people or after all other horses on the premises.

Conditions most conductive to epizootics, unfortunately, are those which commonly occur under most management practices, i.e., the congregation of large numbers of susceptible stressed horses, from diverse locations in poorly ventilated housing.

For prevention and control, steps should be taken to (1) minimize stress so as to decrease reactivation of latent infections in carrier horses, (2) prevent introduction from exogenous sources and isolate new arrivals for at least 3 weeks before placing them with resident horses, (3) avoid formation of large groups of immunologically naive young horses by organizing horses into small epizootically separated units and separating mares and foals into small weaning groups, (4) avoid sudden stressful weaning of large numbers of foals and wean by removing one mare at a time every few days until weaning is completed, (5) separate pregnant mares from weanling and transient horses, (6) provide well ventilated, clean housing.[68,99]

Faced with an outbreak of neurologic disease, dispersal of animals into small isolated groups in separated pastures has been advocated.[91] Although it has been suggested that newly acquired mares be separated from resident pregnant mares for the duration of pregnancy, a 3-week period of isolation is usually more practical and is about twice the period of time that immunologically experienced susceptible mares shed virus after experimental intranasal infection.[90] Control of the disease is likely to remain a problem because of latent infections and management practices that are conducive to infection.

## Prophylaxis

There has been much debate about vaccination schedules for horses. At present there are two vaccines commercially available in the United States—one with an attenuated live virus* and the other containing a formalin inactivated adjuvanted virus.† The former's label claims are limited to use for respiratory disease, although it is used by some veterinarians in brood mares. Neither vaccine contains EHV-4 (EHV-1 subtype 2) antigens but shared antigens result in both producing an-

*Rhinomune, Norden Laboratories, Lincoln, Nebraska
†Pneumabort K, Ft. Dodge Laboratories, Ft. Dodge, Iowa.

tibodies against EHV-4.[68] Protection is not complete and infection and subsequent shedding of EHV-4 may occur in vaccinated horses. In a study in 8- to 12-month-old ponies after 3 doses of the formalin inactivated EHV-1 vaccine, 20% of the ponies had transient fevers and nasal discharge and 66% shed virus following challenge with EHV-4.[70] Frequently, there was only a low response in neutralizing antibody, although this is probably not important as levels did not correlate with immunity unlike CF titers. When the same vaccine was administered to yearling and 2-year-old ponies and pregnant pony mares and the ponies were then exposed to aerosols of EHV-1, they became infected, developed a transient cell associated viremia and shed virus.[88] However, vaccination did decrease the severity and duration of clinical signs as well as quantity and duration of virus shedding for both EHV-1 and EHV-4. When the 2-year-old ponies were rechallenged 2 months after vaccination, their group mean clinical score (numerical scoring of clinical signs) decreased by about 25%; and, when yearlings were challenged 1 month after their third vaccination the mean clinical score was about one third less than that recorded for controls.[88] The recommendation of vaccinating young animals twice at 3- to 4-week intervals and "boosting" 6 months after the second dose does not protect individual horses against infection, although it may decrease the incidence and duration of clinical signs and decrease spread of disease by decreasing the duration and quantity of virus shedding.[70,88] Although abortions may occur despite vaccination, the incidence is decreased in the vaccinated population.[68] Abortion "storms" in vaccinated mares have been associated with infection by a genetically variant virus.[68] For foals, the following vaccination program has been suggested: the first two injections 3 or 4 weeks apart with the second given about 3 weeks prior to weaning and a third given about 6 months later and 3 to 4 weeks prior to the yearling sales or start of training.[66,99] Vaccination does not eliminate the requirement for good management practices to control infection and disease.

Although some clinicians believe that frequent (monthly or biweekly) vaccination decreases the incidence of pharyngeal lymphoid hyperplasia, to my knowledge the efficacy of such a vaccination program in preventing either infection or pharyngeal lymphoid hyperplasia has not been demonstrated. As repeated injections with the inactivated virus vaccine at short intervals can cause local Arthus reactions, a minimum of 60 days between injections has been recommended for all horses except foals.[99] Natural infections may provide better protection against respiratory illness than the vaccine.

Use of a fraction of mycobacterial cell walls plus other adjuvants and stabilizers* was reported to decrease severity and shorten the course of infection in horses with rhinopneumonitis. Of 16 age- and sex-matched horses, the 8 which were treated with the immunostimulant had a shorter illness and were able to return to training much sooner than antibiotic and phenylbutazone treated stablemates.[100] Although EHV-1 was isolated from two horses in each group, vaccination status and antibody levels were not given. At the time of writing, more data are needed. The importance of a well ventilated and clean environment in preventing disease is emphasized by a field study showing that the increase in tracheal exudate associated with EHV-1 infection was much less in a "clean" environment than in a poorly ventilated area with heavy fungus contamination.[89]

## *EHV-2*

EHV-2 or cytomegalic beta herpesvirus is ubiquitous and has been isolated from the respiratory tract, leukocytes, conjunctivae, and other sites in both normal and diseased horses. In a study on Ontario racetracks EHV-2 was the most frequently isolated virus, being recovered primarily in late fall, winter and early spring and not specifically associated with severe outbreaks of respiratory disease.[35] It has the same morphology as EHV-1 but has a slow replication and tends to remain cell associated. It can require up to 28 days to produce cytopathic effects in cell cultures. Both rabbit kidney and equine cell lines

*Equimune, Ragland Research Inc., Athens, GA

are suitable for culture. Infected cells may become enlarged (cytomegaly) and may form intranuclear inclusions.

Indirect immunofluorescent testing provides the most reproducible identification. Neither CF nor VN is suitable.[16] The virus can be shed continuously in healthy horses. The higher percent of positive titers in horses less than 1 year old compared to those between 1 and 9 years of age (98% vs 85%) suggests that it more commonly infects young horses; EHV-1 shows a similar pattern (67% vs 38%).[26]

## Clinical Signs

In addition to infection of the respiratory tract EHV-2 has been isolated from equine cases of keratoconjunctivitis superficialis. Photophobia, blepharospasm, lacrimation, a concentric irregularly limited nonhomogeneous darkening of the cornea with a cloudy ring and an irregular nodular refractile surface were described in all patients.[101] Healing occurred within 8 to 14 days although the nodules took 2 to 4 weeks to regress. Topical steroids caused recrudescence of the lesions and prevented healing. In 2 of 12 horses EHV-2 was isolated from corneal samples. All affected horses had higher VN antibodies to the EHV-2 isolate than their clinically normal stable companions.[101] None showed respiratory illness.

Signs of upper respiratory tract disease—nasal discharge, fever, enlarged lymph nodes, pharyngitis and anorexia—have been seen in foals from which EHV-2 was consistently isolated. Foals sometimes developed "ill thrift" and severe bacterial infections 1 to 6 months later or fatal purpura hemorrhagica. Deaths were seen 2 to 38 days after onset of signs of upper respiratory tract disease. It was proposed that EHV-2 depressed the foals' immune status, permitting severe secondary bacterial infections (Horner, cited in Reference 26).

A subsequent study was done on foals and dams on a farm that had previously had significant respiratory disease attributed to EHV-2.[102] The earliest age at which EHV-2 was recovered was at about 1 month, similar to an earlier report.[103] Chronic virus excretion has been reported previously and is probably due to fluctuating low grade infection of cells in the nasopharynx.[104,105] No positive EHV-2 isolates were found by 9 months of age. At about the time the virus was first isolated 10 of 16 foals showed pyrexia, mucopurulent nasal discharge and swollen lymph nodes. Two foals died at 2 months of age. Bacterial pneumonia, petechial hemorrhages (consistent with bacteremia), pharyngitis and lymphoid depletion of the spleen and thymus were found at postmortem. EHV-2 had been recovered from both foals within 3 weeks of death and was recovered at postmortem from one; various bacteria were also isolated at postmortem. In contrast, none of the mares including 5 from which EHV-2 was isolated, showed any signs other than a serous nasal discharge. Serology showed that all foals had a steady increase in antibodies to EHV-2 until 5 to 6 months of age at which time virus isolation decreased. The mares showed insignificant rises in antibody titers.[103] EHV-1 was also isolated from most of these foals at weaning time (4 to 6 months of age), but not earlier and was, therefore, not the cause of respiratory disease in the young foals. There have been additional reports of severe outbreaks of respiratory disease in 6- to 10-week-old foals that have been attributed to EHV-2 based on virus isolation and rising antibody titers.[106–108] In one group of Arabian foals, no evidence of cellular or humoral deficiency was found to explain increased susceptibility. These foals were not depressed and continued to eat despite a cough, polypnea, and fever. Several foals died and the one that was autopsied had no evidence of secondary bacterial infection. EHV-2 was isolated and gross and histologic studies were diagnostic of viral pneumonia.[107] It is possible that strain variation in EHV-2 accounts for some of the variation in reports on its significance as a respiratory pathogen.

## Diagnosis

Physical examinations do not reveal any signs pathognomonic for EHV-2 and secondary bacterial infections often coexist. Diagnosis is based on viral isolation, immunofluorescent techniques and serologic conversion. Nasal scrapings for immunofluorescent staining for EHV-2 are rapid and cost effective. In one outbreak nasal scrapings obtained from all 4 foals sampled were positive.[107] Transtracheal aspirates may or may not yield positive isolates. If foals die, samples should be saved for virus isolation. Thoracic radiographs have shown interstitial and alveolar lung disease in multifocal or lobar distribution, but these changes also could be seen with bacterial, parasitic or allergic disease.[107,109]

### Prophylaxis and Treatment

There are no specific prophylactic measures and treatment is symptomatic.

# Picornaviruses

## *Rhinovirus*

The role of this RNA virus as a pathogen in horses remains controversial and it has been suggested that rhinovirus infections become clinically apparent only when a horse is stressed by other factors.[110] It may be isolated with other viruses and synergism is possible. Rhinovirus has been isolated from normal horses as well as those showing signs of respiratory disease, and serologic surveys have revealed antibodies in horses with no signs of disease.[110] Over an 18-month period it was recovered 8 times from one horse that showed no clinical abnormalities and the horse had only a low constant antibody level.[16] In a survey of horses in Ontario where nasopharyngeal swabs were collected from horses with signs of respiratory disease and from clinically normal horses, equine rhinovirus subtype 2 was the most frequently isolated virus; 28 of 92 diseased horses and 7 of 38 normal horses yielded isolates.[111] Also, seroconversion with a 4-fold rise in antibody titer was seen in 19 of 92 affected and 5 of 38 normal horses. Although there was a similar seroconversion to rhinovirus subtype 1 in both groups, no isolates were made.[111] No isolates of equine rhinopneumonitis were obtained although seroconversion occurred, only five isolates of equine influenza virus type 2 and no isolates of equine adenovirus or equine viral arteritis virus were made, leading the authors to suggest that equine rhinoviruses are involved in outbreaks of respiratory disease.[111] Many serotypes are known to cause upper respiratory tract disease in man and three equine serotypes have been identified.[7,112] Serotype 1 is strain NM-11 and serotype 2 is P1436/71. The two strains differ in pH stability. A third serotype P313/75 differs from ERV-2 in acid lability.[112,113]

### Clinical Signs

The first isolation of an equine rhinovirus (ERV) was reported in 1962.[114] The virus was recovered from feces and later experimental infection of both horses and a human being caused upper respiratory tract infection. The horses developed a fever and mucoid or mucopurulent pharyngitis and nasal discharge plus a viremia of 4 to 5 days' duration. The single infected person developed fever, rhinitis, pharyngitis, swollen pharyngeal lymph nodes, and viremia. Neither the horses nor the person coughed and there was no spread to contact controls. Since then other studies have associated clinical signs with both types 1 and 2 rhinoviruses.[111-113] Isolates have been made from horses with definite signs of upper respiratory tract disease but only one strain has been associated with an outbreak in a stable.[113] In contrast, experimental infections in both conventional and gnotobiotic foals caused no clinical signs.[113] Signs which have been associated with virus isolation have ranged from none to ulcerative rhinitis; coughing at rest; enlarged submandibular lymph nodes with or without coughing at rest; nasal discharge or fever; and fever, anorexia and coughing at rest.[113] On the basis of serologic studies, rhinovirus has been implicated as causing both nonfebrile pharyngitis in 6- to 9-month-old foals and acute pharyngitis in mature horses.[110]

It appears that type 1 infections are most frequent when young horses are transported and concentrated in large groups, and type 2 infections may be acquired during the suckling stage and are not associated with transport and concentration of horses.[115] In one study within a small group of foals, no ERV-1 antibodies were found but two had ERV-2 antibodies, supporting the hypothesis of type 1 infection occurring when horses are clustered together and stressed and ERV-2 being acquired during suckling. Antibodies to ERV-2 were detected in 1- to 3-month-old foals but at 7 to 9 months of age these foals were all negative.[110] As mentioned previously, ERV-2 has been associated with outbreaks of respiratory disease in horses older than 1 year.[111]

Rhinovirus serotype 1 may be continuously shed for long periods. It was isolated for up to 1 month from the pharynx of some horses following infection and strain 4442 (which fits into neither serotype 1 nor 2), was isolated repeatedly from an asymptomatic pony.[113,114]

### Diagnosis

Diagnosis of rhinovirus infection is based on virus isolation and examination for CF antibodies. However, the high antibody titers in acute phase sera are often confusing and they may decrease during convalescence, reaching preinfection levels by 1 to 2 months following their peak. Interpretation of antibody titers without concomitant virus isolation becomes difficult. In one survey it was not possible to correlate clinical signs with either virus isolation or rising antibody titers.[112] Serologic surveys in Europe showed antibodies to both ERV-1 and ERV-2 more frequently in grouped horses than in solitary horses.[112]

### Treatment

Treatment is often unnecessary. Comments made previously regarding other viral infections apply. As it is debatable that picornaviruses pose a health threat to horses, no specific prophylaxis is recommended.

## Equine Viral Arteritis

The virus causing EVA is an RNA togavirus that was first identified in 1953. Infection occurs in various horse populations worldwide, but it is not considered an important cause of respiratory disease. Its primary importance is its potential to cause abortion. Limited antigenic variation among isolates of the single serotype has been reported.[116] Pathogenicity varies greatly as some infections are inapparent and others severe. Although serologic surveys revealed widespread infection, until the 1984 epizootic in Kentucky, there was little concern abut the significance of EVA.[117,118] The ratio of clinical disease to inapparent infection is much higher in mares bred to EVA affected stallions than in those bred to a presumed chronic carrier asymptomatic stallion.[118] Infection rates are much higher in Standardbreds with 70 to 90% testing seropositive for antibodies compared to only 2 to 3% of Thoroughbred mares.[119]

The virus is transmitted by aerosolized respiratory tract secretions, via contaminated fomites and venereally.[118,120] Transmission can occur horizontally or laterally. Also, although the convalescent carrier state lasts only a few weeks following recovery from the clinical disease, the chronic carrier state can persist for years in stallions. Carrier stallions constantly shed virus in their semen but not in respiratory tract secretions or urine.[118,120] Mares bred to carrier stallions may develop inapparent infections and shed virus into the respiratory tract and perhaps urine, thereby serving to transmit the virus horizontally during their convalescence. However, based on current evidence the frequency of a naturally acquired carrier state in the mare is low or nonexistent.[118] When horses inhale virus particles, virus may be recovered from the nasopharynx for as long as 14 days. It is postulated that in horses infected via inhalation, the virus enters the bronchial lymph nodes and then the circulation.[121] The incubation period is 7 to 19 days.

### Clinical Signs

Signs are highly variable, but most characteristic is a high fever up to 41°C (106°F) which may persist for 5 to 9 days.[120] Other signs include serous nasal discharge and rhinitis, conjunctivitis, lacrimation and palpebral and periorbital edema, limb edema, anorexia and depression, abortion in the pregnant mare, preputial and scrotal edema in the stallion, weakness, diarrhea and sometimes coughing and respiratory distress.[120] Horses are profoundly lymphopenic. Recovery is usual and mortality has been reported only in experimental infection with an unattenuated strain.

## Pathology

Subcutaneous edema and increased pleural and pericardial fluid are usual. Necrosis of the media of the small muscular arteries and acute panvasculitis are seen and, in the cecum and colon, thrombosis and neutrophilic infiltration occur in the submucosa along with infarction and necrosis of the mucosa.

Diagnosis is based on clinical signs, demonstration of a 4-fold rise in virus neutralizing antibody titers in paired sera collected 10 to 14 days apart, and virus isolation.

## Treatment and Prophylaxis

Treatment is symptomatic. Antibiotics against secondary bacterial infections of the respiratory tract are rarely needed. Affected or exposed animals should be isolated for 3 weeks to minimize the likelihood of transmission. The virus is susceptible to most disinfectants and detergents. Specific guidelines have been provided regarding control in breeding animals.[118–120] Restriction of movement of breeding stock and closing the breeding sheds plus vaccination should be implemented if an outbreak threatens.[118,119]

Vaccination has been highly effective. A modified live vaccine is available and although it has a high degree of safety, its use is not recommended in foals less than 6 weeks of age or in pregnant mares. The vaccine will not prevent reinfection or limit replication of challenge virus but it does decrease both duration and amount of virus shed from the nasopharynx.[117] A small percentage of horses vaccinated for the first time reportedly developed mild postvaccinal febrile reactions and transient lymphopenia.[118]

# References


1. Mumford JA, Rossdale PD. Virus and its relationship to the "poor performance" syndrome. Equine Vet J *12*:3, 1980.
2. Gerber H. Clinical features, sequelae, and epidemiology of equine influenza. In: Proceedings of 2nd International Conference on Equine Infectious Disease, Paris (1969). JT Bryans and H Gerber (eds). Basel, S. Karger, 1970, p 63.
3. Plateau E, Jacquet A, Cheyroux M. A study of the serological response of horses to influenza vaccination: Comparison of protocols and types of vaccines. In: Proceedings of 5th International Conference on Equine Infectious Disease. DG Powell (ed). Lexington, The University Press of Kentucky, 1988, p 94.
4. Tumova B. Equine influenza—a segment in influenza virus ecology. Comp Immun Microbiol Infect Dis, *3*:45, 1980.
5. Ada GJ, Jones PD. The immune response to influenza infection. Curr Topics Microbiol Immunol, *128*:1, 1986.
6. Mitchell DM, McMichael AJ, Lamb JR. The immunology of influenza. Br Med Bull *41*:80, 1985.
7. Fenner F, Bachmann PA, Gibbs EPJ, et al. Veterinary Virology. Orlando, Academic Press, 1987.
8. Bayly WM, Liggitt HD, Huston LJ, et al. Stress and its effect on equine pulmonary mucosal defenses. In: Proceedings of 32d Annual Meeting of American Association of Equine Practitioners, 1986, p 253.
9. Anderson NV, DeBowes RM, Myrop KA, et al. Mononuclear phagocytes of transport-stressed horses with viral respiratory tract infection. Am J Vet Res *46*:2272, 1985.
10. Traub-Dargatz JL, McKinnon AO, Bruyninckx WJ, et al. Effect of transportation stress on bronchoalveolar lavage fluid analysis in female horses. Am J Vet Res *49*:1026, 1988.
11. Degre M. Interaction between viral and bacterial infections in the respiratory tract. Scand J Infect Dis *49*:140, 1986.
12. Jakab GJ. Viral bacterial interactions in the lung. In: Advances in Veterinary Science and Comparative Medicine, *26*:154. CE Cornelius and CF Simpson (eds). New York, Academic Press, 1982.
13. Woodside KH, Denas SM, Smith KL, et al. Inhibition of pulmonary macrophage function by airway mucus. J Am Physiol Soc *54*:94, 1983.
14. Cohen D. Epidemiology of virus diseases. In: Basic Medical Virology. JE Prier (ed). Baltimore, Williams & Wilkins, 1966, p 185.
15. England JJ, McChesney AE, Chow TL. Isolation and identification of equine adenoviruses. In: Proceedings of 4th International Conference on Equine Infectious Disease, Lyon (1976). JT Bryans and H Gerber (eds). Princeton, Veterinary Publications, Inc., 1978, p 147.
16. Mumford JA, Thomson GR. Serologic methods for identification of slowly growing herpesviruses isolated from the respiratory tract of horses. In: Proceedings of 4th International Conference on Equine Infectious Disease, Lyon (1976). JT Bryans and H Gerber (eds). Princeton, Veterinary Publications, Inc., 1978, p 49.
17. Wood JM, Mumford JA, Folkers C, et al. Studies with inactivated equine influenza vaccine. 1. Serological responses of ponies to graded dose of vaccine. J Hyg Camb *90*:371, 1983.
18. Hannant D, Mumford JA, Jessett DM. Duration of

circulating antibody and immunity following infection with equine influenza virus. Vet Rec *122*:125, 1988.
19. Beech J, Merryman GS, Spencer PA. Effect of dimethylglycine on antibody response to influenza vaccination in horses. Equine Vet Sci *7*:62, 1987.
20. Mumford JA, Wood JM, Scott AM, et al. Studies with inactivated equine influenza vaccine. 2. Protection against experimental infection with influenza virus A/equine/Newmarket/79 (H3N8). J Hyg Camb *90*:385, 1983.
21. Burrows R, Goodridge D. Observations of picornavirus, adenovirus, and equine herpesvirus infections in the Pirbright pony herd. In: Proceedings of 4th International Conference on Equine Infectious Diseases, Lyon (1976). JT Bryans and H Gerber (eds). Princeton, Veterinary Publications, Inc., 1978, p 155.
22. Ditchfield WJB. Rhinoviruses and para-influenza viruses of horses. J Am Vet Med Assoc *155*:384, 1969.
23. Todd JD. Comments on rhinoviruses and parainfluenza viruses of horses. J Am Vet Med Assoc *155*:387, 1969.
24. Horner GW, Hunter R. Isolation of two serotypes of equine adenovirus from horses in New Zealand. NZ Vet J *30*:62, 1982.
25. Studdert MJ, Blackney MH. Isolation of an adenovirus antigenically distinct from equine adenovirus type 1 from diarrheic foal feces. Am J Vet Res *43*:543, 1982.
26. Jolly PD, Fu ZF, Robinson AJ. Viruses associated with respiratory disease of horses in New Zealand: An update. NZ Vet J *34*:46, 1986.
27. Kamada M, Akiyama Y, Sato K, et al. Isolation of adenovirus from adult Thoroughbred horses. Jpn J Vet Sci *39*:661, 1977.
28. Powell DG, Burrows R, Goodridge D. Respiratory viral infections among Thoroughbred horses in training during 1972. Equine Vet J *6*:19, 1974.
29. Gleeson LJ, Studdert MJ, Sullivan ND. Pathogenicity and immunologic studies of equine adenovirus in specific pathogen free foals. Am J Vet Res *39*:1636, 1978.
30. Kamada M. Comparison of four serological tests for detecting antibodies against equine adenovirus. Exp Rep Equine Health Lab *15*:91, 1978.
31. Sugiura T, Matsumura T, Imagawa H, et al. A seven year serological study of viral agents causing respiratory infection with pyrexia among racehorses in Japan. In: Proceedings of 5th International Conference on Equine Infectious Disease. DG Powell (ed). Lexington, The University Press of Kentucky, 1988, p 258.
32. McChesney AE, England JJ. Equine adenoviral infection: Pathogenesis of experimentally and naturally transmitted infection. In: Proceedings of 4th International Conference on Equine Infectious Disease, Lyon (1976). JT Bryans and H Gerber (eds). Princeton, Veterinary Publications, Inc., 1978, p 141.
33. McChesney AE, England JJ, Whiteman CE, et al. Experimental transmission of equine adenovirus in Arabian and non-Arabian foals. Am J Vet Res *35*:1015, 1974.
34. Kawaoka Y, Bean WJ, Webster RG. Origin of the A/equine/Johannesburg/86 (H3N8) Virus: Antigenic and genetic analysis of equine-2 influenza A hemagglutinins. In: Proceedings of 5th International Conference on Equine Infectious Disease. DG Powell (ed). Lexington, The University Press of Kentucky, 1988, p 47.
35. Ingram DG, Sherman J, Mitchell WR, et al. The epidemiology and control of respiratory disease at Ontario racetracks. In: Proceedings of 4th International Conference on Equine Infectious Disease, Lyon (1976). JT Bryans and H Gerber (eds). Princeton, Veterinary Publications, Inc., 1978, p 329.
36. Couch RB. Viruses and indoor air pollution. Bull NY Acad Med, Second Series *57*:907, 1981.
37. Kudo H, Ohde H, Yamanaka T, et al. Hemagglutination-inhibiting antibodies to equine influenza viruses in Japanese horses and antigenic variation of the viruses. Kitasato Arch Exp Med *59*:49, 1986.
38. Baker DJ. Rationale for the use of influenza vaccines in horses and the importance of antigenic drift. Equine Vet J *18*:93, 1986.
39. Powell DG, Burrows R, Spooner P, et al. Field observations on influenza vaccination among horses in Britain 1971–1976. Dev Biol Stand *39*:347, 1977.
40. Hinshaw VS, Naeve CW, Webster RG, et al. Analysis of antigenic variation in equine 2 influenza A viruses. Bull WHO *61*:153, 1983.
41. Gibson CA, Daniels RS, McCauley JW, et al. Hemagglutinin gene sequencing studies of equine-1 influenza A viruses. In: Proceedings of 5th International Conference on Equine Infectious Disease. DG Powell (ed). Lexington, The University Press of Kentucky, 1988, p 51.
42. Webster RG, Hinshaw VS, Bean WJ, et al. Influenza transmission between species. Philos Trans R Soc Lond (Biol) *288*:439, 1980.
43. Webster RG. The evolution of epidemic influenza viruses. In: Proceedings of 4th International Conference on Equine Infectious Disease, Lyon (1976). JT Bryans and H Gerber (eds). Princeton, Veterinary Publications, Inc., 1978, p 305.
44. Rouse BT, Ditchfield WJB. The response of ponies to myxovirus influenza A/equi-2. III. The protective effect of serum and nasal antibody against experimental challenge. Res Vet Sci *11*:503, 1970.
45. Aquilina AT, Hall WJ, Douglas RG Jr, et al. Airway reactivity in subjects with viral upper respiratory tract infections: the effects of exercise and cold air. Am Rev Respir Dis *122*:3, 1980.
46. Hall WJ, Douglas RG, Hyde RW. Pulmonary mechanics after uncomplicated influenza A infection. Am Rev Respir Dis *113*:141, 1976.
47. McQueen JL, Davenport FM, Keeran RJ, et al. Studies on equine influenza in Michigan 1963. II. Epizootiology Am Epidem *83*:280, 1965.
48. Hannant D, Jessett DM, O'Neill T, et al. Nasopharyngeal tracheobronchial and systemic immune responses to vaccination and aerosol infection with equine-2 influenza A virus (H3N8). In: Proceedings of 5th International Conference on Equine Infec-

tious Disease. DG Powell (ed). Lexington, The University Press of Kentucky, 1988, p 68.
49. Hugoson G, Klingeborne B, Hedberg P. A countrywide test of trotters for possible capacity reducing effects of influenza vaccination. In: Proceedings of 3rd International Symposium on Veterinary Epidemiology and Economy, Virginia, USA. Edwardsville, Kansas, Veterinary Publications, Inc., 1983, p 210.
50. Thomson GR, Mumford JA, Spooner PR, et al. The outbreak of equine influenza in England—January 1976. Vet Rec *100*:465, 1977.
51. Higgins WP, Gillespie JH, Holmes DF, et al. Surveys of equine influenza outbreaks during 1983 and 1984. J Equine Vet Sci *6*:15, 1986.
52. Kemen MJ, Frank RA, Babish JB. An outbreak of equine influenza at a harness horse racetrack. Cornell Vet *75*:277, 1985.
53. Raphel CF, Beech J. Pleuritis secondary to pneumonia or lung abscessation in 90 horses. J Am Vet Med Assoc *181*:808, 1982.
54. Graber CD, Goust JM, Glassman AD, et al. Immunomodulating properties of dimethylglycine in humans. J Infect Dis *143*:101, 1981.
55. Evans DR, Hartgrove TB, Rollins JB, et al. Inactivated propionibacterium acnes (Immunoregulin[TM]) as adjunct to conventional therapy in the treatment of equine respiratory diseases. Equine Pract *10*:17, 1988.
56. Beech J. Topics in treating respiratory disease. In: Proceedings of 32nd Annual Convention of American Association of Equine Practitioners, Nashville, 1987, p 299.
57. Burki F. Serum antibody titers and nasal immunity following repeated parenteral influenza vaccinations in horses. In Proceedings of 4th International Conference on Equine Infectious Disease, Lyon (1976). JT Bryans and H Gerber (eds). Princeton, Veterinary Publications, Inc., 1978, p 191.
58. Bryans JT. Control of equine influenza. In: Proceedings of 26th Annual Convention of American Association of Equine Practitioners, Anaheim, California, 1980, p 279.
59. Wood JM, Mumford JA, Dunleavy U, et al. Single radial diffusion potency tests for equine influenza vaccines. In: Proceedings of 5th International Conference on Equine Infectious Disease. DG Powell (ed). Lexington, The University Press of Kentucky, 1988, p 74.
60. Holmes DF, Lamb LM, Anguish LM, et al. Live temperature-sensitive equine-1 influenza A virus vaccine: efficacy in experimental ponies. In: Proceedings of 5th International Conference on Equine Infectious Disease. DG Powell (ed). Lexington, The University Press of Kentucky, 1988, p 88.
61. Burrows R, Spooner PR, Goodridge D. A three year evaluation of four commercial equine influenza vaccines in ponies maintained in isolation. Develop Biol Stand *39*:341, 1977.
62. Eagles BW, Higgins AJ. Equine influenza reactions (letter). Vet Rec *116*:478, 1985.
63. Mair TS. Adverse reactions to equine vaccinations: A preliminary survey. Vet Rec *122*:396, 1988.
64. Coombs SL, Webbon PM. Tracheal mucus transport in the horse following equine influenza vaccination. Vet Rec *119*:601, 1986.
65. Beveridge WIB. Influenza in horses. Bull Off Int Epid *70*:171, 1968.
66. Bryans JT, Allen GP. Herpesviral diseases of the horse. In: Herpesvirus Disease of cattle, horses and pigs. G Wittmann (ed). Boston, Kluwer Academic Publishers, 1989, p 176.
67. Allen GP, Yeargan MR, Turtinen LW, et al. Molecular epizootiologic studies of equine herpesvirus 1 infections by restriction endonuclease fingerprinting of viral DNA. Am J Vet Res *44*:263, 1983.
68. Allen GP, Bryans JT. Molecular epizootiology, pathogenesis and prophylaxis of equine herpesvirus-1 infections. Prog Vet Microbiol Immun *2*:78. Pandey R (ed). S Karger, Basel, 1986.
69. Studdert MJ, Simpson T, Roizman B. Differentiation of respiratory and abortigenic isolates of equine herpesvirus by restriction endonucleases. Science *214*:562, 1981.
70. Mumford JA, Bates J. Trials of an inactivated equid herpesvirus 1 vaccine: challenge with a subtype 2 virus. Vet Rec *114*:375, 1984.
71. O'Callaghan DJ, Allen GP, Randall CC. Structure and replication of equine herpesviruses. J Eq Med Surg Suppl[1]:1, 1978.
72. Coignoul FL, Bertram TA, Cheville NF. Pathogenicity of equine herpesvirus/subtype 2 for foals and adult pony mares. Vet Microbiol *9*:533, 1984.
73. Patel JR, Edington N, and Mumford JA. Variation in cellular tropism between isolates of equine herpesvirus 1 in foals. Arch Virol *74*:41, 1982.
74. Bridges CG, Edington N. Innate immunity during equid herpesvirus 1 (EHV-1) infection. Clin Exp Immunol *65*:172, 1986.
75. Scott JC, Dutta SK, Myrup AC. In vivo harboring of equine herpesvirus 1 in leukocyte populations and subpopulation and their quantitation from experimentally infected ponies. Am J Vet Res *44*:1344, 1983.
76. Burrows R, Goodridge D: Studies of persistent and latent equine herpesvirus 1 and herpesvirus 3 infections in the Pirbright pony herd. In: Veterinary Medicine. Wittmann G, Gaskell RM and Rziha HJ (eds). The Hague, Martinus Nijhoff, 1984, p 307.
77. Ardans AA. Immunoprophylaxis in the horse. J Am Vet Assoc *181*:1150, 1982.
78. Crandell RA. Selected animal herpesviruses: New concepts and technologies. In: Advances in Veterinary Science and Comparative Medicine, *29*:281. CE Cornelius and CF Simpson (eds). New York, Academic Press, 1985.
79. Edington N, Bridges CG, Huckle A. Experimental reactivation of equid herpesvirus 1 (EHV 1) following the administration of corticosteroids. Equine Vet J *17*:369, 1985.
80. Darlington RW. The role of equine macrophages in resistance or susceptibility to infection by equine

herpesvirus 1. In: Proceedings of 4th International Conference on Equine Infectious Disease, Lyon (1976). JT Bryans and H Gerber (eds). Princeton, Veterinary Publications Inc., 1978, p 129.

81. Campbell TM, Studdert MJ. Equine herpesvirus type 1 (EHV). Vet Bull *53*:135, 1983.
82. Burrows R, Goodridge D. Experimental studies on equine herpesvirus type 1 infections. J Reprod Fert (Suppl) *231*:611, 1975.
83. Thomson GR, Mumford JA, Plowright W. Immunological responses of conventional and gnotobiotic foals to infectious and inactivated antigens of equine herpesvirus type 1. In: Proceedings of 4th International Conference on Equine Infectious Disease, Lyon (1976). JT Bryans and H Gerber (eds). Princeton, Veterinary Publications, Inc., 1978, p 103.
84. Burrows R, Goodridge D. In vivo and in vitro studies of equine rhinopneumonitis strains. In: Proceedings of 3rd International Conference on Equine Infectious Disease, Paris (1972). JT Bryans, H Gerber (eds). Basel, S Karger, 1973, p 306.
85. Kohn CW. Recognition and management of equine viral respiratory diseases. Comp Cont Ed *3*:S101, 1981.
86. Burrows R. The general virology of the herpesvirus group. In: Proceedings of 2nd International Conference on Equine Infectious Disease, Paris (1969). JT Bryans and H Gerber (eds). Basel, S Karger, 1970, p 1.
87. Burki F. Equine rhinopneumonitis. Arch Vet Ital, *23*:73, 1972.
88. Burrows R, Goodridge D, Denyer MS. Trials of an inactivated equid herpesvirus 1 vaccine: challenge with a subtype 1 virus. Vet Rec *114*:369, 1984.
89. Clarke AF, Madelin TM, Allpress RG. The relationship of air hygiene in stables to lower airway disease during an outbreak of equid herpesvirus 1 infection. In: Proceedings of 5th International Conference on Equine Infectious Disease. DG Powell (ed). Lexington, The University Press of Kentucky, 1988, p 268.
90. Bryans JT. On immunity to disease caused by equine herpesvirus 1. J Am Vet Med Assoc *155*:294, 1969.
91. Greenwood RES, Simson ARB. Clinical report of a paralytic syndrome affecting stallions, mares and foals on a Thoroughbred stud farm. Equine Vet J *12*:113, 1980.
92. Jackson TA, Cordy DR, Osburn BI, et al. Equine herpesvirus 1 infection of horses: Studies on the experimentally induced neurologic disease. Am J Vet Res *38*:709, 1977.
93. Jackson TA, Kendrick JW. Paralysis of horses associated with equine herpesvirus 1 infection. J Am Vet Med Assoc *158*:1351, 1971.
94. Mumford JA, Edington N. EHV-1 and equine paresis. Vet Rec *196*:277, 1980.
95. Edington N, Bridges CG, Patel JR. Endothelial cell infection and thrombosis in paralysis caused by equid herpesvirus 1: Equine stroke. Arch Virol *90*:111, 1986.
96. Prickett ME. The pathology of disease caused by equine herpesvirus 1. In: Proceedings of 2nd International Conference on Equine Infectious Disease, Paris, (1969). JT Bryans and H Gerber (eds). Basel, S. Karger, 1970, p 24.
97. Thomson GR, Mumford JA, Campbell J, et al. Serological detection of equid herpesvirus infections of the respiratory tract. Equine Vet J *8*:58, 1976.
98. Kelsey DK, Olsen GA, Overall JC, et al. Alterations of host defense mechanisms by murine cytomegalovirus. Infect Immun *18*:765, 1977.
99. Bryans JT. Application of management procedures and prophylactic immunization to the control of equine rhinopneumonitis. In: Proceedings of 26th Annual Convention of American Association of Equine Practitioners, Anaheim, California, 1980, p 259.
100. Leneau H, Steinmeyer P, Ragland WL. Immunotherapy of equine infectious rhinopneumonitis. In: Proceedings of 32nd Annual Convention of American Association of Equine Practitioners, Nashville, 1987, p 615.
101. Thein, P. The association of EHV-2 infection with keratitis and research on the occurrence of equine coital exanthema (EHV-3) of horses in Germany. In: Proceedings of 4th International Conference on Equine Infectious Disease, Lyon (1976). JT Bryans and H Gerber (eds). Princeton, Veterinary Publications, Inc., 1978, p 33.
102. Fu ZF, Robinson AJ, Horner GW, et al. Respiratory disease in foals and the epizootiology of equine herpesvirus type 2 infection. NZ Vet J *34*:152, 1986.
103. Wilks CR, Studdert MJ. Equine herpesviruses. Epizootiology of slowly cytopathic viruses in foals. Aust Vet J *50*:438, 1974.
104. Turner AJ, Studdert MJ, Peterson JE. Equine herpesvirus 2. Persistence of equine herpesviruses in experimentally infected horses and the experimental induction of abortion. Aust Vet J *46*:90, 1970.
105. Blakeslee JR, Olsen RG, McAllister ES. Evidence of respiratory tract infection induced by equine herpesvirus type 2 in the horse. Can J Microbiol *21*:1940, 1975.
106. Palfi V, Belak S, Molnar T. Isolation of equine herpesvirus type 2 from foals showing respiratory symptoms. Brief report. Zbl Vet Med *B25*:165, 1978.
107. Ames TR, O'Leary TP, Johnston GR. Isolation of equine herpesvirus type 2 from foals with respiratory disease. Comp Cont Ed Eq *8*:664, 1986.
108. Sugiura T, Fukuzawa Y, Kamada M, et al. Isolation of equine herpesvirus type 2 from foals with pneumonitis. Bull Equine Res Inst *20*:148, 1983.
109. Farrow CS. Equine thoracic radiology. J Am Vet Med Assoc *179*:776, 1981.
110. Hofer B, Steck F, Gerber H. Virological investigations in a horse clinic. In: Proceedings of 4th International Conference on Equine Infectious Disease, Lyon (1976). JT Bryans and H Gerber (eds). Princeton, Veterinary Publications, Inc., 1978, p 475.
111. Willoughby RA, Huber L, Viel L. Culture and serological results in acute upper respiratory infec-

tions in horses. In: Proceedings of 7th ACVIM Forum, San Diego (1989). G Pidgeon (ed). Madison, Omnipress, 1989, p 604.

112. Steck F, Hofer B, Schoeren B, et al. Equine rhinoviruses: New serotypes. In: Proceedings of 4th International Conference on Equine Infectious Disease, Lyon (1976). JT Bryans and H Gerber (eds). Princeton, Veterinary Publications, Inc., 1978, p 321.
113. Mumford JA, Thomson GR. Studies on picornaviruses isolated from the respiratory tract of horses. In: Proceedings of 4th International Conference on Equine Infectious Disease, Lyon (1976). JT Bryans and H Gerber (eds). Princeton, Veterinary Publications, Inc., 1978, p 419.
114. Plummer G, Kerry JB. Studies on an equine respiratory virus. Vet Rec *74*:967, 1962.
115. Holmes DF, Kemen MJ, Coggins L. Equine rhinovirus infection—serologic evidence of infection in selected United States horse populations. In: Proceedings of 4th International Conference on Equine Infectious Disease, Lyon (1976). JT Bryans and H Gerber (eds). Princeton, Veterinary Publications, Inc., 1978, p 315.
116. Fukunaga Y, McCollum WH. Complement-fixation reactions in equine viral arteritis. Am J Vet Res *38*:2043, 1977.
117. Timoney PJ, McCollum WH, Roberts AW. Detection of the carrier state in stallions persistently infected with equine arteritis virus. In: Proceedings of 32nd Annual Convention of the American Association of Equine Practitioners, Nashville, 1987, p 57.
118. Timoney PJ, McCollum WH. Equine viral arteritis—epidemiology and control. Equine Vet Sci *8*:54, 1988.
119. Timoney PJ, McCollum WH, Roberts AW. Current strategies for the control of equine viral arteritis. In: Proceedings of 92nd Annual Meeting of U.S. Animal Health Assoc, Little Rock Arkansas, 1988, p 211.
120. Timoney PJ, McCollum WH. Equine Viral Arteritis. Can Vet J *28*:693, 1987.
121. McCollum WH, Prickett ME, Bryans JT. Temporal distribution of equine arteritis virus in respiratory mucosa, tissues and body fluids of horses infected by inhalation. Res Vet Sci *12*:459, 1971.

# CHAPTER 12

# INFECTIONS CAUSED BY BACTERIA, MYCOPLASMAS, PARASITES, AND FUNGI

*JILL BEECH and CORINNE R. SWEENEY*

## Streptococcal Infections

The two streptococcal species of primary importance in equine respiratory disease are Streptococcus zooepidemicus and S. equi, both beta-hemolytic Lancefield Group C members.[1] Strains of S. equi appear to be antigenically homogeneous, but S. zooepidemicus is antigenically heterogeneous with at least 15 different serotypes. The relevance of the different types to clinical disease and immunity is not yet known. The significance of the alpha-hemolytic Streptococcus pneumoniae as an equine pathogen is unclear at present.[2,3]

### *Streptococcus Zooepidemicus*

Streptococcus zooepidemicus is probably the most common equine bacterial isolate. It can be isolated from the upper respiratory tract mucosa of healthy horses[4] and occasionally from healthy horses' tracheobronchial aspirates.[5] It has also been isolated postmortem from the trachea.[6] It cannot invade intact mucous membranes, and therefore pre-existing damage is necessary for infection. Streptococcus zooepidemicus is probably most important as a secondary invader when host susceptibility is increased by viral infection and possibly by stress such as transport or intense exercise. Severe respiratory diseases such as pleuropneumonia have been shown to occur more frequently following transport or other stress.[7–9] Studies on the influence of long distance transport on pulmonary defense in horses have been conflicting; one study showed a decrease in numbers of alveolar macrophages, neutrophils and lymphocytes in the bronchoalveolar lavage fluid following transport,[10] whereas another study did not show this decrease.[11] Alveolar macrophage intracellular oxidative metabolism which is related to antimicrobial activity is decreased for 3 days following intense activity, and this could increase susceptibility to infection.[12] Other studies on the effect of exercise on macrophages showed exercise decreased phagocytosis and cell viability.[13] These effects of exercise could predispose horses to infection and partially explain why severe respiratory infections are more common in intensely exercising horses than in less stressed similarly aged horses.

When a susceptible horse inhales streptococci, infections of the upper respiratory tract such as sinusitis and lymph node abscesses may occur. The lower respiratory tract can become infected, leading to diffuse or focal pneumonia, abscesses and/or pleuritis (Figs. 12–1 to 12–3). Clinical signs depend on the horse's immune status, the severity of infection and whether the upper or lower respi-

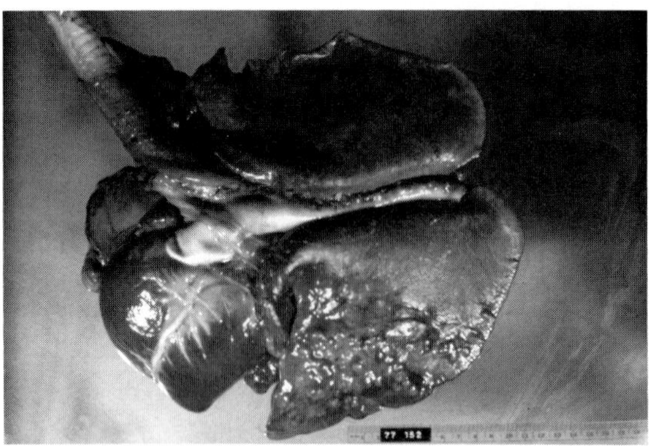

**FIG. 12–1.** Abscesses and pneumonia in the anterior and ventral portion of a foal's left lung.

ratory tract is more adversely affected. Neonatal infections may occur via the umbilicus and cause septicemia.[1]

## Clinical Signs and Diagnosis

Depression, fever, anorexia, and mucopurulent nasal discharge are common signs causing a client to request veterinary attention. A complete physical examination will reveal whether there is palpable lymphadenopathy, whether sinuses are dull on percussion, indicating loss of air filled space, and whether there is evidence of airway disease, pneumonia, consolidation, or pleural fluid. If thoracic percussion is dull, audible air movement is decreased, or there are increased large airway sounds ventrally, one should suspect the presence of pleural effusion or lung consolidation. When airways are narrowed, wheezes may be heard and rales or crackles and clicks occur when they contain fluid or exudate. The pattern and rate of respiration usually give some information about the severity of the process, which may be obstructive, restrictive or both. Isolation of the organism from the site(s) of infection is the basis for diagnosis. The organism is easily grown in the laboratory. Gram stains of material allow a presumptive diagnosis of a streptococcal infection but do not differentiate among streptococci. (S. zooepidemicus appears the same as S. equi, for example.)

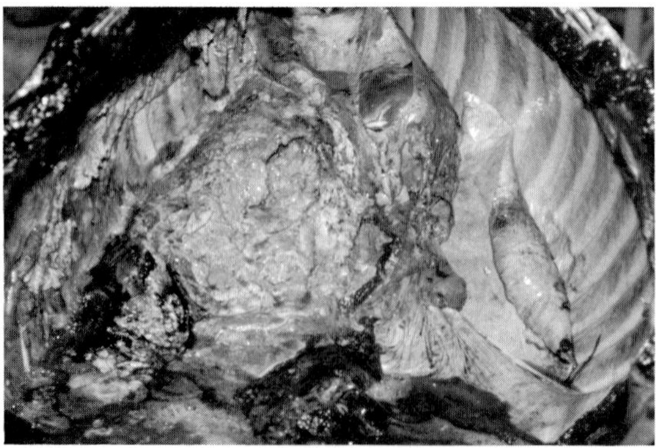

**FIG. 12–2.** Postmortem appearance of a horse with pleuritis and pneumonia. The left pleural cavity is normal, but the right parietal and visceral pleura are covered by thick fibrin ("bread and butter"). Orange fluid had filled about one fifth of the pleural space, and some remains in the lower left aspect of the photograph. The horse's carcass is on its back with the sternum dorsally and the horse's right side is on the viewer's left.

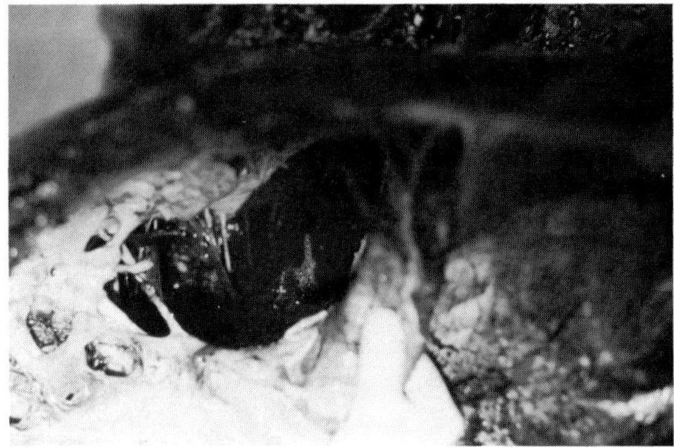

**FIG. 12–3.** Close-up view of pleural adhesions as viewed by a prosector cutting the diaphragm from the abdominal surface. There is considerable pleural fluid as well as multiple adhesions. Clinical signs of pleuritis and pneumonia had existed for longer than 6 weeks prior to necropsy.

## Treatment

When treating an infected horse, sensitivity testing of streptococci is advisable. Streptococci are usually sensitive to penicillin; however, pus and an acid pH decrease the efficacy of penicillin. Erythromycin is effective and an additional advantage is its penetration of lung and pleural fluid and neutrophils. Other drugs which may be effective include chloramphenicol, cephalosporins, trimethoprim-sulfonamide combinations, and synthetic penicillins. Erythromycin, penicillin and many of its synthetic forms, chloramphenicol and trimethoprim sulfa are available as oral preparations, thereby increasing ease of medication. Diarrhea may occasionally occur in association with oral antibiotic medication but usually ceases when the drug is discontinued. In a rare horse, diarrhea may become severe and necessitate treatment and fluid replacement.

In addition to appropriate antibiotic therapy, drainage of any accessible infected areas is important. Flushing of infected areas, such as the sinuses or guttural pouches, with isotonic sterile saline solution may also be helpful. Potentially irritating solutions should be avoided. Persistent streptococcal infections of the sinuses or guttural pouches may require multiple repeated lavages and prolonged treatment (see Chapters 18 and 19). Whether immune modulating drugs such as levamisole or products such as Propionibacterium acnes* or a mycobacterial cell wall product † are useful in enhancing an affected horse's immune responses and shortening the treatment period remains to be determined. Local hot pack application may aid treatment of abscesses. Infected horses should not be transported or otherwise stressed. Nonsteroidal anti-inflammatory drugs may improve the horse's attitude and appetite, but their antipyretic action hinders monitoring the temperature as a guide to therapeutic efficacy of selected antibiotics. Duration of therapy may exceed several months when there is persistent infection or severe pleuritis and/or pneumonia. Nursing care and maintenance of the patient's appetite and good attitude are important in contributing to a favorable outcome.

## *Streptococcus Equi*

Streptococcus equi causes the contagious upper respiratory tract disease commonly referred to as "strangles."[1,14–21] Site of entry of the organism is the upper respiratory tract, especially the soft palate and tonsillar area. Strangles can occur in horses of any age, but horses between 1 to 5 years old are predisposed. Clinical signs usually (but not always) appear 2 to 20 days following exposure.[14] In experimental infection the incubation period is 3 to 6 days and usually 3 to 10 days in natural infection.[1,20,21] Infection is by ingestion or by inhalation and is spread directly between horses or via feed, water buckets or other fomites, or areas contaminated with secretions from infected horses. Human beings can act as fomites and spread infection. Although premises are said to harbor the infection for more than a year,[17] the duration of survival for the organism has not been clearly defined. Unless protected by moist exudate it survives only briefly in the environment.[20] Carrier animals have been documented and could serve to maintain the organism within a herd. Ponies affected with atypical strangles were found to remain infected for at least 8 months and be a source of infection for foals with which they commingled 4 months after they returned to clinical normality.[16] Another study documented shedding that persisted for 10 months in one mare.[22] Although such shedders could explain interepizootic maintenance of infection and some outbreaks, they are unusual, and in most horses nasal shedding ceases by 6 weeks.[23] Infection is usually introduced into a group by a horse that is incubating the disease or is asymptomatic.[24]

Three forms of strangles have been identified: typical, atypical and "bastard" strangles.[16,17,23,25] When cultured on blood agar, atypical streptococci initially have a wet mucoid appearance but then develop an atypical matt morphology within 24 hours of incubation.[16,17,23] The typical form produces golden honey-colored mucoid colonies on blood agar.[23] Both forms are similar in terms of mouse virulence and production of specific M protein.[23] The loss of capsule of the atypical form may render the organism more susceptible to phagocytosis and therefore less virulent.[23] Although the atypical form has been associated with the atypical, less severe form of strangles,[17,23,26,27] both mucoid and matt forms have been associated with atypical mild strangles, and it has also been suggested that the horse's immune status is important in determining expression of the disease.[25] The importance of host factors is also emphasized by the report of an outbreak of severe strangles in foals commingling with ponies that harbored the atypical disease.[27]

The morbidity rate may reach 100%, but this is highly variable depending on the im-

*Immunoregulin, Immunovet, Inc., Tampa, FL.
†Equimune, Ragland Research, Inc. Athens, GA

mune status of horses in the group.[21,28] One study showed attack rates of 17.6% for broodmares, 47.5% for 1-year-old horses, and 37.5% for foals.[29] Mortality rate is usually low although in one outbreak involving a group of poorly managed horses (weanlings) less than a year of age, it reached 10%.[28] In another study, 6 of 74 affected horses died or were euthanatized because of complications, giving a mortality rate just under 3% (6 of 235).[29]

## Clinical Signs and Diagnosis

Clinical signs are variable depending on the form, and expression of the disease is greatly affected by the horse's immune status and presence of antibodies from earlier exposure. In a nonimmune horse, the organism can survive well in neutrophils following phagocytosis.[16]

Fever, depression, anorexia, a serous nasal (and sometimes ocular) discharge which becomes mucopurulent, and abscessed submaxillary, submandibular and retropharyngeal lymph nodes characterize horses affected with typical strangles. Coughing is sometimes a feature. Lymph node enlargement may obstruct respiration and affect swallowing and horses may appear dysphagic or "stiff" or painful in the "throatlatch" area. Lymphadenopathy may be so severe as to cause asphyxiation ("strangles"). Retropharyngeal lymph nodes may rupture and drain externally or internally. Aspiration pneumonia or guttural pouch empyema may result.[18,28,30] Nerves within the guttural pouches or the recurrent laryngeal nerve may be affected. Periorbital abscesses may cause marked eyelid swelling.[21] Myocarditis has been reported. Lactating mares may become agalactic. In the atypical form, horses may or may not be febrile or anorexic, and lymphadenopathy is variable even in horses with profuse purulent nasal discharge.[23]

Duration of clinical signs may range from less than 1 week to more than 2 months. In the majority of horses with strangles, after the lymph nodes abscess, rupture and drain naturally, the disease runs its course and the horses recover uneventfully. A number of complications have been reported to occur, however.[28,29] In one study 20% of the affected horses had complications following strangles.[29] The most common complication is "bastard strangles," the metastasis of S. equi to lymph nodes other than the submaxillary, submandibular or retropharyngeal lymph nodes. While abscesses can occur anywhere in the body, most common locations reported are the lungs, mesentery, liver, spleen, kidney, and brain.[20,28] Abscesses also may occur in the skin. Septic arthritis and tenosynovitis may occur.[19,21] Anemia of chronic disease, weight loss and lethargy may be sequels. Although the prevalence of "bastard strangles" is reported to be low, when the disease does occur, it is difficult to treat successfully and often results in death of the affected horse. There is no conclusive evidence as to what factors contribute to the metastases. Some authors have suggested that it occurs because penicillin alters the streptococcus organism, resulting in an inadequate immune response.[1] To our knowledge, there are no reported experimental or clinical data to support this theory. In burros, abscessation of abdominal lymph nodes and organs and death due to chronic debilitation without signs of acute strangles or any respiratory disease have been reported.[31]

Purpura hemorrhagica can be a serious, sometimes fatal sequel. The condition is characterized by fever, edema of the limbs and frequently of the head, ventral abdomen and thorax and prepuce, and variable depression. Petechial hemorrhages on mucosae are inconsistently seen. Wheals may occur. Glomerulonephritis has occasionally been reported.[32] Colic associated with hemorrhage, edema and necrosis of the intestinal wall due to vasculitis which resembles anaphylactoid purpura (Henoch-Schönlein disease) in man has also been reported.[33] Thrombocytopenia is not a characteristic of this form of purpura. There is evidence, based on both microscopic findings and demonstration of circulating immune complexes, that purpura hemorrhagica is an immune complex mediated disease.[33,34] The immune complexes in sera from horses with poststrangles purpura contain IgA and S. equi specific antigens and horses with purpura hemorrhagica have elevated levels of serum IgA with normal levels of IgG and IgM.[34]

Diagnosis of strangles is based on the presence of classical clinical signs (lymphadenopathy with fever ± nasal discharge) or isolation of the organism. Chains of streptococci may be seen on direct smears of exudate, but these cannot be differentiated from other streptococcal species. Despite great variation in numbers of organisms shed and duration of shedding, nasal swabs are more likely to yield positive cultures from infected horses than are pharyngeal swabs.[14] Lymph node swabs are the most likely specimens to culture positively: in one study, draining lymph nodes were positive 50% of the time. In the same study, when nasal and pharyngeal swab specimens were obtained simultaneously from horses, the former were twice as likely to be positive,[14] and when culture results differed between the two sites, more often the nasal swab was positive and the pharyngeal sample negative.[35] This difference may reflect the more restricted sampling site for the pharyngeal swab while, theoretically, nasal exudate should include material from the entire upper respiratory tract, including the guttural pouches.[31] A selective transport medium, Strepswab* aids laboratory personnel by reducing the contamination by other nonstreptococcal organisms but does not increase the prevalence of isolation compared to use of a Culturette.†[14] Diagnosis is more difficult when there is no readily available source of exudate for culture. Inspissated pus in the guttural pouches can occur without nasal discharge, and internal abscesses may be impossible to diagnose even with radiography, ultrasonography and internal palpation per rectum. An elevated serum fibrinogen or globulin, anemia of chronic disease, and neutrophilia are nonspecific indications of infection. In horses with these abnormalities, historical exposure to "strangles" is often the basis for a tentative diagnosis of S. equi infection.

## Treatment and Control

Control of the disease necessitates quarantining affected horses and preventing exposure of new ones. Separation of horses in different pastures should help, but even when horses are in separate pastures with no contact with one another, spread can occur, most probably via handlers.[29] As degree of nasal shedding is not related to signs of clinical disease, infected horses showing no abnormal signs may serve to spread disease. Also, shedding may be intermittent and heavy or light.[16] Months after it has seemingly recovered, the same horse may have repeated attacks.[15] It has been shown that the atypical form of infection may be maintained within a group of ponies for at least 8 months.[16] In a group of 31 horses with "strangles," 6 (19.4%) had positive cultures from the nares for up to 34 days after clinical signs of the disease had ended.[29] Another study identified four carrier mares, one of which had intermittent serous to mucoid nasal discharge and positive nasal swab cultures for 10 months.[22] These horses could be moved into susceptible herds of horses and serve as a source of S. equi. Since these horses may be clinically normal, neither farm managers nor veterinarians would be alerted to the need for their prolonged isolation.

In general, isolation of affected horses should not terminate when clinical signs are gone but should be maintained for 4 to 5 weeks. It has been recommended that at least three culture negative nasal swab specimens taken several days or a week apart should be obtained to try to ensure that a horse is not shedding S. equi.[22,29] Attendants may transmit the disease among animals; if possible, those caring for sick horses should not work with healthy horses. If this is impossible, conscientious rigorous hand washing, use of disposable gowns, and use of footwear that can be disinfected should be instituted. Obviously, buckets, grooming materials, tack and other potential fomites should not be shared among horses.

Treatment of exposed horses or foals can prevent clinical disease during the period of therapy, but clinical signs can develop if the animals are exposed when antibiotics are discontinued. One study showed a significant decrease in foal morbidity when benzathine penicillin (900,000 IU IM every 48 hours for 21 days) was used.[14] Trimethoprim sulfonamide combinations, ampicillin, and oxytetracycline have also been used[20] and erythro-

*Medical Wire and Equipment Co., Cleveland, OH.
†Marion Scientific, Kansas City, MO.

mycin would also probably be effective. However, it has been suggested that trimethoprim sulfonamide combinations are less effective than penicillin G or ampicillin.[21] Adequate dosage regimens must be used and medication continued beyond the time when clinical signs have resolved. Monitoring serum fibrinogen may help in deciding when to discontinue treatment. When to use antibiotics depends on the severity of clinical signs and numbers and ages of exposed horses. Ease of administration and dosage interval are also factors, especially when large numbers of horses are affected. Systemic antibiotics are not usually indicated for mild infections localized to the lymph nodes or upper respiratory tract. Pneumonia, pleuritis, sinusitis, synovitis, guttural pouch empyema, and other systemic manifestations of the infection should be treated and may require long-term therapy. Pneumonia has been the most common fatal sequel, and any horses suspected of having lower respiratory tract infections should be rigorously treated. Sensitivity testing should be performed to aid in choice of the appropriate drug. Current evidence indicates that horses are not predisposed to "bastard strangles" by use of antibiotics, and one should not avoid their use because of this potential sequel to the disease.[14]

Occasionally surgical drainage is needed for guttural pouch empyema, sinusitis, or retropharyngeal lymph node abscessation. Premature lancing of lymph nodes is contraindicated and may cause fistulous tracts which are slow to heal.[21] Other important contributions to recovery from S. equi infection are nursing care, hot packing abscessed lymph nodes, providing palatable easily swallowed food, and in cases unable or unwilling to eat, feeding by nasogastric tube. A tracheotomy may be needed if a horse is dyspneic and handlers should always be alerted to check for respiratory difficulty that could indicate its requirement. Judicious use of drugs such as flunixin meglumine* may help in reducing pain and fever and improving appetite.

Purpura hemorrhagica can be a severe complication often requiring long-term therapy with antibiotics and anti-inflammatory drugs. High doses of dexamethasone† (30 to 50 mg/450 kg horse s.i.d.) may be required initially. One should try to use the lowest dose possible and not prolong use of high doses if they are not required. It is our impression that dexamethasone is more effective than prednisolone at dosages usually employed. If other factors contraindicate use of steroids, one could try using flunixine meglumine; however, there is no documentation of efficacy.

Commercial vaccines are available. None is completely effective in preventing the disease, but both the M protein extract (Strepvax)‡ and an adjuvanted concentrated purified enzyme extract (Strepguard)§ reportedly reduce the incidence of infection and attack rate in susceptible herds and the duration of clinical signs if a vaccinated horse develops "strangles."[1,36,37] A field evaluation of a commercial M protein vaccine in foals in a feedlot showed that foals vaccinated three times were less than half as likely to develop cervical lymphadenopathy or nasal discharge than unvaccinated foals, but a single vaccination had no effect.[38] However, outbreaks have occurred in herds in which repeated vaccinations have been performed.[24] Another study showed no apparent effect on the incidence of disease when a vaccine program was instituted.[29] Large challenge doses may overcome immunity. Although yearly booster vaccinations are recommended, immunity may be of shorter duration, as clinical signs of "strangles" were reported in yearlings within 6 months of their being vaccinated with M protein vaccine or bacterin.[18] In one study, horses developed strangles 8 to 10 months after vaccination[39] and, in an outbreak, booster vaccination of 1-year-old horses within 12 to 20 weeks of exposure to strangles did not prevent clinical disease.[29] Duration of immunity following natural infection is unknown; some clinicians claim several years, while others claim less than 6 months.[14,15] There is no practical way to determine whether a horse is immune. Measurement of bactericidal antibodies is not help-

*Banamine, Schering Corp., Kenilworth, NJ.

†Azium, Schering Corp., Kenilworth, NJ.

‡Strepvax II, Coopers Animal Health, Kansas City, KS.

§Haver, Mobay Corp., Animal Health Division, Shawnee, Kansas.

ful as levels do not correlate with protection.[24,39] Horses with strong serum bactericidal activity have become infected both naturally and experimentally, and horses recently recovered from strangles were resistant to reinfection despite not yet having developed significant bactericidal antibodies.[24,39] Protection does correlate with concentration of antibodies in the nasopharyngeal mucus, but this is not useful as a clinical diagnostic test.[40] Current efforts are directed to the production of a vaccine delivered by the oral or nasal route that will produce local antibody. Intranasal inoculation with a nonencapsulated avirulent strain of S. equi elicits local antibody production and renders immunized horses resistant to challenge by virulent S. equi.[24,39] Use of such a vaccine would also avoid the undesirable side effects and local reactions sometimes associated with intramuscular strangles vaccines. In one study using commercial M protein vaccine, 44% of young horses were reported to develop injection site swellings, which were often severe.[38]

Foals born from immune mares are resistant to strangles up to 3 months of age.[41] Passive antibody protection is thought to be derived by direct coating of the oral and upper respiratory mucosa by antibodies in milk and by secretion of absorbed colostral immunoglobulins onto the nasopharyngeal mucosa. Radiolabelling has demonstrated that passively acquired circulating IgA is rapidly transported onto the neonatal foal's nasal mucosa.[41] Antibodies persist on the foal's respiratory mucosa during its first 2 months of life.[41]

## *Streptococcus Pneumoniae*

This alpha-hemolytic streptococcus exists in the upper respiratory tract of human beings and, although it is often carried asymptomatically, it is also a recognized pathogen. The human carrier state ranges from 5 to 60% depending on season and environmental conditions.[42] It has been isolated sporadically from horses, but its importance in this species remains unclear.[2,3] There has been a report of pneumococcal septicemia in a foal, and a single serotype of the organism has also been isolated from tracheobronchial aspirates from adult horses and a foal, and from an adult horse's pleural fluid.[2,43] Three of the mature horses had pneumonia and one also had pleuritis and pericarditis; other pathogens (streptococci, pasteurella sp and actinobacillus) were concurrently isolated. Chronic cough existed in two other horses; three had decreased exercise tolerance, and one had exercise-induced pulmonary hemorrhage (EIPH); in only two was S. pneumoniae the sole isolate, and its role in causing or contributing to the clinical signs is speculative. Horses that were treated with antibiotics to which all isolated pathogens were sensitive recovered.[2]

In another study in England, where 26 2- to 3-year-old Thoroughbred horses had sequential tracheobronchial aspirates obtained via an endoscope over a 1 to 18 month interval, S. pneumoniae (capsule type 3) was recovered on one or more occasions from 18 horses and 1 of the horses cultured positive 13 of the 17 times sampled.[3] Horses with clinical signs of respiratory tract infection and positive S. pneumoniae cultures had a rise in antibody titers to S. pneumoniae type 3 for 2 to 4 weeks following onset of clinical signs. However, the bacterium was never demonstrated unequivocally to be a primary cause of clinical disease.[3] Only one horse had a pure culture of S. pneumoniae; in all the others, Streptococcus zooepidemicus and other bacteria were also isolated. Seroconversion was also seen in asymptomatic horses and some horses that had positive cultures never seroconverted. The source of infection was never identified, and it is unknown if infected horses pose a hazard to humans. Although no association was made between infected horses and people with S. pneumoniae infections, horses could potentially transmit the organism to susceptible human beings. Therefore, immunocompromised people should not expose themselves to known infected horses.

As the organism has never been demonstrated to be a primary cause of respiratory disease in horses, infected horses are usually treated for co-existing pathogens.

## Rhodococcus Equi Infection

R. equi, formerly called Corynebacterium equi, causes pneumonia in foals and rarely in older horses.[44–48] Initially reported as a cause of foal pneumonia in 1923,[49] it has remained an important pathogen. Signs are seen primarily in foals between 1 and 6 months of age. Recently, morbidity rates of 5 to 17% worldwide and mortality rates of up to 80% have been reported.[50] Mortality rates have been greatest in foals about 2 months of age. Management and environmental conditions play major roles in determining the magnitude of the challenge to the foal, and therefore affect the prevalence of disease. In addition to its isolation from horses, the organism has also been isolated from lymph node abscesses in swine and ulcerative lymphangitis in cattle.

The main routes of infection are the respiratory and alimentary tracts. Ingestion of the organisms is probably the chief route of exposure in all foals, but is thought rarely to lead to respiratory disease. Intragastric challenge infection can produce lesions in the intestinal tract, but they are not consistent.[51–53] Although there is a report of lung abscesses developing in foals following multiple intragastric challenges,[52] most experimental intragastric infections have failed to cause pneumonia.[51,53,54] In the former study, infected foals were held in yards together, and aspiration from the pharynx or inhalation of R. equi from feces with documented profuse growth of the organism could not be eliminated as possible routes of lung infection. The different quantities of inocula used and variation in ages of foals among the trials may account for some of the inconsistent results from experimental alimentary tract infections. Inhalation of aerosolized rhodococcus or intranasal challenge results in abscesses and pyogranulomatous pneumonia, which mimic the natural disease.[53–55]

Although foals with pneumonia may have coexistent lymphadenitis of gut-associated lymph nodes and sometimes intestinal mucosal lesions, they rarely show clinical signs of intestinal disease. Those foals with intestinal lesions causing clinical signs rarely show signs of respiratory dysfunction.[56]

When R. equi is ingested, it causes mucosal ulceration, which is most extensive in the cecum and colon, and penetrates the epithelium overlying Peyer's patches. Pyogranulomatous inflammation occurs within Peyer's patches. Macrophages ingest the bacteria and probably serve to transport them to lymph nodes. Further dissemination could then occur via lymphatics and the thoracic duct to the pulmonary circulation.[51] R. equi has also been cultured from blood of both experimentally and naturally infected foals. However, there is no evidence to support lung infection via hematogenous spread from the intestines as a significant mechanism in natural infections.[54]

Two clinical forms of naturally occurring R. equi pneumonia have been recognized. The subacute form is characterized by diffuse miliary pyogranulomatous pneumonia, and affected foals usually die within several days of showing respiratory distress; despite the subacute clinical course, lesions are chronic. In the chronic form, pneumonia and sometimes unthriftiness progress for weeks to months, and the few foals that do survive may have pulmonary fibrosis and decreased respiratory capacity.[54] Although infection is thought to occur in the neonatal period signs are often not noticed until the foal is greater than a month old. The umbilical route has also been suggested as a rare route of infection.[54]

Response to experimental infection varies greatly among foals, and susceptibility to the natural disease also appears to vary. Foals under 2 weeks of age are more susceptible, at least to experimental infection.[54,57] Foals with defective immune defenses or those whose maternal immunity has waned prior to their being capable of generating an immune response are most susceptible. Viral infections or stresses that adversely affect the immune system could increase susceptibility. In vitro interaction of R. equi with alveolar macrophages from foals has been studied.[58,59] Foals less than 20 days old had low numbers of alveolar macrophages determined by bronchoalveolar lavages and the foal macrophage could ingest significant numbers of R. equi in vitro only in the presence of immune serum.[53] A defect in microbicidal activity of the macrophages was postulated to allow establishment of disease. In a study on alveolar macrophage function of foals between 2 and 8 months of age, macrophages from nonexposed foals killed only 61% of an infective dose of R. equi versus a 94% killing rate in exposed foals.[59] Opsonization of R. equi with antibodies and lymphocyte factors from sensitized lymphocytes enhanced killing capacity. Other studies employing both ultrastructural morphologic criteria and in vitro bactericidal assays have revealed defective killing.[60,61] In vitro studies showed that 60 to 75% of phagocytosed R. equi remained viable after 24 hours' incubation.[60] Electron microscopic studies of alveolar macrophages showed a lack of phagosome-liposome fusion following ingestion of R. equi, persistence and multiplication of the organism, and irreversible damage of the cell with release of intracellular R. equi into the surrounding medium.[61]

Investigation of interaction of R. equi and polymorphonuclear leukocytes (neutrophils or PMN) and comparison of PMN from foals versus mature horses have yielded conflicting data.[62–66] Neutrophils from 2- to 4-month old foals showed decreased function (phagocytosis of S. aureus and lower oxygen-dependent microbicidal activity) than those of mature mares, suggesting that, like that of human neonates, young foals' neutrophil function is decreased.[63] A study in mature horses indicated that R. equi inhibited PMN bactericidal activity,[62] yet another study showed no difference in bactericidal activity in sick versus normal foals or normal foals versus mature horses.[66] Other studies have also shown that PMN from young and mature horses can phagocytize and kill R. equi in the presence of specific opsonizing antibody.[64,65] In one study comparing neonatal foals (mean age 3.3 days) with foals with a mean age of 36 days and mature mares, there was no significant difference among the groups; however, several individual neonates had significantly decreased bactericidal PMN activity.[64] Therefore, decreased PMN activity may be important in rendering certain foals more susceptible to R. equi infection. Inconsistent findings among the studies can probably be explained not only by different ages of foals studied but also by the bacterial challenge dose, whether equine serum was used, and other differences in methodology. Failure of passive transfer may be a predisposing factor, but there is no documentation of the value of passive transfer of immunity.

The role of humoral factors and possible alteration in foals causing them to be more susceptible to R. equi remains to be elucidated. There is increasing evidence that humoral immunity is important. Enhancement of killing of R. equi by neutrophils and by alveolar macrophages by specific opsonizing antibody has been demonstrated.[59,64] R. equi specific antibody in vitro can interfere with R. equi's ability to block normal alveolar macrophage function,[59] and a similar in vivo action could be very important in the immune response to R. equi. Lymphocytic factors may also enhance the bactericidal activity of alveolar macrophages.[59]

Although there have been earlier reports of apparent beneficial effects of plasma and serum,[67,68] documentation of the prophylactic efficacy of passive humoral immunotherapy is recent.[57] It has been suggested that the protection resulting from use of plasma or serum is superior to that which could be accomplished from use of colostrum or gamma globulin because of nonspecific factors such as fibronectin, interferons, lymphokines, monokines, and complement components in addition to opsonizing and neutralizing antibodies.[64] Fibronectin, for example, can increase bacterial binding capacity of phagocytic cells and increase phagocytosis in the presence of complement and antibody.[64] To our knowledge, there are no published trials on the prophylactic efficacy of colostrum from mares immunized with R. equi.

The habitat of R. equi and the epidemiology of R. equi infections have been subject to debate. The bacterium has been recovered from a variety of soil types. It can be isolated from both the intestinal contents and feces of herbivores,[69–75] and is probably maintained in the horse as normal flora of the intestinal tract. In one study, 65% of 106 horses had the organism in their feces.[72] It can multiply in normal horses' feces providing an important potential source of exposure for young foals, which are commonly coprophagic.[73] Young foals may excrete large numbers of organisms during their first 8 weeks of life, but this later decreases as the anaerobic conditions of the intestines of weaned horses inhibit multiplication.[76] The rapidity with which R. equi multiplies in fresh feces is a function of prevailing environmental temperatures.[77] The organism grows better in soil that is enriched with manure, probably because of the latter's simple organic acids, which enhance growth.[77] Superficial soil has greater numbers of organisms than deep soil.

On some farms R. equi is isolated in large quantities from the soil independent of whether horses are present, whereas on other farms it has been isolated only from areas with horses.[70–71] In another study, culture results from various sites on the same farm differed significantly and the numbers of foals with clinical R. equi infections correlated with the numbers of bacteria cultured from the stable area but not from elsewhere.[69] Also, soil infection at all sites (paddocks, stables, and pastures) correlated with the presence of horses.[71] Number of organisms in pasture soil depends on the length of time the pasture has been in use. Temperature is an important factor and numbers of organisms isolated from both soil and air samples increase with rising temperatures. Below 10°C (50°F), R. equi does not grow, and it grows best at 30°C (86°F). Exposure potential, therefore, increases in spring and early summer in temperate climates. Endemic farms have greater numbers of R. equi in stable soil compared to nonendemic farms, and the number of cases of R. equi pneumonia tends to correlate with the numbers of R. equi/g of soil.[78] Environmental strains appear to be less virulent than those isolated from infected foals' lungs.[77]

Prevalence of the disease appears to increase with dusty environments and dry weather. The number of R. equi that could be isolated from the air of stalls increases as environmental temperature, dryness and windiness increases.[79] The number of organisms isolated from the air decreases on rainy days.[78] Even when pasture soil numbers of R. equi are high, foals grazing on grass pastures seem to be at less risk than foals around stables where there is more chance of environmental dust.[71] The importance of inhalation as the route of infection for the respiratory form is substantiated by the fact that ingestion of R. equi most commonly results in a self-limiting intestinal infection.[80]

## Clinical Signs and Diagnosis

Clinical signs of R. equi respiratory tract infection vary.[48,70,81,82] Some foals are found dead in the field with no antecedent signs; postmortem examination reveals diffuse lung abscesses. Other foals suddenly develop a high fever, a rapid respiratory rate and dyspnea with flared nostrils, and a heaving type of respiratory pattern. The abdominal component to expiration may be quite marked. Foals often appear anxious and may be cyanotic. Dyspnea may be sufficient to deter suckling, and foals may appear reluctant to lie down because of the additional compromise to their respiration. They may appear weak, almost ataxic, and may appear disoriented. Despite exudate in the lower airways, nasal discharge and coughing are inconsistent. Auscultation may reveal rattles, clicks, squeaks, and wheezes in the lungs, or there may be only an increase in coarseness and loss of soft vesicular sounds. These severely affected foals often die within several days despite treatment. Postmortem examination usually reveals lung abscesses as well as a more diffuse pneumonia. Other foals have a more chronic course over weeks. Pleural effusion may occur, but is rare. Chronically affected foals are febrile, depressed, often dyspneic and tachypneic, have tachycardia, and usually lose condition and look unthrifty. Cough and nasal discharge are variable. When a cough is present, it is usually soft and deep. Auscultation may reveal only coarse sounds or large airway sounds suggesting consolidation, or there may be rales, wheezes, clicks, and crackles. When consolidated areas are extensive and superficial in the lungs, it may be possible to percuss them as areas of dullness. Foals are usually severely exercise-intolerant, and minor stresses can precipitate rapid deterioration including collapse. A chronic, active, nonseptic synovitis is not uncommon and results in fluid distention of several joints with no or mild lameness. Foals may also have evidence of uveitis (cloudiness to the aqueous and/or vitreous, miosis, and fibrin, or pus in the aqueous may be seen). Despite postmortem evidence of intestinal involvement in many R. equi-infected foals, clinical signs of the intestinal form of R. equi infection rarely accompany the pulmonary disease.[81]

There are rare reports of mature horses with R. equi infection; they have shown weight loss, fevers, coughing, and dyspnea.[46] One horse had rapidly progressive pneumonia and pleuritis and another had ulcerative lymphangitis. The first horse was 28 years old and reportedly had polyuria, polydipsia, and glucosuria. Although not mentioned in the report, he may have had a pituitary adenoma which increased his susceptibility to infections and predisposed him to R. equi infection.

Clinical laboratory tests usually reveal a nonspecific leukocytosis and increased fibrinogen. One study showed no difference in the leukogram or fibrinogen of survivors versus nonsurvivors,[83] whereas another showed nonsurvivors had significantly higher serum fibrinogen concentrations and leukocyte counts.[84] Because of overlap in ranges of the values, neither test is helpful for prognostication for an individual animal. A study on experimentally induced R. equi infection in foals suggested that serum caeruloplasmin oxidase activity and serum copper concentrations could be useful in early identification of foals as concentrations rose about a week preceding onset of fever or coughing.[53] However, elevations are not specific for R. equi infection as reports in other animals show changes in other infections. Also, there is some overlap of values and a single sample, unless the concentration is extremely elevated, would be difficult to interpret. The degree of elevation did not reflect the severity of infection.[53] Currently, the most helpful diagnostic techniques are tracheobronchial aspirates and thoracic radiographs. Gram-positive pleomorphic rods are often seen on direct microscopic evaluation of transtracheal aspirates. Tracheobronchial aspirates from infected foals usually culture positive for R. equi, but false-negative results may occur as shedding may be episodic and the bacterium is often intracellular and may not grow in culture.[54] Multiple other pathogens may be isolated along with R. equi.[83,84] Radiographs are especially helpful diagnostically when cultures are negative. A prominent alveolar pattern with ill-defined regional consolidation is commonly seen.[84] Nodular lung lesions and lymphadenopathy are almost pathognomonic in foals in this age range, but they may not be present on initial examination. Lesions may become cavitary. A prominent interstitial pattern may be seen in acute or less severely affected foals. Radiographic evidence of tracheobronchial lymphadenopathy was reported to be useful prognostically as it was seen more commonly in foals that did not recover.[84] However, radiographs should not be used as the sole criterion for prognostication and possible euthanasia because foals with severe lesions can recover. Ultrasonography is helpful when lung involvement includes peripheral areas, but abscesses with overlying aerated lung will not be detected because aerated areas prevent passage of the ultrasound beam. Although blood cultures are not routinely performed, and therefore the percentage of positive isolates is unknown, we have obtained a positive blood culture from one severely affected foal who died despite treatment. Whether blood cultures would be an accurate prognostic index remains to be determined.

Lymphocyte immunostimulation tests were shown to be useful diagnostically in foals less than or 2 months of age, as infected foals have a high stimulation ratio compared to normal foals. As some normal foals older than 2 months have higher stimulation ratios than infected foals, in this age group the test is only helpful when negative (stimulation ratio $\leq$ 0.6) as this eliminates R. equi as the cause of pneumonia.[85] As this is not an inexpensive or easily performed test, it is usually not applicable to clinical practices. Evaluation of cell-mediated response by intradermal skin testing with R. equi has not been helpful diagnostically.[86]

Humoral responses have been tested by various techniques as the need for a diagnostic test which will be useful in early detection of infection has long been recognized. Agar gel immunodiffusion and precipitating and hemagglutinating antibody testing have not been useful. An enzyme-linked immunoabsorbent assay (ELISA) was reported to be useful in detecting the presence of specific antibodies against R. equi.[87] However, results have been variable. Ellenburger et al could find no apparent association between the ELISA titers to R. equi and clinical history and found that all adult animals tested had antibody titers to the organism.[88] Hietala et al. examined serum of 22 horses with R. equi infection confirmed by tracheal wash or direct isolation from tissues and found titers ranging from well above to well below normal.[89] A study on experimentally infected foals also suggested that the humoral response could be affected by the route and extent of R. equi exposure as well as the strain.[90] Combining use of an ELISA to detect antibody and quantitative examination of feces for R. equi organisms has been suggested for early diagnosis of infection.[87] Detection of antibodies to equi factor may be useful in diagnosing infected foals; however, some foals with clinical disease do not seroconvert.[91,92] Also, seropositive status can be due to subclinical infection.[92] One study on two farms with endemic R. equi pneumonia suggested that R. equi-specific antibody may play a role in protection against infection because increased clinical severity of pneumonia correlated with a lower specific antibody response. IgM was found to rise 2 weeks before and IgG 2 weeks after the onset of clinical disease.[93] The value of measuring IgM as an aid in the early diagnosis has not, to our knowledge, received further evaluation.

## Treatment and Control

It is generally accepted that a number of antibiotics are effective against R. equi in vitro, yet the drugs may not be effective in vivo. One study showed the following minimum inhibitory concentrations of antibiotics for 90% of isolates tested: penicillin (2 to ≥4 μg/ml), ampicillin (2 to 8 μg/ml), methicillin (>16 μg/ml), cephalothin (8 to 64 μg/ml), clindamycin (1 to 2 μg/ml), kanamycin (2 to 8 μg/ml), neomycin (0.2 μg/ml), amikacin (≤1 to 2 μg/ml), gentamicin (≤0.8 μg/ml), trimethoprim sulfa (4/76 to 34/608 μg/ml), tetracycline (1 to 4 μg/ml), chloramphenicol (8 to 16 μg/ml), erythromycin (≤0.2 μg/ml), and rifampin (0.049 μg/ml).[94,95] Another study showed similar susceptibilities for some of the same drugs.[96] In terms of minimal inhibitory concentrations against R. equi, rifampin is 5 times as potent as gentamicin and 90 times as potent as penicillin, while erythromycin is almost twice as potent as gentamicin and 30 times the potency of penicillin.[97,98] By combining erythromycin and rifampin, a synergistic effect is produced.[95,97] Results of several studies show that erythromycin and rifampin provided the most successful antimicrobial treatment, probably due to the low MIC of these drugs and good tissue and macrophage penetration.[83,95,97,98] The pharmacokinetics of rifampin have been studied in the horse and an oral dose of 5 to 10 mg/kg b.i.d. suggested for treating R. equi infection.[83,95,99] Intramuscular injection is not advised because of inflammation and side effects (pain and sweating). As bacteria rapidly mutate to develop rifampin resistance, the drug should be used only in combination with other antimicrobials.[100] The pharmacokinetics of erythromycin have been studied in the foal and a dose of 25 to 30 mg/kg orally q.i.d. suggested.[101] Both an acid-stable estolate and ethyl-succinate ester forms are available. Erythromycin is widely distributed throughout the body, achieving high levels in lung tissue and bronchial secretions. Like rifampin, erythromycin is highly lipid-soluble and is concentrated within macrophages and neutrophils. Erythromycin is bactericidal at high dose levels. Although diarrhea may occur in horses to which erythromycin is administered, we feel that if diarrhea develops, it is usually self-limiting and rarely requires therapy, ceases when the antibiotic is discontinued, and does not preclude the drug's use. However, severe cases of diarrhea occasionally have been reported in adult horses.[102] These require treatment.

Although reports of MIC and antibiotic susceptibilities indicate that gentamicin might be effective in the treatment of R. equi pneumonia, clinical success with this drug has been limited. One study reported successful treatment of 4 of 5 affected foals using the combination of penicillin and gentamicin,[70] but another study showed that none of 17 foals treated with this combination survived.[83] The ionized nonlipophilic nature of penicillin and gentamicin decreases their ability to penetrate cells and may be one reason for their lack of success in cases where there are large numbers of organisms within macrophages. We do not recommend the use of penicillin and gentamicin for treatment of R. equi, and gentamicin should not be given with erythromycin or rifampin because of antagonistic interactions.[97]

Although R. equi is reported not to be susceptible to concentrations of trimethoprim-sulfadiazine available in tissues with use of the standard dosage, clinical success in foals with mild or early pneumonia has been reported using 6.6 mg trimethoprim/kg t.i.d., p.o., in fixed combination with sulfamethoxazole (Wilson WD, cited in reference 95).

There are two reports on using plasma and serum to treat R. equi infections,[67,68] and a recent report of successful prophylaxis with immune plasma in experimentally infected foals[57] has kindled interest in therapeutic use of immunoprophylaxis. Whether use of immune plasma would benefit an established case of pneumonia remains to be determined.

Nursing care, provision of adequate nutrition, and maintenance of excellent ventilation are important. The authors have not seen any definitive consistent clinical benefit from use of bronchodilators or drugs such as aminophylline that decrease work of breathing. Aminophylline should be used cautiously in patients on erythromycin because the latter delays clearance and elevates blood levels of aminophylline, thus potentiating toxicity. Concurrent theophylline medication has also been shown to decrease serum concentrations of erythromycin ($\geq$30%).[103] Numerous other drugs, including cimetidine and rifampin, also interact and could have therapeutic consequences.[104] Excitement and seizures may occur if theophylline levels rise into the midteens. In addition, human neonates appear to be more sensitive to its cardiovascular effects; tachycardia has been reported even at plasma levels of 13 mg/L.[105] Although there are pharmacokinetic data available for healthy mature horses,[106,107] there is no published information on foals. We do not currently advise use of aminophylline or beta-2-adrenergic bronchodilators (such as albuterol or clenbuterol) because of insufficient data on foals. If aminophylline is used, blood levels should be monitored. Some clinicians use cimetidine or ranitidine plus sucralfate as prophylaxis for gastric ulcers. Local therapy of the distended joints is not indicated since the joint swelling disappears with no permanent effect as the pneumonia resolves. Uveitis should be treated with topical mydriatics (1% atropine or 3% if miosis is persistent) as needed and topical steroids. Systemic flunixin meglumine should also be given at a low dosage to decrease ocular inflammation.

The disease is difficult to prevent or control. Its insidious nature often prevents early detection and the isolation of infected foals. The probable major contributory factors, poor ventilation and dusty conditions, are often the most difficult or impossible to alter. It is important to house foals in well-ventilated dust-free areas and avoid dirt paddocks and crowding, especially around congested stable areas. Stalls should be disinfected with 0.5% formalin, phenol, or similar disinfectants. Manure should be removed from paddocks and other enclosures and composted. If possible, foals should be moved off endemic farms or at least dispersed so that large numbers are not concentrated together. Pastures should be rotated to decrease both dust and exposure. Any sandy or dirt areas should be planted with grass or made "off limits" to foals. Sick foals should be isolated. Breeding practices that result in mares foaling in winter months also should help decrease the disease incidence as environmental challenge will be minimized during the foal's most susceptible age period. Stress and drugs that decrease immune function should be avoided. On one endemic farm, twice-weekly assessment of the temperature, pulse and respiration rates, and lung sounds of foals from birth to 4 months of age allowed early detection and lowered mortality rates.[91] Although monitoring of temperatures may be one of the best ways to detect infections in foals, normal fluctuations must also be considered. It is important to record all findings and have a consistent protocol. Complete blood counts are usually not helpful. Positive bacterial cultures of respiratory tract secretions or feces are not diagnostic of disease as healthy foals may have positive cultures. In some cases the value of the foal(s) may warrant radiography

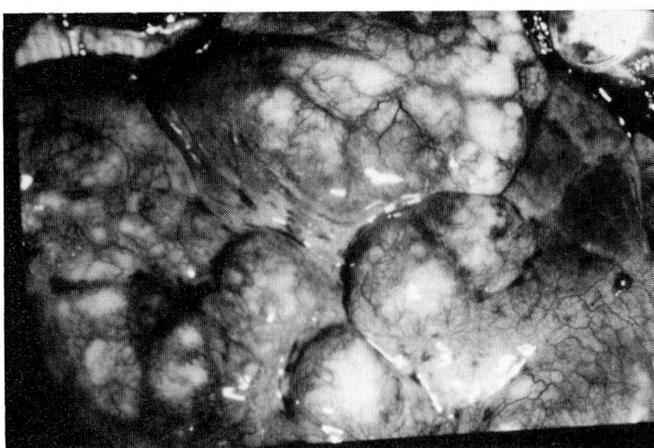

**FIG. 12–4.** Close-up view of a lung surface with multiple abscesses protruding from the parenchyma.

as radiographic evidence of infection may precede clinical signs.

Any foals that die should be necropsied. Postmortem examination findings vary depending on severity of infection and whether the infection was confined to the lungs (Fig. 12–4). Rooney described one form as that of diffuse multiple small parenchymal foci of inflammation with intervening areas of alveolar emphysema and edema and another form as being a mixture of these two changes.[47] Tracheobronchial lymph nodes are usually enlarged and abscessed and/or edematous. Between 45 and 57% of foals with suppurative pneumonia have concomitant multifocal ulcerative colitis and typhlitis and about 75% of these have mesenteric or colonic lymphadenitis.[81,82] Histologically, the lymph nodes and spleen have hyperplasia of the T-dependent paracortical areas, suggesting stimulated cell-mediated immune processes. In the lungs, macrophages and neutrophils fill airways and alveoli, and there is necrosis and granulomatous reaction. R. equi are often numerous and primarily located within macrophages.

## Bordetella Bronchiseptica Infection

Bordetella bronchiseptica, a gram-negative bacterium, is a respiratory pathogen in other species, but its role in equine respiratory diseases has yet to be defined. In species in which it has recognized pathogenicity, it has been found to attach to airway surfaces, cause acute inflammation, stimulate mucus secretion, and alter mucociliary clearance. In our clinic it is rarely cultured from transtracheal aspirates, and is even more rarely a pure isolate. Low frequency of isolation is unlikely to be due to unusual culture requirements. Although growth may require 48 hours of incubation, the bacterium grows easily on commonly used media. In other geographic areas it has been more commonly cultured both as a pure isolate and with other bacteria. A hospital outbreak of respiratory disease in 9 horses was associated with isolation of B. bronchiseptica.[108] In one survey of 80 foals less than 6 months of age with pneumonia, B. bronchiseptica was isolated from up to 28% of the aspirates from which respiratory pathogens were cultured.[109] Of those 61 foals from which one or two pathogens were cultured, B. bronchiseptica was the third most common isolate. All isolates were sensitive to gentamicin, 90% to amikacin, kanamicin, ticarcillin, and chloramphenicol, and 75% to trimethoprim-sulfadiazine and tetracycline. The same authors also reported that erythromycin was effective.[109]

When the organism is isolated from horses with clinical disease, appropriate antibiotic therapy should be started and should cover any other pathogenic bacteria that are isolated.

## Other Bacterial Infections

Of the other bacteria that cause pneumonia, the more common isolates include Klebsiella sp, Escherichia coli, Pasteurella sp, Actinobacillus equili, Staphylococcus sp, and Pseudomonas sp. Mixed populations of bacteria are not uncommonly isolated from horses with pleuropneumonia or aspiration pneumonia. Rarely, Salmonella sp may cause pneumonia. Septicemic foals may have pneumonia as a component of their generalized infection.

Anaerobes may also be important pathogens in infections of the lower respiratory tract, especially in necrotizing pneumonia, lung abscesses, or pleuritis and pneumonia.

As normal horses have anaerobes in the pharynx, positive anaerobic cultures from this site are not significant. Successful isolation of anaerobes requires special culture techniques, and samples should be transferred to the laboratory using a special medium.* Use of this medium is suitable for both aerobic and anaerobic culture. Routine culture swabs are not suitable. Anaerobes most commonly isolated are Bacteroides sp, followed by Clostridium sp.[110] Although a putrid odor is characteristic of anaerobic infections and indicates a poor prognosis in horses with pleuropneumonia, the absence of odor does not exclude the presence of anaerobes. Of 21 horses that had anaerobes cultured from either a tracheobronchial aspirate or pleural fluid, 8 had no evidence of a putrid odor.[110] Anaerobic infections of the lower respiratory tract have a poorer prognosis than aerobic infections.

Antimicrobial treatment of these miscellaneous bacterial infections should be based on Gram stain and culture and sensitivity results and knowledge of which drugs are most likely to reach therapeutic levels at the site of infection. Examination of Gram stains of aspirates helps in choosing an antibiotic prior to receiving the culture result. Broad coverage is usually selected initially. When presence of anaerobes is suspected, penicillin is a good choice and is often combined with a drug effective against gram-negative bacteria. Resistance of many gram-negative bacteria seems to have increased, and selection of appropriate drugs, especially aminoglycosides, is likely to vary among different clinics or in different areas. One study of 260 gram-negative isolates from horses showed that significantly more E. coli, Klebsiella, Enterobacter, and Proteus sp were susceptible to amikacin than to gentamicin, but there was no significant difference in the susceptibility of Pseudomonas sp.[111] However, direct extrapolation to clinical medicine without knowing MIC of the causative organism or patient's blood or tissue levels of antibiotic is difficult as the Kirby Bauer technique using susceptibility discs does not evaluate equal drug concentrations. (The MIC equivalent to a "susceptible reading" is $\leq 16\ \mu g/ml$ for amikacin and $\leq 4\ \mu g/ml$ for gentamicin.) Ticarcillin-clavulanic acid combination* is broad spectrum and may be especially useful in patients in which aminoglycosides are contraindicated. It should be administered IV; IM injection causes pain and in foals may cause transient recumbency.[112] Metronidazole is an excellent antibiotic for treating anaerobic infections and is effective against those Beta-lactamase producing anaerobes which are penicillin resistant. It can be given intravenously or orally, and present dosage recommendations are 15 to 25 mg/kg orally 4 times daily.[113] The same supportive care, maintenance of hydration, drainage of exudate when it is accessible, etc. are indicated in all respiratory infections regardless of the cause.

*Port-A-Cul, BBL Microbiology System, Becton Dickinson and Co., Cockeysville, MD.

*Timentin 3.1, Beecham Laboratories, Bristol, TN.

## Mycobacterial Infections

Mycobacteria are acid-fast, nonmotile, nonsporulating rods, relatively resistant to staining by water soluble dyes but positive for acid fast stains such as Ziehl Nielson.

Tuberculosis is extremely rare in horses especially in the United States. Horses appear to have a high natural resistance. Earlier reports indicated infection was usually with the bovine type (Mycobacterium bovis) and not the avian (Myco. avium) or human type (Myco. tuberculosis).[114] However, a more recent study found that 55 of 69 mycobacterial isolates from horses were of avian type.[115] Generalized avian tuberculosis has been reported.[116] Morphologically the different types cannot be distinguished one from the other. Granulomatous pneumonia, histopathologically resembling mycobacterial infection but without identifiable acid-fast organisms, has been reported.[117–119]

The organism is usually ingested, although primary respiratory infection may occur. The organisms may cause primary lesions in pharyngeal or intestinal lymph nodes. Hematogenous spread may occur and involve other organs, especially lymph nodes and spleen. Miliary tubercles or scattered nodules may result. The lungs may be most severely affected when the spread is miliary, and multiple diffuse small nodules occur. Miliary lesions are reported to cause more rapid progression of disease because organ function is more rapidly compromised.

In horses, the most frequent presenting complaint is chronic weight loss with ensuing weakness and lethargy. Horses terminally affected by the pulmonary form are febrile and dyspneic and have a cough. Abnormal lung sounds may be ausculted and there may be signs of pleural pain.[116] Dyspnea may be inspiratory and expiratory. Osteomyelitis of the cervical vertebrae and associated signs also have been reported.[120]

Radiographs of the thorax may be helpful in defining the pattern and distribution of lesions, but biopsy of these lesion(s) would be necessary for a definitive diagnosis. Diagnosis requires isolation of the organism and demonstration of its presence cytologically or histologically. In making a diagnosis of infection, culture is more sensitive and specific than staining. Acid-fast mycobacterium have been found in nasal swabs from normal horses, and culture was needed to identify the strains, most commonly the rapidly growing members of the Fortuitum group.[121] Despite granulomatous inflammation and the presence of giant cells, acid-fast stains may be negative even in tissue from which the organism is isolated. However, culturing may take 3 to 8 weeks and, at least in human beings, shedding may be intermittent and a number of specimens may be required for a diagnosis. Biopsies are often used for diagnosis, but histologic differentiation from other granulomatous lesions may be difficult. However, caseation is characteristic. Culture of a transtracheal wash and cytologic evaluation may help, and when tuberculosis is suspected, an acid-fast stain should be used. If collection is not sterile, special transport medium such as 10% HPC (cetyl pyridinium chloride) is needed. As not all laboratories process cultures for isolation of these mycobacteria, when one suspects a case and anticipates the need for culture, he/she should identify an appropriate laboratory and follow that laboratory's protocol for sample handling. The intradermal skin test is not reliable and should not be used as a diagnostic tool. Up to 70% of clinically normal horses have been found to have positive tests.[122]

## Treatment

Treatment is not usually attempted, especially because of the associated risk of transmission to man. However, this risk is probably low as tuberculosis is not highly infectious. The greatest risk would occur by sharing an enclosed environment in which the organism could be aerosolized by sneezing, coughing, or perhaps whinnying. In man, risks of contagion are minimal if smears of respiratory tract secretions are negative for the organism. Human beings are regarded as infective only if they have an untreated cavitary lesion, a positive sputum smear, and a productive cough.[123] The organisms are sensitive to sunlight and ionic detergents, but they can remain viable for a long time in feces or sputum, putrifying material, or in the dark where lethal effects of sunlight or disinfectants would not reach them. Immune-suppressed animals and human beings would be at increased risk.

If the horse is to be treated, rifampin and isoniazid should be used. Isoniazid has been used in horses for conditions other than tuberculosis at an oral dosage of 5 to 15 mg/kg orally twice daily.[124] A study on rifampin pharmacokinetics in horses recommended using 5 mg/kg orally twice daily for R. equi infections.[99] In human beings, isoniazid has caused hepatitis and less commonly peripheral neuropathy, dizziness, muscle twitching, and other CNS effects.[125] Streptomycin may also be used, and a dosage regimen of 15 mg/kg/day for 1 month followed by 15 mg/kg twice weekly for 3 months has been suggested for horses.[126] Whether such long-term administration would cause any undesirable side effects such as vestibular deficits or renal compromise is unknown. In humans, streptomycin is routinely used only in conjunction with other drugs and never alone because of the development of resistance.[127] Use of any single drug for treating tuberculosis would favor development of resistance. We know of no published reports on treating horses with tuberculosis.

If treatment is undertaken, the horse

should be isolated with precautions taken to prevent spread of disease. In humans, although sputum smears may continue to be positive for at least 2 months, the patients cease to be infectious after 10 to 14 days of initiating an adequate treatment regimen. In humans, the currently suggested treatment regimen is 9 months of combined rifampin and isoniazid administration. Periodic cultures and sensitivity testing should be performed. If there are radiographic lesions, periodic radiographs may be helpful in revealing any change. Bacillus Calmette-Guérin (BCG) vaccine has been used in humans undergoing potential exposure, but whether it would be beneficial in increasing resistance of exposed horses or other animals to tuberculosis infection is unknown. If a horse is to be treated, consultation with the handler's physician and/or public health officials is advisable, as it is a reportable disease in other species.

## Mycoplasma Infections

The significance of mycoplasma as a cause of respiratory disease in horses is not well defined. Mycoplasmas have been isolated from the respiratory tracts and serum antibodies detected from both normal horses and those with acute respiratory disease.[128–138] Seven strains which have been isolated to date are: Acholeplasma laidlawii, A. equifoetale, A. oculi, M. equirhinus, type N14 related to M. pulmonis, type N29 related to M. felis (M. equipharyngis), type N3 related to M. mycoides group.[131] M. felis is usually isolated only from older horses' tracheas and not from young horses. In one study, M. felis, commonly isolated from old horses, was never found in nasopharyngeal swabs from young Thoroughbreds in racing stables.[131] In one survey of 163 aged horses, 77 yielded positive isolates. M. felis has been cultured from horses with pleuritis and also has been shown experimentally to cause pleuritis.[131,132]

### Diagnosis

Variability in numbers of reported positive isolates may be partly due to sampling technique. Wet preincubated swabs are reported to be more likely to yield mycoplasmas than swabs carried in the dry state. Also, slow-growing strains may not be isolated in the presence of fast-growing strains.[131] Type of culture medium is important, as is site of culture. Mycoplasmas were isolated most frequently from the tonsils, about one third as frequently from the turbinates, one fourth as frequently from the trachea and one seventh as frequently from the bronchus.[131] In horses with pleuritis, positive culture is much more likely from the supernatant than from the sediment.[133,134] Also, subculturing to a range of media at intervals can increase the detection rate.[132]

In one study on older horses, mycoplasmas were isolated from 47% of the horses and isolates tended to be more common in those with confirmed postmortem lung lesions of resolving pneumonia, focal abscesses, exudative tracheitis and/or bronchitis and emphysema compared to those with no lesions; however, this was statistically insignificant. Nasal swab samples taken from 43 horses, 18 of which had clinical signs of respiratory disease, yielded mycoplasmas from 2 of the latter.[130] In one study in Ontario, M. equirhinus was cultured from nasopharyngeal swabs obtained from 55 of 92 horses showing signs of respiratory disease and from 19 of 38 normal horses. In the same two groups of horses, M. felis was isolated from 6 of 92 affected and 1 of 38 normal horses.[132] Horses with exudate in their tracheas or bronchi have been reported to be 3 to 4 times more likely to yield positive mycoplasma isolates than horses without exudate.[129] In young horses in training, mycoplasmas were isolated on at least one occasion from the nasopharynx of 47 of 51 (92%) horses or from 66% of the 227 swabs. In about 10% of the swabs obtained from 15 different horses, more than one mycoplasma was isolated.[131] However, when consecutive isolates were made from the same horse, there was frequently a change in species isolated.

Transmission among horses is highly likely. Serology has been used in diagnosing mycoplasma infection/exposure. Two serologic tests, the indirect hemagglutination inhibition (IHA) and metabolism inhibition test

(MIT), are used. Reproducibility of the MIT requires addition of fresh guinea pig serum to the growth medium. One study showed that the two tests may vary considerably; the prevalence of antibodies to M. felis was 36.6% by MIT and only 5.1% by IHA. The significance of antibody titers is debatable as some studies have shown no association with disease.[135] One study of normal horses and those with respiratory disease in which sequential serum antibody titers and nasopharyngeal cultures were obtained showed that seroconversion occurred in 14 of 92 and 3 of 38 horses in each respective group.[137]

Serologic testing of horses in Britain showed that at some time during a year's sampling period, every one of 92 young horses in race training that were sampled had antibodies to M. equirhinus and N3 strain. Of 835 samples, 73% had CF antibodies to both antigens, 17% had antibodies to N3 only, 4% solely to M. equirhinus, and only 6% had no antibodies. There was considerable interstable and individual horse variation, and in most cases antibodies developed within 1 to 2 months of a horse entering the racing stable.[136] However, infection of ponies with either N3 or M. equirhinus never resulted in clinical signs, and infection could only be established with M. equirhinus. This may have been due to pre-existing antibodies to N3.[132]

As mycoplasmas may inhibit phagocytic function of neutrophils in human beings, cattle, mice, and rabbits, and could thereby predispose the host to secondary bacterial infection, a study on the effect of M. felis on the ability of equine neutrophils to engulf and kill Staphylococcus epidermidis was conducted: bactericidal activity was not impaired, suggesting that this is probably not a mechanism predisposing to secondary bacterial infection in horses.[138]

There is a case report of a 7-year-old horse with pleuritis, showing the usual clinical signs and having a pleural effusion with an increased cell count with 80% mildly degenerated neutrophils, 20% macrophages and erythrophagocytosis. No bacteria were isolated, but M. felis was isolated on Hayflick's medium from the supernatant of a centrifuged sample. The horse had a significant rise in serum antibody titers (256 to 1024 on days 3 and 14 after admission respectively). It recovered following relatively low-dose chloramphenicol treatment.[134] An experimental pony was subsequently inoculated intrapleurally with M. felis and developed signs of pleuritis and pleural effusion with return to normal by day 8 without medication. This experimentally infected pony did have signs of pleural infection at postmortem and also had a rise in serum IHA to M. felis.[134]

In the case of a diagnosis of mycoplasma infection (with elimination of other possible causes) one should select antimicrobial agents effective against the organism. At present, as there are no conclusive data that mycoplasmas are important major equine respiratory tract pathogens, there are no recommendations for prophylaxis or control. When selecting antimicrobial therapy, efficacy against any coexistent microorganisms is important. Erythromycin and tetracycline are effective against mycoplasmas.

## Nocardiosis

Nocardia species belong to the family Actinomycetaceae and are soil saprophytes. N. brasiliensis is a primary pathogen and has rarely been identified as a cause of equine lung disease. It is less widely distributed than N. asteroides, which is a more frequently identified opportunist. The organism may be inhaled, ingested, or mechanically introduced. Nocardia sp cause pyogranulomatous inflammation and have been isolated from horses with pneumonia.

Progressive fatal pneumonia and pleuritis occurred in one horse from which Streptococcus sp were also isolated.[139] Although no organisms were seen in histologic sections of the lung, this is not uncommon. The characteristic postmortem lesions of a copious thick reddish pleural exudate with sulphur granules, pleural adhesions and fibrinopurulent pleuritis and dorsal lung abscesses were found.[139]

Prognosis for recovery is poor. Long-term sulfonamides with or without concurrent penicillin administration are the antimicrobial treatment of choice. Adequate drainage of pleural exudate and supportive care are also needed.

## Parasitic Infections

## *Dictyocaulus Arnfieldi*

Dictyocaulus arnfieldi, the equine lungworm, is generally thought to be uncommon in North American horses. However, clinical disease which is indistinguishable from chronic obstructive pulmonary disease may be seen in horses pastured with donkeys, mules, or asses, the usual reservoir hosts. In horses, signs have been seen in autumn following exposure to mules in midsummer.[140] The reservoir hosts are asymptomatic even when infected with large worm burdens. After second-stage larvae are ingested, they migrate through the lymphatics to the lungs, mature there, and after 13 weeks commence egg-laying in equids that harbor patent infections. The eggs are transported via mucociliary clearance to the pharynx, swallowed, and then passed out in the manure. In the horse or pony, infection is usually but not always nonpatent. The first-stage larvae can live up to 7 weeks in warm soil, but cannot overwinter or withstand cold. The infrequency of patent infections makes the Baermann fecal flotation technique unreliable for use in horses; however, it is usually reliable in donkeys, mules, and asses.

### Clinical Signs and Diagnosis

Diagnosis is usually based on clinical signs of severe coughing and obstructive lung disease and a history of signs starting in late summer or autumn after exposure to donkeys, mules, or asses, or housing in an area where the latter had also been kept without an intervening winter to kill any infective larva. Eosinophils may be seen on a transtracheal aspirate but are not pathognomonic for parasitism. Rarely, the larvae or parasite may be found in a transtracheal wash and occasionally have been seen on endoscopic examination.[140,141] In one report, the fifth-stage larva was seen on direct examination of centrifuged mucus but could not be found on fixed and stained slides. The authors suggested that direct cytologic evaluation of unstained unfixed mucus should always be performed.[140] However, use of iodine to stain the larvae may be helpful.

The Baermann fecal flotation technique should be performed on the patient and any potential reservoir hosts (donkeys, mules, asses). Negative findings do not negate the presence of an infection, and even in hosts with patent infections, egg-laying may be variable. If the horse is negative but in contact with positive donkeys, mules, or asses, the horse should be considered infected. Whether radiographs would be helpful in horses has not been determined. Calves with D. viviparus infections have a diffuse mottling and loss of translucency around the terminal portions of the diaphragmatic bronchi.[142] If animals are necropsied, the adult parasites may be found in the peripheral bronchi and larvae may be found when lung tissue is subjected to the Baermann flotation method. Circumscribed pale overinflated areas may be found in lung parenchyma particularly in the caudal lung regions.

### Treatment and Control

Prophylaxis means avoiding housing horses where donkeys, mules, or asses are or were present unless the weather is cold. Thiabendazole (440 mg//kg/orally) given on two consecutive days has been claimed to be effective in the horse.[140,143] In one horse in which larvae were seen in mucus from a transtracheal aspirate, no inflammatory cells or lungworms were recovered on a subsequent lavage following this treatment.[140] Side effects of thiabendazole treatment have included transient anorexia and fever. Studies on treated and control donkeys showed that 5 days of oral mebendazole (15 to 20 mg/kg/day) was effective in decreasing worm burdens and larval counts.[144] Fenbendazole (15 mg/kg orally/day) has reportedly caused a remission of coughing but, at least in donkeys, fecal larval counts were only transiently suppressed.[144] Ivermectin is reported to be effective.[145,146] To our knowledge, there has not been a good comparative study on the efficacy of these various treatments in horses with clinical signs of Dictyocaulus infection, but at present ivermectin appears to be the drug of choice.

## *Parascaris Equorum*

Although larvae of this parasite migrate through the lungs of foals and young horses, the clinical significance has never been well defined. Clinical respiratory disease has been reported in foals at 2 to 4 weeks of age and in horses between 8 to 10 months old following experimental infection.[147,148] Clinical cases of mild pneumonia and coughing in 2- to 4-month-old foals, characterized by presence of eosinophils and no evidence of sepsis in transtracheal aspirates, no exposure to donkeys, and response to 5 days of fenbendazole (10 mg/kg orally/day) support the suspicion that the parasite is of clinical importance.

When parascaris eggs are ingested, larvae can be found 7 to 14 days later in the lungs, where they incite an eosinophilic reaction in airways and alveoli and mucus exudation and focal hemorrhage.[148] The transitory eosinophilic reaction probably occurs because the larva's cuticle degranulates mast cells, releasing eosinophilic chemotactic factor. Within 3 weeks, lymphocytes replace eosinophils and these lymphocytic nodules usually regress by 73 days.

### Clinical Signs and Diagnosis

Foals infected at a young age cough, have a mucoid or mucopurulent nasal discharge for about 10 days, and sometimes have an increased respiratory rate. They remain afebrile unless secondary infections occur. Copious exudate may be seen on endoscopic examination of the trachea. When horses are affected at 8 to 10 months of age, within 2 weeks they develop a cough, hyperpnea, inappetance, depression, and a serous or somewhat mucoid nasal discharge, and they lose condition. Signs may persist for 3 to 4 weeks, and affected horses may fail to show normal weight gain.[147,148]

Diagnosis is difficult and often based on ruling out other causes of respiratory disease. Lack of evidence of sepsis and the presence of eosinophils in transtracheal aspirates support the diagnosis. Although eosinophils may be found in transtracheal aspirates from clinically normal foals, it has not been determined whether this is due to ascarid migration.[149] Fecal examination for ascarid eggs may not be helpful as clinical signs occur early in the prepatent period prior to egg laying.

### Treatment

As the disease is usually self-limiting, treatment may not be necessary. However, larvicidal fenbendazole may be helpful, and ivermectin would probably be efficacious.

## *Pneumocystis Carinii*

Pneumocystis carinii is an ubiquitous sporozoan that causes interstitial pneumonia in man, especially in infants, aged people or those suffering from primary or secondary immunodeficiency. There have been sporadic reports of it occurring in foals usually in association with Rhodococcus equi but also with Bordetella bronchiseptica.[150] Clinical signs reflect the bacterial pneumonia.

Diagnosis has been at postmortem, although in humans, lung and endobronchial brush biopsies and tracheobronchial aspirates have provided the diagnosis. Silver staining (Gomori methanamine silver) is needed to reveal the organism as it is not easily recognized using routine hematoxylin and eosin staining. It is seen as a cup- or crescent-shaped structure in alveoli and is associated with acidophilic material and mononuclear cell infiltration.

The antimicrobial agent of choice for treatment and for prophylaxis of Pneumocystis carinii is trimethoprim sulfamethoxazole. It is important to treat the primary or coexistent disease with appropriate drugs, and combinations of antibiotics may be necessary. If the affected foal is suspected to have a primary immunodeficiency, it is important to confirm or negate this possibility as its existence will alter the prognosis and treatment.

## Fungal Pneumonias

Fungi are ubiquitous in nature, and constant aerosol exposure of respiratory tissue is inevitable. In most samples of stable air, over 90% of particles visible under a light microscope are spores of fungi or actinomycetes.[151] It has been reported that with a horse standing quietly in its stable without access to hay, the mean concentration of dust particles is low, approximately 12 particles (>0.5 cm in diameter)/cm$^3$, but when the bedding is disturbed during the normal "bedding down" operation, the concentration of respirable dust increases sixfold.[152]

Pulmonary disease due to fungi is caused by inhalation as sporular diameter is sufficiently small to allow penetration into the distal airways and alveoli. Except for pathogenic fungi such as Coccidioides immitis, Histoplasma capsulatum, and Cryptococcus neoformans, tissue invasion usually occurs only in the immunocompromised host, although on occasion the normal individual may be afflicted. Important predisposing factors include qualitative and especially quantitative granulocyte abnormalities and the presence of devitalized tissue. Geographic location is probably important in determining disease incidence.

Few cases of histoplasmosis have been described in horses, and most were 2 years old or less. Signs often did not indicate a primary lung infection, despite lung pathology. There is a report of one horse having a fever, depression, nasal discharge, dyspnea, tachypnea, abnormal lung sounds, and weight loss.[153] Thoracic radiographs revealed a severe diffuse miliary pattern compatible with fungal pneumonia and a transtracheal aspirate revealed yeasts and pyogranulomatous inflammation. A needle aspirate of the lung confirmed the presence of Histoplasma capsulatum.[153]

Fungal pathogens that generally infect only equine patients with abnormal host defenses to infection are called "opportunistic fungi" and include Aspergillus sp, the Phycomycetes (Mucor; Rhizopus), and Candida sp. In vitro studies support the critical role of phagocytic cells in host defense against opportunistic fungi. For example, in the immunocompromised patient, Aspergillus sp may produce a fulminant invasive pulmonary infection. Pulmonary aspergillosis in a 2-year-old female with myelomonocytic leukemia has been reported.[154] Although physical examination showed no definitive signs of respiratory tract disease, thoracic radiographs revealed diffuse interstitial pulmonary infiltrate and postmortem examination revealed many raised firm nodules (1 to 35 mm in diameter) from which Aspergillus sp was isolated.[154]

In a survey of approximately 25 horses with fungal pneumonias diagnosed at postmortem examination at the George Widener Hospital, University of Pennsylvania, the majority of horses had a serious primary problem such as enterocolitis, peritonitis, nephritis, endotoxemia, or septicemia. Many horses showed no clinical signs of respiratory disease and the diagnosis of fungal pneumonia was made solely by postmortem examination. Most had been on antimicrobial therapy for a varying length of time for their primary problem.

### Diagnosis

Clinicians must be careful in attributing significance to the presence of fungal elements in a transtracheal aspirate or the isolation of fungus from these samples. Fungal hypha are often present either free or in large mononuclear cells in tracheal aspirates from healthy horses.[155] Sixteen percent of healthy horses were reported to have fungal growth on bacterial culture plates of their transtracheal aspirates.[156] None of these horses had evidence of fungal pneumonia. Another study showed that horses in old wooden barns had 7 times more fungi isolated than horses in a new equine hospital.[157] To be significant, cytologically the fungal elements should be in large numbers and be involved in the inflammatory process within the lung. If fungal pneumonia is suspected, a percutaneous lung biopsy might confirm the diagnosis. However, as the lesions, though multiple and diffuse, are usually small in size and not detectable by ultrasound examination, biopsying is done "blindly" and may not sample an affected site. The biopsy can be examined cytologically, histologically, and by culture.

In patients with suspected aspergillus infection, careful examination of the nose and paranasal sinuses may be rewarding. In human beings, biopsy of a nasal erosion or ulcer that reveals organisms histologically is highly predictive of concomitant or future invasive pulmonary aspergillosis.[158] Serology is not helpful as normal horses as well as those with chronic obstructive pulmonary disease can have titers to aspergillus (J. Hall, personal communications, 1988).

Clinical signs suggestive of pulmonary aspergillosis include coughing and hemoptysis. Radiographs of affected patients may reveal virtually any infiltrative pattern. Although miliary patterns are seen, the most common initial radiographic finding is reported to be a patchy bronchopneumonia.[159] Multiple focal sites are common, and lesions tend to be peripheral in distribution.

### Treatment

As most equine cases of fungal pneumonia occur secondary to a severe primary disease (e.g., liver failure, enterocolitis, and sometimes neoplasia), which is often responsible for the death of the horse, there are few clinical data on treatment regimens. The drug of choice depends on the opportunistic fungus involved. Specific antifungal agents include amphotericin B, ketaconazole, miconazole, 5-fluorocytosine, and iodides. Oral iodides at a dose of 20 g/450 kg (1000 lb) horse SID have been used in a horse and clinically caused regression of fungal lesions of the upper respiratory tract. Ketaconazole administered orally at 30 mg/kg BID is absorbed in horses and mean peak serum levels of approximately 3.8 μg/ml have been reported.[160] Pneumonia caused by Aspergillus has been successfully treated with intravenous amphotericin B using the following regimen: Day 1: 0.3 mg/kg BW; Day 2: 0.4 mg/kg BW; Day 3: 0.5 mg/kg BW; Day 4: no drug; Day 5: 0.5 mg/kg BW. This dose is given every 2 days for 1 month. Renal function must be monitored carefully and the drug stopped for 5 days if signs of renal dysfunction are apparent.[161] Successful treatment of a horse with histoplasmosis has been reported using the following dosage regimen of IV amphotericin B: 0.3, 0.45, and 0.6 mg/kg on days 1, 2, and 3 respectively, 4 days without treatment, then doses of 0.6 mg/kg every other day until a total cumulative dose of 6.75 mg/kg of amphotericin B had been administered.[153] For each dosage, amphotericin B was mixed in 1 L of 5% dextrose in water and administered over 1 hour via a 14 g 5 inch intravenous catheter. Side effects included transient polyuria and polydypsia during the fourth week, an intermittent fever during the first 2 weeks, and lethargy lasting 18 to 24 hours after every treatment. The drug is not approved for use in horses.

Prevention of invasive fungal pneumonia is difficult. Avoidance of large inhaled inocula is impossible in horses because of their environmental conditions. Horses recumbent for long periods inhale even greater numbers of spores even in well-ventilated stables. Improving ventilation and minimizing exposure to inspired spores would be most beneficial. Although air filters are sometimes placed in stables, they are frequently inadequate for the size of the stable and/or inadequately maintained. Negative ionizers may enhance killing of airborne bacteria but do little to lower levels of fungal spores from moldy hay.[162,163] At present, the most important method of disease prevention is decreasing environmental exposure, prompt effective treatment of predisposing illnesses, and possibly judicious avoidance of overuse of corticosteroids and broad spectrum antibiotics.

## References

1. Bryans JT, Moore BO. Streptococcus and Streptococcal Diseases: Recognition, Understanding and Management. Wannamaker LE and Matson JM (eds). New York, Academic Press, 1972, p 327.
2. Benson CE, Sweeney CR. Isolation of *Streptococcus pneumoniae* type 3 from equine species. J Clin Microbiol, *20*:1028, 1984.
3. Mackintosh ME, Grant ST, Burrel MH. Evidence of *Streptococcus pneumoniae* as a cause of respiratory disease in young Thoroughbred horses in training. Proceedings of 5th International Conference on Equine Infectious Disease. DG Powell (ed). Lexington, University Press of Kentucky, 1988, p 41.
4. Kasai K, Nobata R, Rya E. On the incidence of *Streptococcus hemolyticus* in the normal tonsils of horses

and the typing of equine tonsillar streptococci. Jpn J Vet Sci, *6*:116, 1944.

5. Sweeney CR, Beech J, Roby KAW. Bacterial isolates from tracheobronchial aspirates of healthy horses. Am J Vet Res, 46:2562, 1985.
6. Kamada M, Akujama Y. Studies on the distribution of *Streptococcus zooepidemicus* in the equine respiratory tract. Exp Rep Equine Health Lab, *12*:53, 1975.
7. Smith B. Pleuritis and pleural effusion in the horse: A study of 37 cases. J Am Vet Med Assoc, *170*:208, 1977.
8. Raphel CF, Beech J. Pleuritis secondary to pneumonia or lung abscessation in 90 horses. J Am Vet Med Assoc, *181*:808, 1982.
9. Mair TS, and Lane JG. Pneumonia, lung abscesses, and pleuritis in adult horses: A review of 51 cases. Equine Vet J, *21*:175, 1989.
10. Bayly WM, Liggitt HD, Huston LJ, et al. Stress and its effect on equine pulmonary mucosal defenses. Proceedings of 32nd Annual Convention of American Association of Equine Practitioners, 1986, p 253.
11. Traub-Dargatz JL, McKinnon AO, Bruyninckx WJ, et al. Effect of transportation stress on bronchoalveolar lavage fluid analysis in female horses. Am J Vet Res, *49*:1026, 1988.
12. Wong CW, Thompson HL, Thong YH, et al: Effect of strenuous exercise on chemiluminescence response of equine alveolar macrophages. Equine Vet J, *22*:33, 1990.
13. Huston LJ, Bayly WM, Liggitt HD, et al. Alveolar macrophage function in Thoroughbreds after strenuous exercise. In: Equine Exercise Physiology 2. Gillespie JR and Robinson NE (eds). Davis, CA, ICEEP Publications, 1987, p 243.
14. Sweeney CR, Benson CE, Whitlock RH, Meirs D. *Streptococcus equi* infection in horses, Parts I and II. Compend Contin Ed, *9*:689 and 845, 1987.
15. Clabough D. *Streptococcus equi* infection in the horse: A review of clinical and immunological considerations. Equine Vet Sci, *7*:279, 1987.
16. Timoney JF. Shedding and maintenance of *Streptococcus equi* in typical and atypical strangles. Proceedings of 5th International Conference on Equine Infectious Disease. DG Powell (ed). Lexington, University Press of Kentucky, 1987, p 28.
17. Woolcock JB. Studies in atypical *Streptococcus equi*. Res Vet Sci, *19*:115, 1975.
18. Sweeney CR, Whitlock RH, Meirs DA, Whitehead SC, et al. Complications associated with *Streptococcus equi* infection on a horse farm. J Am Vet Med Assoc, *191*:1446, 1987.
19. Blood DC, Radostits OM, Henderson JA. Veterinary Medicine. Philadelphia, Lea & Febiger, 1989, p 562.
20. Yelle MT. Clinical aspects of *Streptococcus equi* infection. Equine Vet J, *19*:158, 1987.
21. Wilson WD. *Streptococcus equi* infections (strangles) in horses. Equine Pract, *10*:12, 1988.
22. George JL, Reif JS, Shideler RK, et al. Identification of carriers of *Streptococcus equi* in a naturally infected herd. J Am Vet Med Assoc, *183*:80, 1983.
23. Prescott JF, Srivastava SK, deGannes R, et al. A mild form of strangles caused by an atypical *Streptococcus equi*. J Am Vet Med Assoc, *180*:293, 1982.
24. Timoney JF. Protecting against strangles: A contemporary view. Equine Vet J, *20*:392, 1988.
25. Todd AG: Strangles. J Comp Pathol Ther, *23*:212, 1910.
26. Mahaffey LW. Respiratory conditions in horses. Vet Rec, *74*:1295, 1962.
27. Timoney JF, Timoney PJ, Strickland KL: Lysogeny and the immunologically reactive proteins of *Streptococcus equi*. Vet Rec, *115*:148, 1984.
28. Ford J, Lokae MD. Complications of *Streptococcus equi* infection. Equine Pract, *2*:41, 1980.
29. Sweeney CR, Benson CE, Whitlock RH, et al. Description of an epizootic and persistence of *Streptococcus equi* infections in horses. J Am Vet Med Assoc, *194*:1281, 1989.
30. Knight AP, Voss JL, McChesney AE, et al. Experimentally induced *Streptococcus equi* infection in horses with resultant guttural pouch empyema. VM/SAC, *70*:1194, 1975.
31. Wisecup WG, Schroeder C, Page NP. Isolation of *Streptococcus equi* from burros. J Am Vet Med Assoc, *150*:303, 1967.
32. Roberts MC, Kelly WR. Renal dysfunction in a case of purpura hemorrhagica in a horse. Vet Rec, *110*:144, 1982.
33. Gunson DE, Rooney JR. Anaphylactoid purpura in a horse. Vet Pathol, *14*:325, 1977.
34. Galan JE, Timoney JF. Immune complexes in purpura hemorrhagica of the horse contain IgA and M antigen of *Streptococcus equi*. J Immunol, *135*:3134, 1985.
35. Sweeney CR, Benson CE, Whitlock RH, et al. Unpublished data, 1987.
36. Bryant S, Brown KK, Lewis S, et al. Protection against strangles with an enzymatic *Streptococcus equi* extract. Vet Med, *80*:58, 1985.
37. Reif JS, George JL, Shideler RK. Recent developments in strangles research: Observations on the carrier state and evaluation of a new vaccine. Proceedings of 27th Annual Convention of American Association of Equine Practitioners, New Orleans, 1981. p 33, 1982.
38. Hoffman A, Staempfli H, Viel L, et al. Field evaluation of a commercial M protein vaccine (Strepvax II) in a feedlot for foals with epidemic strangles. Proceedings of Seventh Annual Veterinary Medicine Forum. Am Coll Vet Intern Med, 1989, p 1027.
39. Timoney JF, Eggers D. Serum bactericidal responses to *Streptococcus equi* of horses following infection or vaccination. Equine Vet J, *17*:306, 1985.
40. Galan JE, Timoney JF, Curtiss III R. Mucosal nasopharyngeal immune response of horses to protein antigens of *Streptococcus equi*. Infect Immun, *47*:623, 1985.
41. Galan JE, Timoney JF, Lengemann FW. Passive transfer of mucosal antibody to *Streptococcus equi* in the foal. Infect Immun, 54:202, 1986.
42. Austrian R, Thorn G. Pneumococcal infections. In: Principles of Internal Medicine. Harrison (ed). New York, McGraw-Hill Book Co., 1979, pp 802–808.

43. Harms FR. Pneumokokkeninfektion beim Rohlen. Dtsch Tieraerztl Wochenschr, *49*:10, 1941.
44. Ellenberger MA, and Genetzky RM. *Rhodococcus equi* infections. Literature review. Comp Cont Ed, *8*:5414, 1986.
45. Bain AM. *Corynebacterium equi* infections in the equine. Aust Vet J, *39*:116, 1963.
46. Roberts MC, Hodgson DR, Kelly WR. *Corynebacterium equi* infection in an adult horse. Aust Vet J, *56*:96, 1980.
47. Rooney JR. Corynebacterium infection in foals. Mod Vet Pract, *47*:43, 1986.
48. Hillidge CJ. Review of Corynebacterium *(Rhodococcus equi)* lung abscesses in foals: Pathogenesis, diagnosis and treatment. Vet Rec, *119*:261, 1986.
49. Magnusson H. Spezifische infektiose pneumone beim fohlen. Einneurer eitenger beim pferd. Arch Wiss Prakt Tiescheilk, *50*:22, 1923.
50. Elissalde GS, Renshaw HW, Walberg JA. *Corynebacterium equi:* An interhost review with emphasis on the foal. Comp Immunol Microbiol Infect Dis, *3*:433, 1980.
51. Johnson JA, Prescott JF, Markham RJF. The pathology of experimental *Corynebacterium equi* infection in foals following intragastric challenge. Vet Pathol, *20*:450, 1983.
52. Wilks CR, Barton MD, Allison JF. Immunity to and immunotherapy for *Rhodococcus equi*. J Reprod Fertil Suppl, *32*:497, 1982.
53. Barton MD, Embury DH. Studies of the pathogenesis of *Rhodococcus equi* infection in foals. Aust Vet J, *64*:332, 1987.
54. Martens RJ, Fiske RA, Renshaw HW. Experimental subacute foal pneumonia induced by aerosol administration of *Corynebacterium equi*. Equine Vet J, *14*:111, 1982.
55. Johnson JA, Prescott JF, Markham RJF. The pathology of experimental *Corynebacterium equi* infection in foals following intrabronchial challenge. Vet Pathol, *20*:440, 1983.
56. Cimprich RE, Rooney JR. *Corynebacterium equi* enteritis in foals. Vet Pathol, *14*:95, 1977.
57. Martens RJ, Martens JG, Fiske RA. *Rhodococcus equi* foal pneumonia: protective effects of immune plasma in experimentally infected foals. Equine Vet J, *21*:249, 1989.
58. Zink MC, Johnson JA, Prescott JF, et al. The interaction of *Corynebacterium equi* and equine alveolar macrophages in vitro. J Reprod Fert Suppl, *32*:491, 1982.
59. Hietala SK, Ardans AA: Interaction of *Rhodococcus equi* with phagocytic cells from *R. equi* exposed and nonexposed foals. Vet Microbiol, *14*:307, 1987.
60. Zink MC, Yager JA, Prescott JF, et al. In vitro phagocytosis and killing of *Corynebacterium equi* by foal alveolar macrophages during postnatal maturation. Am J Vet Res, *46*:2171, 1985.
61. Zink MC, Yager JA, Prescott JF, et al. Electron microscopic investigation of intracellular events after ingestion of *Rhodococcus equi* by foal alveolar macrophages. Vet Microbiol, *14*:295, 1987.
62. Ellenberger MA, Kaeberle ML, Roth JA. Effect of *Rhodococcus equi* on equine polymorphonuclear leukocyte function. Vet Immunol Immunopathol, *7*:315, 1984.
63. Coignoul FL, Bertram TA, Roth JA, et al. Comparison of polymorphonuclear function in mares and foals. Am J Vet Res, *45*:898, 1984.
64. Martens JG, Martens RJ, Renshaw HW. *Rhodococcus* (Corynebacterium) *equi*: bactericidal capacity of neutrophils from neonatal and adult horses. Am J Vet Res, *49*:295, 1988.
65. Martens RJ, Martens JG, Renshaw HW, et al. *Rhodococcus equi.* Neutrophil chemiluminescent and bactericidal responses to opsonizing antibody. Vet Microbiol, *14*:277, 1987.
66. Yager JA, Duder CK, Prescott JF. The interaction of *Rhodococcus equi* and foal neutrophils in vitro. Vet Microbiol, *14*:287, 1987.
67. Magnusson H. Pyemia in foals caused by *Corynebacterium equi.* Vet Rec, *50*:1459, 1938.
68. Henry JI. *Corynebacterium equi* septicemia in foals: Control and therapy #786. Post-graduate committee in Veterinary Science, University of Sydney, 1979.
69. Robinson RC. Epidemiological and bacteriological studies of *Corynebacterium (Rhodococcus) equi.* Isolates from California farms. J Reprod Fertil (Suppl), *32*:477, 1982.
70. Smith BP, Robinson RC. Studies of an outbreak of Corynebacterium pneumonia in foals. Equine Vet J, *13*:223, 1981.
71. Prescott JF, Travers M, Yager-Johnson JA. Epidemiologic survey of *Corynebacterium equi* infections on five Ontario horse farms. Can J Comp Med, *48*:10, 1984.
72. Woolcock JB, Mutimer MD, Farmer AMT. Epidemiology of *Corynebacterium equi* in horses. Res Vet Sci, *28*:87, 1980.
73. Barton M, Hughes K. *Rhodococcus equi,* a soil organism. J Reprod Fertil Suppl, *32*:481, 1982.
74. Woolcock JB, Farmer AMT, Mutimer MD. Selective medium for *Corynebacterium equi.* J Clin Microbiol, *9*:640, 1979.
75. Barton MD, Hughes KL. Ecology of *Rhodococcus equi.* Vet Microbiol, *9*:65, 1984.
76. Takai S, Ohkura H, Watanabe Y, et al. Quantitative aspects of faecal *Rhodococcus (Corynebacterium) equi* in foals. J Clin Microbiol, *23*:794, 1986.
77. Hughes KL, Sulaiman I. The ecology of *Rhodococcus equi* and physiocochemical influences on growth. Vet Microbiol, *14*:241, 1987.
78. Prescott JF. Control of *Rhodococcus equi* pneumonia in foals. Penn Annual Conference Proceedings, Philadelphia, 1990, p 129.
79. Takai S, Fujimori T, Katsuzaki K, et al. Ecology of *Rhodococcus equi* in horses and their environment on horse-breeding farms. Vet Microbiol, *14*:233, 1987.
80. Prescott JF, Johnson JA, Markham RJF. Experimental studies on the pathogenesis of *Corynebacterium equi* infection in foals. Can J Comp Med, *44*:280, 1980.
81. Yager JA. The pathogenesis of *Rhodococcus equi* pneumonia in foals. Vet Microbiol, *14*:225, 1987.
82. Zink MC, Yager JA, Smart NL. *Rhodococcus equi* infection in horses 1958–1984; a review of 131 cases.

In: Proceedings of Dorothy Havermeyer Foundation Workshop on *Corynebacterium equi (Rhodococcus equi)* Pneumonia of Foals. University of Guelph, Ontario, Canada, June–July, 1986, p 45.

83. Sweeney CR, Sweeney RW, Divers TJ. *Rhodococcus equi* pneumonia in 48 foals: Response to antimicrobial therapy. Vet Microbiol, *114*:329, 1987.
84. Falcon J, Smith BP, O'Brien TR, et al. Clinical and radiographic findings in *Corynebacterium equi* pneumonia of foals. J Am Vet Med Assoc, *186*:593, 1985.
85. Prescott JF, Ogilvie TH, Markham JF. Lymphocyte immunostimulation in the diagnosis of *Corynebacterium equi* pneumonia of foals. Am J Vet Res, *41*:2073, 1980.
86. Woolcock JB, Mutimer MD, Bowles PM. The immunological response of foals to *Rhodococcus equi:* A review. Vet Microbiol, *14*:215, 1987.
87. Takai S, Kawazu S, Tsubaki S. Enzyme linked immunosorbent assay for diagnosis of *Corynebacterium (Rhodococcus) equi* infection in foals. Am J Vet Res, *46*:2166, 1985.
88. Ellenburger MA, Kaeberle ML, Roth JA. Equine humoral immune response to *Rhodococcus equi.* Am J Vet Res, *45*:2428, 1984.
89. Hietala SK, Ardans AA, Sansome A. Detection of *Corynebacterium equi*-specific antibody in horses with enzyme-linked immunosorbent assay. Am J Vet Res, *46*:13, 1985.
90. Takai S, Kawazu S, Tsubaki S. Humoral immune response of foals to experimental infection with *Rhodococcus equi.* Vet Microbiol, *14*:321, 1987.
91. Prescott JF, Mechang'a R, Kiviecien J, et al. Prevention of foal mortality due to *Rhodococcus equi* pneumonia on an endemically affected farm. Can Vet J, *30*:871, 1989.
92. Skalka B. Dynamics of *Equi*-factor antibodies in sera of foals kept on farms with differing histories of *Rhodococcus equi* pneumonia. Vet Microbiol, *14*:269, 1987.
93. Ardans AA, Hietala SK. Studies on endemic *Rhodococcus equi* pneumonia. In: Abstracts, Proceedings of Dorothy R. Havermeyer Foundation Workshop on *Corynebacterium equi (Rhodococcus equi)* Pneumonia of Foals. University of Guelph, Ontario, Canada, June–July, 1986, p 15.
94. Prescott JF. The susceptibility of isolates of *Corynebacterium equi* to antimicrobial drugs. J Vet Pharmacol Therap, *4*:27, 1981.
95. Prescott JF, Sweeney CR. Treatment of *Corynebacterium equi* pneumonia in foals: A review. J Am Vet Med Assoc, *187*:725, 1985.
96. Woolcock JB, Mutimer MD. *Corynebacterium equi:* In vitro susceptibility to twenty-six antimicrobial agents. Antimicrob Agents Chemother, *18*:976, 1980.
97. Prescott JF, Nicholson VM. The effects of combinations of selected antibiotics on the growth of *Corynebacterium equi.* J Vet Pharmacol Ther, *7*:61, 1984.
98. Hillidge CJ. Use of erythromycin rifampin combination in treatment of *Rhodococcus equi* pneumonia. Vet Microbiol, *14*:337, 1987.
99. Burrows GE, MacAllister CG, Beckstrom DA, et al. Rifampin in the horse: comparison of intravenous, intramuscular and oral administration. Am J Vet Res, *46*:442, 1985.
100. Thornsburg C, Hill BC, Swenson JM, et al. Rifampin: spectrum of antibacterial activity. Rev Infect Dis, *5*:5412, 1983.
101. Prescott JF, Hoover DJ, Dohoo JR. Pharmacokinetics of erythromycin in foals and in adult horses. J Vet Pharmacol Ther, *6*:67, 1983.
102. Burrows GE. Pharmacotherapeutics of macrolides, lincomycin and spectinomycin. J Am Vet Med Assoc, *176*:1072, 1980.
103. Paulsen O, Nilsson LG, Bengtsson HI. The interaction of erythromycin with theophylline. Eur J Clin Pharmacol, *32*:493, 1987.
104. Jonkman JHG. Therapeutic consequences of drug interactions with theophylline pharmacokinetics. J Allergy Clin Immunol, *78*:736, 1986.
105. Aranda JV, Chemtob S, Laudignon N, et al. Pharmacologic effects of theophylline in the newborn. J Allergy Clin Immunol, *78*:773, 1986.
106. Kowalczyk DF, Beech J, Littlejohn D. Pharmacokinetic disposition of theophylline in horses after intravenous administration. Am J Vet Res, *45*:2272, 1984.
107. Ayres JW, Pearson EG, Riebold TW, et al. Theophylline and dyphylline pharmacokinetics in the horse. Am J Vet Res, *46*:2500, 1985.
108. Bayly WM, Reed SM, Foreman JH, et al. Equine bronchopneumonia due to *Bordetella bronchiseptica.* Equine Pract, *4*:25, 1982.
109. Darien BJ, Brown CM, Walker RD. *Bordetella bronchiseptica,* a significant respiratory pathogen in foals and weanlings 5th International Conference on Equine Infectious Disease. Lexington, University Press of Kentucky, 1987, poster.
110. Sweeney CR, Divers TJ, Benson CE. Anaerobic bacteria in 21 horses with pleuropneumonia. J Am Vet Med Assoc, *187*:721, 1985.
111. Orsini JA, Benson CE, Spencer PA, et al. Resistance to gentamicin and amikacin of gram-negative organisms isolated from horses. Am J Vet Res, *50*:923, 1989.
112. Sweeney RW, Beech J, Simmons RD. Pharmacokinetics of intravenously and intramuscularly administered ticarcillin and clavulanic acid in foals. Am J Vet Res, *49*:23, 1988.
113. Sweeney RW, Sweeney CR, Soma LR, et al. Pharmacokinetics of metronidazole given to horses by intravenous and oral routes. Am J Vet Res, *47*:1726, 1986.
114. Griffith AS. Types of tubercle bacilli in equine tuberculosis. J Comp Pathol, *50*:159, 1937.
115. Muser R. Tuberkulose, Tuberkulinreakton und Mycobakterien bein Pferd. Inaugural dissertation, Tierargh Fak, München, 1961.
116. Mair TS, Taylor FGR, Gibbs C, et al. Generalized avian tuberculosis in a horse. Equine Vet J, *18*:226, 1986.
117. Derksen FJ, Slocombe RF, Brown CM, et al. Chronic

restrictive pulmonary disease in a horse. J Am Vet Med Assoc, *180*:887, 1982.

118. Buergelt CD, Hines SA, Cantor G, et al. A retrospective study of proliferative interstitial lung disease of horses in Florida. Vet Pathol, *23*:750, 1986.
119. Winder C, Ehrensperger F, Hermann M, et al. Interstitial pneumonia in the horse: Two unusual cases. Equine Vet J, *20*:298, 1988.
120. Nielson SW, Sprating FR. Tuberculous spondylitis in a horse. Br Vet J, *124*:503, 1968.
121. Mair TS, Jenkins PA. Isolation of mycobacteria from the nasal cavity of horses. Equine Vet J, *22*:54, 1990.
122. Konyha LD, Kreier JP. The significance of tuberculin tests in the horse. Am Rev Resp Dis, *103*:91, 1971.
123. Mangura BT and Reichman LB. Pulmonary tuberculosis. In: Respiratory Infections: Diagnosis and Management. Pennington JE (ed). New York, Raven Press, 1983, p 397.
124. Roberts WD. Isoniazid in equine therapy. Proceedings of 17th Annual Convention of American Association of Equine Practitioners, 1971, p 33–34.
125. Wlodaver CG, MacGreor RR. Mycobacteria. In: The Pneumonias. Levinson ME and Wright J (eds). Boston, PSG, Inc., 1984, p 390.
126. Peel JE. Tuberculosis. In: Current Therapy in Equine Medicine. Robinson NE (ed). Philadelphia, W.B. Saunders Co., 1983.
127. Kendig EL. Tuberculosis disorders of children. In: Disorders of the Respiratory Tract in Children. Kendig EL and Chernig V (eds). 4th Ed. Philadelphia, W.B. Saunders Co., 1983, p 662.
128. Windsor DG. The isolation of mycoplasma from horses. Vet Rec, *93*:593, 1973.
129. Allam WD, Powell DG, Andrews BE, Lemcke RE. Letter: The isolation of *Mycoplasma* sp from horses. Vet Rec, *93*:402, 1973.
130. Moorthy ARS, Spradbow PB. Isolation of mycoplasmas from the respiratory tract of horses in Australia. Vet Rec, *98*:235, 1976.
131. Poland J, Lemcke R. Mycoplasmas of the respiratory tract of horses and their significance in upper respiratory tract disease. Proceedings of 4th International Conference on Equine Infectious Disease. Princeton, Veterinary Publications, Inc., 1978, p 437.
132. Willoughby RA, Huber L, Viel L. Culture and serological results in acute upper respiratory infections in horses. Proceedings of 7th Annual Veterinary Medical Forum (ACVIM). San Diego, 1989, p 604.
133. Rosendal S, Blackwell TE, Lunsden JH, et al. Detection of antibodies to *Mycoplasma felis* in horses. J Am Vet Med Assoc, *188*:292, 1986.
134. Ogilvie TH, Rosendal, S, Blackwell TE, et al. *Mycoplasma felis* as a cause of pleuritis in horses. J Am Vet Med Assoc, *182*:1374, 1983.
135. Kirchhoff H, Ammar AM, Heitmann J, et al. Serological investigation of horse sera for antibodies against mycoplasmas and acholeplasmas. Vet Microbiol, 7:147, 1982.
136. Hooker JM, Butler M. Studies on the occurrence and development of equine mycoplasma antibodies. Proceedings of 4th International Conference on Equine Infectious Disease. Princeton, Veterinary Publications, Inc, 1978, p 437.
137. Doster IR, Lin BC. Identification of Mycoplasma hyopneumoniae in formalin-fixed porcine lung using an indirect immunoperoxidase method. Am J Vet Res, *49*:1719, 1988.
138. Rosendal S, Lunsden JH, Viel V, et al. Phagocytic function of equine neutrophils exposed to *Mycoplasma felis* in vitro and in vivo. Am J Vet Res, *48*:758, 1987.
139. Deem DA, Harrington DD: Nocardia brasiliensis in a horse with pneumonia and pleuritis. Cornell Vet, *70*:321, 1980.
140. George LW, Tanner ML, Robertson E, et al. Chronic respiratory disease in a horse infected with *Dictyocaulus arnfieldi*. J Am Vet Med Assoc, *179*:820, 1981.
141. Whitwell KE, Greet TRC. Collection and evaluation of tracheobronchial washes in the horse. Equine Vet J, *16*:499, 1984.
142. Head JR, Suter PF, Ettinger SJ. Lower respiratory tract diseases. In: Textbook of Veterinary Internal Medicine. Ettinger SJ (ed). Philadelphia, W.B. Saunders Co., 1975, *1*:661.
143. Round MC. A study of the natural history of lungworm infection on the Equidae, PhD thesis. University of Cambridge, England, 1972.
144. Clayton HM. Lung parasites. In: Current Therapy in Equine Medicine. Robinson NE (ed). Philadelphia, W.B. Saunders Co., 1983, p 520.
145. Lyons ET, Drudge JH, Tolliver SC. Ivermectin: Treating for naturally occurring infections of lungworms and stomach worms in equids. Vet Med, *80*:58, 1985.
146. Britt DP, Preston JM. Efficacy of ivermectin against *Dictyocaulus arnfieldi* in ponies. Vet Rec, *116*:343, 1985.
147. Clayton HM, Duncan JL. Clinical signs associated with Parascaris equorum infection in worm free pony foals and yearlings. Vet Parasitol, *4*:69, 1978.
148. Nichols JM, Clayton HM, Piril HM, et al. A pathological study of the lungs of foals infected experimentally with Parascaris equorum. J Comp Pathol, *88*:261, 1978.
149. Crane S, Ziemer EL, Sweeney CR. Tracheobronchial aspirates from clinically normal foals: cytologic and bacteriologic evaluation. Am J Vet Res, *50*:2042, 1989.
150. Shively JN, Dellers RW, Buergelt CD, et al. Pneumocystis carinii pneumonia in two foals. J Am Vet Med Assoc, *162*:648, 1973.
151. Clark AF, Madelin T. Technique for assessing respiratory health hazards from hay and other source materials. Equine Vet J, *19*:442, 1987.
152. Webster AJF, Clark AF, Madelen TM, et al. Air hygiene in stables 1: Effects of stable design, ventilation and management on the concentration of respirable dust. Equine Vet J, *19*:448, 1987.
153. Cornick JL. Diagnosis and treatment of pulmonary histoplasmosis in a horse. Cornell Vet, *80*:97, 1990.

154. Blue J, Perdriget J, Brown E. Pulmonary aspergillosis in a horse with myelomonocytic leukemia. J Am Vet Med Assoc, *190*:1562, 1987.
155. Beech J. Cytology of tracheobronchial aspirates in horses. Vet Pathol, *12*:157, 1975.
156. Sweeney CR, Beech J, and Roby KAW. Bacterial isolates from tracheobronchial aspirates from healthy horses. Am J Vet Res, *46*:2562, 1985.
157. Mansmann RA. Evaluation of transtracheal aspiration in the horse. J Am Vet Med Assoc, *169*:631, 1976.
158. Talbot G. Aspergillus. In: The Pneumonias. Levison ME (ed). Bristol, John Wright and Sons, Ltd., 1984, p 494.
159. Lawson GHK, McPherson EA, Murphy JR, et al. The presence of precipitating antibodies in the sera of horses with chronic obstructive pulmonary disease (COPD). Equine Vet J, *11*:172, 1979.
160. Prades M, Brown MP, Gronwell, RR. Ketaconazole in the horse: Body fluid and endometrial concentrations after repeated oral administration. Vet Surg, *15*:131, 1986.
161. Ruoff WW. Fungal pneumonia in horses. Proceedings of 34th Annual Convention of American Association of Equine Practitioners, 1988, p 423.
162. Phillips GB, Harris GJ, Jones MW. The effect of air ions on bacterial aerosols. Int J Biometeorol, *8*:27, 1964.
163. Edwards JH, Trotman DM, Mason OF. Methods of reducing particle concentrations of Aspergillus fumigatus conidia and moldy hay dust. Sabauroudia, *23*:237, 1985.

# CHAPTER 13

# THORACIC NEOPLASIA

*CORINNE R. SWEENEY and DEBORAH M. GILLETTE*

Surveys of equine neoplasms indicate the low incidence of thoracic neoplasia in the horse. In an abattoir survey in London of 1308 horses, only two had pulmonary tumors (1 granular-cell myoblastoma; 1 bronchiolar adenoma).[1] Two other surveys of 155 and 687 equine necropsies, reported no thoracic neoplasms.[2,3] Gerber in his report on pulmonary disease in the horse states that the practical importance of lung tumors is negligible.[4] In a 20-year period (1968 through 1987), out of 5629 horses examined by the Necropsy Service at the University of Pennsylvania, 35 (0.62%) horses had neoplasia involving the thoracic cavity.

The incidence of primary lung tumors of any type is reported to be less than 1% of all tumors in domestic animals including the horse.[5] This is in contrast to man, in whom there is a much greater frequency of lung tumors related to cigarette smoking and various other environmental or occupational exposures to carcinogens. Metastatic lesions are more common, because of the vulnerability of the lungs to tumor emboli. Gross and microscopic patterns of metastatic pulmonary neoplasia can sometimes be difficult or impossible to distinguish from those of primary lung neoplasia, thus an important factor in the diagnosis is exclusion of possible primary sites elsewhere in the body.

Antemortem diagnosis of thoracic neoplasia first requires the recognition of thoracic disease. As most of the reported cases of thoracic neoplasia involve metastatic disease, and the horse's clinical signs are generally related to the primary site of the neoplasm, the clinician often has no reason to suspect thoracic involvement. When there are signs of abnormal respiratory function such as dyspnea, tachypnea, hemoptysis, coughing, cyanosis, nasal discharge, or epistaxis, relevant diagnostic tests are more likely to be performed.

Primary pulmonary tumors reported in the horse include granular cell tumor,[6–12] bronchial myxoma,[13] pulmonary carcinoma,[14–16] and pulmonary chondrosarcoma.[17,18] Other primary thoracic tumors reported in the horse include pleural mesothelioma,[19,20] thymoma,[21] and lymphosarcoma.[22]

Granular-cell tumor (myoblastoma), the most frequently reported primary pulmonary tumor of the horse, is a neoplasm of mesenchymal origin. Originally thought to be derived from myoblasts, these tumors are now believed to originate from a fibroblast-like cell related to the progenitor of Schwann cells.[16] All 12 granular-cell tumors reported in horses have been confined to the lungs. Nine of these involved only the right lung[6–12] and two involved the left lung only.[8,9] In only one horse were both lungs involved.[9] The neoplasm usually has consisted of multiple, well-defined nodules associated with a major bronchus and often protruding into the bronchial lumen. The main histologic feature of the tumor is lobular aggregation of large, round to polyhedral cells with abundant acidophilic granular cytoplasm. The lobules are surrounded and dissected by fibrovascular stroma. The cytoplasmic granules in the tumor cells are PAS-positive and have characteristic ultrastructural features. Most granu-

**TABLE 13–1.** ***Clinical and Postmortem Data From 16 Horses with Thoracic Neoplasia***

| Diagnosis | Age (yr) | Breed | Sex | Antemortem Diagnosis | Antemortem Examination of TBA | PF | Biopsy | Primary Neoplasia Site | Degree of Involvement in Thorax: Lung | Pleural Cavity | Thoracic Lymph Nodes |
|---|---|---|---|---|---|---|---|---|---|---|---|
| Adenocarcinoma | 10 | AR | M | No | NE | NE | NE | Unknown | Severe | Moderate | Severe |
| Adenocarcinoma | 15 | AR | G | No | NE | NE | NE | Unknown | Severe | – | Severe |
| Adenocarcinoma | 7 | QH | G | No | – | NE | NE | Thyroid | Mild | – | – |
| Adenocarcinoma | 8 | TB | G | Yes | – | – | + | Kidney | Severe | – | – |
| Adenocarcinoma | 6 | SB | M | Yes | – | NE | + | Kidney | Severe | – | – |
| Adenocarcinoma[23] | 18 | X | F | Yes | + | NE | NE | Uterus | Severe | – | Mild |
| Adenocarcinoma[24] | 11 | QH | F | Yes | NE | + | NE | Ovary | – | * | Severe |
| Squamous cell carcinoma | 14 | X | G | Yes | NE | + | NE | Stomach | – | Moderate | Severe |
| Squamous cell carcinoma | 7 | SB | F | Yes | NE | + | NE | Stomach | – | Severe | – |
| Squamous cell carcinoma | 8 | QH | G | No | NE | NE | NE | Oral cavity | Mild | – | – |
| Squamous cell carcinoma | Aged | Pony | F | No | NE | NE | NE | Vulva | Mild | – | – |
| Squamous cell carcioma | 7 | APP | G | No | NE | NE | NE | Prepuce | Mild | – | – |
| Hemangiosarcoma | 9 | TB | G | No | NE | NE | NE | Muscle | Moderate | – | – |
| Hemangiosarcoma[45] | 7 | TB | F | Yes | – | – | + | Unknown | Severe | Severe | – |
| Hemangiosarcoma[44] | 6 | SB | G | No | – | NE | NE | Unknown | Severe | – | Mild |
| Undifferentiated sarcoma | 0.25 | TB | F | No | NE | NE | NE | Unknown | Mild | – | – |

AR - Arabian
QH - Quarter Horse
TB - Thoroughbred
SB - Standardbred
X - Crossbred

APP - Appaloosa
M - Male
G - Gelding
F - Female
NE - Not evaluated

\+ - Positive
* - Effusion
– - No evidence of neoplasia
TBA - Tracheobronchial aspirate
PF - Pleural fluid

lar-cell tumors have been diagnosed only at postmortem examination.

The only two reported primary pulmonary carcinomas in the horse were in a 4-year-old Quarter Horse stallion who was examined because of signs of cardiac failure[14] and a 20-year-old Arabian-Quarter Horse mare.[15] The tumor in the stallion was thought to be of pulmonary or mediastinal origin with metastasis to the heart. The pleural cavity, including the surface of the pleura and mediastinum, was invaded with variably-sized, soft yellow-grey masses. Tumor masses were present throughout the pulmonary parenchyma, packing and occluding many pulmonary vessels. The tumor in the mare involved the right lung and was thought to be of bronchial origin.[15]

Of the 35 horses with thoracic neoplasia at the University of Pennsylvania, 7 (20%) had metastatic adenocarcinoma (Table 13–1). The primary sites of the tumor in these horses included kidney, uterus, thyroid, and ovary and could not be determined in two horses (Fig. 13–1).[23,24] Four of the seven horses had no pleural effusion. Cytologic examination of the fluid from one horse was normal. One horse had 10 L of pleural fluid which was not examined and one had pleural fluid containing neoplastic epithelial cells.

Biopsy of a thoracic mass yielded an antemortem diagnosis of adenocarcinoma in two horses. Bronchoscopy showed a proliferative mass in the trachea of one 14-year-old mare with a primary adenocarcinoma of the uterus, and tracheobronchial aspirates of this same horse revealed neoplastic cells.[23] A 6-year-old Standardbred horse had an adenocarcinoma that occupied 60 to 75% of the pulmonary parenchyma, but the horse was still in active race training within two weeks of euthanasia. In three horses, no clinical signs referable to the respiratory tract were present and the thoracic adenocarcinoma was not diagnosed antemortem. Therefore, in two of these three horses with severe pulmonary neoplasia, no diagnostic tests specific for respiratory tract dysfunction were performed and it is un-

| Examination of Other Organs | | | | | | | | | |
|---|---|---|---|---|---|---|---|---|---|
| *Nonthoracic Lymph Nodes* | *Liver* | *Kidney* | *Spleen* | *Diaphragm* | *GI Tract* | *Pericardium* | *Myocardium* | *Skeletal Muscle* | *Other Sites* |
| + | + | + | − | − | − | − | − | − | Aorta |
| + | + | − | − | − | − | − | − | − | |
| + | + | + | + | − | − | − | + | − | Adrenal; thyroid |
| + | − | + | − | − | − | − | − | − | |
| − | + | + | − | + | − | − | − | − | Vena cava |
| + | − | − | − | − | − | − | − | − | |
| + | − | − | − | − | − | − | − | − | Adrenal |
| + | − | − | − | + | + | − | − | − | |
| + | + | − | + | + | + | + | − | − | Peritoneum; ovary |
| − | − | − | − | − | − | − | − | − | |
| + | − | − | − | − | − | − | − | − | |
| + | − | − | − | − | − | − | − | − | |
| + | − | − | − | − | − | − | − | + | |
| + | − | + | + | + | + | + | + | − | |
| + | + | + | + | + | + | + | + | + | Brain |
| + | − | − | − | − | − | − | + | + | |

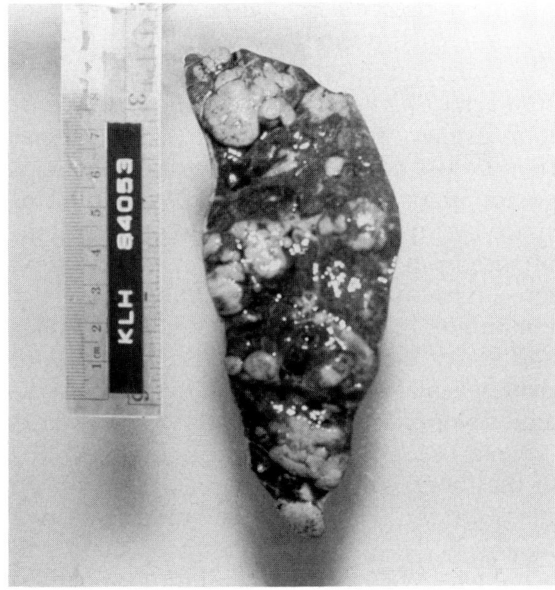

**FIG. 13–1.** Renal papillary adenocarcinoma metastasized to the lung of a 6-year-old Standardbred horse. (Courtesy of Kathleen Hawkins and Laboratory of Large Animal Pathology, New Bolton Center)

known if abnormalities would have been found.

Primary pulmonary chondrosarcoma has been reported in a horse.[17] Cytologic examination of pleural fluid and an antemortem needle aspirate of the pulmonary mass revealed neoplastic cells in this horse. The neoplasm probably originated from cartilaginous tissue of the bronchial tree.[17] Another report describes metastatic chondrosarcoma in the lungs of a horse with a primary tumor in a rib.[18]

A primary bronchial myxoma, a benign connective tissue tumor, was reported in a 25-year-old Arabian mare with a history of intermittent coughing, hyperpnea, and respiratory disease of two years' duration. The irregularly nodular tumor originated from the left cranial lobal bronchus at the carina of the trachea.[13]

Primary pleural tumors are rare, but pleural mesothelioma has been reported in two horses.[19,20] Mesotheliomas arise from the cells of the serous lining of the pleural cavity. They appear as multiple small firm nodules or villous projections on a thickened serosal surface. The tumor is frequently associated with a large volume of pleural effusion. Cytologic examination of the pleural effusion in one horse revealed numerous pleomorphic mesothelial cells. The pleomorphism of these cells ranged from cells containing three or four nuclei to more differentiated cells forming pseudomembranes. Many multinucleated cells were arranged in polypoid nodules of 50 or more cells.[20]

Thymomas are neoplasms of thymic epithelial cells, regardless of the presence or absence of lymphocytes. Thymomas have been reported infrequently in the horse.[21,25–27] A metastatic thymic carcinoma with squamous differentiation was reported in a horse with multiple lung nodules and invasion of the first two ribs on both sides of the chest.[21] Cytology of a needle-biopsy specimen from the mass revealed cells compatible with those of a carcinoma.

Equine lymphosarcoma occurs in mediastinal, alimentary, multicentric, cutaneous, and generalized forms; combinations of one or more of these are not infrequent. In one report of 20 horses with lymphosarcoma, four horses had thoracic involvement,[28] while another paper reports that three of five horses had thoracic involvement.[29] In a 1973 review of 54 cases of equine lymphosarcoma, the lung was involved in 17% of the horses, while the thoracic lymph nodes were involved in 35%.[30] Mair reported on 11 horses with lymphosarcoma involving the thorax.[22] A large intrathoracic tumor that compressed the trachea, causing dyspnea, has been reported in a one-month-old foal; hepatic lymphosarcoma was also found at postmortem.[31] In the University of Pennsylvania survey, thoracic lymphosarcoma was the single most common neoplasm of the thorax and was present in 19 (54%) of the 35 cases of neoplasia. In 14 of those cases a large cranial mediastinal mass was present and appeared to represent coalescence of several grossly enlarged lymph nodes rather than thymus involvement. Horses ranged in age from 3 to 23 years and included many different breeds and both sexes. The most consistent clinical features among horses with thoracic lymphosarcoma were inappetence, weight loss, ventral edema, dyspnea, pleural effusion, and distension of the jugular veins. Massive pleural effusion associated with variable degrees of collapse of the ventral portions of the lungs was also present in 8 of the 11 horses reported in Mair's study.[22] When pleural fluid was examined in horses with thoracic lymphosarcoma, in 8 of 10 reported cases cytology revealed lymphoblasts with mitotic figures.[22,32–34] In the University of Pennsylvania survey pleural fluid cytology was diagnostic in 6 (75%) of the 8 horses that had pleural fluid examined. Diagnosis also has been made by biopsy of a peripheral lymph node.

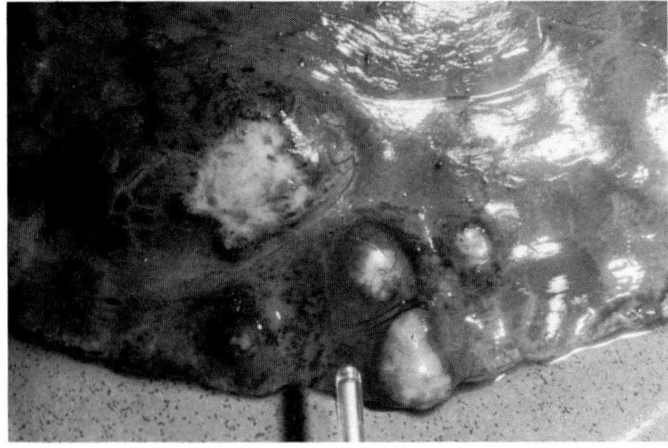

**FIG. 13–2.** Squamous cell carcinoma metastasized to the lung.

Squamous cell carcinomas commonly metastasize to the thoracic cavity either hematogenously or by direct extension from the stomach.[35–38] The stomach is the most common primary tumor site from which metastasis occurs to the pleural cavity. It is suggested that carcinomas reach the pleural space by invasion of the diaphragmatic lymphatics from the peritoneum or by direct extension through the diaphragm. Occasionally the tumor might extend along the thoracic and lower cervical esophagus. Cytology of pleural fluid has provided an antemortem diagnosis of carcinoma in several horses.[35,36]

Metastatic squamous cell carcinoma (SCC) of the thorax was found in 5 (14%) of the 35 cases in the Pennsylvania survey. In two horses, a 7-year-old Standardbred mare and a 14-year-old Crossbred gelding, gastric SCC had spread to the visceral pleural surfaces (Fig. 13–2). In both horses, antemortem cytologic examination of pleural fluid revealed neoplastic cells. The pleural fluid had a mildly elevated white cell count (less than 20,000

WBC/mm$^3$) and an increased protein content (4.1 to 5.7 g/dl). An 8-year-old Quarter Horse gelding had SCC of the oral cavity, an aged pony mare had SCC of the vulva, and a 7-year-old Appaloosa gelding had SCC of the prepuce. None of these horses had an increased volume of pleural fluid nor clinical signs referrable to the thoracic cavity; all had pulmonary metastases discovered at necropsy.

Hemangiosarcoma with pulmonary involvement has been reported previously in five horses.[39–44] The first definitive case of this tumor in a horse was described as a pleural hemangioendothelioma.[39] Hemothorax, anemia, and dyspnea were commonly associated with pulmonary hemangiosarcoma. Signs of disease in most cases were present for less than 3 weeks and death was attributed to hemorrhage. A tentative antemortem diagnosis of hemangiosarcoma was made in only one case using transcutaneous direct thoracoscopy which enabled observation of hemorrhages distributed over the visceral and parietal pleural surfaces.[42]

Three horses (9%) in the Pennsylvania survey had hemangiosarcoma. One horse having no signs of respiratory disease was euthanatized following diagnosis of hemangiosarcoma from surgical biopsies of masses in the shoulder and hind quarter muscles. The horse had no pleural effusion. Pulmonary metastasis was found on postmortem examination but there was no pleural involvement and no other organs were affected. The other two horses were admitted to the hospital with epistaxis of pulmonary origin. Clinical evaluation including two transtracheal washes, ultrasonographic examination, and radiographs of the thorax did not determine the cause of the pulmonary hemorrhage in the 6-year-old Standardbred gelding.[44] The 7-year-old Thoroughbred brood mare had severe hemothorax (54 L) and persistent bleeding into the pleural cavity. Cytologic examination of a transtracheal wash, bronchoalveolar lavage, and pleural fluid showed no evidence of neoplasia. Pleuroscopy revealed greater than 100 small 0.10 to 1.0 cm diameter dark-red nodules on the parietal and visceral pleural surfaces and within the lung parenchyma. A uterine biopsy instrument passed through a stab incision in the intercostal space was used to obtain a specimen of several of these masses which confirmed the diagnosis of hemangiosarcoma. In neither of these two latter cases was the primary site determined, but tumors were present in many organs including lung, muscle, heart, small intestine, small colon, spleen, liver, kidney, pericardium, peritoneum, uterus, lymph nodes, diaphragm, and brain.

In the Pennsylvania survey, a single case of undifferentiated sarcoma involving the lung was found in a 3-month-old Thoroughbred female. The tumor, discovered in the lumbar body wall during surgical correction of an intussusception, also involved multiple skeletal muscles, myocardium, and the iliac lymph nodes. The primary site could not be determined. The two lung metastases were small (0.5 to 2.0 cm).

With the exception of lymphosarcoma, most thoracic neoplasms in the horse are metastatic and frequently clinically inapparent. Cytologic examination of a tracheobronchial aspirate or pleural fluid, or histologic examination of a thoracic mass biopsy may provide an antemortem diagnosis.

## References

1. Cotchin E, Baker-Smith J. Tumours in horses encountered in an abattoir survey. Vet Rec, *97*:339, 1975.
2. Baker JR, Leyland A. Histological survey of tumours of the horse with particular reference to those of the skin. Vet Rec, *96*:419, 1975.
3. Sundberg JP, Burstein T, Page EH, et al. Neoplasms of Equidae. J Am Vet Med Assoc, *170*:150, 1977.
4. Gerber H. Chronic pulmonary disease in the horse. Equine Vet J, *5*:26, 1973.
5. Priester WA, McKay FW. The Occurrence of Tumors in Domestic Animals (Monograph 54). Washington, DC. National Cancer Institute, *56*:67, 1980.
6. Gianelli F. Mioblastoma a cellule granulose nei bronchi di un equino. Acta Biomed Ateneo Parmense, Sezione I, *28*:5, 1957.
7. Alexander JE, Keown GH, Palotay JL. Granular cell myoblastoma with hypertrophic pulmonary osteoarthropathy in a mare. J Am Vet Med Assoc, *146*:703, 1965.
8. Misdorp W, Nauta-vanGelder HL. "Granular-cell myoblastoma" in the horse. A report of 4 cases. Pathologica Veterinaria, *5*:385, 1968.
9. Parodi AL, Tassin P, Rigoulet J. Myoblastome à cel-

lules granuleuses. Recueil de Médecine Vétérinaire, *15*:489, 1974.

10. Parker GA, Novilla MN, Brown AC, et al. Granular cell tumour (myoblastoma) in the lung of a horse. J Comp Pathol, *89*:421, 1979.
11. Nickels FA, Breeze RG. Equine granular cell tumor. Mod Vet Pract, *61*:593, 1980.
12. Turk MAM, Breeze RG. Histochemical and ultrastructural features of an equine pulmonary granular cell tumor (myoblastoma). J Comp Path, *91*:471, 1981.
13. Murphy JR, Breeze RG, McPherson EA. Myxoma of the equine respiratory tract. Mod Vet Pract, *598*:529, 1978.
14. Dill SG, Moise NS, Meschter CL. Cardiac failure in a stallion secondary to metastasis of an anaplastic pulmonary carcinoma. Equine Vet J, *18*:414, 1986.
15. Uphoff CS, Lyncoln JA. A primary pulmonary tumor in a horse. Equine Pract, *9*:19, 1987.
16. Jubb VF, Kennedy PC, Palmer N. Pathology of Domestic Animals. Vol 2, 3rd Ed. London, Academic Press, Inc, 536, 1985.
17. Clem MF, O'Brien TD, Feeney DA, et al. Pulmonary chondrosarcoma in a horse. Comp Cont Ed, *8*:964, 1986.
18. Sullivan DJ. Cartilagenous tumors (chondroma and chondrosarcoma) in animals. Am J Vet Res, *21*:531, 1960.
19. Kolbl VS. Pleuramesothelion also Todesurache bei einem Pferd. Wien tierarztl Mschr 66 Jahrgang Heft, *1*:22, 1979.
20. Kramer JW, Nickels FA, Bell T. Cytology of diffuse mesothelioma in the thorax of a horse. Equine Vet J, *8*:81, 1986.
21. Whiteley LO, Leininger JR, Wolf CB, et al. Malignant squamous cell thymoma in a horse. Vet Pathol, *23*:627, 1986.
22. Mair TS, Lane JG, Lucke VM. Clinicopathological features of lymphosarcoma involving the thoracic cavity in the horse. Equine Vet J, *17*:428, 1985.
23. Gunson D, Gillette D, Beech J, et al. Endometrial adenocarcinoma in a mare. Vet Pathol, *17*:777, 1980.
24. Morris DM, Acland HM, Hodge TG. Pleural effusion secondary to metastasis of an ovarian adenocarcinoma in a horse. J Am Vet Med Assoc, *187*:272, 1985.
25. Blanchard L, Poisson J, Drieux H. Pathologie comparé des tumeurs du thymus. Con interêt pour l'histogénèse. Rec Med Vet, *115*:129, 1939.
26. Moulton JE, Dungsworth DL. Tumors of the lymphoid and hemopoietic tissues. In: Tumors of Domestic Animals. Moulton (ed). 2nd Ed, Berkeley, University of California Press, 1978, p 177.
27. Parker GA, Casey HW. Thymomas in domestic animals. Vet Pathol, *15*:353, 1976.
28. Rebhun WC, Bertone A. Equine lymphosarcoma. J Am Vet Med Assoc, *184*:720, 1984.
29. Theilen GH, Fowler ME. Lymphosarcoma (lymphocytic leukemia) in the horse. J Am Vet Med Assoc, *140*:923, 1962.
30. Neufeld JL. Lymphosarcoma in the horse: A review. Can Vet J, *14*:129, 1963.
31. Seahorn TL, Carter GK, Morris EL, et al. Lymphosarcoma in a foal: A case report. Equine Vet Sci, *8*:317, 1988.
32. Smith BP. Pleuritis and pleural effusion in the horse. A study of 37 cases. J Am Vet Med Assoc, *170*:208, 1977.
33. Thatcher CD, Roussel AJ, Chickering WR, et al. Pleural effusion with thoracic lymphosarcoma in a mare. Comp Cont Ed, *7*:S726, 1985.
34. Genetzky RM, Doctor DM, Hagemoser WA, et al. Mediastinal lymphosarcoma in a gelding. Mod Vet Pract, *63*:972, 1982.
35. Meagher DM, Wheat JD, Tennant B, et al. Squamous cell carcinoma of the equine stomach. J Am Vet Med Assoc, *164*:81, 1974.
36. Meuten DJ, Price SM, Seiler RM, et al. Gastric carcinoma with pseudohyperparathyroidism in a horse. Cornell Vet, *68*:179, 1978.
37. Vaala WE. Pleuritis and pleural effusion in a mare secondary to disseminated squamous cell carcinoma. Comp Cont Ed, *9*:674, 1987.
38. Ford TS, Vaala WE, Sweeney CR, et al. Pleuroscopic diagnosis of gastroesophageal squamous cell carcinoma in a horse. J Am Vet Med Assoc, *190*:1556, 1987.
39. Jackson C. The incidence of pathology of tumours of domestic animals in South Africa: A study of the Onderstepoort collection of neoplasms with special reference to their histopathology. Onderstepoort J Vet Sci Anim Indust, *6*:1, 1936.
40. Gruys E, Kor HAR, Van Der Werff VD. Benauwdheid door intrathoracale verbloeding met haemangiosarcomen bij een paard. Tijdschr Diergeneesk, *6*:310, 1976.
41. Reinacher VM. Hamangioendotheliome in der Skelettmuskulatur eines Pferdes. Berl Munch Tierarztl Wochenschr, *91*:121, 1978.
42. Frye FL, Knight HD, Brown SI. Hemangiosarcoma in a horse. J Am Vet Med Assoc, *182*:287, 1983.
43. Valentine BA, Ross CE, Bump JL, et al. Intramuscular hemangiosarcoma with pulmonary metastasis in a horse. J Am Vet Med Assoc, *188*:628, 1986.
44. Johnston J, Beech J, Saik JE. Disseminated hemangiosarcoma in a horse. J Am Vet Med Assoc, *193*:1429, 1988.
45. Rossier Y, Sweeney CR, Heyer G, et al. Pleuroscopic diagnosis of disseminated hemangiosarcoma in a horse. J Am Vet Med Assoc, *196*:1639, 1990.

## CHAPTER 14

# MISCELLANEOUS LUNG AND PLEURAL INJURIES

*JILL BEECH*

## Pulmonary Edema

Pulmonary edema may be a life threatening complication of other primary diseases. Factors affecting accumulation of fluid within the lung include hydrostatic and colloid osmotic interstitial and vascular forces, the surface area and porosity of the fluid exchanging membranes of the vessels and alveoli, and the muscle contractility and functional integrity of the lymphatics.[1] Pulmonary microvasculature pressure can be increased by any increase in left atrial or pulmonary artery pressure. Pulmonary edema may occur in acute renal failure. Rapid intravenous (IV) fluid administration can also increase the microvascular hydrostatic pressure, enhancing the likelihood of edema. Increases in microvascular permeability may occur with sepsis and disseminated intravascular coagulation (DIC), hypoxic acidosis, and other conditions such as allergic reactions, aspiration pneumonia, near drowning and inhalation of smoke or other noxious fumes when vasoactive substances are released and allow leakage of protein and fluid.

Clinical signs reflect the primary disease plus decreased lung compliance and decreased gas exchange. Both respiratory and metabolic acidosis may ensue.

Diagnosis is based on clinical examination, the presence of a history of predisposing causes, and radiographs. Horses develop a shallow rapid respiratory pattern and may be dyspneic. Fine crackles and even rales may be audible on auscultation. Fluid (clear or slightly yellow or pink tinged) may drip from the nostrils and can increase in volume without necessarily becoming frothy. Progression to this stage warrants a grave prognosis. Radiographic findings are nonspecific but include peribronchial and perivascular cuffing, increased prominence to vessels, and a hazy reticular or lattice-like pattern. Underlying pulmonary disease may obscure signs of edema, and radiographs of sufficiently high quality to show relatively subtle changes may not be obtainable in mature horses.

Treatment consists of correcting the cause, reversing hypoxemia, decreasing plasma volume and left atrial pressure, increasing plasma colloid osmotic pressure, and decreasing patient anxiety. Intranasal oxygen and even ventilation may be needed in severe cases. Diuretics such as furosemide should be used. If the horse is receiving IV fluids, administration should be stopped or the flow greatly decreased. In other species morphine in small doses (0.05 to .1 mg/kg IV every 2 to 3 minutes) has been used to relieve dyspnea and anxiety[2] and divert blood volume from the pulmonary to the systemic circulation, thereby decreasing pulmonary capillary pressure. Its excitatory effects in the horse would probably preclude its use by itself. As one of its beneficial effects is depression of respiratory centers, thereby changing rapid violent respiratory movement to a slow deep rhythm, other drugs such as sedatives which act similarly might be beneficial in some cases.

Furosemide may be given IV or IM at a dose of 1 to 2 mg/kg (.5 to 1 mg/lb) and repeated in 1 hour. If this appears to be helpful, one could then titrate the dosage for each patient. In a normal horse given a dose of 1 mg/kg, approximately 8 L of urine is produced in about 1 hour.[3] A dose of 4 mg/kg elicits maximum response. Although horses respond to a second dose, subsequent doses elicit less response. There have been few studies on furosemide's effects on pulmonary hemodynamics in the horse[4,5] and the effects in horses with pulmonary edema have not been reported. Administration of colloid solutions should be cautious or in conjunction with use of diuretics as they can initially increase vascular pressures. Plasma may be safer than other colloid preparations such as dextrans. Also, if there is an increase in vascular permeability, they will have little beneficial effect in raising intravascular osmotic pressure. Aminophylline may be beneficial.

Drugs with antiprostaglandin activity (flunixin meglumine,* phenylbutazone, aspirin) and antihistamines may help. The use of corticosteroids is controversial and if they are used, antibiotic coverage is probably advisable, especially as edema has been shown to impair pulmonary bacterial defense mechanisms.[6]

## Smoke Inhalation

The effects of smoke inhalation are due to both the direct effect of heat and the damage caused by substances within the smoke. Much of the heat is probably dissipated in the upper respiratory tract thereby exerting most of its effects in the nasal passages, pharynx, larynx, and upper trachea. Many noxious gases such as sulfur and nitrogen oxides, hydrocyanic acid, carbon monoxide, and toxic vapors from plastics can be generated in fires and subsequently inhaled. Irritant gases can combine with water to form corrosive acids. Aldehydes can denature protein and cause pulmonary edema. In addition to their direct effect, toxic gases can also be absorbed on soot particles and carried down to the lungs. Particulate material can induce bronchoconstriction.

Carbon monoxide may be present in sufficiently high concentration to cause poisoning within a short time after exposure. Carbon monoxide shifts the oxyhemoglobin curve to the left, thereby decreasing oxygen release until tissue oxygen levels become low. It also combines with hemoglobin to form carboxyhemoglobin, resulting in hypoxia. The clinical recognition of carbon monoxide poisoning and severely impaired tissue oxygenation is difficult because the patient's blood is bright red and because despite low oxygen content the oxygen tension or $PaO_2$ is not decreased.

Apart from the individual effects of toxic products within the smoke, smoke inhalation can cause bronchiolitis, bronchopneumonia, and interstitial and alveolar edema.[7] The airways may become obstructed with inflammatory cells, necrotic epithelial cells and carbonaceous material, and blood. The upper airway also becomes edematous and inflamed. Areas of atelectasis or air trapping may occur secondary to airway obstruction. Macrophage function is adversely affected and this could predispose the patient to infections.

Clinical signs depend on the amount and type of smoke inhalation and whether specific poisonous gases have been inhaled. The patient may show signs of severe hypoxemia and may be depressed, disoriented or irritable, ataxic or even moribund and comatose. Auscultation may reveal decreased air movement, crackles, rales, or wheezes; but these may not become apparent for 12 to 24 hours. If edema of the airways is sufficiently severe, air flow may be severely obstructed. Edema fluid may be visible at the nostrils and later may be replaced by inflammatory exudate. Fever may occur immediately or after 1 to 2 days. Clinical laboratory evaluation usually reflects the degree of inflammation and blood gases may be helpful in assessing ventilatory function.

Treatment should focus on providing a patent airway, reversing any toxic effects, providing ventilatory support and decreasing any edema. Use of antibiotics is controversial

*Banamine, Schering Corp., Kenilworth, NJ

but should be instituted if there is definite evidence of infection or the patient deteriorates despite supportive therapy. If antibiotics are used, they should provide broad aerobic and anaerobic coverage.

Humidified oxygen may be needed in severe cases. Bronchodilators might be useful in counteracting reflex bronchoconstriction. If there is upper airway obstruction, a tracheostomy and insertion of a tube may be necessary. Furosemide may help decrease any pulmonary edema. Corticosteroids are probably not indicated but use of nonsteroidal anti-inflammatory drugs may be beneficial in decreasing mediator release, thereby limiting or suppressing both inflammation and bronchoconstriction.[1] If the horse has also been burned and requires IV fluids, the lungs should be carefully monitored to ascertain whether pulmonary edema is developing.

## Drowning/Near Drowning

Drowning or near drowning is rare in horses although one might be concerned about a potential increase due to the popularity of swimming horses. Several equine cases of near drowning have been reported.[8,9] Therapy for near drowning is aimed at correcting hypoxemia and abnormal acid base balance, treating associated infection, and in some cases pulmonary edema or circulatory disturbances.

The severity of hypoxemia depends on the duration of submersion and whether aspiration occurs. When the latter occurs, treatment is more complicated because of potential persistent hypoxemia, metabolic acidosis, and infection. If fresh water is aspirated, pulmonary surfactant is altered leading to atelectasis and hypoxemia. If salt water is aspirated, the hypertonic fluid draws in more fluid from the circulation leading to fluid filled alveoli and hypoxemia. Theoretically, aspiration of large volumes of hypertonic fluids could decrease blood volume, and hypotonic fluids such as fresh water would increase it; however, it is unlikely a horse would survive aspirating the volume required to have this effect.

Temperature of water has an important effect on the outcome as hypothermia protects patients due to its prolonging tolerance for hypoxia. Extremely cold temperatures may be deleterious because they can induce cardiac arrhythmias. It is unknown whether horses have a diving reflex like human beings. This reflex of bradycardia, peripheral vasoconstriction, and selective perfusion of the heart and brain occurs when a person's face is immersed in water less than 20°C.[10]

Metabolic acidosis is common but not consistent in near drowned human patients. However, blood gases probably are quite variable depending on the interim between the event and examination; this time period is likely to be longer in horses when floods and storms are the precipitating causes. One reported horse actually had a compensated respiratory alkalosis.[8]

Electrolytes are usually not significantly affected regardless of whether salt or fresh water is aspirated. Nor is hemolysis a significant problem, although aspiration of large volumes of fresh water potentially could cause hemolysis due to low $PaO_2$ and hypotonicity.

Aspiration pneumonia may be a sequel and can be detected by auscultation, an elevated temperature, thoracic radiographs, and cytologic and culture evaluation of a tracheobronchial aspirate. As the pulmonary changes are likely to reflect alveolar densities and interstitial fluid, radiographs are more likely to be helpful than ultrasonographic examination.

Immediate treatment should stabilize the patient.[11] Oxygen should be provided, if possible. Near drowned human patients may look relatively well clinically, yet still be significantly hypoxemic and require oxygen. Arterial blood gas analysis is the only accurate means of assessing blood gas status. Both positive end expiratory pressure (PEEP) and continuous positive airway pressure (CPAP) have been beneficial in human patients in treating hypoxemia and pulmonary edema; however, neither may be available or tolerated in equine patients.

Bronchospasm may occur and should be treated. Aminophylline is frequently used in man and has also been used in horses. In one equine case report a loading dose of 11 mg/

kg aminophylline was given by slow intravenous drip followed by oral dosing of 5 mg/kg orally every 12 hours.[8] One should remember that concurrent use of some drugs can affect levels of unbound aminophylline and potentiate toxicity. For example, erythromycin potentiates toxicity because of increasing free drug levels in the blood.

Intravenous fluids and/or bicarbonate may be needed but administration must be cautious if there is potential or actual pulmonary edema. Use of diuretics is controversial, but drugs such as furosemide may decrease pulmonary edema albeit only transiently.

If there is evidence of infection, broad spectrum antimicrobial therapy to combat aerobes and anaerobes is advisable.

Antifungal drugs are usually not given but depending on the precipitating event one should be concerned about possible fungal pneumonia and aspiration of plant or other foreign material.

Steroids are thought not to be helpful and definitely are contraindicated if there is infection. Flunixin meglumine may be helpful in decreasing inflammation and for its antiendotoxin effect.

Pulmonary surfactant administration has also been suggested as being helpful but it is not usually advocated for use in human near drowning victims.

Prognosis depends on length of immersion, water temperature, amount and type of fluid aspirated, whether foreign material and/or infectious organisms are aspirated, general health and immune function of the horse, and how soon treatment is instituted. However, clinical signs, temperature response, and progressive radiographs can be helpful. Clinical signs may not parallel radiographic signs. If the horse survives the acute stage, then one has to consider possible residual damage. In man, there is concern over residual neurologic deficits; however, these appear to be rare except in comatose patients.[10] Impaired exercise tolerance is always possible if significant lung damage occurs, but this must be assessed on an individual basis.

## Pneumoconiosis

There are few reports of pneumoconiosis in horses. A mild form has been described in ponies working in coal mines. Pathologic studies showed minimal fibrosis and many compact aggregates of coal dust.[12] The best documented cases have been horses from the Monterey-Carmel peninsula of California with silicate pneumoconiosis.[13]

In man, onset of clinical signs of silicosis is usually decades following exposure. Severity of clinical signs depends on genetic factors, the presence of coexisting diseases, the amount and type of silica, and the duration of exposure.[13,14] It is the small 0.5 to 5 $\mu$m particles that are deposited in small airways and alveoli and subsequently phagocytosed that cause the disease. In decreasing order of frequency, fibrosis and cytotoxicity are most likely to occur from the tridymite, cristobalite, quartz, and ceosite forms of silica. In the reported horses cristobalite was the major silica species identified.[13] Usually this form of silica associated with volcanic igneous rocks is a minor component of soils; its high concentration in the Monterey area was unusual. Whether other geographic areas contain a similarly high content has not been reported.

From 1978 to 1980 9 horses were diagnosed as having silicate pneumoconiosis.[13] All horses originated from the Monterey peninsula or Carmel valley. Although in the published report all horses were symptomatic, asymptomatic cases from the same area have been diagnosed on the basis of histopathology.*

All of the affected horses have been afebrile and in good condition with no abnormal nasal discharge or cough. The owners' complaints have been exercise intolerance and sometimes exercise induced respiratory distress (sweating, nostril flaring, abducted elbows, reluctance to move, and shaking). Resting respiratory rates were elevated.

Physical examination revealed a restrictive pattern of breathing. Auscultation revealed harsh breath sounds and some wheezing which was exacerbated by exercise. In only one horse was there evidence of exudate. Hematology was noncontributory to the diagnosis. Transtracheal aspirates were obtained in 6 horses and contained primarily alveolar

*Knight HD, Schwartz LW, Malloy RL. Silicate Pneumoconiosis and Pulmonary Fibrosis in Horses from the Monterey-Carmel Peninsula, Davis, CA. Class notes.

macrophages, some of which had cytoplasmic inclusions. Small numbers of bacteria and/or fungi were isolated. Radiographs of the thoraxes of eight horses revealed miliary interstitial nodular densities which were severe in 6.

Seven of the horses died or were euthanatized and gross pathologic studies revealed interstitial granulomatous pneumonia, and fibrosis and sometimes necrosis. Bronchial lymph nodes also had granulomatous inflammation. Macrophages contained crystalline particles; these were much more obvious on transmission electron microscopic studies than in light microscopic evaluation. X-ray diffraction analysis identified this material as the cristobalite form of silica.

One of the 11 horses was treated with steroids, nonsteroidal anti-inflammatory drugs, bronchodilators, and antimicrobials and showed no apparent response. However, it and three other untreated horses did not progress over the observed time period.

## Hemothorax

Hemothorax may result from hemorrhage from the lungs when there is damaged visceral pleura or from damage to parietal pleural vessels. Trauma, especially if there is a coexisting coagulopathy, rib fractures which lacerate intercostal vessels or lung parenchyma, severe abscess or neoplasia which erodes through vessels of the lung or the visceral pleura, and hemangiosarcoma involving the pleural surfaces, can all cause hemothorax. Rupture of lung parenchymal bullae may be accompanied by hemorrhage as well as pneumothorax. Rupture of any of the great vessels could result in fatal hemothorax.

Diagnosis is based on clinical examination and thoracentesis. A history of trauma or bleeding disorder may increase one's suspicion of a hemothorax. With a bleeding disorder there are usually other sites of hemorrhage. The thorax should be carefully palpated, especially in foals, for any rib fractures or displacement or change in thoracic excursion. Pain and shallow respiration may be exhibited if there is a rib fracture or concurrent pleuritis. Dyspnea is variable depending on the volume of blood in the pleural cavity and the underlying disease condition.

Auscultation reveals a decrease in lung sounds ventrally below the level of blood accumulation. Heart sounds are often muffled or may radiate abnormally widely. Percussion reveals a change from the normal resonance of aerated lung to dullness over the hemothorax. If there is accompanying pneumothorax, dorsal lung sounds may be difficult to hear and percussion sounds are abnormally resonant dorsally. The condition may be unilateral or bilateral depending on the etiology and whether the mediastinum is intact. Thoracocentesis allows evaluation of the type of fluid within the thorax. Fluid should be collected for cell count, packed cell volume (PCV), total protein (TP), and for cytologic evaluation. It should be cultured if there is a possible infectious etiology. When infection is suspected or there is concurrent nasal discharge, a transtracheal aspirate should also be obtained for culture and sensitivity and cytology. Cytologic evaluation should always be performed to determine whether there is evidence of neoplasia or infection, however, absence of neoplastic cells in either pleural fluid or a tracheobronchial aspirate does not eliminate neoplasia as a cause. Radiographs and ultrasonography can be helpful in determining the underlying cause for the hemothorax. A clotting profile and platelet count should be determined if there is evidence of bleeding elsewhere or a coagulopathy is suspected.

### *Treatment*

Treatment consists of treating the underlying cause and removing the blood (and air if there is pneumothorax). If the blood is not removed, it organizes and may result in fibrothorax. Fractured ribs should be stabilized to prevent further trauma. Infections require appropriate antibiotics. Prophylactic broad spectrum antibiotics are advisable even if there is no initial evidence of sepsis, as blood is an excellent culture medium. Repeated thoracocentesis and drainage may be needed if the blood reaccumulates.

The horse's packed cell volume (PCV) and total protein (TP) should be monitored. Intravenous fluid replacement and even whole blood may be required if blood loss is severe.

Prognosis depends on the underlying cause. Cases with uncomplicated trauma should respond well. Certain infections may be extremely difficult to treat and require long-term antibiotics. If trauma is due to a penetrating wound, the prognosis is poor because of the pleuritis that frequently ensues. Neoplasia has an extremely poor prognosis. If clotting disorders are due to hepatic disease, prognosis is likewise poor, but those which are secondary to certain drugs or chemicals may respond well to appropriate therapy and discontinuing administration of the offending agent.

## Pneumothorax

Pneumothorax is rare in horses. Puncture or laceration of the trachea, external penetrating trauma of the thorax, rib fracture and subsequent puncture of the lung, and ruptured esophagus or trachea can be causes. Horses with pleuropneumonia that develop bronchopleural fistulas can develop pneumothorax, although fibrinous adhesions usually localize the leak and pneumothorax does not become generalized. Cellulitis due to gas forming organisms could also extend to involve the thoracic cavity. Pneumothorax caused by a tracheotomy or other tracheal puncture, such as a tracheobronchial aspirate, is usually asymptomatic and only detected incidentally if thoracic radiographs are taken following the procedure. Closed pneumothorax occurs when air is trapped within the pleural space. Open pneumothorax results when there is a wound which allows egress and ingress of air. Tension pneumothorax occurs when a flap of tissue permits more air to enter than escape from the pleural cavity and intrapleural pressure exceeds that of atmospheric air.

Clinical signs may include evidence of an external wound or other trauma, tachypnea, dyspnea, and sometimes cyanosis. Auscultation reveals absence of normal lung sounds in the dorsal thorax when the lung is partially collapsed. The area of abnormality will depend on the extent of pneumothorax and volume of collapsed lung. Percussion reveals hyperresonance over the area of pneumothorax. Co-existent subcutaneous emphysema can complicate interpretation. If a horse with subcutaneous emphysema seems unduly dyspneic or distressed, one should suspect a possible coexistent pneumothorax as the former does not usually cause dyspnea, unless it involves the face and neck, thereby compressing the airway. Radiographs are diagnostic as is aspiration of air from the thoracic cavity. The latter should be done aseptically and carefully so as not to lacerate underlying lung. When pneumothorax is extensive, lung trauma is less likely as the lung surface no longer is adjacent to the thoracic wall.

Treatment consists of relieving the pneumothorax and treating the cause. An open sucking wound should be occluded promptly with a bulky sterile dressing and a chest tube inserted for decompression. The wound can later be debrided and appropriately sutured and the horse placed on broad spectrum antibiotics. A careful search should be made for any residual foreign material which could migrate into the pleural cavity and cause pleuritis. Ultrasonography may be helpful in evaluating the extent of the injury and revealing the presence of foreign material. However, subcutaneous emphysema or air in the deeper tissues or fascial planes may prevent accurate sonographic imaging. If the cause of the pneumothorax requires correction under general anesthesia, the horse must first be stabilized and rendered fit for anesthesia; chest tubes should be inserted for decompression to correct the atelectasis and improve ventilation. Any fractured rib should be stabilized so as to prevent further damage. Tracheal defects should be sutured when possible. If the pneumothorax recurs or continues, one or more tubes should be left in place to allow constant removal of air. The flutter valve system using an indwelling thoracic catheter and a Heimlich chest drainage valve* is safe and effective, allows continuous drainage, and

---

*Heimlich chest drainage valve, Bard-Parker, Div. of Becton, Dickinson Co., Rutherford, NJ

should function for long periods provided it is correctly placed and there is no accumulation of pleural fluid to clog the valve. Regardless of method of drainage, it is advisable to provide broad spectrum antibiotic prophylaxis. In long-standing cases, re-expansion of the lungs should be gradual as rapid re-expansion could result in pulmonary edema.

Prognosis is good provided the leak seals or can be sealed, the air is removed, and complicating infections are treated successfully. Major pulmonary parenchymal lesions resulting in air leakage or esophageal leaks usually cause severe septic pleuritis and have a poor prognosis.

## Chemical-Induced Lung Injury

### *Perilla Frutescens Ketone Poisoning*

Perilla frutescens, purple mint, is common in much of the eastern United States. It contains preformed pneumotoxins. There is one report of natural poisoning in a horse and poisoning has been induced experimentally.[15,16] Affected animals develop a restrictive breathing pattern due to pulmonary edema, proliferation of alveolar epithelial cells, and hyaline membrane formation. Dyspnea may be severe and in the experimentally induced disease, ponies died at 6 to 7 days.[16]

### *Pyrrolizidine Alkaloids*

Pyrrolizidine alkaloids are most widely recognized as hepatotoxins. However, they can also cause alveolar and interstitial edema, proliferation of bronchiolar and alveolar epithelial cells and megalocytosis, interstitial fibrosis and cellular infiltration, congestion, and intra-alveolar hemorrhage.[17] The pneumotoxic effect is due to pyrrolic derivatives of the pyrrolizidine alkaloids. These are formed in the liver by metabolism by the mixed function oxidase (MFO) system, where they cause cell necrosis and megalocytosis and are carried hematogenously to the lungs. Pulmonary vascular endothelial cells are the first to be damaged. In the lung, further MFO metabolism may cause bronchiolar and alveolar epithelial changes. Lung lesions only develop in association wth liver lesions.

Pyrrolizidine alkaloids come from a variety of plants. Crotalaria dura, C. globifera and C. juncea have caused lung disease in horses in Africa. The stems and leaves are eaten in hay or grazed when other feed is scarce.[16]

Signs are fever and dyspnea as well as signs related to hepatotoxicity, and affected animals die. To my knowledge it has not been described in the United States.

### *Three Methyl Indole (3MI) Toxicity*

Experimentally, three methyl indole (3MI) can cause obstructive pulmonary disease.[18,19] This metabolite of the amino acid L tryptophan is found in tobacco smoke and also in the equine gut following oral tryptophan administration.[19] Within several hours of dosing 3MI causes necrosis of small airway epithelium, sparing that of large airways. Ciliated cells are not affected. Inflammatory cells infiltrate the injured bronchioles and the lumina become filled with desquamated epithelial cells. Basement membrane is denuded. Poorly differentiated bronchiolar cells proliferate and may become 2 to 6 cells thick. Granulation tissue and neutrophils and eosinophils thicken the lamina propria. These airway reactions plus the intraluminal necrotic cells and inflammatory cells result in bronchiolar obstruction and acinar overinflation. Alveolar edema has also been described.[19,20] The bronchiolitis obliterans, although lessened, is still extensive at 30 days in animals surviving the acute stages.

Clinical signs include dyspnea, which may become severe, increased expiratory effort, and sometimes cyanosis. Hypoxemia and decreased nitrogen washout times have been measured.[18] Other studies have shown a normal $PaO_2$ but a decreased $PaCO_2$ with decreased dynamic compliance and specific conductance, increased functional residual capacity, and increased minimal lung volume.[20] Clinical signs are most severe from 7 to 10 days post dosing. As it is an experimental disease and no naturally occurring cases are reported, no treatment regimens can be advocated.

## References


1. Mellins RB, Stalcup SA. Pulmonary edema. In: Disorders of the Respiratory Tract in Children. EL Kendig, V Chernick (eds). 4th ed. Philadelphia, WB Saunders Co, 1983, p 458.
2. Davis LE. Management of acute pulmonary edema. J Am Vet Med Assoc, *175*:97, 1979.
3. Tobin T, Roberts BL, Swerczek TW, et al. The pharmacology of furosemide in the horse III: Dose and time response relationships, effects of repeated dosing, and performance effects. J Equine Med Surg, *2*:216, 1978.
4. Muir WW, Milne DW, Sharda RT. Acute haemodynamic effects of furosemide administered intravenously in the horse. Am J Vet Res, *37*:1177, 1976.
5. Dixon PM. Effects of furosemide on pulmonary arterial pressures of normal horses and horses affected with chronic obstructive pulmonary disease (COPD). Equine Vet J, *12*:28, 1980.
6. LaForce FM, Mallane JF, Boehme RF, et al. The effect of pulmonary edema on antibacterial defenses of the lung. J Lab Clin Med, *82*:634, 1973.
7. Mellins RB. Lung injury from hydrocarbon aspiration and smoke inhalation. In: Disorders of the Respiratory Tract in Children. EL Kendig, V Chernick (eds). 4th Ed. Philadelphia, WB Saunders Co, 1983, p 389.
8. Austin SM, Foreman JH, Goetz TE. Aspiration pneumonia following near drowning in a mare: A case report. Equine Vet Sci, *8*:313, 1988.
9. Humber KA. Near drowning of a gelding. J Am Vet Med Assoc, *192*:377, 1988.
10. Gordon BA. Drowning and the diving reflex in man. Med J Aust, *16*:583, 1972.
11. Modell JH. Drowning and near drowning. In: Disorders of the Respiratory Tract in Children. EL Kendig and V Chernick (eds). Philadelphia, WB Saunders Co, 1983, p 396.
12. Heppleston AG. Changes in the lungs of rabbits and ponies inhaling coal dust underground. J Pathol Bacteriol, *67*:349, 1954.
13. Schwartz LW, Knight HD, Malloy RL, et al. Silicate pneumoconiosis and pulmonary fibrosis in horses from the Monterey-Carmel peninsula. Chest, *80*:82S, 1981.
14. Davis GS. The pathogenesis of silicosis: State of the art. Chest, *89*:166S, 1986.
15. Lindley WH. Ergot toxicosis [horse]. Mod Vet Pract, *59*:64, 1978.
16. Breeze RG, Carlson JR. Chemical induced lung injury. In: Advances in Veterinary Science and Comparative Medicine. Vol 26. CE Cornelius, CF Simpson, DL Dungworth (eds). New York, Academic Press, 1982, p 201.
17. McLean EK. The toxic actions of pyrrolizidine (Senecio) alkaloids. Pharmacol Rev, *22*:429, 1970.
18. Breeze RG, Brown CM, Lee HA, et al. Pathophysiology of 3-methylindole in ponies: a model of obstructive pulmonary disease. Second Western Conference on Food Animal Veterinary Medicine, Ft. Collins, CO, 1981, p 6.
19. Paradis MR. MS Thesis, The effects of oral tryptophan, indoleacetic acid and indole in ponies. Washington State University, Pullman, WA, 1980.
20. Derksen EJ, Robinson NE, Slocombe RF, et al. Three methyl indole induced pulmonary toxicosis in ponies. Am J Vet Res, *43*:603, 1982.

## CHAPTER 15

# CHRONIC OBSTRUCTIVE PULMONARY DISEASE

*FREDERIK J. DERKSEN*

Chronic obstructive pulmonary disease (COPD) is one of the most commonly diagnosed conditions affecting the equine lung; since domestication, the disease has plagued horse owners in the temperate parts of the world. It has long been suspected that the disease is associated with improperly cured hay and straw. Already in 1874 Williams wrote, "I have no hesitation in asserting that broken wind is generally due to improper food, more particularly to bad, musty, or coarse hay, containing a large quantity of woody fiber, from being allowed to become too ripe before being cut . . ."[1] Yet little was understood about its pathogenesis and, consequently, management of the disease has been largely ineffective. In the last several years, our knowledge about the pathogenesis of COPD has improved significantly and consequently a more rational treatment regime can be recommended. This chapter will describe our present understanding of COPD and emphasize newer knowledge of its pathogenesis.

COPD is a complex syndrome with clinical signs ranging from exercise intolerance in the performance horse to expiratory dyspnea, chronic purulent nasal discharge, cough, and weight loss in the chronic respiratory cripple.[2] Between these two extremes, a range of clinical signs is recognized. Many synonyms for chronic obstructive pulmonary disease exist in the literature. These include heaves, chronic emphysema, chronic bronchitis, chronic bronchiolitis, recurrent airway obstruction, broken wind, and hay sickness.[3,4] In a clinical setting, the use of pathologic descriptions such as chronic bronchitis, bronchiolitis, or emphysema is probably not warranted because in individual cases the underlying pathologic condition is unknown. In this chapter I will use the term COPD because it indicates the chronic nature of the disease and because the name suggests the presence of airway obstruction.

In the literature, there is a paucity of information on the epidemiology of COPD. However, anecdotal reports suggest that the condition is rare in climates where animals are housed outside all year around and is common in climates where horses are stabled and fed hay for long periods of time. The disease is uncommon in young horses and its incidence increases with age. There is no apparent breed or sex predisposition for chronic obstructive pulmonary disease.[5]

## History and Clinical Signs

Historical information is most important when evaluating horses with COPD. In many cases the disease is seasonal and associated with housing horses indoors.[6] In other cases, onset of clinical signs occurs 1 to 2 weeks after feeding a new batch of hay or moving the horse to a new barn. In some cases COPD has been associated with the presence of birds in the barn where the affected animals are housed.[7] In many instances the onset of the disease is insidious and the owner is unaware of exactly when clinical signs started. In some horses clinical signs of lung disease became apparent following a viral respiratory tract infection from which the horse never fully recovered. This is particularly common in race horses with COPD because race horses commonly suffer from virus infections and because economic pressures often prevent adequate time for recovery following viral infections in these animals. Clinical signs of COPD may be apparent only during exercise. Affected horses show no clinical signs at rest but do not perform adequately. Other clinical signs include chronic intermittent dry or productive cough, intermittent purulent nasal discharge especially after exercise, and expiratory dyspnea. Clinical signs are usually intermittent but, as the disease progresses, clinical signs may become continuous. The increased expiratory effort eventually results in hypertrophy of abdominal musculature and a "heave line" becomes apparent.

## Pathology

Although COPD is a clinical disease recognized in antiquity, the pathologic disease is not clearly described. In part, this is due to the fact that the severity and the type of lesions are variable in horses with clinical signs of COPD and because at the level of the bronchioles and the gas exchange region of the lung, the lesions are not homogeneously distributed. In some areas of the lung, airways may appear nearly normal, while in an adjacent region lesions may be severe. Thus, careful sampling and quantitative pathology are required to accurately describe COPD.

The main lesion of COPD is bronchiolitis characterized by diffuse epithelial hyperplasia, mucus plugging of airways, and neutrophilic, lymphocytic and plasmacytic infiltrates.[8] In some cases eosinophils are an important constituent of the cellular infiltrate but in others eosinophils are rare.[9] Commonly, the lesion extends into the peribronchiolar tissues and peribronchiolar fibrosis is also present. Goblet cells, which are rare in the bronchioles of normal horses, become more numerous in the bronchioles of horses affected with COPD. In horses that are severely affected, the normally single layer of epithelium is hyperplastic and contains numerous PAS positive goblet cells. In contrast, the Clara cells in the bronchioles are decreased in number.[10] The alveoli subserved by obstructed or partially obstructed bronchioles are overinflated (alveolar emphysema).[11] Emphysema, defined as destruction of alveolar walls thereby creating abnormally large air spaces, has been described by some authors as an important feature of COPD.[12] However, it is now clear that emphysema is rare in horses with COPD.[3] In severe cases, emphysema may be found, especially near the pleural surface, but even in these cases, bronchiolitis and not emphysema is the dominant pathologic feature. In other species, chronic lung disease commonly results in increased pulmonary vasculature resistance causing right ventricular (RV) hypertrophy and right heart failure. An abattoir survey of horses diagnosed as suffering from COPD on clinical grounds showed no gross evidence of RV dilatation or hypertrophy.[13] However, another study on clinicopathologically and historically confirmed COPD cases showed the weight ratio between the left and right ventricles was significantly less in affected horses compared to controls, indicating relatively heavier right ventricles.[13] No clinical evidence of right heart failure or postmortem evidence of right heart dilatation was observed.[13] Thus, although right ventricular hypertrophy may occur in horses with COPD, congestive heart failure resulting from cor pulmonale is uncommon.

## Etiology

It appears unlikely that clinical signs of COPD in all horses are caused by one etiologic agent. Several different lung insults may well result in a stereotypic response of the lung to these injuries and clinical signs of COPD. However, in a large subgroup of horses with COPD, the disease clearly has an allergic etiology.

## *Allergy*

The evidence of an allergic etiology of COPD comes from several immunologic, physiologic, and epidemiologic studies.[14–17] In horses with COPD, there is a greater prevalence of serum antibody titers against antigens commonly found in the horse's environment.[14] These antigens include actinomycetes such as Micropolyspora faeni and Thermoactinomyces vulgaris and molds such as Aspergillus fumigatus, Alternaria, Penicillium, and Rhizopus sp. Many affected horses also have a positive skin test against these antigens.[15] However, many horses without clinical signs of COPD also have serum antibody titers and positive skin tests using the same antigens. Conversely, some affected horses do not have serum antibody titers or positive skin tests. Thus, as a group, horses with COPD have serum antibody levels and positive skin tests against several environmental antigens more commonly than control horses. Because considerable overlap exists between normal and affected horses, serum antibody titers and skin testing cannot be used to diagnose COPD in individual horses.

Bronchial provocation tests also suggest an allergic etiology for COPD in horses.[14] Challenge of affected horses with Micropolyspora faeni, Aspergillus fumigatus, or hay dust results in airway obstruction, hypoxemia, gas exchange impairment, and clinical signs of COPD. Bronchoprovocation using these agents has no clinical effect on control horses. Additional evidence suggesting that COPD has an allergic etiology stems from a group of horses and ponies with COPD, in which airway obstruction and gas exchange impairment was repeatedly induced by placing these animals into a barn and feeding them dusty hay. These animals with COPD consistently went into clinical remission within 2 weeks after removal from the barn and pasturing without exposure to hay or straw.[6,16,17] These studies confirm epidemiologic observations that COPD is common in climates where horses are housed indoors and fed hay for long periods of time, while the disease is rare in climates where animals are kept on pasture. However, in the southern U.S.A., a recurrent airway obstructive disease has been reported in pastured animals. These animals enter clinical remission when removed from pasture and housed indoors.[18]

## *Diet*

Many of the epidemiologic data incriminating exposure to hay or straw as an important factor in the etiology of COPD may also be interpreted to suggest that hay or straw contains substances injurious to the lung. It has been demonstrated that 3-methylindole when fed to horses causes clinical signs of lung disease indistinguishable from those of COPD.[19,20] In addition, the pulmonary lesions induced by 3-methylindole in the horse are also characterized by bronchiolitis.[19] 3-methylindole is a metabolite of L-tryptophan, an amino acid commonly found in some hay. Although preliminary evidence suggests that L-tryptophan when fed to horses is not metabolized to 3-methylindole, it appears that under appropriate conditions it may be possible that an oral pneumotoxin such as 3-methylindole could be ingested and be responsible for pulmonary injury characterized by bronchiolitis and clinical signs of COPD.

## *Previous Infection*

Many authors report that COPD commonly follows viral respiratory tract infections.[21] A similar correlation exists between viral respiratory disease and chronic respiratory diseases including asthma in humans.[22] In humans it has been shown that the majority of infants suffering from virus-induced bronchiolitis at an early age will suffer from chronic respiratory illness in later life.[23] The mechanism whereby viruses may induce long-term pulmonary injury is unknown, but virus infections may alter the ratio of alpha and beta-adrenergic receptors in the airways in favor of alpha receptors.[24] This would result in airway narrowing in response to adrenergic agonists which would normally cause airway dilation. This could in part explain the airway hyperresponsiveness observed in asthmatic people and in horses with COPD. Although the role of previous viral infections in the pathogenesis of COPD in horses awaits further investigation, it is clear that viruses may induce long-term pulmonary dysfunction and consequently measures aimed at reducing the incidence of viral infections (e.g., frequent vaccination) appear appropriate.

## Genetic Predisposition

A genetic predisposition to COPD has been suspected for many years. This suspicion is based on the observation that, among horses kept under identical environmental conditions, some individuals develop COPD while others do not. In addition, it has been suggested that COPD is more common in ponies and draft horses. The latter observation could be explained by the lower economic values of ponies and draft horses and the consequently poor management conditions to which these animals may be subjected.[5] Inherited deficiency of serum antiprotease-1-antitrypsin is known to predispose to the development of emphysema in people. Antiprotease-1-antitrypsin functions to protect the lung against lysosomal proteases. Preliminary evidence suggests that horses with COPD have normal serum levels of antiprotease-1-antitrypsin,[25] and therefore deficiency of this enzyme does not appear to be a likely cause of COPD in horses. Thus, although individual horses may be predisposed to develop COPD, a genetic predisposition to the disease remains unproven.

## Pathophysiology

Chronic obstructive pulmonary disease is characterized by hypoxemia, decreased dynamic compliance, increased pulmonary resistance, and prolongation of nitrogen washout, findings compatible with diffuse airway obstruction[26,27] (Fig. 15–1). In part, airway obstruction is the result of plugging of airways with mucus, cellular debris, and exudate. However, because in most horses with COPD airway obstruction may be substantially reduced by administration of atropine, a muscarinic bronchodilator, airway obstruction is also caused by airway smooth muscle contraction.[28] Understanding the mechanism of airway obstruction is important because it suggests that the therapy of horses with COPD should be directed at reducing airway inflammation and relieving smooth muscle contraction. The mechanisms responsible for airway inflammation in COPD are unclear. In ponies with COPD there is an increase in bronchoalveolar lavage IgG concentration 1 week after acute disease exacerbation induced by exposure to hay dust.[29] In addition, there is a marked increase in neutrophil numbers in bronchoalveolar lavage fluid of affected ponies.[29,30] This suggests that a type III reaction of Gell and Coombs may be involved in the pathogenesis of the disease. The large number of neutrophils recruited into the lung may release toxic oxygen radicals or enzymes exacerbating lung injury. Mediators such as histamine, eicosanoids, or platelet activating factor could also play a part in the inflammatory response and result in airway smooth muscle contraction.

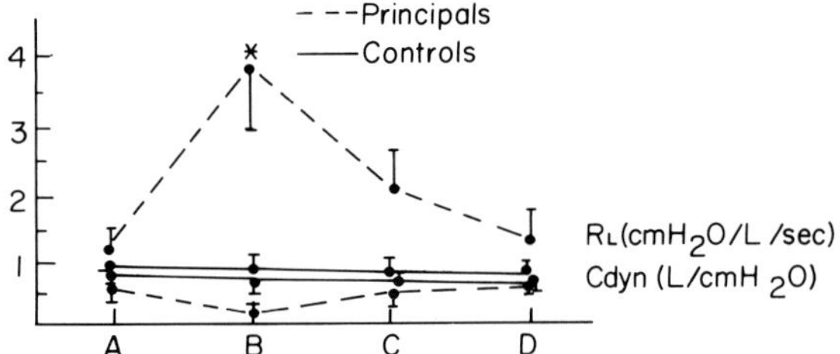


**FIG. 15–1.** Effects of barn exposure on pulmonary function in normal ponies and ponies with a history of COPD (principals). Measurements were made after ponies had been on pasture for 2 months (A), after they had been housed in a barn (B), and after they had been returned to pasture for 1 to 2 weeks (C and D respectively). This treatment had no effect on pulmonary function in control ponies, but barn exposure caused airway obstruction as indicated by an increase in pulmonary resistance (RL) and a decrease in dynamic lung compliance (Cdyn) in ponies with a history of COPD (principals). Airway obstruction in principals was reversed by returning ponies to pasture.

We have recently shown that following exposure to hay dust, plasma thromboxane concentrations are increased in ponies developing recurrent airway obstruction (heaves) but not in control ponies. This suggested a role for cyclooxygenase products in the pathogenesis of heaves. However, this hypothesis was refuted because cyclooxygenase blockade with flunixin meglumine did not prevent airway obstruction and airway hyperresponsiveness in these ponies. These latter results are supported by clinical observations that nonsteroidal anti-inflammatory agents are ineffective in the treatment of COPD. Thus, cyclooxygenase products appear unimportant in the pathogenesis of COPD. 15-Hydroxyeicosatetraenoic acid (15-HETE), a lipoxygenase product of arachidonic acid metabolism, is also increased in plasma of ponies with COPD.[31] The elucidation of the role of the HETES and other leukotrienes in the pathogenesis of COPD will have to await development of specific lipoxygenase enzyme inhibitors.

In ponies with COPD there is an increased number or activity of alpha-adrenergic receptors.[32] The cause of this increased alpha receptor activity is unknown but has been reported in asthmatic persons and several models of experimental lung disease. Because alpha-receptor stimulation results in bronchoconstriction, this change in airway receptors could in part expiain the bronchoconstriction observed in horses with COPD.

In 1947, Obel and Schmitterlow reported that horses with heaves have hyperreactive airways.[33] This finding had potentially important clinical implications because airways that are hyperresponsive to nonspecific stimuli will also respond by bronchoconstriction to irritants such as dust, ammonia fumes, and fungal spores which are common in the horse's environment. In addition, if diseased horses also had hyperresponsive airways during periods of clinical remission, tests of airway responsiveness may have been useful in detecting horses with subclinical COPD. We found that during periods of clinical disease, the airways of horses with COPD are hyperreactive to nonspecific stimuli, including histamine, methacholine, and citric acid.[16,17] Thus, when diseased horses are exposed to aerosolized irritants such as ammonia fumes, dust, or pollutants, airway obstruction will occur. However, airways of horses with COPD are only hyperresponsive during the

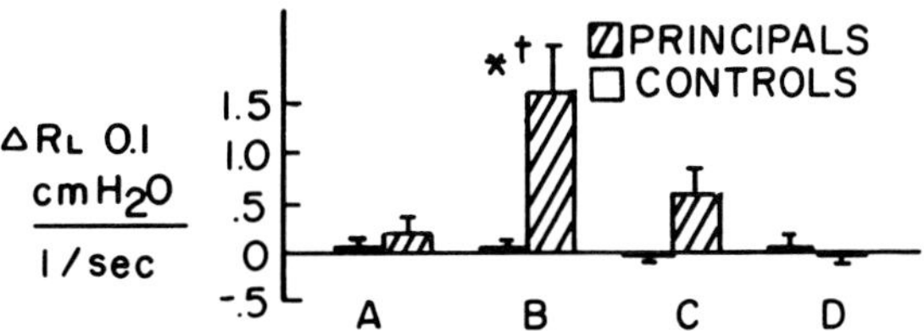


**FIG. 15–2.** A measure of airway responsiveness (ΔRL 0.1) is shown for ponies during clinical remission on pasture (periods A, C, and D) and after housing ponies in a barn which caused airway obstruction in principal ponies (B). Note the marked airway hyper-responsiveness of principal ponies at period B, but not at periods A, C, and D. (From Armstrong PJ, Derksen FJ, Slocombe RF, et al. Airway response to aerosol methacholine and citric acid in ponies with recurrent airway obstruction (heaves). Am Rev Respir Dis, *133*:357, 1986.)

time horses show clinical signs of the disease and not during periods of clinical remission (Fig. 15–2). Airway hyperresponsiveness is also characteristic of human asthma and the mechanism of airway hyperresponsiveness is unknown. Airway hyperresponsiveness in horses with COPD means that inhalation of irritants may exacerbate or prolong clinical signs of COPD in affected horses. Thus, when treating horses with COPD, careful attention should be paid to barn ventilation and air quality.

Coughing is a common clinical sign of horses with COPD. The cough reflex starts with the stimulation of mechanoreceptors in the respiratory system. The lung contains three types of mechanoreceptors able to send information to the central nervous system regarding the status of the lung. These receptors are the slowly adapting stretch receptor, the receptor associated with unmyelinated c fibers, and the irritant receptor.[34] Stimulation of the irritant receptor will result in coughing and bronchoconstriction. The irritant receptor is located beneath the respiratory epithelium and its myelinated afferent fibers travel in the vagus nerve. Irritant receptors respond to mechanical stimulation, deposition of foreign materials such as dust or fungal spores, chemical substances such as ammonia fumes or ozone, mediators of inflammation such as histamine, and bronchoconstriction.[35] Stimulation of irritant receptors results in bronchoconstriction or coughing. Bronchoconstriction following irritant receptor stimulation may be prevented by muscarinic blockade using atropine. In cases when coughing is due to inappropriate bronchoconstriction, bronchodilators may be used to inhibit the cough.

Airway inflammation, as seen in cases of COPD, injures the airway epithelium and exposes the irritant receptors. This in turn may lead to chronic coughing in response to otherwise innocuous stimuli. However, inappropriate irritant receptor stimulation is not responsible for airway hyperresponsiveness, because the latter cannot be prevented by muscarinic blockade.[36]

## Diagnosis

In severe cases, a presumptive diagnosis of COPD may be made based on history and clinical signs. However, in order to confirm a diagnosis of COPD or in mild cases of disease, diagnostic aids may be helpful.

### *Auscultation and Percussion*

In horses with COPD in which the disease is clinically apparent only by a decrease in exercise tolerance, auscultation findings are often normal. However, the chance of finding abnormal lung sounds on auscultation may be increased by the use of a rebreathing bag or by exercising the horse just prior to auscultation. The earliest auscultation abnormality that may be appreciated is loud or harsh breath sounds. Wheezing may be apparent at the end of exhalation when airways are narrowest. In more severely affected animals, a variety of adventitious lung sounds may be heard, including wheezes throughout the respiratory cycle and rarely crackles. It is important to understand that auscultation is a qualitative test only and does not reveal the severity of the lung disease present.[37] Percussion is thought to be useful in the hands of some clinicians, while others de-emphasize its importance. In mild cases of COPD, percussion of the thorax is usually normal. In more advanced cases, percussion may reveal a caudoventral enlargement of the lung field and the presence of more resonant sounds suggestive of pulmonary hyperinflation.

### *Endoscopy*

Endoscopic examination of the upper airway, trachea, and central airways is an important diagnostic aid when evaluating horses with COPD. Endoscopy is especially useful in mildly affected cases when diagnosis is a challenge. In horses with COPD, the upper airway is usually normal, although exudate arising from the trachea may coat the pharynx. Most normal horses allow the passage of the fiberoptic endoscope through the larynx into the trachea without coughing. In horses with COPD, introduction of the endoscope into the trachea may induce coughing, suggesting a hyperirritable airway. In affected horses a variable amount of yellow viscous material may be present in the trachea. Cytologic evaluation confirms that this material is an exudate and not primarily mucus. In some horses, tracheal exudate is only apparent immediately following exercise. With the longer fiberoptic endoscopes now available, the clinician may evaluate airways beyond the carina. In COPD central airways do not appear to be inflamed, but exudate is present in their lumens.

### *Radiography*

Radiography of the adult horse's thorax requires radiographic equipment generally not available to the equine practitioner. Even with the most powerful radiographic equipment available, radiographic detail is poor. In horses with COPD, thoracic radiographs reveal a mixed pattern of radiodensity throughout the lung field. In experimental lung disease in horses it has been shown that extensive pathologic lesions must be present in the lung before radiographic abnormalities are apparent. Thoracic radiographs are helpful in detecting focal or miliary lesions in the lung and distinguishing these cases from cases of COPD. Thoracic radiographs have not been helpful in the detection of early or subclinical cases of COPD.

## Airway Cytology

Transtracheal aspiration has been used in the evaluation of airway cell populations in horses with COPD.[38–41] It has been suggested that in horses with COPD the percentage of neutrophils in transtracheal aspirate fluid is increased. When interpreting transtracheal aspirate cytology, the assumption is made that the tracheal cytology in some manner reflects the pulmonary airway cell population. Recent evidence suggests that this assumption is not valid in horses with COPD and that the transtracheal aspirate cytology correlates poorly with the airway cell population as assessed by histopathology[40] and bronchoalveolar lavage. In addition, the variability in the percentage of neutrophils in transtracheal aspirate fluid of normal horses ranges from 0 to 83%.[40] This large variability in tracheal cell population of normal horses further limits the clinical usefulness of evaluating transtracheal aspirate cytology in cases of chronic lung disease. However, transtracheal aspirate cytology may have some value in distinguishing cases of COPD from parasitic lung disease in which the tracheal cell population contains a large percentage of eosinophils.

In contrast the variability in neutrophils observed in bronchoalveolar lavage fluid cytology of normal horses ranges from 0 to 17%.[42] In addition, there is a good correlation between bronchoalveolar lavage cytology and histopathologic score in horses with COPD.[43] Thus, bronchoalveolar lavage appears to be a more useful technique than transtracheal aspirate when evaluating horses with COPD. The bronchoalveolar lavage cytology of ponies with COPD is normal when ponies are in disease remission. However, during periods of disease exacerbation, there is a marked and consistent increase in the percentage of neutrophils in bronchoalveolar lavage fluid.[29] In some horses with COPD, the eosinophils in bronchoalveolar lavage fluid also increase.[29] Although an increase in BAL neutrophils is not pathognomonic for COPD, pulmonary neutrophilia in BAL fluid may be helpful in detecting airway inflammation and in conjunction with clinical data, confirming a diagnosis of COPD.

## Pulmonary Function Testing

Chronic obstructive pulmonary disease is characterized by airway obstruction. This results in decreased dynamic compliance, increased pulmonary resistance, and prolongation of nitrogen washouts.[26] Pulmonary function tests allow a quantitative assessment of the severity of the lung disease and document the presence of airway obstruction. However, these tests of pulmonary function require equipment generally not available to the equine practitioner. In addition, these tests are not particularly sensitive and are not helpful in the early detection of subclinical cases of COPD. Therefore, these tests of pulmonary function are rarely used in clinical practice.

The primary function of the lung is gas exchange and in horses with COPD this function is impaired resulting in hypoxemia. Measurement of arterial blood gas tension ($PaO_2$) is the simplest and often most helpful test of pulmonary function. This test can be easily performed in the field. Arterial blood may be collected in a syringe coated with heparin. At sea level a $PaO_2$ less than 83 torr is considered abnormal. Because in normal animals $PaO_2$ decreases with altitude, at higher elevations a lower $PaO_2$ may be normal.

# Therapy

## Changes in the Environment

In the majority of cases of COPD, lung injury is the result of exposure of the sensitized respiratory system to organic dust (Fig. 15–3). Therefore, the most important aim of therapy is to prevent this exposure. Damp, dusty barns with poor ventilation tend to exacerbate clinical signs of COPD, while the optimal environment is a pasture with a modest shelter against inclement weather.[44] If pasture is not available, horses with COPD should be

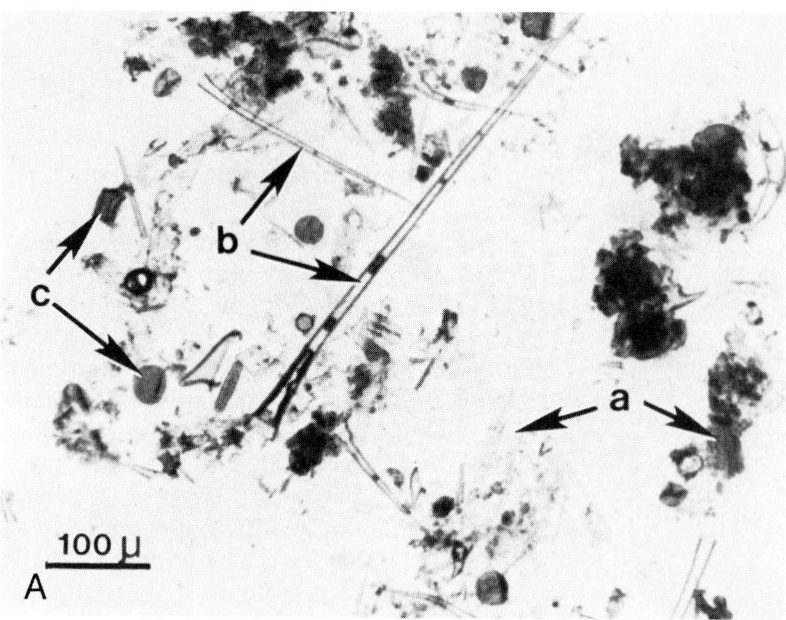


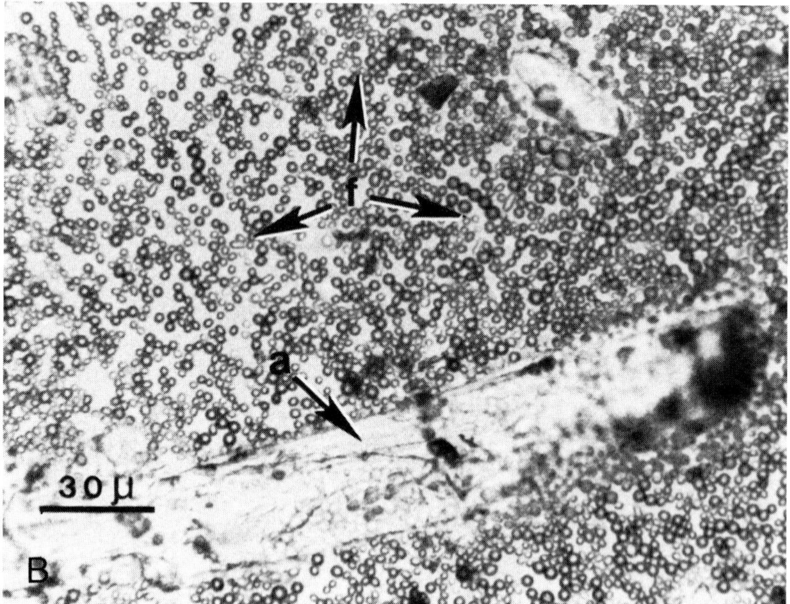


**FIG. 15–3.** A. Photomicrograph of a clean hay sample, the principal dust constituents being of plant origin. (a) fragments of leaves or stalks, (b) plant hair, and (c) pollen grains. B. Photomicrograph of dust collected from heavily molded hay. (a) same as in part A above. Most of the particles are fungal spores (f). They are mostly in the 2 to 5 μm diameter size range and are therefore respirable. (A and B From Clarke AF, Madelin T. Technique for assessing respiratory health hazards from hay and other source materials. Equine Vet J, *19*:442, 1987.)

housed in a well ventilated barn with access to the outside. Animals should be bedded on nondusty material such as moist wood shavings, shredded paper, or clay. Pelleted feed (or hay substitutes) should be fed.

Established management practices are frequently so ingrained that the veterinarian may have difficulty convincing horse owners to keep animals out of their poorly ventilated barns. Consequently, the therapy of horses with COPD is often centered around drug therapy with inevitably poor results and the suggestion that horses with COPD cannot be treated effectively. Therapeutic efforts are nearly always unsuccessful unless the horse's environment is altered and exposure to offending aerosol antigens is eliminated. This fact must be emphasized to owners who might otherwise be reluctant to follow recommendations. In mild cases of COPD involving racehorses, rest appears to be an important part of therapy. Exercise to keep the animal in racing shape could delay the resolution of the inflammatory response.

## *Corticosteroids*

Chronic obstructive pulmonary disease in the horse is characterized by airway inflammation. Reduction of the inflammatory response by corticosteroids will result in the resolution of clinical signs of the disease. However, it is important to emphasize that airway inflammation will return following cessation of therapy if exposure to offending antigens is not prevented. Corticosteroids reduce the inflammatory response by a variety of mechanisms, including the inhibition of phospholipase A, thereby preventing production of metabolites of arachidonic acid including prostaglandins and leukotrienes. Corticosteroids also inhibit cellular migration including the migration of neutrophils into the lungs of horses with COPD. In addition, corticosteroids potentiate the action of beta-2-receptor stimulants resulting in bronchodilation and inhibition of mediator release from inflammatory cells. Corticosteroids are powerful inhibitors of the inflammatory response. However, the undesirable side effects of corticosteroids are also potentially serious and may become apparent weeks after initiation of therapy. Thus, corticosteroids should be used with caution. Therapy should be aimed at optimal therapeutic response with minimal side effects. Corticosteroids at high doses suppress the immune response resulting in increasing susceptibility to respiratory or other infections. Prolonged use of corticosteroids may result in Cushing-like signs such as depression, muscle wasting, a long dry hair coat, hyperglycemia, polydipsia and polyuria. In addition, corticosteroids depress the release of ACTH from the posterior pituitary. Therefore, sudden withdrawal of exogenous administered corticosteroids after prolonged use may result in adrenal insufficiency. The risk of complications associated with corticosteroid usage may be minimized by a proper therapeutic regimen. To prevent steroid dependence, prednisone is administered orally every other day in the morning at a dose of 1 to 2 mg/kg. Endogenous plasma steroid levels peak in the morning and decline to reach their lowest level in the early evening. When the drug is given every other day, sufficient stimulation of the adrenal cortex occurs to prevent steroid dependence. After 2 weeks of steroid therapy, the response to treatment is assessed and the dose level gradually reduced until a minimum effective dose is reached.

## Bronchodilator Therapy

Chronic obstructive pulmonary disease is characterized by airway obstruction caused in part by airway smooth muscle constriction. Therefore, bronchodilators could play an important part in the therapy of COPD. However, little is known about the autonomic receptor populations in horse airways, the pharmacokinetics of bronchodilator drugs, or efficacy of bronchodilation therapy in clinical cases. Much investigation needs to be done before rational use of bronchodilator therapy in equine medicine may be recommended.

Hypoxemia is a common complication of bronchodilator therapy by aerosol or other routes.[45] This paradoxic problem is explained by ventilation-perfusion mismatching caused by preferential deposition of aerosol bronchodilator in well-ventilated lung regions, while in poorly ventilated regions little bronchodilator drug is deposited. In addition, systemically absorbed bronchodilators may cause vasodilation (beta$_2$ effect) in poorly ventilated lung regions. Especially in patients whose $PaO_2$ is below 60 torr, because of the nonlinear shape of the oxyhemoglobin dissociation curve, bronchodilator therapy may decrease $PaO_2$ to critically low levels. In these cases, oxygen therapy is indicated in conjunction with bronchodilator therapy.

## *Sympathomimetic Agents*

Sympathomimetic agents with specific affinity for beta$_2$ receptors belong to the most commonly used group of bronchodilators used in veterinary medicine. Beta$_2$ receptor bronchodilators include norepinephrine, isoproterenol, ephedrine, and clenbuterol. Sympathomimetic agents cause bronchodilation by stimulation of beta$_2$ receptors present in the large and small airways This in turn results in increased intracellular concentrations of cyclic AMP in airway smooth muscle cells and airway smooth muscle relaxation. Sympathomimetic bronchodilators were developed for their specific affinity for $beta_2$ adrenergic receptors present in the airways, vascular beds, and uterus, thereby minimizing their side effects on other organs including the heart, central nervous system, and gastrointestinal system. However, $beta_2$ receptor specificity is not complete and high doses of $beta_2$ receptor agonists will result in side effects including trembling, excitement, sweating, gastrointestinal ileus, colic, and tachycardia. These effects can, in large part, be attributed to the inadvertent stimulation of $beta_1$ receptors.

## Ephedrine

Ephedrine is a sympathomimetic bronchodilator present in several commercially available oral preparations. The drug is derived from an ancient Chinese medicinal obtained from the shrub Ephedra sinica. Ephedrine is a moderately active $beta_2$ receptor stimulant. However, its main mechanism of action is through the release of stored norepinephrine. Because after a few days of therapy these catecholamine stores may become depleted, drug tolerance develops and progressively more drug is needed to maintain bronchodilation. In addition, because norepinephrine does not have $beta_2$ receptor specificity, alpha and $beta_1$ receptors are also stimulated. In human medicine, ephedrine has largely been superseded by newer generations of more specific $beta_2$ receptor agonists.

## Isoproterenol

Isoproterenol is one of the most potent sympathomimetic bronchodilators available. The drug is classified as a catecholamine and has a low affinity for alpha adrenergic receptors but has marked $beta_1$ effects. The lack of $beta_2$ receptor specificity limits the clinical usefulness of this drug as a bronchodilator in lung disease because at therapeutic doses when administered systemically there are serious side effects including tachycardia, tremors, anxiety, and sweating. These side effects are mainly due to $beta_1$ receptor stimulation. In addition, isoproterenol has a short half-life and bronchodilation may last less than 1 hour. Isoproterenol may be useful in the treatment of acute airway obstruction sometimes seen in acute exacerbations of chronic obstructive pulmonary disease. The drug is diluted in saline solution and administered intravenously at a dose of 0.4 μg/kg of body weight. The infusion should be discontinued when the heart rate doubles. Isoproterenol at the same dose may also be delivered by aerosol. Although this route of administration is less convenient, side effects are greatly reduced and effective bronchodilation is achieved. Isoproterenol should not be given orally because absorption is erratic. Because of the cardiovascular side effects, isoproterenol cannot be recommended as a routine therapeutic agent.

## Clenbuterol

Clenbuterol is a specific $beta_2$ agonist as well as an expectorant. In horses, the drug is absorbed well orally and has a greater than 90% bioavailability. The half-life of clenbuterol is long and a twice daily oral or IV dosage regimen maintains blood levels in a therapeutic range. Because of its specificity for $beta_2$ receptors, clenbuterol at the recommended dosage of 0.8 μg/kg of body weight has little effect on the gastrointestinal tract or heart and therefore side effects are minimal. Several reports in the literature suggest that clenbuterol at a dose of 0.8 μg/kg of body weight is an effective bronchodilator in normal horses and horses with chronic obstructive pulmonary disease.[46] However, in a recent study clenbuterol administration at a dose of 1.6 μg/kg of body weight was unable to prevent histamine induced airway obstruction in ponies, suggesting that clenbuterol is not an effective bronchodilator in the horse.[47] Further study is required to resolve the question as to the efficacy of clenbuterol as a bronchodilator in horses. In Europe and Canada the drug has been on the market for many years but in the United States it is presently not available.

## *Anticholinergic Drugs*

Extracts of the plant Atropa belladonna (deadly nightshade) have been used in the treatment of human asthma for centuries. The chief constituent of this plant is atropine. Some of the earliest remedies used in the treatment of heaves in horses also contain anticholinergic agents related to atropine. Atropine is a potent parasympatholytic agent and because of its competive antagonism of acetylcholine blocks muscarinic neural transmission. However, when it is systemically administered, bronchodilation is only one of many possible effects. Other effects of atropine administration include gastrointestinal ileus, tachycardia, mydriasis, and central nervous system excitation, especially in ponies.[48] These many side effects preclude the routine use of systemically administered atropine as a bronchodilator in horses. However, therapeutic selectivity may be obtained by local delivery of the drug. Atropine, when administered by aerosol, is an effective bronchodilator and systemic side effects are greatly reduced. Glycopyrrolate is a synthetic anticholinergic agent with a limited ability to cross the blood-brain and placental barriers. The drug has been used as a preanesthetic agent in the horse at a dose of 0.005 mg/kg and one case report suggests its efficacy in the treatment of COPD at a dose of 0.007 mg/kg.[49] This dose appeared to be effective for 8 hours. However, more information on the use of glycopyrrolate must be available before its use for the treatment of COPD can be recommended. New anticholinergic agents with more specific bronchodilator effects and fewer side effects are presently being evaluated.

## *Phosphodiesterase Inhibitors*

The second messenger cyclic AMP promotes airway smooth muscle relaxation and bronchodilation. Cyclic AMP is metabolized to the inactive 5-AMP by phosphodiesterase. Thus, phosphodiesterase inhibitors like caffeine, theobromine, and theophylline promote bronchodilation by inhibiting the breakdown of intracellular cyclic AMP. Theophylline, the most commonly used bronchodilator in this group, is an effective bronchodilator in horses when blood concentrations are approximately 10 μg/ml.[50] However, excitement may occur at only 15 μg/ml.[50] Thus, in the horse, as in other species, the therapeutic blood level of theophylline is close to the toxic level. In addition, when it is orally administered, absorption of theophylline is erratic, making the drug difficult to use clinically. It is likely that in the future theophylline or related phosphodiesterase inhibitors will play a larger role in bronchodilator therapy in horses as part of a combination of agents acting synergistically.

## Miscellaneous Therapy

Disodium cromoglycate (cromolyn) is able to prevent mast cell degranulation and has been shown to be effective in the treatment of human asthma.[51] The drug has no direct effect on airway smooth muscle and has no known direct antagonist activity against mediators of inflammation. Therefore, cromolyn is only effective prophylactically and is not effective in cases of established disease. Thompson and McPherson[52] administered 80 mg of aerosolized cromolyn to 54 horses with a history of COPD. When they were exposed to natural antigen (dusty straw bedding and hay), a single dose of cromolyn prevented the onset of clinical signs for a mean of 3.6 days, while four successive daily treatments prevented clinical signs of COPD for a mean of 24.3 days. In a more recent study, up to 520 mg of aerosolized cromolyn given on 2 consecutive days was administered to five horses with a history of COPD.[53] Although this therapy somewhat ameliorated the deterioration in pulmonary function induced by subsequent exposure of these horses to barn and hay dust, the effect was of short duration and clinical signs of COPD were not significantly altered.

Most cases of COPD can be kept asymptomatic by ensuring strict environmental control. However, unavoidable exposure to antigen may occur, for example during shipping or at horse shows. In these cases, prophylactic cromolyn therapy may prevent the onset of clinical signs of COPD.

## Immunotherapy

Immunotherapy has been used to treat allergic lung disease in people for many years. Immunotherapy starts with skin testing to identify the offending antigen. Once the antigen is identified, allergens with adjuvant are administered subcutaneously at increasing concentrations at weekly intervals. Therapy is continued indefinitely. Production of blocking IgG antibodies, decreased levels of IgE, and induction of T-suppressor cells have been proposed as mechanisms whereby immunotherapy exerts its effect. In horses, interpretation of skin tests is difficult because the skin of many clinically normal horses responds vigorously to a large number of antigens. Nonetheless, it has been reported that immunotherapy may be effective in the treatment of COPD in some horses.[54]

## References

1. Williams W. Asthma, broken wind. In: The Principles and Practice of Veterinary Medicine. Edinburgh, Maclachlam and Steward, 1874, pp 358–363.
2. Cook WR. Chronic bronchitis and alveolar emphysema in the horse. Vet Rec, *99*:448, 1976.
3. Breeze RG. Heaves. The problem of disease recognition. Vet Clin North Am, *1*:219, 1979.
4. Asmundsson T, Gunnarsson E, Johannesson T. Haysickness in Icelandic horses: Precipitin tests and other studies. Equine Vet J, *15*:229, 1983.
5. McPherson EA, Lawson GHK, Murphy J, et al. Chronic obstructive pulmonary disease (COPD): Factors influencing the occurrence. Equine Vet J, *11*:167, 1979.
6. Derksen F, Robinson NE, Armstrong PJ, et al. Airway reactivity in ponies with recurrent airway obstruction (heaves). J Appl Physiol, *58*:598, 1985.
7. Mansmann RA, Osburn BI, Wheat JD, et al. Chicken hypersensitivity pneumonitis in horses. J Am Vet Med Assoc, *166*:673, 1975.
8. Thurlbeck WM, Lowell FC. Heaves in horses. Am Rev Respir Dis, *89*:82, 1964.
9. Van den Ingh TSGAM. Morphologic aspects of bronchitis and bronchiolitis in the horse. In: Lung Function and Respiratory Diseases in the Horse. E Deegen and RE Beadle (eds). Hanover, Germany, 1986, pp 13–15.
10. Drommer W, Kaup FJ, Iregui C, et al. Transmission and scanning electron microscopic findings in the tracheobronchial tree of horses with chronic obstructive pulmonary disease. In: Lung Function and Respiratory Diseases in the Horse. E Deegen and RE Beadle (eds). Hanover, Germany, 1986, pp 16–19.
11. Kaup FJ, Drommer W, Iregui C, et al. Morphologic alterations of the alveolar region in horses with chronic obstructive pulmonary disease. In: Lung Function and Respiratory Diseases in the Horse. E Deegen and RE Beadle (eds). Hanover, Germany, 1986, pp 20–22.
12. Gillespie JR, Tyler WS. Chronic alveolar emphysema in the horse. Adv Vet Sci Comp Med, *13*:59, 1969.
13. Dixon PM, Nicholls JM, McPherson EA, et al. Chronic obstructive pulmonary disease. Anatomical cardiac studies. Equine Vet J, *14*:80, 1982.
14. McPherson EA, Lawson GHK, Murphy JR, et al. Chronic obstructive pulmonary disease (COPD) in horses: Aetiologic studies: Response to intradermal and inhalation antigen challenge. Equine Vet J, *11*:159, 1979.
15. Halliwell REW, Fleischman JB, Mackay Smith M, et al. The role of allergy in chronic pulmonary disease of horses. J Am Vet Med Assoc, *174*:277, 1979.
16. Armstrong PJ, Derksen FJ, Slocombe RF, et al. Airway response to aerosol methacholine and citric acid in ponies with recurrent airway obstruction (heaves). Am Rev Respir Dis, *133*:357, 1986.
17. Derksen FJ, Scott BS, Robinson NE, et al. Intravenous histamine administration in ponies with recurrent airway obstruction (heaves). Am J Vet Res, *46*:774, 1985.
18. Beadle RE. Summer pasture associated obstructive pulmonary disease. In: Current Therapy in Equine Medicine. NE Robinson (ed). Philadelphia, WB Saunders Co., 1983, 512–516.
19. Breeze RG, Lee HA, Grant BD. Toxic Lung Disease. Mod Vet Prac, *59*:302, 1978.
20. Derksen FJ, Robinson NE, Slocombe RF, et al. 3-methylindole-induced pulmonary toxicosis in ponies. Am J Vet Res, *43*:603, 1982.
21. Gerber H. Chronic pulmonary disease in the horse. Equine Vet J, *5*:26, 1973.
22. Witting HJ, Granford NJ, Glaser Y. The relationsip between bronchiolitis and childhood asthma: A follow-up study of 100 cases of bronchiolitis in infancy. J Allergy, *30*:19, 1959.
23. Rooney JC, Williams HE. The relationship between proven viral bronchiolitis and subsequent wheezing. J Pediatr, *79*:744, 1971.
24. Burse WW. Decreased granulocyte response to isoproterenol in asthma during upper respiratory infections. Am Rev Respir Dis, *115*:783, 1977.
25. Matthews AG. Identification and characterization of the major antiproteases in equine serum and an investigation of their role in the onset of chronic obstructive pulmonary disease (COPD). Equine Vet J, *11*:177, 1979.
26. Willoughby RA, McDonell WN. Pulmonary function testing in horses. Vet Clin North Am, *1*:171, 1979.
27. Muylle E, Oyaert W. Lung function tests in obstruc-

tive pulmonary disease in horses. Equine Vet J, *5*:37, 1973.

28. Murphy JR, McPherson EH, Dixon PM. Chronic obstructive pulmonary disease (COPD): Effects of bronchodilator drugs on normal and effected horses. Equine Vet J, *12*:10, 1980.
29. Derksen FJ, Scott JS, Slocombe RF, et al. Bronchoalveolar lavage in ponies with recurrent airway obstruction (heaves). Am Rev Respir Dis, *132*:1066, 1985.
30. Deconto I. Cytomorphologic findings in tracheobronchial secretions from horses with acute or chronic pulmonary disease. In: Lung Function and Respiratory Diseases in the Horse. E Deegen and RE Beadle (eds). Hanover, Germany, 1986, pp 23–24.
31. Gray PR, Derksen FJ, Robinson NE, et al. Increased plasma 15-hydroxyeicosatetraenoic acid (15-HETE) concentrations during acute airway obstruction in ponies. FASEB J, *2*:A1184, 1988.
32. Scott JS, Broadstone RV, Derksen FJ, et al. Alpha 1 adrenergic induced airway obstruction in ponies with recurrent pulmonary disease. J Appl Physiol, *64*:2324, 1988.
33. Obel NJ, Schmetterlow CG. The action of histamine and other drugs on the bronchial tone in horses suffering from alveolar emphysema (heaves). Acta Pharmacol, *4*:71, 1948.
34. Paintal AS. Vagal sensory receptors and their reflex effects. Physiol Rev, *53*:159, 1973.
35. Mills JE, Sellick H, Widdicombe JG. Activity of lung irritant receptors in pulmonary micro-embolism, anaphylaxis and drug induced bronchoconstriction. J Physiol (Lond), *203*:337, 1969.
36. Broadstone RV, Scott JS, Derksen FJ, et al. Effects of atropine on lung function and airway reactivity in ponies with chronic airway disease (heaves). J Appl Physiol, (in press).
37. Kotlikoff MI, Gillespie JR. Lung sounds in veterinary medicine. Part I. Terminology and mechanisms of sound production. Comp Cont Ed, *5*:634, 1983.
38. Burch GE, Jensen B. The use of cytology in the diagnosis of equine respiratory infections. Equine Pract, *9*:7, 1987.
39. Beech J. Cytology of tracheobronchial aspirates in horses. Vet Pathol, *12*:157, 1975.
40. Larson VL, Busch RH. Equine tracheobronchial lavage: Comparison of lavage cytology and pulmonary histopathologic findings. Am J Vet Res, *46*:144, 1985.
41. Whitwell KE, Greet TRC. Collection and evaluation of tracheobronchial washes in the horse. Equine Vet J, *16*:499, 1984.
42. Derksen FJ, Brown CM, Sonea I, et al. Comparison of transtracheal aspirate and bronchoalveolar lavage cytology in 50 horses with chronic lung disease. Equine Vet J, *21*:23, 1989.
43. Viel L. Structural functional correlations of the lung in horses with small airway disease. PhD Thesis, University of Guelph, Guelph, Canada, 1983.
44. Clarke AF, Madelin TM, Allpress TG. The relationship of air hygiene in stables to lower airway disease and pharyngeal lymphoid hyperplasia in two groups of Thoroughbred horses. Equine Vet J, *19*:524, 1987.
45. Ziment I. Pharmacology of sympathomimetic agents. In: Respiratory Pharmacology and Therapeutics. Philadelphia, WB Saunders Co, 1978, pp 147–189.
46. Sasse HL, Hajer R. NAB365, a beta$_2$-receptor sympathomimetic agent: Clinical experience in horses with lung disease. J Vet Pharmacol Ther, *1*:241, 1978.
47. Derksen FJ, Scott JS, Slocombe RF, et al. Effect of clenbuterol on histamine induced airway obstruction in ponies. Am J Vet Res, *48*:423, 1987.
48. Duscharme N, Fubini S. Gastrointestinal complications associated with the use of atropine in horses. J Am Vet Med Assoc, *182*:229, 1983.
49. Goetz TE. Successful management of equine chronic obstructive pulmonary disease. Vet Med, *79*:1073, 1984.
50. McKiernan BC, Scott J, Koritz GD, et al. Efficacy of aminophylline in ponies with chronic obstructive lung disease. Proc Comp Resp Soc, 1986, p 8.
51. Eggleston PA, Breiman CW, Poison WE. A double blind trial of the effect of cromolyn sodium on exercise-induced bronchospasm. J Allergy Clin Immunol, *50*:57, 1972.
52. Thomson JR, McPherson EA. Prophylactic effects of sodium cromoglycate on chronic obstructive pulmonary disease in the horse. Equine Vet J, *13*:243, 1981.
53. Soma LR, Beech J, Gerber NH. Effects of cromolyn in horses with chronic obstructive pulmonary disease. Vet Res Commun, *11*:339, 1987.
54. Beech J, Merryman GS. Immunotherapy for equine respiratory disease. J Eq Vet Sci, *6*:6, 1986.
55. Clarke AF, Madelin T. Technique for assessing respiratory health hazards from hay and other source materials. Equine Vet J, *19*:442, 1987.

# CHAPTER 16

# EXERCISE-INDUCED PULMONARY HEMORRHAGE

*JOHN R. PASCOE*

The original intent in suggesting the name "exercise-induced pulmonary hemorrhage" (EIPH) was to link the readily identifiable features, exercise and lung hemorrhage, of an apparently common clinical problem and suggest an association, as a reference point for further discussion.[1] This term was felt to provide a more accurate description of the problem than earlier descriptive terms such as "blood vessel breaking, bleeders, epistaxis and sporadic idiopathic epistaxis." Perhaps equally importantly its use was intended to focus on the lung as the primary site of hemorrhage.[1] Without knowledge of the coexisting respiratory pathologic changes a more specific description was not possible. Even in the light of recent detailed descriptions of the morbid changes in the lungs of horses known to experience EIPH, a more specific description is not forthcoming. Thus, while I recognize that exercise-induced pulmonary hemorrhage is in all likelihood a clinical sign rather than a disease per se, this terminology and its acronym, EIPH, will continue to be used in this chapter since it serves its function as a useful reference point for discussion. Consideration of the morbid lung changes and thoughtful contemplation of the various hypotheses proposed as mechanisms to explain the genesis of EIPH should alert the reader that our knowledge of this problem is still in its infancy.

Recently it has been suggested that EIPH is not a disease entity or a syndrome, but rather it is a clinical sign of other respiratory disease.[2] Proponents of this philosophy argue that recurrent laryngeal neuropathy is the primary disease and that EIPH, rather than abnormal respiratory noise and/or impaired performance, is the principal clinical sign. Since there is evidence to suggest that recurrent laryngeal neuropathy may in fact be part of a more generalized distal axonopathy in horses,[3] it could be argued that recurrent laryngeal neuropathy is itself a clinical sign and not a disease. Thus, if the facts were known, the argument could be extended to the specific disease causing the axonopathy, which currently is unknown, so that the axonopathy would also in fact be merely a sign of disease.

## Historical Background

As alluded to in the introductory comments, mankind's desire to label and categorize observations for the purpose of discussion and learning yields a variety of chronologically related synonyms that variously reflect our understanding, or lack thereof, of disease processes. It is not certain when the initial observations of EIPH were made or even if they were recorded. Perusal of the early literature of farriery and veterinary medicine suggests that epistaxis and its association with exercise have been recognized in horses for at least 4 centuries.[4]

*Of Bleeding at the Nofe.*

MAny horfes, (efpecially young horfes) are oft fubject to this bleeding at the Nofe, which I imagine proceedeth either from the much abundance of Blood, or that the vein which endeth in that place is either broken fretted, or opened. It is opened many times by means that blood aboundeth too much, or that it is too fine, or too fupple, and fo pierceth through the vein. Again, it may be broken by fome violent ftrain, cut, or blow; and laftly, it may be fretted and gnawn through by the fharpnefs of the blood, or elfe by fome other evil humour contained therein. The cure is, according to the antient Farriers, to take the juyce of the roots of Nettles, and fquirt it up into the horfes Noftrils, and lay upon the nape of the horfes neck a wad of Hay dipt in cold water, and when it waxeth warm, take it off, and lay on a cold one. Other Farriers ufe to take a pint of red wine, and put therein a quartern of Bole-Armonick beaten into fine powder, and being made luke-warm, to pour the one half thereof the firft day into his Noftril that bleedeth, caufing his head to be holden up, fo as the Wine may not fall out, and the next day to give him the other half.

Others ufe to let the horfe blood on the breaft vain, on the fame fide that he bleedeth, at feveral times: then take of Frankincenfe one ounce, of Aloes half an ounce, and beat them into fine powder, and mingle them throughly with the whites of three Eggs untill it be as thick as Honey, and with foft Hares hair thruft it up into his noftrils, filling the hole full of Afhes, Dung, or Hogs-dung, or Horfes dung mixt with Chalk and Vinegar.

Now for mine own part, when none of thefe will remedy or help (as all have failed me at fome time) then I have ufed this, take two fmall whip-cords, and with them garter him exceeding hard about fome ten or twelve inches above his knees of his fore-legs, and juft beneath his Elbows, and then keep the nape of his neck as cold as may be, with moift Cloaths, or wet Hay, and it will ftaunch him prefently.

**FIG. 16–1.** Reproduction of Gervase Markham's 1681 description "Of bleeding at the nose."

Gervase Markham (1681) provided an early description of epistaxis and some rather colorful cures (Fig. 16–1).[4] Professor William Robertson in his text on the Practice of Equine Medicine published in 1883 describes in detail the problem of pulmonary congestion.[5] This was defined as "a hyperaemia condition of the pulmonary capillary vessels, sometimes attended with extravasation from these into the air-sacs, and interconnective-tissue." He noted that "active congestion, the most frequently occurring form in the horse, may be observed to a certain extent, but not to that of disease, accompanying all active exertion" and "in horses of any class this may occur when put to severe exertion or prolonged work, for which they are unprepared by a certain amount of previous work and by proper feeding."[5]

Another English writer, J.B. Robertson, investigating the possible heritable basis of "blood-vessel breaking" in Thoroughbred horses confirmed the association of epistaxis with exercise and provided an amusing anecdote of the stigma associated with this condition. He reported that one of the earliest known bleeders was a horse called Bleeding Childers, so named because of his frequent episodes of epistaxis. Retired to stud because of training difficulties related to frequent bleeding episodes he was tactfully renamed Bartlet's Childers and is noted as the grandsire of Eclipse.[6] Robertson's description of the stallion Herod who raced in the Great Subscription Purse at York in 1766 "but broke a blood vessel and was beaten off" and whose "form was at times unaccountably bad and it is significant that the first and only time he met a number of runners he showed the weakness (bleeding)" serves to illustrate that epistaxis was recognized in young horses and that it was associated with poor performance.[6]

Perhaps even more enlightening is Robertson's notation that "If the lesion occurs high up in the nasal cavity and close to the pharynx whilst the horse is doing a gallop, not infrequently some of the blood is forced by the inspired air into the glottis, and so gains access to the lungs. When this happens, the horse may fall suddenly, and, on regaining his feet, cough up the blood which has reached the bronchial tubes. Very occasionally he never regains his feet and dies almost immediately from asphyxia."[6] That these changes were interpreted incorrectly should caution each of us to view current interpretations with an open mind.

Surprisingly, earlier pathology texts are, in general, devoid of descriptions of morbid changes associated with epistaxis and although some such as Huytra, Marek and Manninger (1926) describe pulmonary hemorrhage as occurring "in horses after overheating in rapid running or in consequence of hard work, also as part of the clinical picture of heart disease,"[7] there are no detailed descriptions of any associated histologic changes. Perusal of the literature between 1900 and 1974 suggests that opinion varied between the vasculature of the lung and the nose as the source of bleeding.

In 1974, Cook dispelled many of these earlier notions and, based on careful clinical deduction, identified a group of horses that bleed from the lungs during or after competitive exercise.[8] This seminal work provided the framework for endoscopic studies, conducted 4 years later, that identified the high prevalence of EIPH and largely have provided the most recent impetus for further investigation.[1]

## Clinical Signs

The predominant clinical sign of EIPH is blood within the tracheobronchial airways. Epistaxis occurs relatively infrequently and has been observed in 1 to 10% of horses with endoscopic evidence of blood in the airways.[9,10] In some horses there may be blood-staining of the neck and chest and blood may be spattered on the rider. More commonly, epistaxis, varying in character from slight blood tinged respiratory secretions to a trickle of blood from the nostril, is observed only after the horse is allowed to lower its head. With normal "cooling out" and postexercise watering procedures, this may not occur until the horse is released in its stall.

Other signs are variable and depend to a large extent on the degree of coexisting respiratory disease. Since, in most instances, EIPH occurs as a consequence of strenuous exercise other reported signs are likely to be related to performance. Thus indicators of impaired or poor performance such as slowing or stopping in a race or training gallop may be reported by the rider. Abnormalities in respiratory pattern, effort, or sound may also be reported. A variety of colorful terms—"bobbling," "gurgling," and "choking"—are often used to describe these signs. Since these descriptive terms are relatively nonspecific and convey different meanings to different persons, their observation requires thorough clinical examination to elucidate their origin.

Clearance of blood from the larynx may initiate increased frequency of swallowing and this sign is occasionally noted by astute grooms and trainers.[1,9] Although coughing can occur in association with EIPH it is a relatively non-specific sign and, in general, is usually indicative of stimulation of airway irritant receptors. Endoscopic observation of coughing horses with EIPH often reveals either an inflamed respiratory mucosa or the presence of inhaled particulate matter, especially dirt or grass from the racing surface, adhered to the pharyngeal mucosa or within the tracheobronchial airways.[1] With coughing, blood present in the trachea is often sprayed circumferentially around the lumen rather than being located ventrally.

Difficult or labored breathing may occur fairly soon after exercise in some horses with EIPH. Inappropriate breathing patterns suggest that extensive hemorrhage has occurred either within the lung parenchyma, subpleurally, or into the pleural space. Occasionally, horses with impending respiratory infection, especially pneumonia and pleuropneumonia, will show exaggerated respiratory effort shortly after exercise. In these instances, the horses often exhibit variable signs of distress and immediate medical attention is warranted.

## Diagnosis

Confirmation of EIPH requires either direct observation of blood in the tracheobronchial airways following exercise or identification of hemosiderophages in respiratory secretions.[1,9] Hemosiderophages may also be seen in other conditions associated with bleeding into the airways and/or alveoli and are not specifically diagnostic for EIPH.

### *Endoscopy*

While observation of epistaxis during or after exercise is strongly suggestive of EIPH careful endoscopic examination of the airways is important to rule out other sources of hemorrhage. In the absence of a visible source of bleeding in the airways rostral to the trachea, observation of blood in the tracheobronchial airways in the immediate post-exercise period is considered definitive evidence of EIPH. Most EIPH positive horses will have blood visible for at least 90 minutes after exercise although in some horses traces of blood will still be visible after 4 to 6 hours. Temporal variations occur and depend on the time of onset of bleeding relative to examination, the volume of blood loss and the efficiency of the mucociliary escalator in clearing the blood from the lower airways. Because of this it has generally been recommended that horses be examined within 30 to 90 minutes after exercise.[9] Most treatment efficacy studies have used 60 minutes as the standard postexercise interval for examination.[11–13] If it is strongly suspected that a horse bled but there is no evidence on the initial examination, re-examination 30 minutes later is advised. Horses with epistaxis should be examined as soon as possible after exercise to determine the origin of hemorrhage especially if the bleeding is suspected to originate from a site rostral to the larynx.

## Cytology

When endoscopy is not possible, cytologic examination of tracheobronchial secretions for hemosiderophages is recommended.[9] Identification of hemosiderophages (Fig. 3–2, p 46) can be enhanced by the use of special stains such as Sano's trichrome stain or Perl's Prussian Blue stain which selectively stains iron pigment.[14,15] It has been reported that most (>90%) horses in training have hemosiderophages in their respiratory secretions.[15] Considering that these cells can be found in large numbers in alveoli and lung connective tissue septa of EIPH horses, and are apparently cleared slowly from the lung, their recovery in respiratory secretions might be anticipated for prolonged periods after a bleeding episode.[16] Hemosiderophages have been recovered from transtracheal aspirates collected from horses that have not exercised for at least 150 days after a known episode of EIPH.[17]

Neutrophils and eosinophils have also been reported to be more common in the respiratory secretions of horses known to have experienced EIPH.[15] The interrelationship of these three cell types in EIPH is unknown but it is assumed that the presence of neutrophils and eosinophils reflects coexisting lung inflammation. Lung sections from EIPH positive horses have confirmed the presence of accumulations of eosinophils in alveolar spaces and in connective tissue spaces around alveoli, airways, and vessels but in most instances these cells were located in regions remote from those containing large accumulations of hemosiderophages.[16]

In some racing jurisdictions in North America, a signed affidavit from a licensed veterinarian stating that hemosiderophages were identified in respiratory secretions is considered proof of EIPH, for the purpose of administering permitted prerace medication for EIPH.

## Radiographic Findings

Attempts to correlate radiographic and pathologic findings in EIPH have been disappointing. The predominant radiographic feature evident on thoracic radiographs is an increased bronchointerstitial pattern particularly in the dorsocaudal lung field.[18] Although this pattern correlates with the distribution and type of morbid lung change observed, the specificity of interpretation in any individual horse is limited.[18] Other studies have described relatively discrete regions of increased parenchymal density in the same thoracic location and it is likely that these markings represent lung consolidation either as a sequela of hemorrhage, pneumonia, or lung abscess.[19,20] In other horses diffuse increases in soft tissue density are noted in the dorsocaudal lung field and based on the rapidity with which these changes resolve it is likely that they represent extensive parenchymal hemorrhage (Fig. 16–2).[19] In horses with EIPH and without other clinical evidence of lung disease, thoracic radiographs taken prerace, within 60 minutes of racing, and again 24 hours after racing failed to detect changes suggesting that in most horses the blood loss into the parenchyma and airways associated with EIPH is not detectable with thoracic radiographs.[21]

## Lung Ventilation–Perfusion Scans

Imaging the airways with aerosolized $^{99m}$Tc-DTPA and the pulmonary circulation with intravascular $^{99m}$Tc macroaggregated albumin can provide functional images of lung ventilation and perfusion.[22] Lung regions with di-

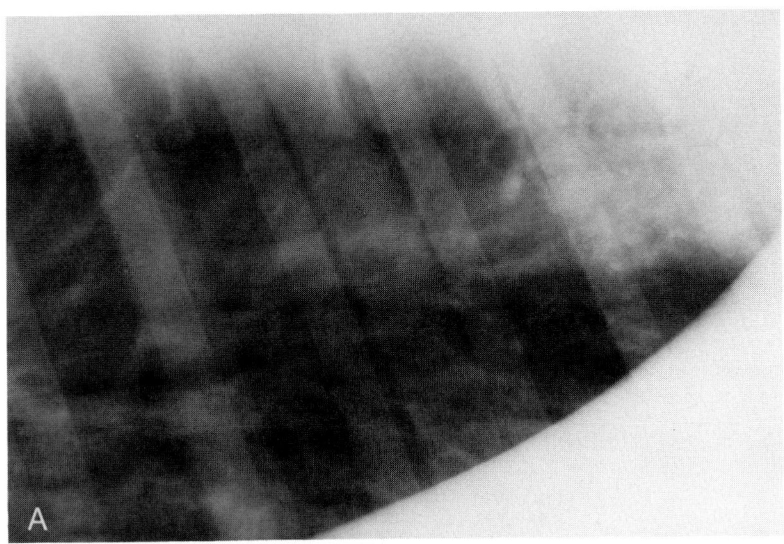


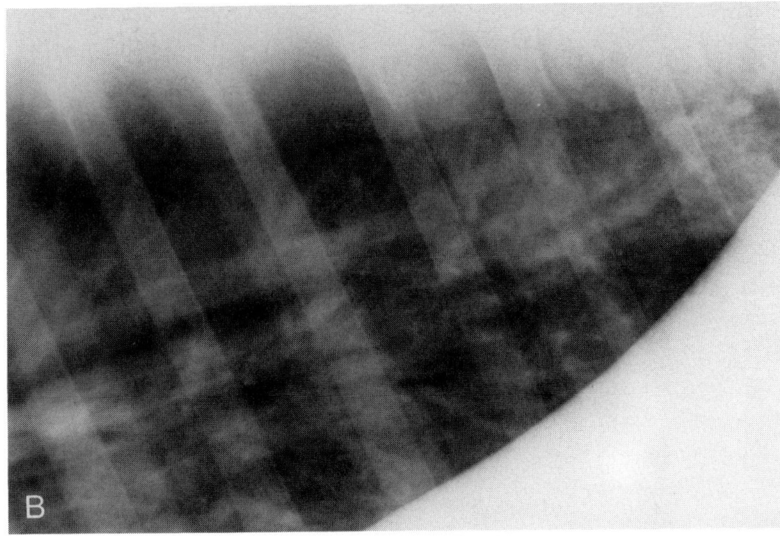


**FIG. 16–2.** Lateral thoracic radiograph of the caudodorsal lungfield. Note (A) the homogeneous increase in density in the thoracophrenic angle at 24 hours after EIPH and (B) the resolution of this pattern 5 days later. Although the location of this radiographic pattern is coincident with the location of the principal pathologic changes in the lung, it is not a consistent radiographic finding in the lungs of horses known to experience EIPH.

minished air and blood flow will acquire less radiolabel and thus be evident as regions of reduced intensity on the lung images. Studies in horses with a history of EIPH and radiographic changes in their lungs indicate loss of perfusion and a variable reduction in ventilation to affected lung regions (Fig. 16–3).[22] Although loss of pulmonary perfusion was evident, it is probable from subgross observation of EIPH lungs after vascular injections that these regions were receiving collateral supply from the bronchial circulation.[23] Additional studies are needed to confirm this apparent alteration in lung perfusion in horses with EIPH.

## Coagulation Profiles

In the absence of other systemic disease, EIPH is not usually associated with changes in clinical clotting profiles.[9] Changes in adenosine phosphate induced platelet aggregation have been reported in five horses with a prior history of EIPH, 5 minutes after a 1.2 km gallop at maximal speed.[24] None of the five

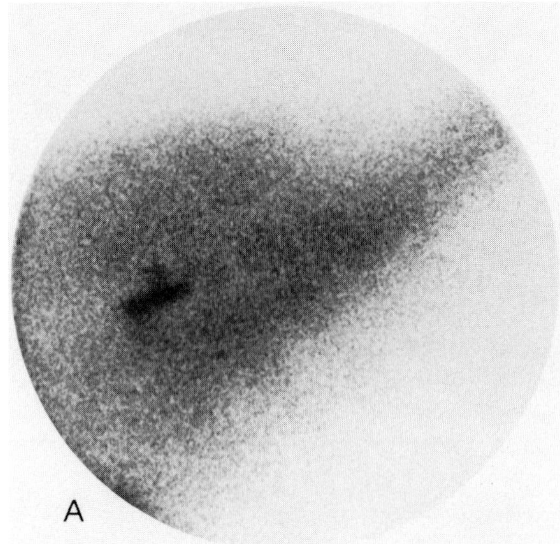


**FIG. 16–3.** A. Lateral pulmonary perfusion scan with 99m Tc macroaggregated albumin. B. Lateral thoracic radiograph of the dorsocaudal lung field in the same horse. Note the perfusion deficit in the dorsocaudal lung field corresponding with the increased density identified on lateral thoracic radiograph.

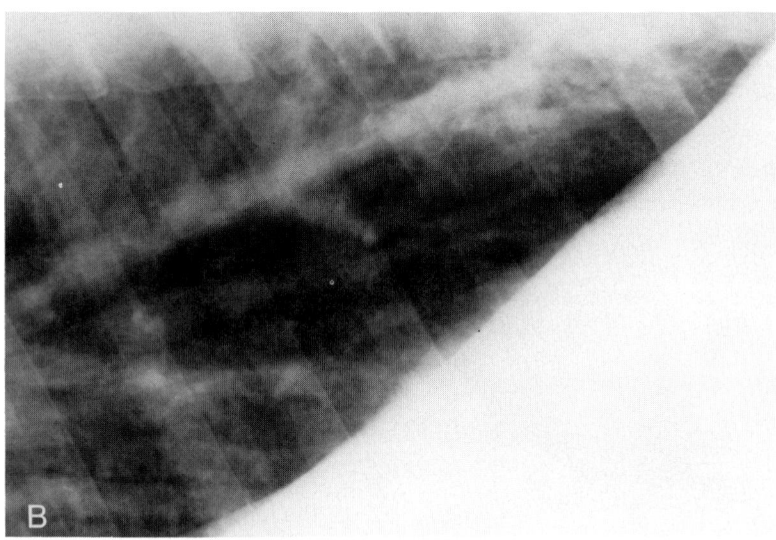


horses had EIPH after this gallop so the significance of this change in platelet aggregability is unknown.

## Epidemiologic Features

### *Prevalence*

Endoscopic surveys have indicated that EIPH occurs in horses used for a variety of different competitive activities.[25] Flat racing horses, particularly Thoroughbreds, have been studied extensively and the reported frequency of EIPH in racing Thoroughbreds, Quarter Horses, and Appaloosas has varied between 43 and 75%.[9,34] Surveys in Thoroughbred horses used for steeplechase, timber races, and jumping indicate a similar frequency of EIPH.[25] About 30% of Standardbreds (pacers and trotters) experience EIPH and a limited study of polo ponies indicated that the frequency in this group was 11%.[9,26] Two separate studies in horses (primarily

Arabians and Anglo-Arabians) used for endurance riding failed to detect EIPH at the end of 50 and 100 mile races.[9]

The results of cytologic studies suggest that most, if not all, Thoroughbred horses in race training experience EIPH after moderately strenuous exercise.[15] The minimum level of exercise necessary to induce EIPH is unknown, but based on available survey data it would seem that EIPH occurs soon after training begins, especially after galloping (>14m/s), and continues to occur in association with moderately strenuous exercise throughout the remainder of the horse's racing career. Short sudden bursts of activity such as starting from a racing gate, barrel racing, and steer roping have induced EIPH (unpublished observations) but the frequency in horses used for these events is unknown. Similarly it is not known if "pulling competitions" in draft breeds can induce EIPH.

Collation of published data suggests that there is little geographic variation in the incidence of EIPH within and between countries.[9,10,17,27] Similarly there appears to be no difference in prevalence between horses raced at sea level and at altitude. The frequency in Thoroughbred racehorses in Bogota, Colombia (elevation 3000 m) has been reported as 67% (R. Bennincore, personal communication) similar to that reported for Thoroughbreds racing at sea level in North America.

## *Age and Sex*

With the exception of one study in racing Quarter Horses,[28] there is no apparent sex difference in the frequency of EIPH. It has been suggested that in Quarter Horses, EIPH occurs more often in stallions than geldings.[28] Most studies have reported that older horses are more likely to bleed. It is believed that this reflects the chronic and apparently progressive nature of the lung injury.[9]

## *Performance*

The influence of EIPH on performance is variable, being apparently incapacitating in some horses and having no apparent influence in others.[21] Endoscopic surveys have indicated no association between race finishing position and EIPH.[1,9] Analysis of racing times standardized for distance and adjusted for track variations indicates that in most instances times were adversely influenced in the race in which EIPH was recognized.[29] Similar findings were reported for horses with epistaxis that were not examined with an endoscope. However, it is unknown if any of these horses bled during earlier races, nor was there any information concerning other factors such as musculoskeletal injury that may have been contributing factors.

## Necropsy Findings

Gross examination of the collapsed lung in situ reveals slightly raised, blue-brown colored areas distributed dorsally and laterally within the dorsal half of the caudal lobe (Fig. 16–4).[30] No involvement has been noted in the cranial, middle, or accessory lobes.[30] In more severely affected lungs there is apparent confluence of the lesions to produce involvement of most of the dorsocaudal portion of the caudal lobe. Also, in severely affected lungs there appears to be patchy distribution of parenchymal staining along the dorsum of the lung toward but not rostral to the cardiac notch. On closer inspection, the subpleural vasculature is more prominent in association with the discolored regions which also have a firmer consistency than the surrounding normal colored lung.[30] The prominent subpleural vessels appear to originate from branches of the bronchoesophageal arteries in the pulmonary ligaments (Fig. 16–5).

When the lungs are removed, examination of the costal surfaces reveals bilaterally symmetric parenchymal staining (Fig. 16–6A). In severe cases, the diaphragmatic surface usually has a single roughly circular area of staining (Fig. 16–6B). With lung inflation, the discolored areas become light brown or bronze in color and have a fine reticular pattern that seems to be confined to lobules (Fig. 16–7).

Transverse (dorsoventral) sections of fixed

lung show that the rust colored staining extends from the surface into the parenchyma and that the degree of parenchymal staining diminishes toward the hilum.[23] The stained areas of lung appear to be preferentially distributed in dorsal bronchopulmonary segments, with the dorsobasal bronchopulmonary segment being most involved. Examination of transverse slices from lungs with colored latex injected into the pulmonary and bronchial arterial circulations indicates an increase in bronchial arterial vessels within stained lung areas.[23] These vessels are particularly prominent around diseased small airways and in lung regions with distorted parenchymal architecture (Fig. 16–8).[23] Correlated subgross and microangiographic examinations demonstrate the complexity of the bronchial arterial neovascularization of diseased lung regions (Fig. 16–9).[31]

Microscopic findings include bronchiolitis, increased fibrous connective tissue in interlobular septa, around airspaces, and around diseased airways and some vessels (Fig. 16–10).[16] Large accumulations of macrophages and giant cells containing iron pigments are found in alveoli, airways, and within connective tissue around airspaces and vessels.[16] Although bronchiolitis is observed in lung regions without hemosiderophages, the converse does not appear to be true. Focal accumulations of eosinophils are noted in some regions with hemosiderophages, but in general are located in regions remote from the hemosiderophages and other structural changes.[16] Increased numbers of vessels are noted around diseased airways and within regions of interstitial fibrosis. Some of these muscular arteries have apparent duplication and fragmentation of the internal and external elastic lamina.[16]

## Pathogenesis

The cause and pathogenesis of EIPH are unknown. At least five hypotheses have been proposed to explain the mechanisms that might be involved in EIPH. In chronologic order, these include (1) asphyxia,[32] (2) bronchiolitis,[8] (3) lung stresses in response to small airway disease,[33] (4) lung stresses during strenuous exercise,[34] and (5) recurrent laryngeal neuropathy.[2] It is not intended to discuss these concepts in detail and the interested reader is referred to the source material for further contemplation.

The identification of consistent morbid changes in the lungs of horses known to have experienced EIPH provides a reference point that reasonable hypotheses must include if they are to be accepted.

Before pursuing this argument further it should be realized that the reported pathologic changes originated from a group of older Thoroughbred racehorses, known to have had EIPH or epistaxis, that had been retired from racing.[17] This point is emphasized because gross changes in the lungs of younger horses are not nearly as marked (unpublished observations). Also the interval from last race or EIPH episode to necropsy in the study group was sufficiently long that repair processes may have obliterated some important early changes in these lungs. Nevertheless, when attempting to develop an hypothesis to explain the pathogenesis, the predominant changes that warrant consideration are the specific regional location, hemosiderophage sequestration, bronchiolitis, interstitial fibrosis, and bronchial arterial neovascularization.

Bronchial arterial neovascularization is known to occur in response to inflammation and is considered an integral part of the pulmonary repair process.[35] Bronchiolitis was observed in most lung sections but the cellular response was more pronounced in those dorsocaudal regions with hemosiderophage accumulations.[16] It is not known if pre-existing bronchiolitis was more severe in these regions or if the observed response had been exacerbated by hemorrhage. The consistent regional location suggests that structural features may predispose to the observed patterns. Most of the affected lung appeared to be distributed dorsal to the principal bronchus with the most severely affected region corresponding to the dorsobasal bronchopulmonary segment. This segment is subtended by the terminal divisions of the principal bronchus and because of its axial alignment with the principal bronchus it is likely that this segment would be the favored site for

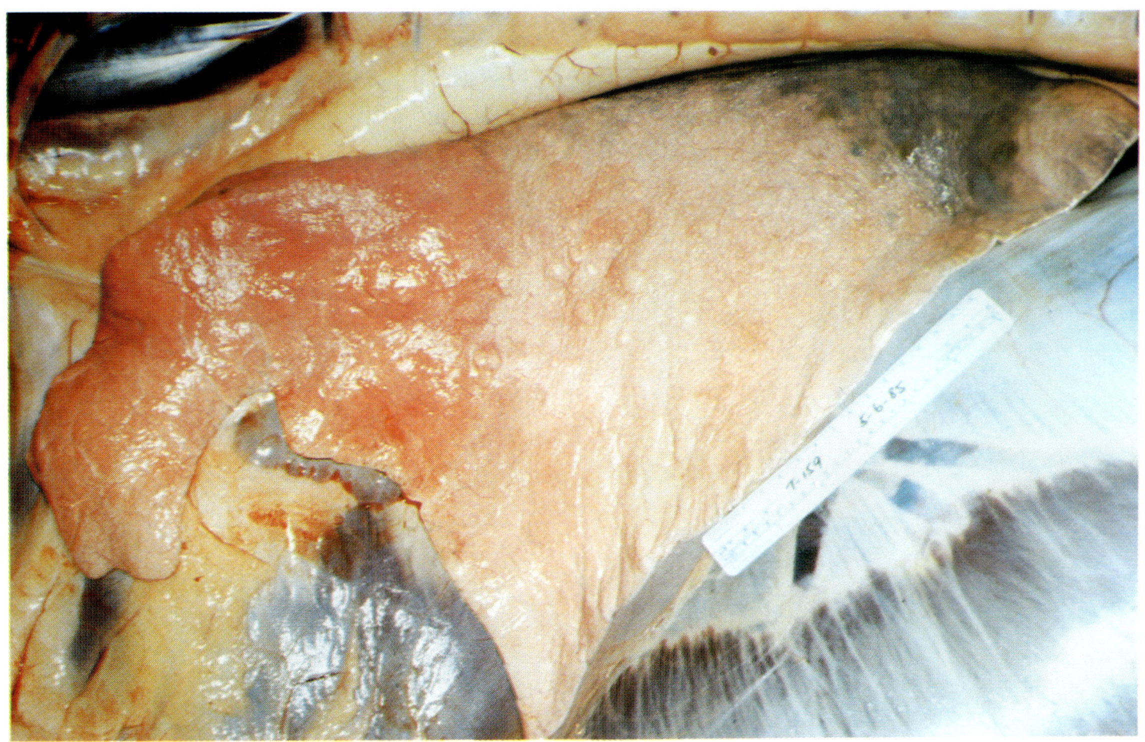


**FIG. 16–4.** Left thoracic cavity. Note the blue-brown areas of parenchymal staining in caudodorsal lung and the associated increase in prominence of the subpleural vessels.

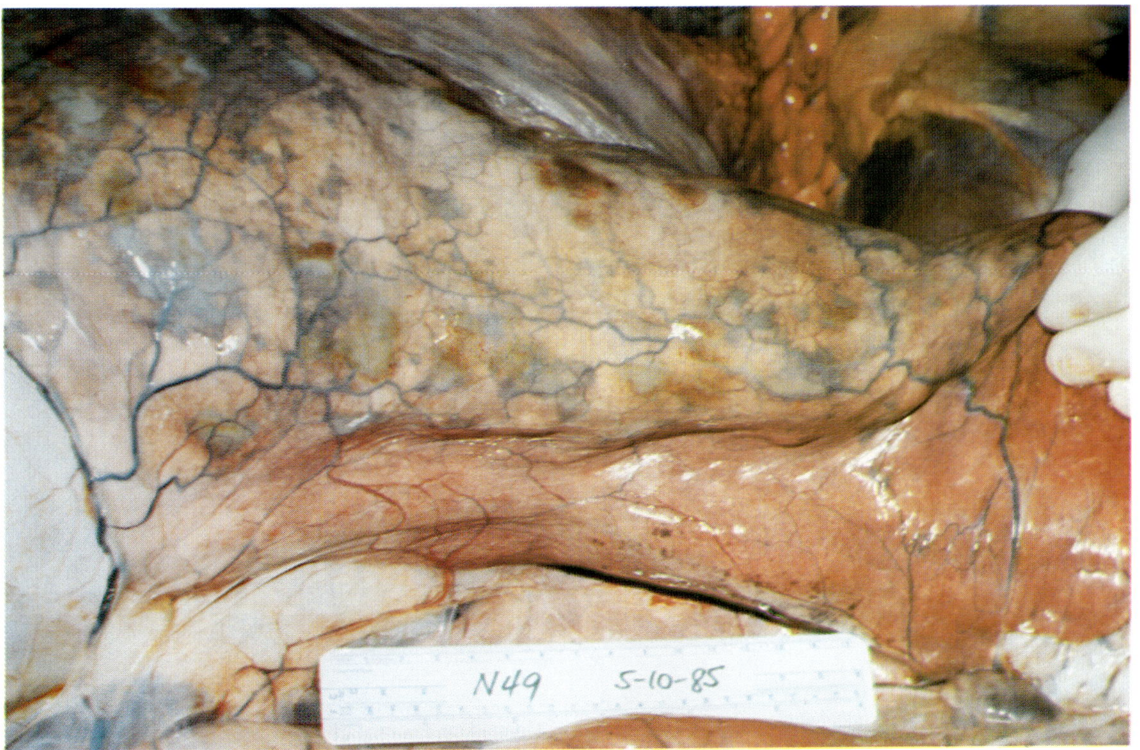


**FIG. 16–5.** The prominent subpleural vessels originate from the branches of the bronchoesophageal arteries in the pulmonary ligament.

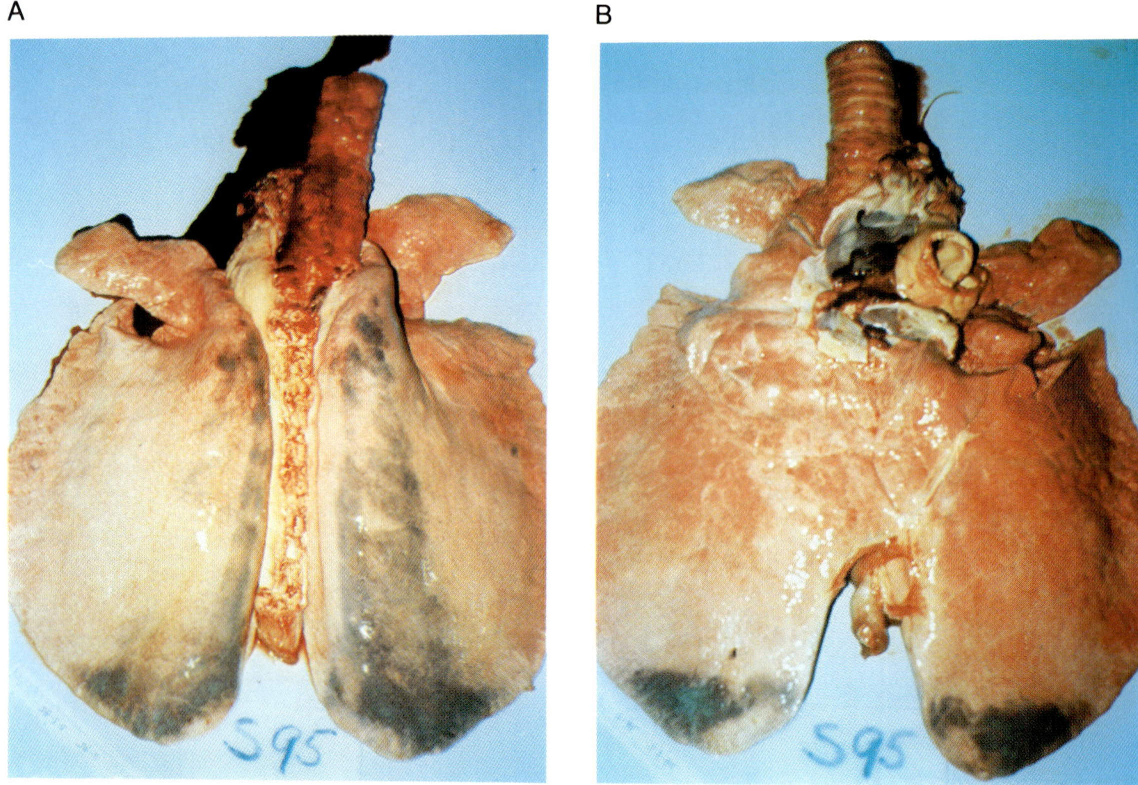


**FIG. 16–6.** Costal (A) and diaphragmatic (B) surfaces of the lungs showing the distribution of parenchymal staining.

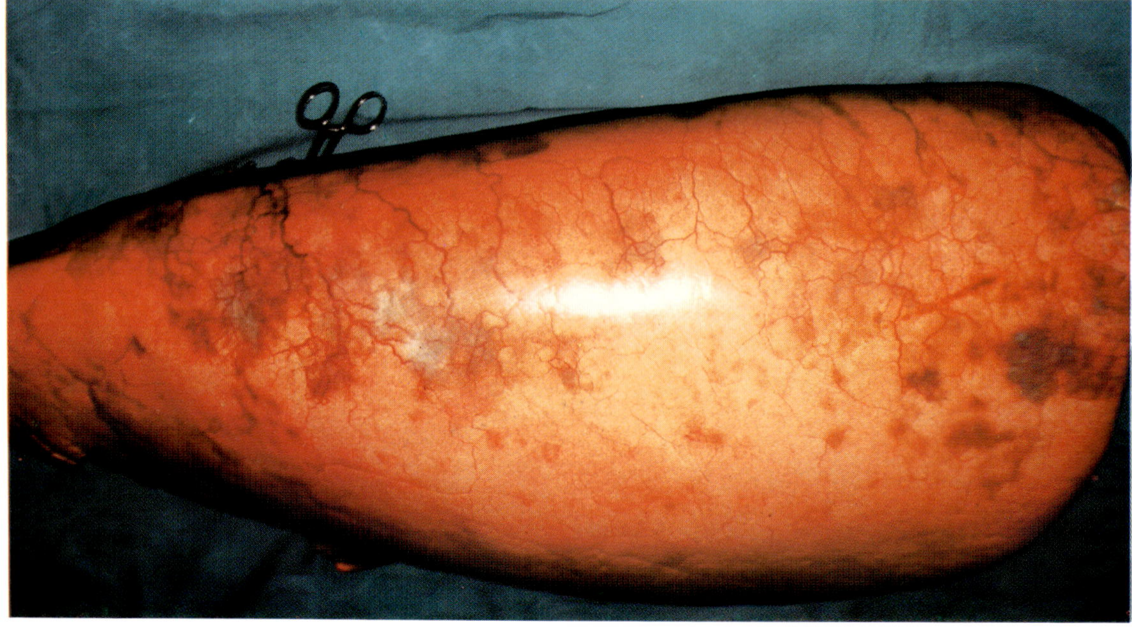

**FIG. 16–7.** Appearance of stained areas after lung inflation. Staining is light brown to bronze in color and appears to be confined to lobules.

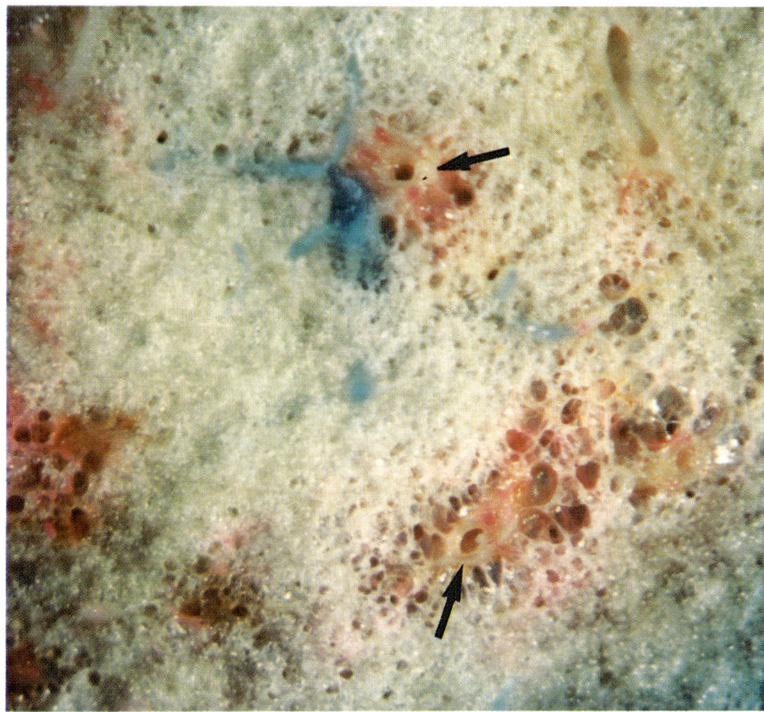

**FIG. 16–8.** Prominent bronchial arteries (red) are noted around abnormal small airways (arrows) and in regions with parenchymal distortion, where airspaces were enlarged.

inhaled particle deposition. Similarly the other dorsal bronchopulmonary segments have short straight bronchial divisions compared with the ventral bronchopulmonary segments.[36] Clearly studies of aerosol and particle deposition in the equine lung during resting breathing and various exercise loads are indicated.

The increased interstitial fibrosis evident in interlobular septa and interalveolar septa and around airways and vessels would likely contribute to a loss of pliability of the lung tissues in affected regions. This reduced regional compliance means that affected lung regions will be more difficult to expand than the surrounding normal lung. Because all lung regions are interconnected, nonuniform expansion of regions is likely to result in shear forces at the interface of regions with different compliance.[33] Depending on their magnitude, these forces could conceivably cause tissue disruption.[37] If airflow to this region of reduced compliance is also decreased because of small airway disease, then the distending forces from the expanding normal regions will be increased, further increasing shear stresses at the interface. It has been argued that horses may be more susceptible to these mechanical influences in the presence of small airway disease because their collateral ventilation is poor and pressure equalization in expanding partially obstructed segments may not occur within the inspiratory phase of the respiratory cycle during strenuous exercise.[33] Similar arguments can be developed to suggest that pulmonary alveolar capillary transmural pressure in poorly expanding segments may increase sufficiently to cause capillary rupture.[33]

The exact source of hemorrhage, pulmonary or bronchial circulation, has not yet been determined, nor is the type of vessel known. It has been widely assumed that the bleeding occurs from capillaries, but there is no proof of this concept. From subgross and microangiographic studies it seems likely that bleeding probably occurs from the developing collateral circulation once this is established; however, this also remains unproven. There are many unanswered questions concerning the distribution of the bronchial circulation in healthy and diseased horse lungs. The importance of bronchopulmonary anastomoses and their contribution to control of blood flow

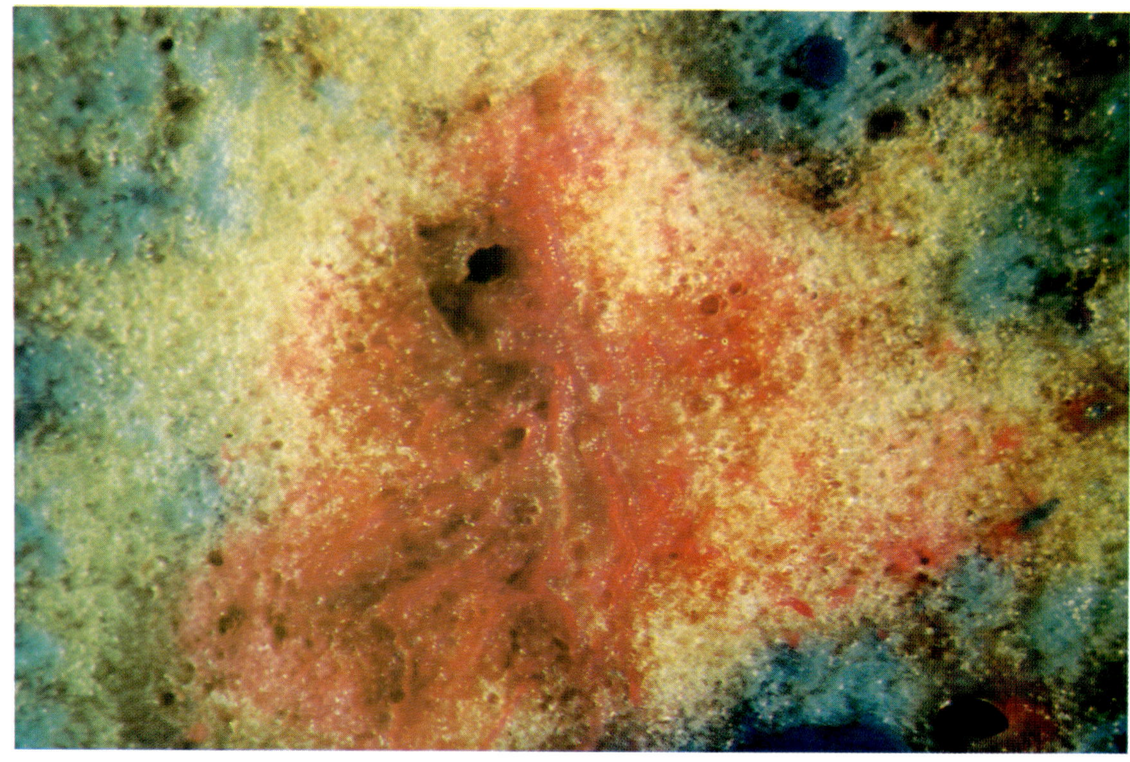

A

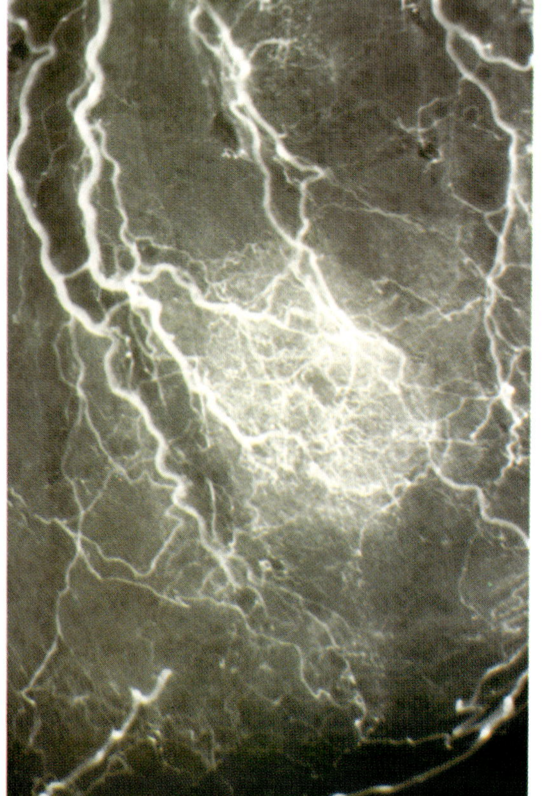

B

**FIG. 16–9.** Gross (A) and microangiographic (B) appearance of bronchial arterial neovascularization in stained regions of lung. The neovascularization appears to be centered around small airways.

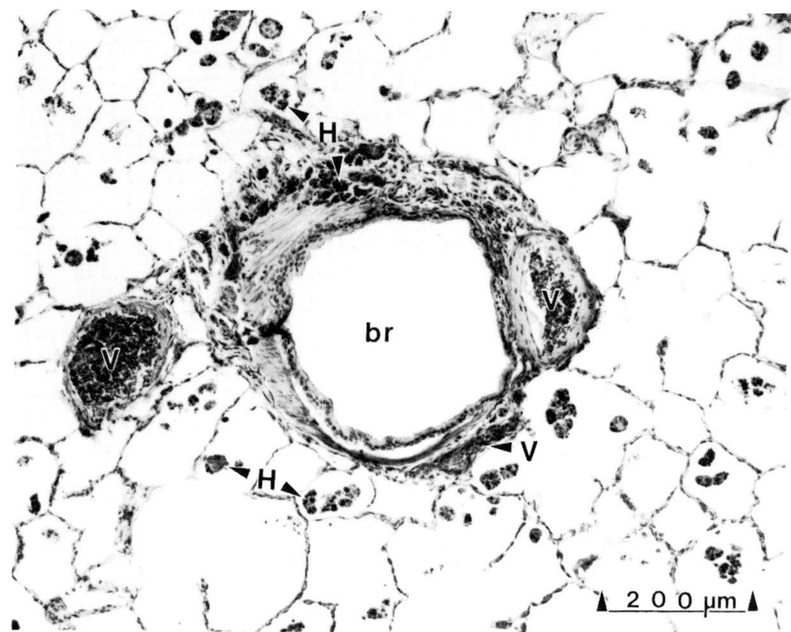


**FIG. 16–10.** Light micrograph showing the predominant histologic features of lungs from a horse with EIPH. Transverse section of a bronchiole (br) with increased peribronchiolar connective tissue and numerous adjacent vessels (V). Many macrophages containing hemosiderin (hemosiderophages, H) are identified within the airspaces and within the connective tissue. Hematoxylin and eosin. (Reprinted with permission from Equine Veterinary Journal 1987; *19*:411–418).

under different conditions are also unknown.[38]

Suffice it to say that EIPH is a topic that generates lively discussion and tempts speculation about its etiopathogenesis. It is also evident that considerably more investigation is needed before the credence of any of these ideas can be fully established.

## Treatment

The plethora of treatments in current use include diuretics, β-2 agonists, hormones, coagulants, hematinics, citrus pulp, bee pollen, and heated saturated water vapor. The diversity of these agents attests to the paucity of our knowledge about EIPH, the inventiveness of the prescribers, and the general frustration experienced by clinicians and horsemen in coping with this problem. Unfortunately there are few published efficacy studies on which to base reasonable judgments about the value of these different treatments. Given the chronic and apparently progressive nature of the lung lesions observed in horses with EIPH it is difficult to envisage a curative treatment and palliation of the signs without impairment of performance may be the best that can be achieved.

### *Furosemide*

Without doubt, furosemide is the most widely used and most controversial approved prerace medication for horses that experience EIPH.[11,39] Its origins as a treatment for EIPH are obscure but it is believed that it was originally prescribed on the assumption that EIPH might occur as a consequence of pulmonary edema. To date there is no evidence that maximally exercising horses experience pulmonary edema.

Initially the controversy over the use of furosemide concerned the influence of diuresis on the chemical detection of prohibited medications or their metabolites that are excreted in urine. With increased sophistication in drug testing methodology, this no longer presents a major problem and the controversy continues to focus on the influence of furosemide on performance.[39] Furosemide (1 mg/kg IV) did not improve performance in normal Standardbreds,[39] but has been shown to improve performance in Thoroughbred horses known to experience EIPH.[29] Although performance improved, it did not increase beyond their pre-EIPH performance level, based on racing times standardized for distance and adjusted for track differences.[29] The influence of furosemide on the performance of horses known not to experience EIPH is currently being investigated (CR Sweeney, personal communication).

Furosemide (0.3 to 0.6 mg/kg IV), if permitted, is given 3 to 4 hours prior to racing as mandated by state racing authorities. At least 50% of furosemide treated horses continue to experience EIPH and while furosemide may decrease the amount of bleeding it is not effective in preventing EIPH in most horses.[11,12] Furosemide (1 mg/kg IV) induces transient mild changes in cardiovascular performance in both resting and exercising horses.[40,41] Studies in treadmill exercised ponies 10 and 120 minutes after furosemide (1 mg/kg IV) administration have shown similar mild influences on cardiovascular function.[42] Mean aortic and pulmonary artery pressures are slightly attenuated at 120 minutes and these changes have been attributed to volume contraction with diuresis.[42,43] Unfortunately a study to mimic the drug's use under racetrack conditions with respect to dose and time of administration has not been performed. Considering the mild response noted with more acute study intervals it is doubtful that additional benefits might be obtained at the longer intervals mandated in racetrack practice.

Efficacy studies have reported some beneficial effect of furosemide in limiting EIPH in 50% of the horses studied.[11] Assuming that these were not false negative observations, by what other mechanisms might furosemide effect cardiorespiratory function? Renal release of prostaglandins has been reported after furosemide administration in other species. It has been speculated that if this occurred in horses and if the prostaglandins released were capable of inducing bronchodilation then some beneficial effect may ensue.

## *Hesperidin-Citrus Bioflavinoids*

Fed as a supplement, hesperidin-citrus bioflavinoid (28 g daily for 85 to 100 days) was not effective in preventing EIPH in 38 of 45 horses.[12]

## *Heated, Saturated Water Vapor*

This therapy evolved from the use of oxygen-enriched, heated, saturated water vapor as an adjunctive treatment for cystic fibrosis in children. The hot water vapor acts as a mucolytic to aid in the removal of respiratory secretions. Despite initial marketing claims to the contrary, this therapy has proven ineffective in controlling or reducing EIPH in Thoroughbreds.[13]

## Ancillary Management Considerations

Some trainers favor the practice of "drawing" a horse before a race. This includes restricting the intake of hay or hay and water the morning of the race and muzzling the horse if straw bedding is used. The intent of this practice is to reduce the mass of ingesta within the large intestine and theoretically reduce pressure on the diaphragm. It is unknown whether this practice reduces EIPH and the mechanical influences of this practice on respiratory function are also unknown.

Cook (1971) also advocated avoiding excessive tightening of the girth.[44] Normally the girth is positioned far cranially and its influence on chest wall mechanics and ultimately on lung function in horses is unknown.

## References

1. Pascoe JR, Ferarro GL, Arthur RM, et al. Exercise-induced pulmonary hemorrhage in racing Thoroughbreds: A preliminary study. Am J Vet Res, *42*:703, 1981.
2. Cook WR, Williams RM, Kirker-Head CA, et al. Upper airway obstruction (partial asphyxia) as the possible cause of exercise-induced pulmonary hemorrhage in the horse: An hypothesis. J Equine Vet Sci, *8*:11, 1988.
3. Cahill JI, Goulden BE. The pathogenesis of equine laryngeal hemiplegia—A review. NZ Vet J, *35*:82, 1987.

4. Markham G. Of Bleeding at the Nose. Chapter XX, Of Cures Chyrurgical. In: Markham's Masterpiece. London, 1681, pp 184–185.
5. Robertson W. A Text-Book of the Practice of Equine Medicine. London, Bailliere, Tindall and Cox, 1883, pp 484–491.
6. Robertson JB. Biological search-light on racehorse breeding. VI. The heredity of blood-vessel breaking in the Thoroughbred. Bloodstock Breeder's Review, *2*:265, 1913.
7. Hutyra F, Marek J. Pulmonary hemorrhage. In: Special Pathology and Therapeutics of the Diseases of Domestic Animals. Mohler JR and Eichhorn A (eds). Third authorized American edition, Vol. II. Chicago, Eger, 1926, pp 624–627.
8. Cook WR. Epistaxis in the racehorse. Equine Vet J, *6*:45, 1974.
9. Pascoe JR, Raphel CF. Pulmonary hemorrhage in exercising horses. Comp Cont Ed, *4*:S411, 1982.
10. Raphel CF, Soma LR. Exercise induced pulmonary hemorrhage in Thoroughbreds after racing and breezing. Am J Vet Res, *43*:1123, 1982.
11. Pascoe JR, McCabe AE, Franti CE, Arthur RM. Efficacy of furosemide in the treatment of exercise-induced pulmonary hemorrhage in Thoroughbred racehorses. Am J Vet Res, *46*:2000, 1985.
12. Sweeney CR, Soma LR. Exercise-induced pulmonary hemorrhage in Thoroughbred horses: Response to furosemide or hesperidin-citrus bioflavinoids. J Am Vet Med Assoc, *185*:195, 1984.
13. Sweeney CR, Hall J, Fisher JRS, et al. Efficacy of water vapor-saturated air in the treatment of exercise-induced pulmonary hemorrhage in Thoroughbred racehorses. Am J Vet Res, *44*:1705, 1988.
14. Beech J. Cytology of tracheobronchial aspirates in horses. Vet Pathol, *12*:157, 1975.
15. Whitwell KE, Greet TRC. Collection and evaluation of tracheobronchial washes in the horse. Equine Vet J, *16*:499, 1984.
16. O'Callaghan MW, Pascoe JR, Tyler WS, et al. Exercise-induced pulmonary haemorrhage in the horse: Results of a detailed clinical, postmortem and imaging study. V. Microscopic observations. Equine Vet J, *19*:411, 1987.
17. O'Callaghan MW, Pascoe JR, Tyler WS, et al. Exercise-induced pulmonary haemorrhage in the horse: Results of a detailed clinical, postmortem and imaging study. I. Clinical profile of the horses. Equine Vet J, *19*:384, 1987.
18. O'Callaghan MW, Pascoe JR, Tyler WS, et al. Exercise-induced pulmonary haemorrhage in the horse: Results of a detailed clinical, postmortem and imaging study. VI. Radiological/pathological correlations. Equine Vet J, *19*:419, 1987.
19. Pascoe JR, O'Brien TR, Wheat JD, et al. Radiographic aspects of exercise-induced pulmonary hemorrhage in racing horses. Vet Radiol, *24*:85, 1983.
20. O'Callaghan MW, Goulden BE. Radiographic changes in the lungs of horses with exercise-induced epistaxis. NZ Vet J, *30*:117, 1982.
21. Pascoe JR. Why does exercise-induced pulmonary haemorrhage occur? Equine Vet J, *17*:159, 1985.
22. O'Callaghan MW, Hornof WJ, Fisher PE, et al. Exercise-induced pulmonary haemorrhage in the horse: Results of a detailed clinical, postmortem and imaging study. VII. Ventilation/perfusion scintigraphy in horses with EIPH. Equine Vet J, *19*:423, 1987.
23. O'Callaghan MW, Pascoe JR, Tyler WS, et al. Exercise-induced pulmonary haemorrhage in the horse: Results of a detailed clinical, postmortem and imaging study. III. Subgross findings in lungs subjected to latex perfusion of the bronchial and pulmonary arteries. Equine Vet J, *19*:394, 1987.
24. Bayly WM, Meyers KM, Keck MT, et al. Effects of exercise on the hemostatic mechanism of Thoroughbred horses displaying post-exercise epistaxis. J Equine Vet Sci, *3*:191, 1983.
25. Sweeney CR, Soma LR. Exercise-induced pulmonary hemorrhage in horses after different competitive exercises. In: Equine Exercise Physiology. Snow DH, Rose RJ, Persson SGB (eds). Cambridge, Granta 1982, pp 51–56.
26. Voynick BT, Sweeney CR. Exercise-induced pulmonary hemorrhage in polo and racing horses. J Am Vet Med Assoc, *188*:301, 1986.
27. Apel GA. Untersuchungen zum Vorkommen belastungsinduzierten Lungenblutens beim Rennpferd in Westdeutschland. Inaugural Dissertation, Hanover, 1988.
28. Hillidge CJ, Whitlock TW. Sex variation in the prevalence of exercise induced pulmonary hemorrhage in horses. Res Vet Sci, *40*:406, 1986.
29. Soma LR, Laster L, Oppenlander F, et al. Effects of furosemide on the racing times of horses with exercise-induced pulmonary hemorrhage. Am J Vet Res, *46*:763, 1985.
30. O'Callaghan MW, Pascoe JR, Tyler WS, et al. Exercise-induced pulmonary haemorrhage in the horse: Results of a detailed clinical, postmortem and imaging study. II. Gross pathology. Equine Vet J, *19*:389, 1987.
31. O'Callaghan MW, Pascoe JR, Tyler WS, et al. Exercise-induced pulmonary haemorrhage in the horse: Results of a detailed clinical, postmortem and imaging study. IV. Changes in the bronchial circulation demonstrated by CT scanning and microradiography. Equine Vet J, *19*:405, 1987.
32. Rooney JR. The lungs. In Autopsy of the Horse: Technique and Interpretation. Baltimore, Williams & Wilkins, 1970, pp 113–119.
33. Robinson NE. Functional abnormalities caused by upper airway obstruction and heaves: Their relationship to the etiology of epistaxis. Vet Clin N Am: Large Anim Pract, *1*:17, 1979.
34. Clarke AF. Review of exercise induced pulmonary hemorrhage and its possible relationshlip with mechanical stress. Equine Vet J, *17*:166, 1985.
35. Deffebach ME, Charan NB, Lakshminarayan S, et al. The bronchial circulation: Small, but a vital attribute of the lung. Am Rev Resp Dis, *135*:463, 1987.
36. Hare WCD. The respiratory system. In: Sisson and Grossman's The Anatomy of the Domestic Animals, 5th Ed. R Getty (ed). Vol 1. Philadelphia, WB Saunders Co, 1975, pp 498–523.
37. Mead J, Takishima T, Leith D. Stress distribution in the lungs: A model of pulmonary elasticity. J Appl Physiol, *25*:596, 1970.

38. O'Callaghan MW, Pascoe JR, Tyler WS, Mason DK. Exercise-induced pulmonary haemorrhage in the horse: Results of a detailed clinical, postmortem and imaging study. VIII. Conclusions and implications. Equine Vet J, *19*:428, 1987.
39. Tobin T, Roberts BC, Swerczek TW, et al. The pharmacology of furosemide in the horse. III. Dose and time relationships, effects of repeated dosing and performance effects. J Equine Med Surg, *2*:216, 1978.
40. Muir WW, Milne DW, Skarda RT. Acute hemodynamic effects of furosemide administered intravenously in the horse. Am J Vet Res, *37*:1177, 1976.
41. Milne DW, Gabel AA, Muir WW, et al. Effects of furosemide on cardiovascular function and performance when given prior to simulated races: A double-blind study. Am J Vet Res, *41*:1183, 1980.
42. Manohar M. Effect of furosemide administration on systemic circulation of ponies during severe exercise. Am J Vet Res, *47*:1387, 1986.
43. Goetz TE, Manohar M. Pressures in the right side of the heart and esophagus (pleura) in ponies during exercise before and after furosemide administration. Am J Vet Res, *47*:270, 1986.
44. Cook WR. The cause of ear, nose and throat disease in the horse. British Racehorse, August 1971, p 327.

# CHAPTER 17

# NASAL PASSAGES

*DAVID E. FREEMAN*

Diseases that obstruct the nasal passages are rare in horses but are poorly tolerated because they have a profound effect on air flow. In addition, diagnosis and treatment of lesions in the caudal nasal passages are difficult because of the latters' inaccessibility and because of the complex anatomy of this part of the upper respiratory tract.

## Anatomy

The horse has large, widely spaced nostrils that are supported medially by the alar cartilages. Fibrous tissue and, in some horses, a joint connects each alar cartilage medially to the nasal septum and allows it to undergo considerable movement.[1] Dorsal to the lamina of the alar cartilage, the nostril leads into a blind cutaneous pouch, called the nasal diverticulum or false nostril. This diverticulum is separated ventrally from the true nostril or vestibule by a thick fold of skin, the alar fold.[1] Medially, the alar fold is continuous with the skin and mucosa of the nostrils and nasal passages and its lateral edge is free and curved ventrally so that the separation of the nasal diverticulum from the nasal cavity is incomplete.[1]

The nasal cavity is divided into two halves by the nasal septum and vomer bone. The septum is composed of hyaline cartilage that blends with the perpendicular plate of the ethmoid bone at the caudal end of the nasal cavity.[1] Its ventral border rests in a groove of the vomer bone caudally and on the palatine processes of the incisive bones rostrally and the dorsal margin is attached to the frontal and nasal bones.[1] The ventral part of the nasal septum is covered by an abundant venous plexus.[1]

The lateral aspect of each nasal cavity is divided longitudinally into the dorsal, middle and ventral meati by the dorsal and ventral conchae[2] (Fig. 17–1). The conchae are composed of delicate scrolls of bone that are attached laterally and coil in opposite directions medially toward the middle meatus.[2] The largest is the dorsal concha and its caudal part is in direct communication with the frontal sinus[2] (Fig. 17–1). Its rostral part is divided by septa into several independent cells or cavities, each with separate openings into the middle nasal meatus.[2] The ventral conchal sinus is similar in design, with its caudal part in direct communication with the rostral maxillary sinus and its rostral part divided into cells[2] (Fig. 17–1). At the level of the first cheek tooth, both conchae are attached rostrally by prominent folds of mucous membranes[1] (Fig. 17–1). These folds and the ventral part of the ventral nasal concha contain a dense submucosal plexus of veins.[1]

The ethmoidal labyrinth projects rostrally from the cribriform plate into the nasal cavity on both sides of the perpendicular plate of the ethmoid (Fig. 17–1). It is a complex structure made up of numerous, delicate, scroll-like bones, called the ethmoturbinates or ethmoidal conchae.[2]

The ventral meatus is the largest of the three nasal meati[1] (Fig. 17–1). It combines with the common nasal meatus, which is the

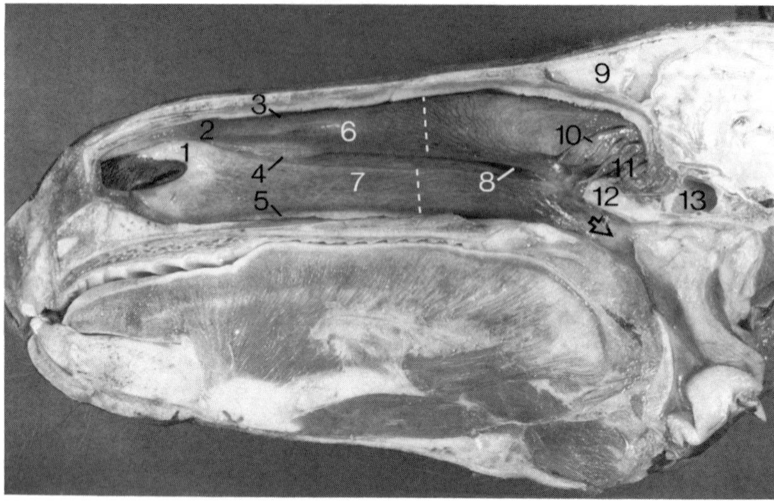


**FIG. 17–1.** Sagittal section of horse's head. 1 = Junction of alar fold and ventral nasal concha; 2 = dorsal conchal fold; 3 = dorsal nasal meatus; 4 = middle nasal meatus; 5 = ventral nasal meatus; 6 = dorsal concha; 7 = ventral concha; 8 = approximate location of the nasomaxillary opening, which is concealed by the dorsal concha; 9 = septum between frontal sinuses; 10 = middle nasal concha; 11 = ethmoturbinates; 12 = vomer bone; 13 = sphenopalatine sinus. Arrow is passing through the right choana into the nasopharynx. Broken lines mark the separation between scrolled portions of the dorsal and ventral conchae rostrally from the caudal parts that communicate with the frontal and maxillary sinuses.

narrow, vertical channel between the nasal septum and conchae, to form the principal respiratory passage.[1] The ventral nasal meatus also provides the most convenient route for passage of instruments through the upper respiratory tract; however, failure to maintain instruments along the floor of the ventral meatus can cause copious hemorrhage from injury to submucosal veins on the nasal septum and ventral concha. The ventral nasal meatus leads directly into the nasopharynx through the choanae.[1,2] Each choana is an almost horizontally disposed opening caudal to the caudal edge of the hard palate and separated from the other by the vomer bone[1,2] (Fig. 17–1).

The skin of the nostrils and vestibule is continued within the nasal cavity by a pseudostratified columnar ciliated epithelium which contains numerous goblet cells. Many mucoserous glands are contained within the mucosa of the nasal cavity. The caudal, dorsal parts of the nasal cavity are covered by a thick, olfactory epithelium.

## Function

Functions of the nasal cavity are olfaction and warming, moistening, and filtering inspired air. It is a major conduit for inspired air during strenuous activity because the horse is limited to nasal breathing.[3] Upper airway resistance constitutes a significant fraction of total airway resistance in the horse and 80 to 90% of this fraction can be attributed to the nasal cavity.[3,4] Resistance is usually greater during inspiration than during expiration and most resistance from the nasal cavity arises from within the nostrils.[3] Resistance at this site can be attributed to collapse of soft tissue structures during inspiration and this collapse is opposed by dilatation of the nostrils during strenuous breathing.[3] Air flow through the meati encounters little if any change in resistance[3] and may be enhanced by vasoconstriction of vessels in the ventral conchae and the nasal septum.[5]

## Examination

One should attempt to obtain a history regarding the duration of the problem, previous trauma or surgery, the response to any previous treatment, the nature of abnormal respiratory noises, and the effect of the problem on the horse's exercise tolerance. The nostrils and external parts of the nasal passages should be viewed from directly in front of the horse to determine any asymmetry in size and shape and, during strenuous breathing, for any asymmetry in movement. Any nasal discharge should be noted for color, consistency, odor, and presence of any blood. Differences in air flow between each nostril should be compared by placing the palms of both hands over them during normal breathing. Each nostril can be closed manually and air flow then noted from the other side during this procedure.[6] The nostrils, alar fold, and alar cartilages should be palpated and the nasal vestibule should be examined by careful digital palpation. The examination should be performed with the horse at rest and again shortly after exercise.

## Endoscopy

The nasal passages can be examined by means of a 10- to 12-mm diameter colonoscope. Because the floor of the nostril is higher than the floor of the ventral meatus,[5] gentle downward pressure should be applied to the endoscope during insertion to ensure that it is directed ventrally. The tip of the endoscope should be advanced along the floor of the ventral meatus until it is in the nasopharynx. From that point, it is slowly withdrawn and the tip turned dorsally to view as much of the nasal passage as possible. When an abnormality is found, the distance from it to the nostril is measured by markings on the endoscope. Other parts of the upper respiratory tract should be examined also to rule out diseases that can cause similar clinical signs. The opposite nasal passage should be examined and any difference in width noted. Marked encroachment of the nasal septum or conchae into the nasal passage can be seen on endoscopic examination but subtle changes are difficult to assess. If nasal obstruction is so severe that the endoscope cannot be passed up the involved side, it should be inserted in the other side and the tip turned caudally around the vomer bone to examine the caudal aspect of the affected nasal passage.

In order to detect lesions on the dorsal aspect of the ventral concha, a pediatric endoscope with a 7-mm diameter tip should be directed into the middle meatus. However, many horses resent this procedure and may struggle and traumatize the nasal mucosa and induce copious hemorrhage. Heavy sedation or even general anesthesia may be required for adequate safe examination of fractious horses.

## Radiography

The nasal passages are air-filled cavities that provide a natural negative contrast medium for surrounding bone and cartilage and soft tissue densities. Satisfactory lateral radiographs of the horse's head can be obtained by using portable equipment with the horse conscious but sedated. A rope halter without metal fittings is used to eliminate confusing radiopacities. A short exposure time is required to eliminate motion and this can be accomplished by using ultrafast rare earth screen/film combinations. Grids are unsuitable for skull radiographs on the standing horse because they prolong exposure time and are difficult to position.

The normal cartilage of the nasal septum and associated soft tissues are radiolucent on lateral radiographs;[7] however, on dorsoventral projections, the nasal septum and its mucosal coverings are radiodense and are not obscured by overlying bones.[7] Although the dorsoventral projection is the most useful radiographic method of evaluating the nasal passages of the horse, special techniques and powerful units may be required to obtain sufficiently diagnostic radiographs.[8] Care must be taken to center the beam on the midline because the nasal passages and septum cannot be adequately evaluated on oblique views.[8]

## Biopsy

Portions of lesions on the rostral end of the nasal passage can be removed for biopsy under direct view through the nostrils. A portion of the tissue can be cultured and the remainder examined histologically. Samples should be submitted for culture on Sabouraud's or similar fungal culture medium when fungal infection is suspected. A portion of the lesion can be digested in potassium hydroxide and examined on a wet mount after staining with lactophenol cotton blue or similar stain for fungal elements.

If the lesion is located in the caudal part of the nasal cavity, a uterine biopsy forceps can be used to remove a portion of it under endoscopic guidance; however, care should be taken during this procedure because of the risk of inducing copious hemorrhage. The biopsy forceps of the fiberoptic endoscope remove only a superficial portion of the lesion, and this may not provide diagnostic information.

## Diseases of the Nasal Passages

### *Atheroma*

An atheroma, which is actually misnamed, is a sebaceous cyst that forms a firm, subcutaneous, spherical swelling caudal to the dorsal commissure of the nostril in the nasoincisive notch.[9–13] The condition is usually but not exclusively unilateral and is usually seen in young horses.[9–12] The lesion is painless and, although it can progressively enlarge with time, rarely causes upper airway obstruction.[9] Contents of an atheroma vary from a thin watery fluid in small lesions to a thick, greasy, dark gray substance in larger ones.[13]

***Treatment.*** Surgical removal of an atheroma is usually requested as a cosmetic procedure.[14] Surgery can be performed on the standing, conscious horse with local anesthetic infiltration of the surgery site or an infraorbital nerve block.[11] A longitudinal skin incision is made over the cyst and it is carefully dissected from the surrounding subcutaneous tissues.[14] The skin edges are then apposed with nonabsorbable suture material.[14] To avoid formation of a scar on the nostrils, the cyst can be removed through an incision on its undersurface, by approaching it through the false nostril or nasal diverticulum.[11,14] Alternatively, the cyst may be drained into the nasal diverticulum and the cavity thoroughly swabbed with tincture of iodine.[13] Recurrence is more likely after this method than after excision.[12]

### *False Nostril Noises*

An abnormal noise heard during work and less frequently at rest can be attributed to abnormal alar folds in some horses.[15] It is not possible to characterize the alar fold abnormality in every case but the condition has been attributed to excessive or thickened alar folds[9] or to a functional problem, possibly involving the transversus nasi muscle, which elevates the alar cartilages and closes the opening into the nasal diverticulum during deep breathing.[15] The condition is seen most often in young horses when first placed into work.[9] In male horses under 3 years of age, the unerupted upper canine teeth may also reduce width of the nasal vestibule and thereby exacerbate the problem.[9]

***Clinical Signs.*** During work, a low keyed, harsh whistling or snoring noise can be heard on inspiration and to a greater extent on expiration.[9,15] In some horses, the noise that is heard at rest is similar to that heard in tranquilized horses, especially those under the influence of xylazine.[9] Although the problem seldom reduces exercise tolerance,[9] flaccid alar folds that are drawn passively into the nasal passages during inspiration can increase upper airway resistance.[3,4]

***Diagnosis.*** Diagnosis is based on history and clinical signs, especially an evaluation of the noise as heard under normal working conditions. The noise is similar to that made by a horse with laryngeal hemiplegia but is primarily heard during expiration and has an obvious external origin.[15] The first step of the examination should be digital palpation of the alar fold, false nostrils, and the vestibule of the nostrils. Frequently, it is difficult to palpate any abnormality in these areas and the normal, ventral curve of a free edge of an alar fold should not be confused with excessive tissue. Subjective accurate assessment of the size of the alar folds is difficult. Some affected horses have a slightly abnormal and pinched appearance to the nostrils with collapse of the alar cartilages and a deep nasal diverticulum.[15] The abnormal noise should not be confused with the rattling noise that some horses make with the nasal diverticulum during expiration, called "high blowing."[10,11] "High blowing" is largely due to excitement and should disappear as the horse is worked.[11]

The most satisfactory diagnostic step is to maintain the alar cartilages and the fold in the fully dilated position by means of a temporary suture and to work the horse while this is in place.[9] Local anesthetic is infiltrated and a heavy suture material is placed in mattress fashion through the alar folds, caudal to the alar cartilages.[6,9] It is tied over the nasal bones so that the nostrils are fully dilated.[6,9] If the suture reduces or eliminates the noise at work, a diagnosis of abnormal alar folds can be made.[9]

***Treatment.*** If the preceding diagnostic step eliminates the noise, the horse may benefit from resection of the alar folds.[15] This procedure is performed with the horse under general anesthesia. The skin and hair are cleaned with a mild antiseptic soap externally and within the nasal diverticulum and nostril.[14] The alar fold is then uncurled and its edges are grasped with two or more Allis tissue forceps along the free margin.[15] The lateral margin of the nostril is also retracted from the surgical field. The incision is started caudal to the alar cartilage toward the medial attachment of the alar fold and is then continued caudally to remove as much of the fold as possible, including some of the accessory cartilage at the most rostral limit of the ventral concha.[14,15] Heavy surgical scissors or electrocautery are preferable to sharp dissection because the area is quite vascular and hemorrhage is pronounced from the resected end of the ventral concha.[14,15] The incised edges of skin and mucosa are sutured together dorsally and ventrally along the line of resection with a continuous pattern of absorbable suture material.[14,15] The horse is then turned over so that the procedure can be performed on the other side. The procedure can be completed more easily if the lateral walls of the nasal diverticulum are incised.[14,15] However, this is undesirable in show horses because the skin incision may leave a blemish over the nostrils. If an incision is made over the lateral wall of the nasal diverticulum, this should also be sutured in a continuous pattern starting along the inner lining of the wall first and then continuing along the external edges.

***Prognosis.*** Healing is usually rapid and by first intention. The horse can resume training in 1 to 2 weeks after surgery and the prognosis is generally favorable.

## *Laceration of the Nostrils*

If wounds of the nostrils are allowed to heal by second intention, the resulting scar formation can cause stenosis and restrict movement of the alar cartilage.[11,16] Consequently, air flow is restricted and exercise tolerance reduced.[11,16] Therefore, first intention healing should be the aim and can be accomplished by careful debridement and apposition of the wound edges with the horse sedated or following regional anesthesia of the infraorbital nerve. After surgery, the horse may have to be put in cross-ties to prevent it from rubbing the wound against a wall or in a cradle to prevent it from rubbing the wound against its forelegs.[11] If healing is by second intention and the nostrils become stenotic, the opening can be enlarged by double apposing Z-plasty.[16]

Treatment of wounds associated with fractures of the nasal and frontal bones and fistulas into the nasal passages or sinuses is described in Chapter 18.

## *Foreign Bodies and Concretions*

Occasionally, foreign bodies such as grass seeds, twigs or thorn branches become lodged in the nasal passages.[10] These cause considerable discomfort, head shyness and epistaxis but clinical signs usually resolve rapidly after removal.[10,11,17] For example, a mineralized concretion firmly embedded in the nasal mucosa of 1 horse caused a foul smelling, slight mucopurulent nasal discharge with recurrent epistaxis over a 3-year period, but clinical signs disappeared shortly after surgical removal.[17] Diagnosis is usually based on endoscopic examination but may sometimes require radiography or xeroradiography.

## *Paralysis of the Nostrils*

Muscles that retract the walls of the nostrils and collapse the nasal diverticulum by retraction of the alar folds are innervated by the 7th cranial (facial) nerve.[1,11] Any injury to this nerve at a part other than the lower buccal branch will result in nasal asymmetry at rest and failure to dilate the nostrils during deep inspiration.[11] Damage to both nerves or a central lesion causes bilateral paralysis and collapse of both nostrils so that air flow is markedly reduced.[11] Traumatic injuries to the facial nerve may be ameliorated by treatment with anti-inflammatory agents during the acute stages.[6]

The paralysis can resolve with time but, if present for 6 weeks or more, carries an unfavorable prognosis.[6] In these cases, the chances of return to athletic performance can be improved by removing skin over the nostrils along the edges of the nasoincisive notch and removing the alar folds. Although this method may restore air flow to normal, the resulting defects in the nostrils are unsightly and may be considered undesirable by some owners.

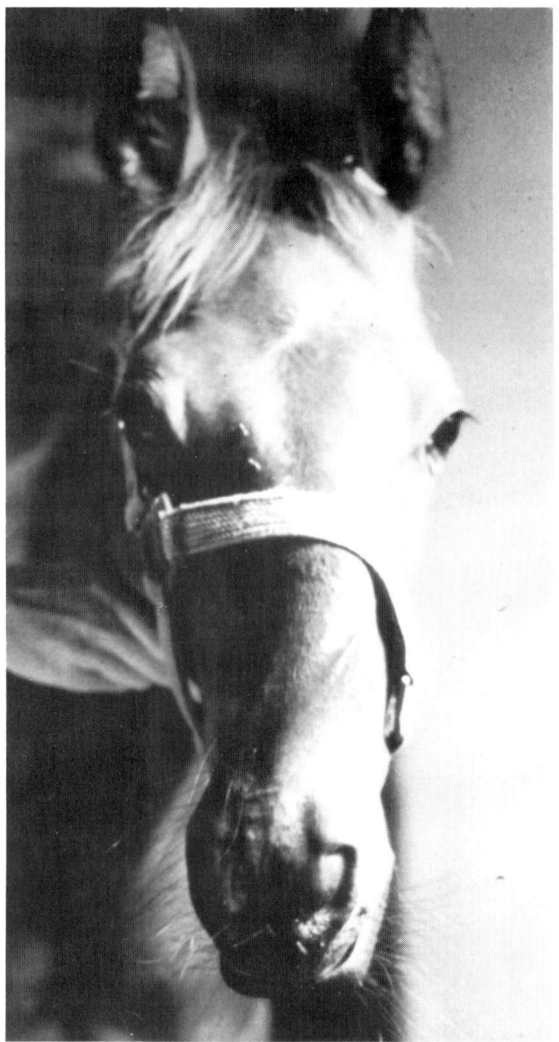

**FIG. 17–2.** Yearling with severe wry nose. Treatment was not attempted.

## *Wry Nose*

Wry nose is a congenital defect characterized by marked deviation of the maxilla, nasal bone, incisive bone, and nasal septum to one side and a sigmoid appearance and dorsal hump of the opposite side[18] (Fig. 17–2). There may also be a corresponding but milder deviation of the most rostral part of the mandible[19] and a foal with severe wry nose can also have a cleft of the soft and hard palate.[20] Affected horses make an abnormal noise on both inspiration and expiration but may not have difficulty with mastication or prehension of food, in spite of a severe malocclusion of the incisor teeth.[18,21] The cause is unknown, but an unfavorable intrauterine position[19,21] or genetic and other factors may be involved.

Surgical treatment can improve the facial contour and air flow through the nasal passages[18,21] but at least two surgical procedures may be required. The first involves an intraoral approach and a transverse osteotomy of the incisive bone, realignment of the upper incisor teeth with the lower incisors and augmentation of the short segment of incisive bone with an autogenous rib graft.[18] Steinmann pins are inserted across the osteotomy lines to stabilize the repair. In a second surgical procedure, the nasal septum is removed and the nostrils are enlarged by cosmetic surgery.[18,21] Although surgery can produce some improvement,[18,21] the procedure is difficult and expensive, the horse may not be capable of strenuous activity afterward, and the final appearance of the nose may not be normal.[18,21] Some improvement can be expected over time without surgery[21] and can be complete in mild cases.[19]

## Amyloidosis

Amyloidosis is the deposition of glycoprotein fibrils in various organs, apparently in response to continued immunologic or other stimulation of the reticuloendothelial system.[22] Case examples are horses used for antiserum production.[23] It is believed that the liver produces a serum protein in response to chemical mediators liberated during chronic inflammation and that macrophages process this protein into amyloid fibrils.[22–24] The actual cause of amyloidosis is unknown[22] and a primary disease or stimulus cannot be identified in all cases.[22–24]

In horses, the upper respiratory tract seems to be a common site of amyloidosis.[22–24] In this rare disease, amyloid deposits are usually found in the nostrils, on the alar folds, along the septum and conchae, and, in exceptional cases, in the pharynx, guttural pouches, larynx, and lymph nodes of the head.[22–24]

***Clinical Signs.*** Clinical signs of amyloidosis include nasal discharge, reduced exercise tolerance, dyspnea, epistaxis, weight loss, and the presence of raised, firm, nonpainful, nodular or plaque-like swellings on the nostrils, nasal septum, and floor of the nasal cavity (Fig. 17–3).[23,24] Nodules are usually smooth-walled but ulcerate and bleed easily when traumatized.[24] Even long-standing nodules have only a moderate degree of associated inflammation.[24] There is no evidence for predisposition due to age, breed, or sex.[24]

***Diagnosis.*** Nodules in the most rostral end of the nasal passages can be seen through the nostrils.[24] Proliferative masses extending farther caudally along the nasal passages and in the pharynx and larynx can be seen on endoscopic examination.[24] The diagnosis is established on histopathologic examination of biopsy specimens from the nodules.[24] Paraffin-embedded sections stained with Congo red have light green birefringence.[22–24] If these sections are treated with dilute sulfuric acid and potassium permanganate before staining with Congo red, they lose their congophilia and much of the light green birefringence.[22,24]

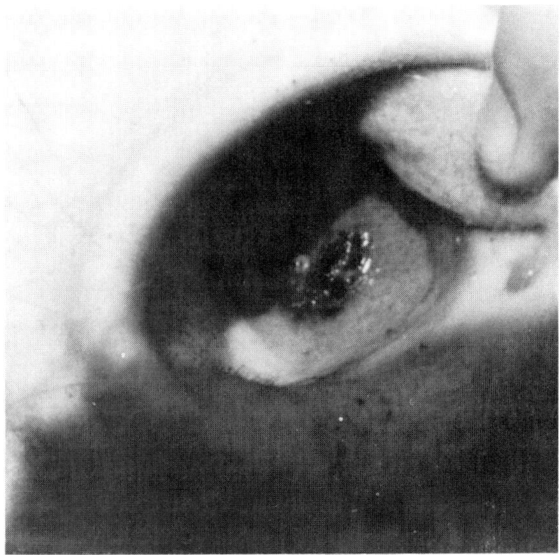

FIG. 17–3. Amyloidosis. Raised brownish green plaque with a slightly roughened surface on the mucosa of the rostral nasal septum.

***Treatment and Prognosis.*** In one series of four horses, treatment with topical and systemic corticosteroids, either alone or in combination, was unsuccessful.[24] However, surgical removal of the nodules in all four horses, along with the alar folds when these structures were involved, was effective and allowed the horses to return to their former use without recurrence over a 1-year follow-up period.[24]

## Fungal Diseases

Fungal diseases of the upper respiratory tract in horses are rare and sporadic. Many of them are difficult to treat because they are frequently extensive and available antifungal agents are too expensive, too toxic or ineffective against the causative organisms. Also, the true relationship between some fungi and the infection is unclear because these are opportunistic invaders that can flourish in a host with impaired resistance or in wounds or tissues that are devitalized by an existing lesion. However, predisposing causes are rarely identified. Direct transmission of a fungal disease to other animals is rare.[25]

Because fungal diseases in horses frequently differ by site of distribution, difficulty

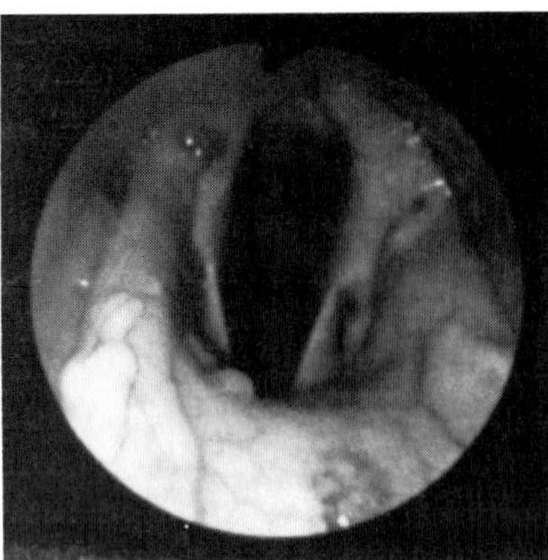

**FIG. 17–4.** Phycomycosis affecting the larynx. Granulomatous and ulcerated lesions are present on the arytenoids and epiglottis. (Photograph courtesy of Dr. James Schumacher.)

of treatment and prognosis, they will be discussed separately.

## Phycomycosis

Phycomycosis is one of the most frequently reported fungal infections in the nasal passages of horses,[26–29] with most cases in the United States originating from Texas.[25] The organism involved in phycomycosis of the nasal passages (rhinophycomycosis) is Conidiobolus coronata, an inhabitant of soil and decaying vegetation.[25,26] The disease is more common in swampy areas or hot climates.[27,28] The organism has a high affinity for skin of the nostrils and nasal passage mucosa, where it causes granulomatous and ulcerated lesions with hard, pale, elongated masses of necrotic tissue. Lesions may also occur on the larynx (Fig. 17–4). These masses are called "leeches"[25] or "kunkers"[28] and contain hyphae.

The infection can be focal or systemic, but the upper respiratory form is usually confined to the primary site.[25,29] Although phycomycosis on the limbs of horses may develop at the site of a previous injury,[25] trauma may not be required to initiate rhinophycomycosis.[26–28]

***Clinical Signs.*** Rhinophycomycosis can cause dyspnea[27,28] and may be severe enough to occlude the nostrils.[26,29] The lesion is usually confined to the rostral part of the nasal cavity, where it can be seen protruding from the nostril and septum as a mass of granulating nodules.[27–29] "Leeches" may protrude from the surface.[27] The lesion can cause intense pruritus that provokes the horse to mutilate it and cause surface ulceration and hemorrhage.[25,27,28] The lesion may expand into the oral cavity and in severe cases may distort the lips and impair eating, resulting in weight loss.[27,29] The condition can be unilateral or bilateral[26] and may extend caudally into the nasal passages.[29]

***Diagnosis.*** Rhinophycomycosis can be recognized by clinical signs and appearance of the lesion. Endoscopy can be used to determine the most caudal limits of lesions in the nasal passages.[27–29] The elongated, gray to yellow, hard necrotic nodules within the granulation tissue are diagnostic features.[29] The lesion can be confused grossly with squamous cell carcinoma, habronemiasis, or sarcoid.[28] A biopsy should be taken and primary isolation attempted on Sabouraud's dextrose agar. Masses of hyphae can be seen in wet mounts prepared from leeches after they have been digested in 20% KOH[26] or in sections stained with silver and periodic-acid Schiff stains.[28] Leeches must be included in biopsy samples because the surrounding granulation tissue may not contain hyphae.[25]

***Treatment.*** Complete surgical excision of the masses of granulation tissue may be successful[28] and can be combined with postoperative topical treatment.[26] Recurrence is common. Usually the lesion is so advanced at the time of diagnosis that treatment is difficult. Amphotericin B injected intralesionally and applied topically with DMSO is reported to have been successful.[27] However, topical treatment may be of little value in extensive lesions because of inadequate penetration.[26] Intravenous amphotericin B has been successful against phycomycosis at other sites.[30]

## Cryptococcosis

This rare disease is caused by Cryptococcus neoformans, a yeast-like saprophyte that is distributed widely in nature and can be found in barnyard soil and manure.[25] In horses, infection is most common in the nasal cavity,[31] and the lips, lungs, and meninges are less common sites.[25] Pulmonary and neurologic infections have an acute fulminating course,[25] whereas infections in the nasal cavity are chronic.[32] Infections that begin as nasal granulomas can extend to the lungs and small intestine[32] and can involve the paranasal sinuses[30] and orbit, the nasopharynx, ethmoturbinates,[33] nasal septum, and dorsal and ventral conchae.[34,35] Lesions can cause considerable bony erosion, disruption, and compression of adjacent sinus walls and nasal septum.[32–35]

***Clinical Signs.*** Signs are determined by the site of infection. Intranasal lesions cause mucopurulent, malodorous, blood-tinged unilateral nasal discharge and dyspnea.[32–35] Horses with severe, protracted infections can lose weight.[34] Dysphagia has been reported in a horse with a large mass that extended into the nasopharynx and impinged on the soft palate.[31] If visible, the lesion can be recognized as a large, lobulated, firm swelling[25,32] and may contain numerous cysts.[35] External deformation of the sinuses and periorbital tissues may be severe and blindness has occurred due to a postorbital mass.[33]

***Diagnosis.*** Early diagnosis is important because the disease poses a potential human health hazard.[31,33] Biopsy specimens can be taken from lesions in the most caudal parts of the nasal cavity by means of the biopsy instrument of the fiberoptic endoscope or through trephine openings into the nasal openings or sinuses. On histopathologic examination of a biopsy specimen, organisms can be seen stained with hematoxylin and eosin and periodic acid-Schiff reagent[31] and can be grown on a culture of the nasal discharge.[32] Also, if material is suspended in India ink and examined microscopically, the organisms can be recognized as budding yeast cells with a thick mucoid capsule.[25,31,35] On radiographs, smooth, well-demarcated masses may be seen in the nasal passages and sinuses.[32] Masses can be seen in the caudal part of the nasal passages on endoscopic examination.[32] Immunologic techniques are useful for presumptive diagnosis and for prognosis in human beings[36] and animals with cryptococcosis.[37,38] There are no reports of their use in horses.

***Treatment.*** Amphotericin B may be effective against this organism but infection is usually too advanced to treat by the time the diagnosis is made. In one case that involved the frontal and maxillary sinuses, treatment with IV amphotericin B daily for 33 days was unsuccessful but cryotherapy eliminated the infection.[30] Oral ketoconazole has been used successfully in treatment of nasal cryptococcosis in cats.[37] This drug is strongly fungicidal against Cryptococcus neoformans in vitro and could be considered for treatment of nasal cryptococcosis in horses.[39] In horses, 30 mg/kg orally twice daily was not reported to cause undesirable side effects over several days but absorption was variable.[40] Neither the effects of long-term therapy in horses nor its efficacy in fungal infections have been reported. Immunologic tests may be a valuable noninvasive means of assessing the response to medical and surgical treatment[36–38] but, as previously mentioned, have not been described for the horse.

## Coccidioidomycosis

Coccidioides immitis occurs in the soil and may be endemic in some areas of the southwestern United States and in South America.[25,41] Infection can cause disseminated disease or localized nodules and granulomas in man and animals, including horses.[25,41] Localized coccidioidal granulomas have been reported in the nasal cavity of horses, originating from the cribriform plate, frontal bone, and ethmoturbinate region and extending to the sinuses and nasopharynx.[41,42] Infection is usually confined to these sites, where it causes considerable damage.[41,42]

***Clinical Signs.*** This disease can present as a slowly developing, chronic disease.[41,42] Clinical signs include mucopurulent nasal discharge, epistaxis, reduced exercise tolerance, and abnormal respiratory noise, even at rest in some cases.[41,42]

***Diagnosis.*** Endoscopic examination is usually required to make the diagnosis because lesions are most commonly found in the caudal part of the nasal passages.[41] The lesion can be recognized as a smooth-walled, glistening mass protruding into the nasal passages.[41] On radiographs, it appears as a smooth-walled, soft tissue density in the nasal passages.[41] Chronic pyogranulomatous reactions with thick layers of fibrous tissue and typical Coccidioides immitis spherules can be seen on histopathologic examination of biopsies.[41,42] Immunologic methods of diagnosis have been used in other animals for this infection[38] and various methods of detecting Coccidioides antigen or antibody to the organism are available,[36] but their use in horses has not been described.

***Treatment.*** Surgical removal is the treatment of choice,[41,42] but infection has been known to recur subsequently at different sites.[42] To approach the lesion, trephine holes may have to be placed through the nasal bone and into the nasal cavity or into the maxillary sinus if this is involved.[41] Oral ketoconazole has been used successfully for treatment of coccidioidomycosis in other species[43] and could be considered for this disease in horses.[40]

## Aspergillosis

Aspergillus fumigatus has been isolated from mycotic plaques in the middle meatus and on the ventral concha of horses.[44]

***Clinical Signs and Diagnosis.*** Affected horses have foul-smelling, scanty nasal discharge and less consistent findings are intermittent epistaxis and submandibular lymph node enlargement.[44] The lesion may be obscured in the recess of the middle meatus, making endoscopic diagnosis difficult.[44] Biopsy material and purulent nasal discharge can be removed through the endoscope and the organisms identified on cultures and smears.[44] Immunologic methods used to diagnose aspergillosis in other animals[38] have been unreliable for nasal aspergillosis in horses.[44]

***Treatment.*** Topical natamycin infused through the endoscope or nystatin powder insufflated on the affected nasal passage for 3 to 11 days has been reported to be successful and recovery can be enhanced by debridement of the mycotic plaque with the biopsy instrument of the endoscope prior to topical treatment.[44] The apparently favorable response to treatment in this report should be interpreted with full awareness that the efficacy of these drugs against Aspergillus species is controversial.[45–50] Topical amphotericin B, miconazole and ketoconazole have each been reported to be effective in treatment of keratomycosis due to Aspergillus species.[47,48] Although in vitro sensitivity testing has been suggested for aid in selecting optimal therapy,[46] in vitro testing itself is imprecise.[47]

## Rhinosporidiosis

The organism responsible for rhinosporidiosis in animals and man, Rhinosporidium seeberi, is considered a fungus based on morphologic features but it cannot be grown successfully on artificial media.[25,51] Rhinosporidiosis is a rare disease that is seen sporadically in the southern United States and in other countries.[25] One or several sessile or pedunculated small polyps can be seen at the opening of the nostril around the nasal septum but other clinical signs are rare.[25,51] Diagnosis is based on histopathologic examination of biopsy specimens.[51] Surgical removal is frequently successful but must be complete to avoid recurrence, and additional lesions may develop at adjacent sites.[25,51]

## Mycetomas

Mycetoma (maduromycosis or maduromycotic mycetoma) is a term used to denote infections characterized by local, lobulated swellings, and granulomas that contain abscesses and draining tracts, and are caused by the higher fungi.[25] Lesions can be single or multiple and develop on skin and mucous membranes in several sites with some evidence that a wound or repeated irritation is required to start infection.[25] Pseudallescheria boydii causes human mycetoma and was isolated from a superficial, calcified mass on the conchae, frontal and sphenopalatine sinuses of a horse.[52] Horses with nasal infection have a mucopurulent nasal discharge and epistaxis.[52] Endoscopy is required to assess lesions deep in the nasal passages.[52] A biopsy of the lesion should be submitted for histopathologic examination and culture. Lesions that are well circumscribed can be removed surgically[25] and can be treated topically with a drug effective against the organism involved.[52]

## Miscellaneous

Small, superficial mycotic plaques can develop on the most rostral end of the nasal septum in young horses and cause mild, intermittent epistaxis but rarely other clinical signs. No single organism has been isolated consistently from cases seen at this clinic and, in some horses, more than one fungus and several bacteria can be found in representative biopsy specimens. Treatment by curettage of the plaques, chemical debridement by vigorous rubbing with sponges soaked in Lugol's iodine, topical treatment with antifungal agents or thiabendazole, alone or in combination, have been used successfully. However, treatment may have to be applied for several weeks before lesions regress fully. It is unknown if untreated lesions would spread or resolve spontaneously.

## *Diseases of the Nasal Septum*

Diseases of the nasal septum are rare.[53] Most are congenital abnormalities that usually remain undetected until the horse is worked, unless associated with external signs such as facial asymmetry or abnormal shape of the nasal bones.[9] Traumatic injury to the nasal septum (Fig. 17–5) includes accidents during nasogastric intubation, falls, collision with solid objects, and kicks from other horses.[53] "Cystic" degeneration of the septum can be congenital or can develop following severe respiratory infections.[53] Other less common causes of nasal septum disease are hyperplasia of the nasal cartilage associated with edematous tissue and reactive cartilage,[7] amyloidosis,[24] fungal diseases,[25,34,35] and squamous cell carcinoma.[54] Failure to change a foal's halter can cause a permanent defect in the septum because the nose becomes compressed as it outgrows the noseband.[6]

***Clinical Signs.*** The most common clinical signs of nasal septum thickening or deviation are low-pitched stertorous breathing and dyspnea during exercise, usually in young horses.[53] The abnormal respiratory noise is usually louder on inspiration[9] and can be evident at rest in some horses.[53] Facial deformity such as deviation or prominence of the nasal bones may be evident but is not consistent.[9]

***Diagnosis.*** History of recent or past injury to the nose indicates the need for thorough examination of the nasal passages and the nasal septum in particular. Septal abnormalities in the most rostral end can be detected by palpation and can be seen through the nostril.[53] History may reveal difficulty in passage of a nasogastric tube through one nasal passage.[53]

On endoscopic examination, the extent and severity of septal injury can be determined. A flexible fiberoptic endoscope is used for this purpose. Dorsoventral radiographs are more useful than lateral views and radiographic changes include deformity, deviation, and thickening of the radiopaque outline of the cartilage (Fig. 17–6). Biopsies of any nodules or discrete and localized lesions on the septum may help to identify tumors, amyloidosis or fungal infections. Information obtained from radiographs and from endoscopy should be combined to determine the surgical approach and the amount of nasal septum that must be removed to eliminate the lesion.[53]

***Treatment.*** Treatment involves resection of the abnormal nasal septum. Blood loss of 4 to 8 L can be expected during surgery; although transfusions are infrequently required, a blood donor identified by crossmatch should be available. Intravenous balanced polyionic electrolyte solutions should be given during surgery at an average rate of 8 to 10 L per hour.[53]

The horse is placed under general anesthesia in lateral recumbency and a tracheotomy is performed. The dorsal aspect of the face is prepared for aseptic surgery and an 18-mm circular trephine hole is made in the midline of the nose immediately rostral to the frontal sinus (Fig. 17–7). This point is identified as the level at which the nasal bones diverge from a parallel course towards the medial canthus of the eyes (Fig. 17–7). The nasal septum is then compressed by a Doyen intestinal forceps or similar instrument inserted through the trephine hole.[13] The most rostral end of the nasal septum is incised from top to bottom with a hardbacked or cartilage scalpel at least 5 cm caudal to the most rostral end, provided that transection at this level is sufficient to remove all the lesion.[13] The cut end of the septum is grasped with vulsellum forceps and, because hemorrhage at this time is quite profuse, it is important to proceed rapidly.

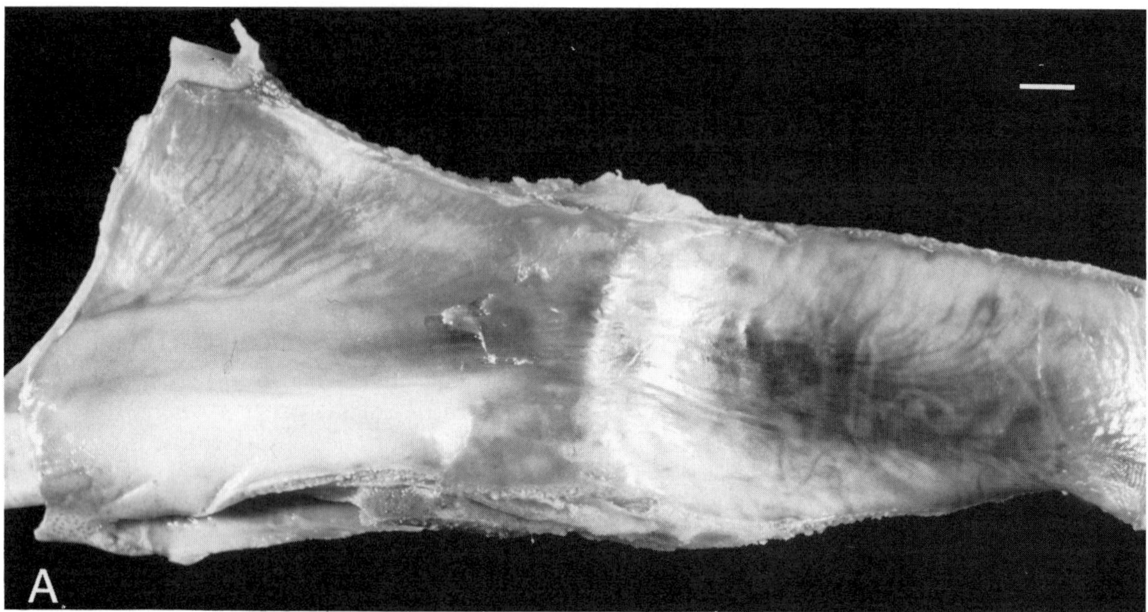


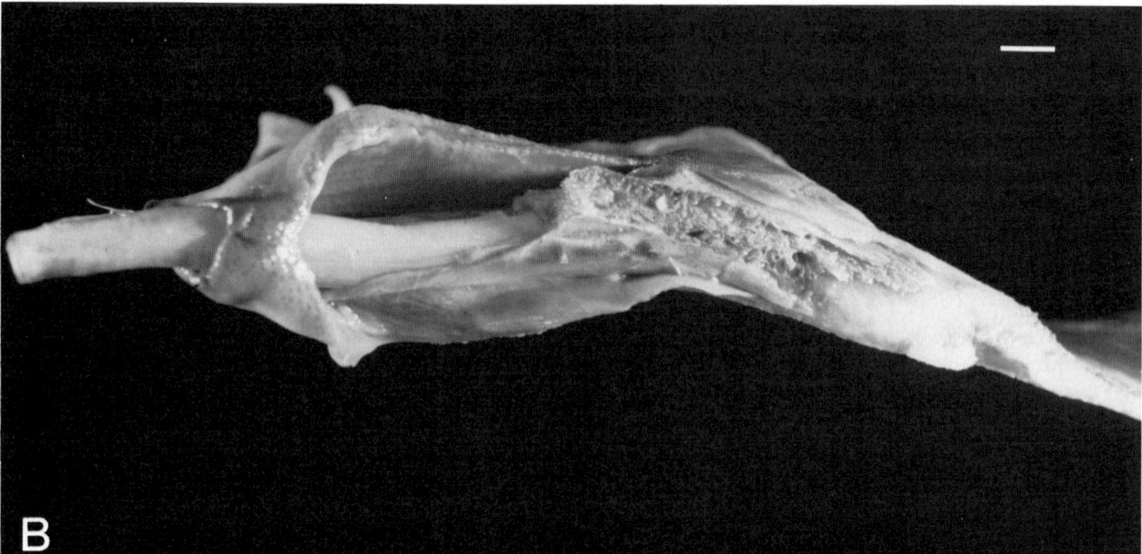


**FIG. 17–5.** Septum removed from the horse in Figure 17–6A. A. Side view of septum removed by technique with obstetrical wire (see text). The septum is buckled and thickened as a result of previous blunt trauma to the face. The bar is 1 cm. B. Ventrodorsal view showing deviation and thickening of the septum. The bar is 1 cm.

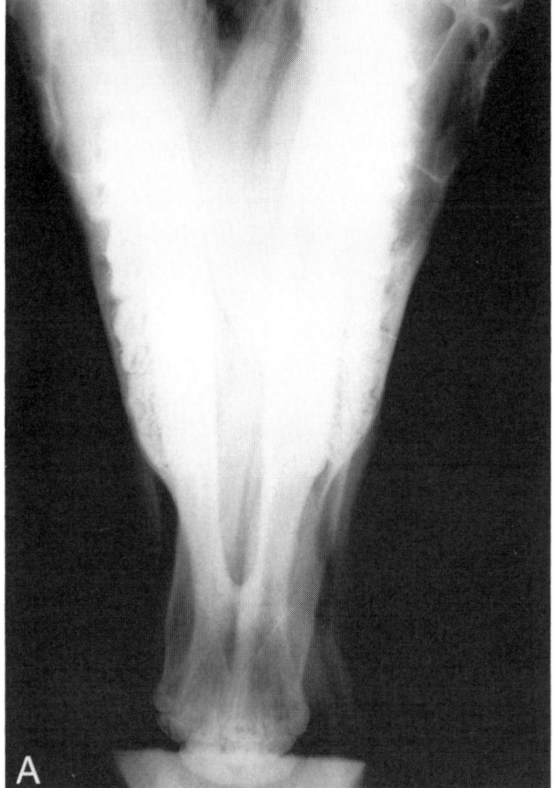


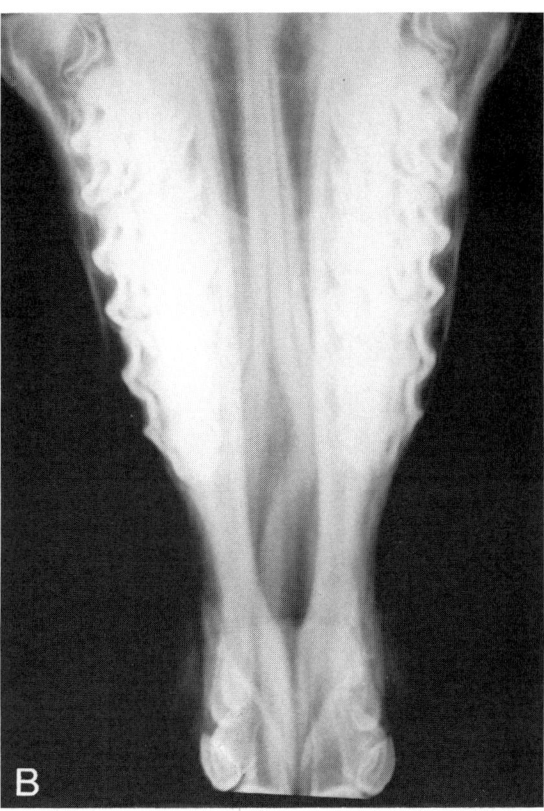


**FIG. 17–6.** Dorsoventral radiographic views of nasal septum deformities in horses. A. Horse with severe, trauma-induced septal thickening and deviation (see Fig. 17–5). The entire length of the nasal septum is involved and the nasal passages are occluded. The upper respiratory obstruction was reduced by surgical removal of the septum. (Courtesy of Dr. Peter Bousum.) B. Yearling with septal deviation possibly caused by fracture. (Courtesy of Dr. Peter Bousum.)

Tension is applied to the forceps and a guarded chisel is used to sever the dorsal and ventral attachments back to the level of the intestinal clamp.[13,53] An osteotome or a wide screwdriver with a sharp concave notch ground into its tip can be used to cut the nasal septum flush with the intestinal forceps.[53] Traction is applied through the vulsellum forceps to extract the severed nasal septum through the nostrils. To control the copious hemorrhage that ensues, the nasal passages are packed with the sterile gauze soaked in 1:10,000 epinephrine solution. This is sutured to the nostrils to retain the tampon of gauze in position for the next 48 to 72 hours when it is removed.[13]

A limitation of the preceding method is failure to remove any diseased portion that is behind the most caudal line of resection[53] (Fig. 17–8). Also, when the caudal incision in the septum is directed vertically from the trephine hole, the raw edge of remaining septum is at a point approximately 10 mm from the ventral conchae[53] (Fig. 17–8). If excessive granulation tissue subsequently forms on this edge, it will reduce the width of the nasal passage and can adhere to the adjacent conchae.[53]

A method was therefore devised to place a caudal incision in the septum at a 120° angle to the nasal bones and directed toward the most rostral extent of the sphenopalatine sinus[53] (Fig. 17–8). The purpose of this is to remove any diseased segment in the caudal part of the nasal septum and to place the cut surface of remaining septum at a wide segment of nasal passages where subsequent swelling is unlikely to disrupt air flow.[53] The trephine hole is placed as described and a 10-F catheter is then inserted along the dorsal

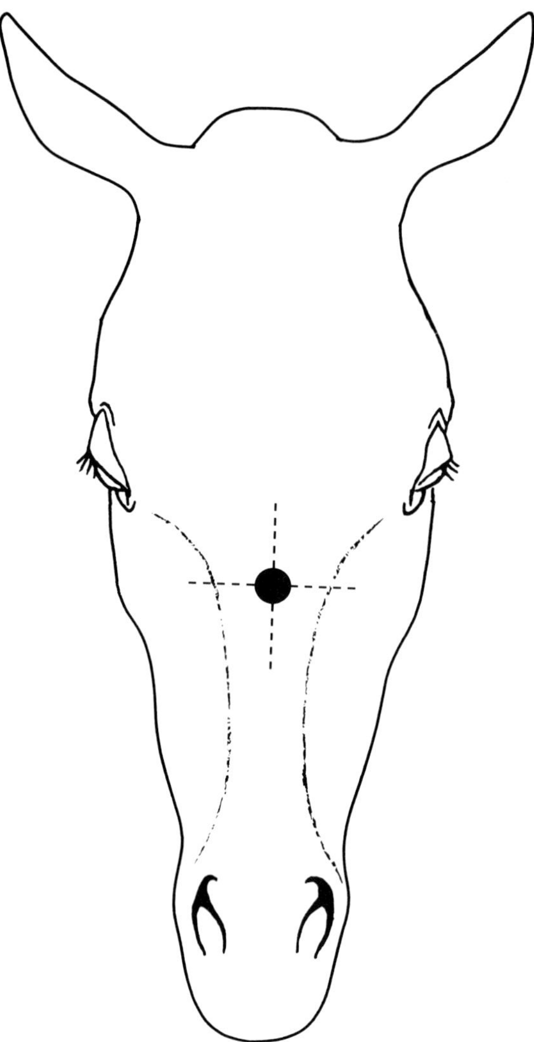

**FIG. 17–7.** Location of trephine hole in the skull at intersection of midline with a line through the point where nasal bones diverge toward the eyes. For septum removal, the caudal cut in the septum is made through this hole (see text for details).

meatus on one side until its tip can be seen at the trephine hole. A long segment of obstetrical wire is then passed through the catheter and retrieved through the trephine hole. This end of the wire is then passed through the trephine hole on the opposite side of the nasal septum and threaded in a rostral direction until it can be retrieved through the nostril (Fig. 17–9). Another length of obstetrical wire is passed along the ventral meatus of one nasal passage as far caudally as possible and the horse is extubated.[53] A hand is then passed through the mouth and the end of the obstetrical wire is retrieved by fingers passed around the caudal edge of the soft palate (Fig. 17–10). The retrieved end of wire is brought through the mouth around the caudal edge of the soft palate (Fig. 17–10). This procedure is repeated on the other side with another length of obstetrical wire. The two free ends of the obstetrical wire that extend from the mouth are spliced together by means of 1 in. adhesive tape (Fig. 17–10). Then, the free end of a wire that extends from the nostril on one side is slowly withdrawn to pull the spliced ends back through the mouth, over the soft palate and through the nasal passage on that side (Fig. 17–10). When the spliced ends are brought through the nostril, they are disconnected and handles are applied to the free ends of the single wire that extend from each nostril (Fig. 17–10). The rostral incision is then made in the nasal septum as described.[53] The dorsal and ventral attachments of the septum are severed using the obstetrical wires to the level of the rostral incision.[53] A caudal incision is made at a 120 degree angle to the nasal bones using an osteotome fashioned from a standard wide screwdriver with a v-shaped notch ground into its tip.[53] The septum is then removed and the nasal passage packed as described.

In addition to the advantages described, the wires cut the nasal septum attachments cleanly, whereas several cuts may be required with a chisel when the septum is markedly deviated or thickened.[53] In addition, the guarded chisel can traumatize adjacent conchae.[53] In a small horse or foal, the biopsy instrument of the flexible fiberoptic endoscope may have to be used to retrieve the free end of the obstetrical wire in the pharynx.[53] If only the rostral end of the nasal septum is involved, it may be possible to excise the involved portion through a longitudinal incision in the dorsal aspect of the nasal diverticulum.[53]

Postoperative care includes parenteral antibiotics and nonsteroidal anti-inflammatory agents. The packing is removed 48 to 72 hours after surgery and, on the following day, the nasal cavity is flushed with warm water from a hose through the trephine opening to remove dried blood, debris and small fragments of tissue and bone. The tracheotomy tube is

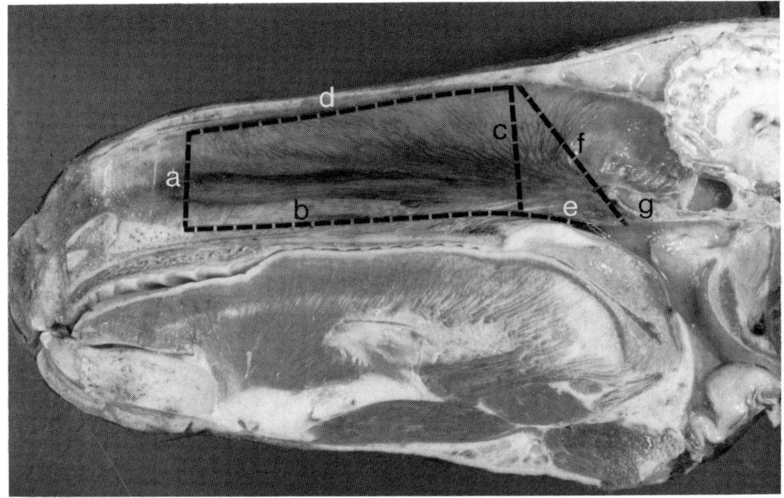


**FIG. 17–8.** Sagittal section of head to show portions of septum removed by guarded chisel technique (lines a,b,c, and d) and by obstetrical wire technique with angled caudal cut (lines a,be,f and d). With the latter technique, lines be and d are cut with obstetrical wire as described in text. Line f forms a 120° angle with the nasal bones. g = Sphenopalatine sinus.

removed at the same time. The open incisions, such as the tracheotomy and the trephine site, are cleaned daily and can be coated with antibiotic ointments with or without corticosteroids (to prevent exuberant granulation tissue). These treatments are continued for approximately 2 weeks, by which time all incisions have healed by second intention. Horses are rested for approximately 2 months before they return to normal activity.[53]

***Prognosis.*** In a survey of 22 horses that underwent removal of the nasal septum, 13 of 18 with followup information (72%) did not make a respiratory noise at rest; however, 16 (90%) made a noise during work, although this was considered less than before surgery.[53] Nine horses (50%) did not have respiratory difficulties during work and 7 of these returned to their original use, including racing.[53] Thirteen horses had excellent cosmetic results but 5 had some flattening of the nose at the level of the nasal diverticulum.[53] This could be attributed to removal of too much of the rostral end of the nasal septum, thereby leaving inadequate support for the bridge of the nose and nasal diverticula.[53] This problem seems to be most common in foals under 6 months of age.[53,55] In some horses with nasal flattening, the alar fold was later removed to increase airway size.[53]

## *Neoplasia and Neoplasia-like Lesions*

Neoplasia of the nasal passages is rare. In a 9-year survey of tumors in nasal passages and sinuses in domestic animals from 13 university hospitals in the United States and Canada over a 9-year period, 13 neoplasms in horses were in the nasal passages and 9 in the sinuses.[56] In an 8-year survey from a single university hospital, 16 neoplasms were found in these sites and twice as many were found in the sinuses as the nasal passages.[21] The percentage of these tumors that are malignant in horses has been reported as approximately 50% in one study[21] and 68% in another.[56] Horses 15 years of age or older are at higher risk than young horses.[56] Tumors of the nasal passages can metastasize to other sites, usually to adjacent lymph nodes, but most are confined to the primary site where they cause considerable destruction and infiltration of surrounding tissues.[54,57] Although most tumors in the paranasal sinuses and the nasal cavities are sporadic, endemic tumors were described in Norway and Sweden in the early part of this century.[58] Viruses can cause nasal tumors in other species,[58] but limited attempts to implicate them in horses have been unsuccessful.[59,60]

Squamous cell carcinoma is the most common tumor in the sinuses and nasal passages of horses.[54,56,58] Other types of tumors in the nasal passages include fibromas, hemangiosarcoma, adenocarcinoma, chondroma, fibrosarcoma,[56] myxomas,[61] poorly differentiated carcinomas,[21,57] neurofibroma, mast cell tumors,[21] and lymphosarcoma.[62,63] Fibrous dysplasia is not a tumor but a benign fibro-osseous lesion of bone of unknown cause,

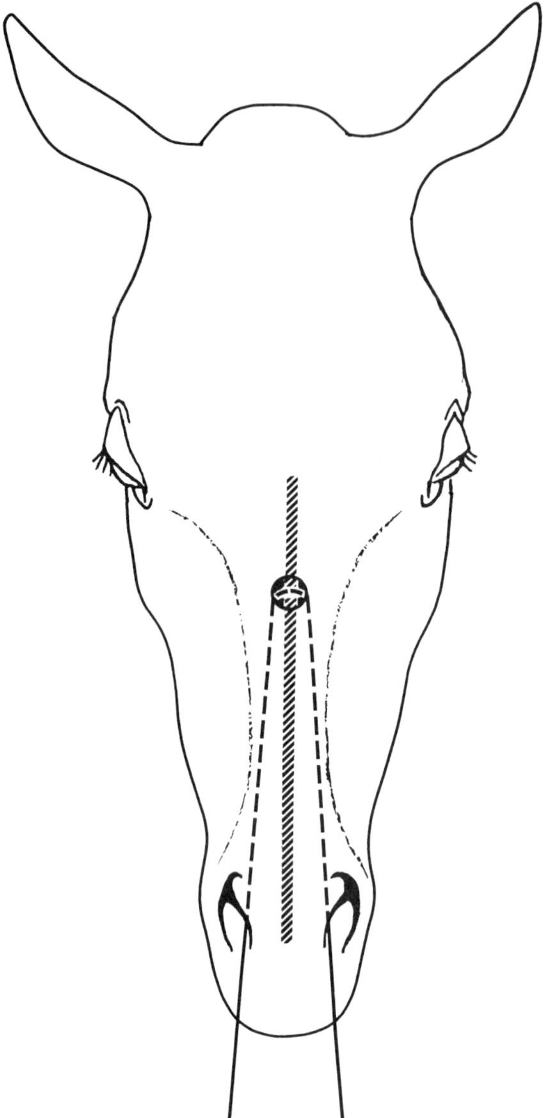

FIG. 17–9. Placement of obstetrical wire to make cut in nasal septum along line d in Figure 17–8. The wire is placed over the septum through the trephine hole (see text for details).

and it has been described in the ventral meatus of a 7-month-old colt.[64]

***Clinical Signs.*** Tumors of the nasal passages cause chronic disease similar to chronic sinusitis. The horse may be in poor condition, have unilateral or bilateral mucopurulent nasal discharge, sometimes stained with blood, abnormal respiratory noise at rest or during work, dyspnea, and facial deformity. The lesion may be externally visible if it involves the rostral part of the nasal passages.[54]

***Diagnosis.*** Tumors of the nasal passages can be difficult to differentiate from polyps, ethmoid hematomas, osteodystrophy, congenital abnormalities of the teeth and sinuses, fungal infections, and sinusitis. If a part of the lesion is accessible through the nostrils, a biopsy can be used to make a histopathologic diagnosis. Radiographs and endoscopic examination can be used to show the extent and the severity of the lesion.

***Treatment.*** If the tumor is localized, it may be possible to resect it and part of the tissues from which it originates. However, the condition is usually too advanced with too much tissue destruction by the time the diagnosis is made. The anatomy of the nasal passages is also complex and part or all of the tumor may not be readily accessible through most surgical approaches. The high risks of recurrence and the possibility of metastasis to other organs also worsen the prognosis for recovery after surgical treatment.[57]

## Nasal Polyps

A nasal polyp is a pedunculated growth that arises from the mucosa of the nasal cavity and also from the nasal septum or tooth alveolus.[9] Polyps are usually unilateral and single, but bilateral cases and multiple growths can develop.[9,65] They form as a result of hypertrophy of the mucous membrane or as exuberant proliferation of fibrous connective tissue in response to chronic inflammation.[57,65] The cause is unknown and they can develop in horses of any age, breed, or sex.[65]

***Clinical Signs.*** Nasal polyps can cause nonspecific clinical signs such as dyspnea, unilateral mucopurulent nasal discharge with a foul odor, and occasionally epistaxis.[9,13,65] As the polyp enlarges, it may extend rostrally until it protrudes beyond the nostrils. It is round, ovoid or pedunculated, with a firm or rubbery consistency and a smooth, slimy surface, sometimes interrupted with roughened areas and ulcerations.[65] It is usually white but some areas may be pink to red.[13,65,66] The size varies but a polyp up to 30 cm in length has been described.[13]

***Diagnosis.*** Diagnosis is not difficult if the most rostral end of the polyp can be seen

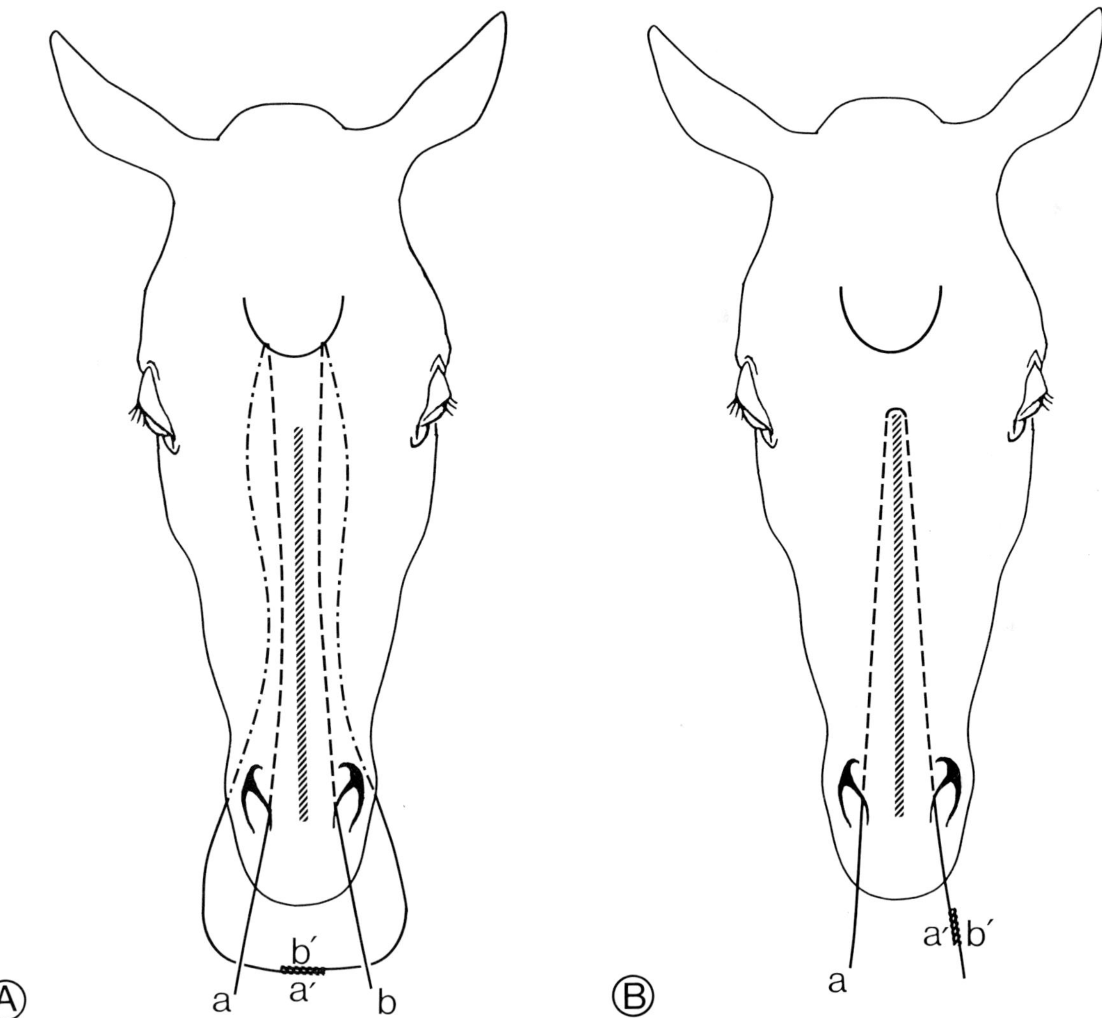


**FIG. 17–10.** Placement of obstetrical wires to make cut along line be in Figure 17–8. A. Wire a is passed through the right nasal passage and its end, a′, is retrieved around the caudal edge of the soft palate by a hand passed through the mouth. Wire b is inserted in a similar fashion and its end, b′, is also brought out through the mouth. The ends a′ and b′ are spliced together with adhesive tape. Segments of wires in nasal passages are represented by broken lines and segments in the mouth are represented by broken and dotted lines. B. Wire b is gently pulled through the left nasal passage, drawing the intraoral loop formed by both wires around the edge of the soft palate and into the left nasal passage. Continued withdrawal of wire b brings the spliced ends of both wires, a′, b′, through the left nostril. In this way, wire a is looped completely around the ventral edge of the vomer bone and is seated against the junction of the vomer with the hard palate. At this point, a′ is disconnected from b′ and wire aa′ is used to make cut be in Figure 17–8.

through the nostrils. On histologic examination, polyps are found to be composed of mature and immature fibrous tissue that is sparsely cellular and edematous, well-vascularized and covered with cuboidal and columnar epithelium.[65] There may be evidence of recent hemorrhage, superficial erosion, infection, and granulation tissue.[57,65]

Polyps that are still contained deep within the nasal passages can be seen on endoscopic examination, almost completely filling the ventral meatus. If the endoscope is passed up the opposite nostril, the caudal border of the mass can be seen, in some cases extending around the caudal edge of the nasal septum.[66] The extent and possibly the origin of the mass may be determined on radiographic examination.[9]

***Treatment.*** Polyps are removed surgically with the horse in lateral recumbency under general anesthesia with the affected side uppermost. If the mass originates from the rostral ¼ of the nasal passage, it can be exposed through an incision in the roof of the false nostril extending caudally to the nasoincisive notch.[14] The polyp is then bluntly dissected from the underlying mucosa and the site of attachment should be curetted to remove any remaining abnormal tissue.[14] Hemorrhage from the site of attachment is profuse and necessitates packing of the nasal passage with sterile gauze soaked in 1:10,000 epinephrine solution. This can be removed after 48 hours.[14]

If the mass is attached further caudally in the nasal passage, a trephine opening should be made over the approximate point of attachment and sufficiently lateral to the midline so that the nasal septum will not be injured.[13] If necessary, the trephine openings can be enlarged with rongeurs or by combining several trephine openings.[14] The polyp is then removed as described above. It can also be removed through a sinus bone flap.[21]

A polyp can be removed by cutting its stalk with a wire snare inserted through the nostrils and guided by a hand inserted through the mouth.[66] Recurrence is likely after this because it is difficult to remove all the abnormal tissue.[66]

## Choanal Atresia

A bucconasal membrane separates the primitive buccal or oral cavity from the nasal pits during embryologic development of mammals.[67] Rupture of this membrane establishes a communication between the caudal nasal cavity and the pharynx. Failure to rupture causes choanal atresia. Both bilateral and unilateral cases have been described in the horse.[68–70] The partition between the nasal passages and nasal pharynx can be a complete or partially thin or opaque membrane[68] and can contain cartilage, bone, and nasal epithelium.[69]

***Clinical Signs and Diagnosis.*** Clinical signs become evident immediately after birth in bilateral cases because the foal experiences severe dyspnea and air cannot be detected passing through the nostrils.[68–70] A nasogastric tube passed through the ventral meatus will be obstructed at the level of the medial canthus of the eye. If the condition is unilateral, the foal can survive but may subsequently have partial airway obstruction.[70] On endoscopic examination, it is evident that the tip of the endoscope can only be advanced to the caudal end of the nasal passages at which level it encounters an obstruction.[69] If radiographs are taken after liquid contrast material is instilled into the caudal part of the nasal passages, it will coat the obstructing membrane but will not pass into the nasopharynx.[69]

***Treatment.*** Bilateral complete choanal atresia is a life-threatening condition and a tracheotomy must be performed immediately after birth to save the foal's life.[68–70] Definitive treatment can be undertaken when the foal becomes stable. Forceful rupture of the membrane is not recommended because this could damage the cribriform plate and the brain in a foal.[68,69] It may be possible to perforate a thin membrane by electrocoagulation or by the laser, but these have not been used in the horse for this purpose.[68] In one foal, successful surgical treatment involved an approach to the caudal nasal passage through bilateral flaps centered along the midline followed by removal of the obstructing tissue and bone by combinations of sharp and blunt dissection.[69]

In addition, the caudal 2 to 3 cm of the nasal septum was removed and the nasal cavity was packed with gauze to reduce postoperative hemorrhage.[69] Indwelling stents, such as canine endotracheal tubes of 12-mm internal diameter or indwelling polyvinyl tubes or tubes of similar material should be inserted through both choanae and left in place for 6 weeks. Otherwise, the new opening in the choanae will fill in by fibrosis and the condition will recur.[69]

***Prognosis.*** In one case in which surgical treatment was attempted, the foal made an abnormal but acceptable respiratory noise during exercise.[69] It also had malocclusion with caudal displacement of the upper incisors and cheek teeth attributed to incongruous growth of the jaws caused by surgical damage to suture lines.[69] Before surgery is performed, foals should be evaluated for the presence of other congenital abnormalities.[69]

## *Necrosis of the Conchae*

This condition usually develops secondary to infection in the ventral conchal sinus, especially if the process is confined to that cavity and the purulent contents cannot drain into the adjacent rostral maxillary sinus and from there through the nasal maxillary opening.[13] In some cases, the dorsal conchal sinus may also be involved[11,71] and infection can spread through the intervening thin plates of bone to involve the rostral parts of the dorsal and ventral conchae.[71] This condition is described more fully in Chapter 18.

***Clinical Signs and Diagnosis.*** Clinical signs are similar to those of sinusitis. The conchae may undergo metaplasia and extensive mineralization with enlargement and complete loss of the normal pattern on dorsoventral radiographs.[72] On endoscopic examination, foci of inspissated purulent material may be seen along the caudal part of the middle meatus.[11]

***Treatment.*** In this condition, the involved bone and membrane are necrotic and can be readily detached if they are grasped with a uterine biopsy instrument inserted through the nasal passage under endoscopic guidance.[11] The area can then be copiously lavaged with warm water to dislodge any remaining necrotic material and pus.[11] Alternatively, a trephine opening can be made through the nasal bone slightly lateral to the midline and at the level where the nasal bones diverge towards the medial canthus of the eye.[13] An osteotome or similar instrument can be used to detach the necrotic bone at the level of the trephine and the most rostral attachments can be severed by cutting them with an osteotome inserted through the nostrils[13] or through an incision in the skin over the nasoincisive notch.[71] Intraoperative hemorrhage is profuse and the nasal cavity should be packed with sterile gauze soaked in 1:10,000 epinephrine solution. Prior to surgery a potential blood donor should be identified by crossmatch and made available.

## References


1. Hare WCD. Equine respiratory system. In: Sisson and Grossman's The Anatomy of the Domestic Animals. 5th ed. R Getty (ed). Philadelphia, WB Saunders Co, 1975, p 498.
2. Hillman DJ. Skull. In: Sisson and Grossman's The Anatomy of the Domestic Animals. 5th Ed. R Getty (ed). Philadelphia, WB Saunders Co, 1975, p 318.
3. Robinson NE, Sorenson PR. Pathophysiology of airway obstruction in horses: A review. J Am Vet Med Assoc, *172*:299, 1978.
4. Robinson NE, Sorenson PR, Goble DO. Patterns of airflow in normal horses and horses with respiratory disease. Proc Am Assoc Eq Pract, *21*:11, 1975.
5. Cook WR. Clinical observations on the anatomy and physiology of the equine upper respiratory tract. Vet Rec, *79*:440, 1966.
6. Goble DO, Geiser DR, Jones RD. Examination, diagnosis and treatment of equine upper respiratory disorders: Part I. J Equine Med Surg, *3*:162, 1979.
7. Stilson AE, Herring DS, Robertson JT. Contribution of the nasal septum to the radiographic anatomy of the equine nasal cavity. J Am Vet Med Assoc, *186*:590, 1985.
8. Lattimer JC. Equine nasal passages, sinuses, and guttural pouches. In: Textbook of Veterinary Diagnostic Radiology. DE Thrall (ed). Philadelphia, WB Saunders Co, 1986, p 64.
9. Boles C. Abnormalities of the upper respiratory tract. Vet Clin North Am, *1*:89, 1979.
10. Greet TRC. The respiratory tract. In: Equine Surgery and Medicine, Vol. 1. J Hickman (ed). New York, Academic Press, 1985, p 247.
11. Cook WR. Diseases of nose; horse. Int Encyclopedia Vet Med, *5*:2082, 1966.
12. Pascoe JR, Summers PM. Clinical survey of tumours

and tumour-like lesions in horses in south east Queensland. Equine Vet Jour, *13*:235, 1981.
13. Frank ER. Veterinary Surgery Notes. Minneapolis, Burgess Publishing Co, 1944, p 85.
14. Boles C. Treatment of upper airway abnormalities. Vet Clin North Am, *1*:127, 1979.
15. Foerner JJ. The diagnosis and correction of false nostril noises. Proc Am Assoc Eq Pract, *17*:315, 1971.
16. Bowman KF, Swaim SF, Vaughan JT. Double opposing Z-plasty for correction of stenotic naris in a horse. J Am Vet Med Assoc, *180*:772, 1982.
17. Phillips TN, Morrissey RL. Nasal concretion in a horse. Ill Vet, *8*:29, 1965.
18. Valdez H, McMullan WC, Hobson HP, et al. Surgical correction of deviated nasal septum and premaxilla in a colt. J Am Vet Med Assoc, *173*:1001, 1978.
19. Vandeplassche M, Simoens P, Bouters R, et al. Aetiology and pathogenesis of congenital torticollis and head scoliosis in the equine foetus. Equine Vet J, *16*:419, 1984.
20. Radke B. Ein Faill von rechtsseitiger Cheilognathopalatoschisis lateralis bei einem Fohlen (A case of cheilognathopalatoschisis lateralis in a foal). DTW, *87*:264, 1980.
21. Boulton CH. Equine nasal cavity and paranasal sinus disease. A review of 85 cases. Eq Vet Sci, *5*:268, 1985.
22. Jakob W. Spontaneous amyloidosis of mammals. Vet Path, *8*:292, 1971.
23. van Andel ACJ, Gruys E, Kroneman J. Amyloid in the horse: A report of nine cases. Equine Vet J, *20*:277, 1988.
24. Shaw DP, Gunson DE, Evans LH. Nasal amyloidosis in four horses. Vet Pathol, *24*:183, 1987.
25. Bridges CH. Systemic Mycoses. In: Equine Medicine and Surgery. 2nd Ed. EJ Catcott and JF Smithcors (eds). Wheaton, American Veterinary Publications, Inc., 1972, p 119.
26. Miller RI. Equine Phycomycosis. Comp Cont Ed Pract Vet, *9*:S472, 1983.
27. Hanselka DV. Equine nasal phycomycosis. VM/SAC, *72*:251, 1977.
28. Hutchins DR, Johnston KG. Phycomycosis in the horse. Aust Vet J, *48*:269, 1972.
29. Bridges CH, Romane WM, Emmons CW. Phycomycosis of horses caused by *Entomophthora coronata*. J Am Vet Med Assoc, *140*:673, 1962.
30. Joyce JR, McMullan WC, Burns SJ. The use of amphotericin B in late pregnancy in mares. J Eq Med Surg, *1*:256, 1977.
31. Corrier DE, Wilson SR, Scrutchfield WL. Equine cryptococcal rhinitis. Comp Cont Ed Pract Vet, *9*:S556, 1984.
32. Roberts MD, Sutton RH, Lovell DK. A protracted case of cryptococcal nasal granuloma in a stallion. Aust Vet J, *57*:287, 1981.
33. Scott EA, Duncan JR, McCormack JE. Cryptococcosis involving the postorbital area and frontal sinus in a horse. J Am Vet Med Assoc, *165*:626, 1974.
34. Carrig CB. What is your diagnosis? J Am Vet Med Assoc, *153*:1206, 1968.
35. Wätt DA. A case of cryptococcal granuloma in the nasal cavity of a horse. Aust Vet J, *46*:493, 1970.
36. Penn RL, Lambert RS, Goerge RB. Invasive fungal infections. The use of serologic tests in diagnosis and management. Arch Intern Med, *143*:1215, 1983.
37. Pentlarge VW, Martin RA. Treatment of cryptococcosis in three cats, using ketoconazole. J Am Vet Med Assoc, *188*:536, 1986.
38. Jackson JA. Immunodiagnosis of systemic mycoses in animals: A review. J Am Vet Med Assoc, *188*:702, 1986.
39. Gabal MA. Antifungal activity of ketoconazole with emphasis on zoophilic fungal pathogens. Am J Vet Res, *47*:1229, 1986.
40. Prades M, Brown MP, Gronwall RR, et al. Ketoconazole in the horse: body fluid and endometrial concentrations after repeated oral administration. Vet Surg (Abstr), *15*:131, 1986.
41. Reed SM, Boles CL, Dade AW, et al. Localized equine nasal coccidioidomycosis granuloma. J Equine Vet Med Surg, *3*:119, 1979.
42. Hodgin EC, Conaway DH, Ortenburger AI. Recurrence of obstructive nasal coccidioidal granuloma in a horse. J Am Vet Med Assoc, *184*:339, 1984.
43. Moriello KA. Ketoconazole: Clinical pharmacology and therapeutic recommendations. J Am Vet Med Assoc, *188*:303, 1986.
44. Greet TRC. Nasal aspergillosis in three horses. Vet Rec, *109*:487, 1981.
45. Reynolds JEF (ed). Martindale the Extra Pharmacopoeia. 28th Ed. London, The Pharmaceutical Press, 1982, p 728.
46. Coad CT, Robinson NM, Wilhelmus KR. Antifungal sensitivity testing for equine keratomycosis. Am J Vet Res, *46*:676, 1985.
47. O'Day DM. Selection of appropriate antifungal therapy. Cornea, *6*:238, 1987.
48. Johns KJ, O'Day DM. Pharmacologic management of keratomycoses. Surv Ophthalmol, *33*:178, 1989.
49. Stamm AM, Dismukes WE. Current therapy of pulmonary and disseminated fungal diseases. Chest, *83*:911, 1983.
50. Utz JP. Chemotherapy of the systemic mycoses. Symposium on antimicrobial therapy. Med Clin North Am, *66*:221, 1982.
51. Myers DD, Simon J, Case MT. Rhinosporidiosis in a horse. J Am Vet Med Assoc, *145*:345, 1964.
52. Brearley JC, McCandlish IAP, Sullivan M, et al. Nasal granuloma caused by *Pseudallescheria boydii*. Equine Vet J, *18*:151, 1986.
53. Tulleners EP, Raker CW. Nasal septum resection in the horse. Vet Surg, *12*:41, 1983.
54. Schuh JCL. Squamous cell carcinoma of the oral, pharyngeal and nasal mucosa in the horse. Vet Pathol, *23*:205, 1986.
55. McIlwraith CW, Turner AS. Equine Surgery Advanced Techniques. Philadelphia, Lea & Febiger, 1987, pp 244–249.
56. Madewell BR, Priester WA, Gillette EL, et al. Neoplasms of the nasal passages and paranasal sinuses in domesticated animals as reported by 13 veterinary colleges. Am J Vet Res, *37*:851, 1976.
57. Leyland A, Baker JR. Lesions of the nasal and par-

anasal sinuses of the horse causing dyspnoea. Br Vet J, *131*:339, 1975.

58. Cotchin E. Spontaneous neoplasms of the upper respiratory tract in animals. In: Cancer of the Nasopharynx. Muir C, Shanmugarantnam K (eds). UICC Monograph Series, Vol. 1, 30, 203, Munksgaard, Copenhagen, 1967, p 203.
59. Hultgren BD, Schmotzer WB, Watrous BJ, et al. Nasal-maxillary fibrosarcoma in young horses: a light and electron microscopic study. Vet Pathol, *24*:194, 1987.
60. Acland HM, Orsini JA, Elkins S, et al. Congenital ethmoid carcinoma in a foal. J Am Vet Med Assoc, *184*:979, 1984.
61. Rahko T, Alitalo I, Paatsama S. Myxoma in the nasal cavity of the Finnish-bred horse: A report on three cases recently observed in Finland. Acta Vet Scand, *13*:131, 1972.
62. Meschter CL, Allen D. Lymphosarcoma within the nasal cavities of an 18-month-old filly. Equine Vet J, *16*:475, 1984.
63. Firth EC. Horner's syndrome in the horse: Experimental induction and a case report. Equine Vet J, *10*:9, 1978.
64. Livesey MA, Keana DP, Sarmiento J. Epistaxis in a Standardbred weanling caused by fibrous dysplasia. Equine Vet J, *16*:144, 1984.
65. Moulton JE (ed). Tumors in Domestic Animals. Berkley, University of California Press, 1978, p 241.
66. Stickle RL, Jones RD. Excision of a nasal polyp. VM/SAC, *71*:1453, 1976.
67. Balinksy BI. An Introduction to Embryology. 5th Ed. Philadelphia, Saunders College Publishing, 1981, p 448.
68. Crouch GM. Bilateral choanal atresia in a foal. Comp Cont Ed Pract Vet, *5*:206, 1983.
69. Goring RL, Campbell M, Hillidge CJ. Surgical correction of congenital bilateral choanal atresia in a foal. Vet Surg, *13*:211, 1984.
70. Sprinkle FP, Crowe MW, Swerczek TW. Choanal atresia in foals. Mod Vet Prac, *65*:306, 1984.
71. DeMoor Von A, Verschooten F. Empyem und Nekrose der Nasenmuscheln beim Pferd (Empyema and necrosis of the nasal conchae in a horse). DTW, *89*:275, 1982.
72. Gibbs C, Lane JG. Radiographic examination of the facial, nasal and paranasal sinus regions of the horse. II. Radiological findings. Equine Vet J, *19*:474, 1987.

## CHAPTER 18

# PARANASAL SINUSES

*DAVID E. FREEMAN*

The horse's sinuses are large and not readily accessible by most methods of examination and sinus diseases are usually well advanced before clinical signs become apparent. For these reasons, they are difficult to treat. Although sinus diseases are generally considered common in horses, a recent survey in one university hospital over an 8-year period found the prevalence to be only 1.06% of all cases examined.[1]

## Anatomy

### *Maxillary Sinus*

The maxillary sinus, composed of both caudal and rostral parts, is the largest paranasal sinus in the adult horse.[2] Its dorsal margin is a line drawn from the medial canthus of the eye to the nasoincisive notch (Fig. 18–1). Its rostral limit is a line drawn at right angles to the dorsal margin to meet the most rostral end of the facial crest (Fig. 18–1). The floor is parallel and slightly ventral to the facial crest and a line drawn directly from the middle of the orbit to the facial crest marks the most caudal limit (Fig. 18–1). In horses under 5 years, the maxillary sinuses are largely filled with embedded parts of the 3rd to 6th cheek teeth (4th premolar, 1st, 2nd and 3rd molars). As the reserve crowns of cheek teeth become shorter with age, the maxillary sinus enlarges and its rostral limit approaches the infraorbital foramen.[2,3]

Position of the bony septum that divides the maxillary sinus into rostral and caudal parts is variable, but it is usually directed obliquely across the roots of the 4th and 5th cheek teeth, approximately 5 cm from the end of the facial crest[2] (Fig. 18–1). The dorsal part of the septum is formed by the bulla of the ventral conchal sinus and is delicate and cribriform (Fig. 18–2). Rarely, an opening can be found dorsally.[2]

The rostral maxillary sinus is bounded laterally by the maxilla and medially by the infraorbital canal. It opens into the middle nasal meatus through a compressed passageway that leads to the nasomaxillary opening. It communicates with the ventral conchal sinus through a long, slit-like communication, the conchomaxillary opening, which is dorsal to the infraorbital canal (Fig. 18–3).

The caudal maxillary sinus is larger than the rostral.[2] It has a large opening into the sphenopalatine sinus caudal and medial to the infraorbital canal and a small opening medially into the middle conchal sinus (Fig. 18–1). Dorsally, it communicates with the frontal sinus through the large oval (approximately 4 by 3 cm) frontomaxillary opening, at the level of the medial canthus (Fig. 18–1). A compressed passageway between the rostral edge of the frontomaxillary opening and the conchal bulla leads from the caudal maxillary sinus, through the nasomaxillary opening, into the middle nasal meatus (Fig. 18–2).

### *Frontal Sinuses*

The right and left frontal sinuses are separated along the midline by a complete sep-

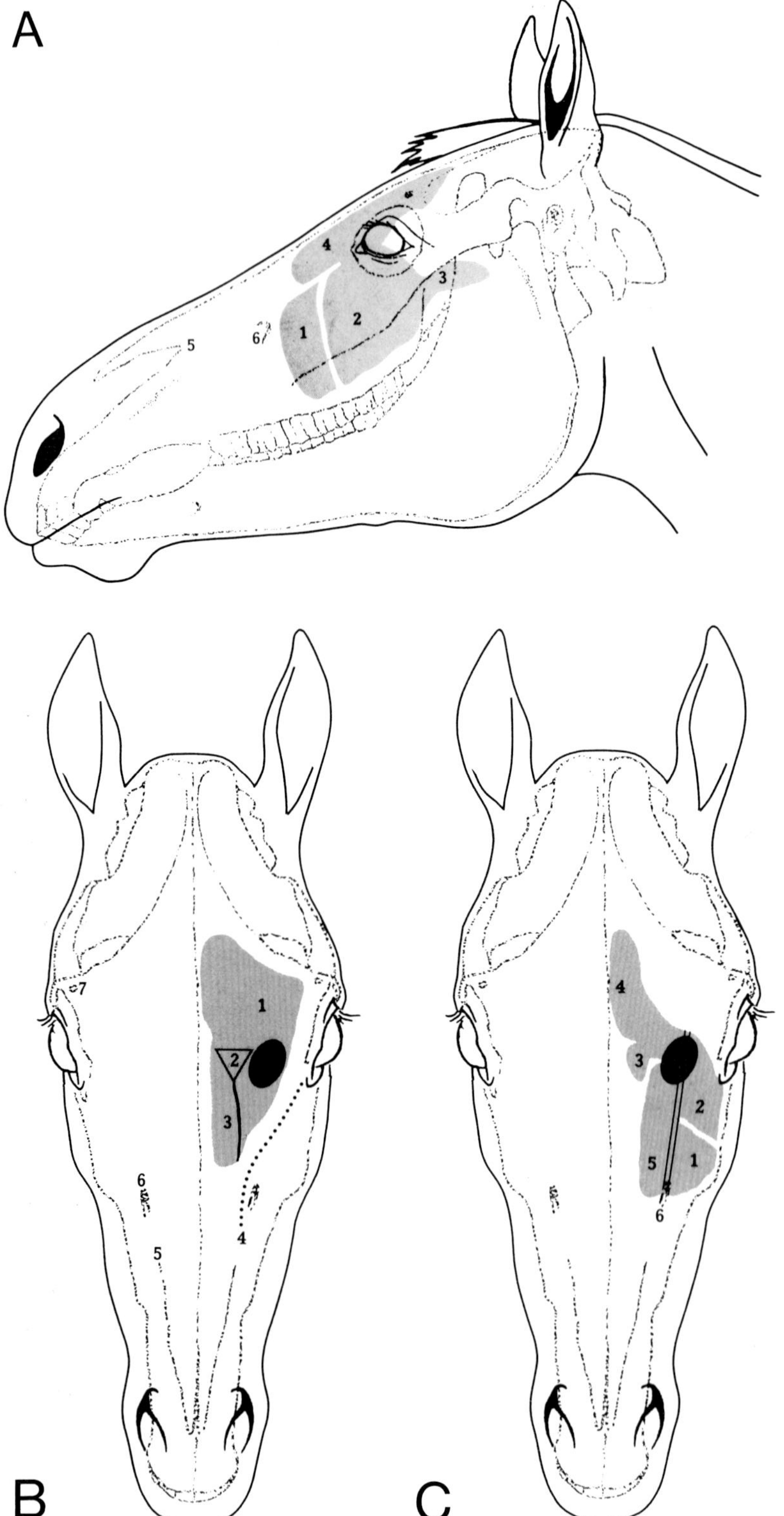


**FIG. 18–1.** Outlines of the paranasal sinuses of the horse. A. Lateral view. 1 = Rostral maxillary sinus; 2 = caudal maxillary sinus (note septum between 1 and 2); 3 = sphenopalatine sinus; 4 = frontal sinus; 5 = nasoincisive notch; 6 = infraorbital foramen. B. Dorsal view of conchofrontal sinus. 1 = Frontal sinus; 2 = ethmoid labyrinth; 3 = dorsal conchal sinus; 1 and 3 = conchofrontal sinus; 4 = course of nasolacrimal duct (dotted line); 5 and 6 as in 1A; 7 = supraorbital foramen. Black oval = frontomaxillary opening. C. Dorsal view of maxillary sinus. 1 = Rostral maxillary sinus; 2 = caudal maxillary sinus; 3 = middle conchal sinus; 4 = sphenopalatine sinus; 5 = ventral conchal sinus; 6 = infraorbital foramen leading into infraorbital canal (parallel lines).

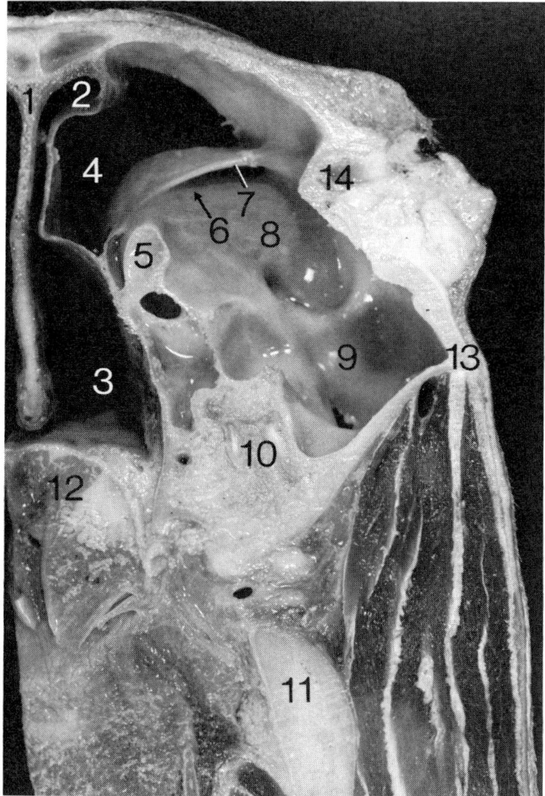


**FIG. 18–2.** Transverse section through the head of an adult horse at the level of the medial canthus of the eye and viewed from back to front. 1 = Nasal septum; 2 = dorsal nasal meatus; 3 = ventral nasal meatus; 4 = dorsal conchal sinus; 5 = infraorbital canal; 6 = compressed passageway leading from the caudal maxillary sinus to the middle nasal meatus; 7 = rostral edge of the frontomaxillary opening; 8 = caudal bulla of the ventral conchal sinus; 9 = septum between rostral and caudal maxillary sinuses; 10 = root of sixth cheek tooth (third molar); 11 = mandible; 12 = soft palate; 13 = facial crest; 14 = opening of nasolacrimal duct.

tum. The caudal margin of the frontal sinus is a line rostral to the temporomandibular joint in an adult horse (Fig. 18–1) and level with the orbit in the young foal.[4] The lateral margin of the frontal sinus is a line drawn from the medial canthus of the eye to the nasoincisive notch (Fig. 18–1). The rostral extent of the sinus is a line drawn at right angles from the midline to midway between the medial canthus and the infraorbital foramen or ⅔ the distance from the medial canthus to the rostral end of the facial crest (Fig. 18–1). This corresponds to the point at which the nasal bones lose their parallel course and diverge towards the orbit. The convex surface of the ethmoidal labyrinth projects into the floor of the frontal sinus between the orbits. At its rostral end, the frontal sinus has a large medial and ventral communication with the dorsal conchal sinus, with which it combines to form the conchofrontal sinus (Figs. 18–1 and 18–3).

## *Middle Conchal and Sphenopalatine Sinuses*

The middle conchal sinus is small and projects medially into the nasal passage and

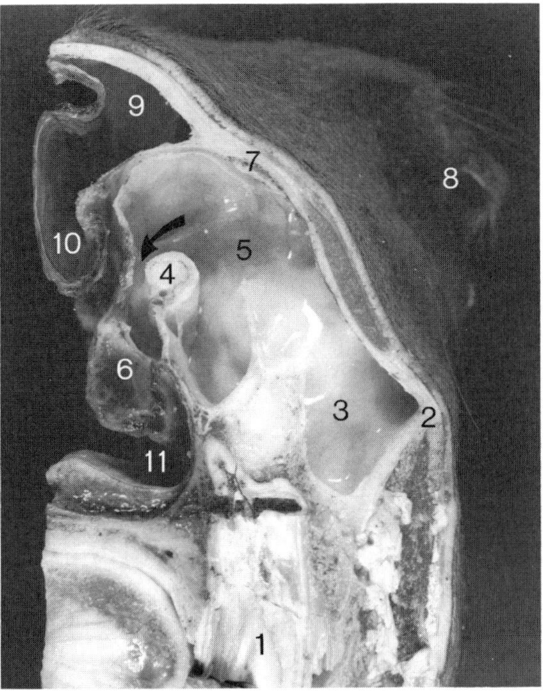


**FIG. 18–3.** Transverse section through the head of a 10-year-old horse at the level of second molar (fifth cheek tooth), viewed from front to back, left side. 1 = Second molar; 2 = facial crest; 3 = rigid bony septum between caudal and rostral maxillary sinuses; 4 = infraorbital nerve in infraorbital canal; 5 = rostral maxillary sinus (plate of bone behind numeral 5 is the conchal bulla); 6 = ventral conchal sinus; 7 = nasolacrimal duct; 8 = medial canthus of eye; 9 = frontal sinus; 10 = dorsal conchal sinus (9 and 10 combined form the conchofrontal sinus); 11 = ventral nasal meatus. The arrow indicates the conchomaxillary opening, which is the communication between the rostral maxillary sinus and the ventral conchal sinus.

opens laterally into the caudal maxillary sinus (Fig. 18–1). The sphenopalatine sinus lies beneath the ethmoidal labyrinth[2] (Fig. 18–1).

## *Mucosa and Blood Supply*

The paranasal sinuses are lined by respiratory mucous membrane, composed largely of pseudostratified columnar ciliated epithelium and goblet cells.[5] The mucosa is pale over much of its surface because underlying vessels are sparse, but the submucosa of the ventral nasal concha contains a rich venous plexus.[5] Blood flow to the frontal sinus is provided largely by the ethmoidal artery and the maxillary sinus is supplied by branches of the sphenopalatine artery.[5]

## *Cheek Teeth*

The premolars appear as both deciduous and permanent teeth and the molars are permanent. The embedded part of the tooth is united to a bony alveolus by the alveolar periosteum, a vascular layer of connective tissue.[6] As the exposed or functional crown of the tooth is worn down, the embedded part or reserve crown continues to erupt so that the occlusal surfaces of the teeth are maintained in apposition.[6] The tooth roots are not formed completely until after eruption and this allows the cheek teeth to grow for some time after they come into wear.[3] The deciduous premolars are short and much of the alveolar bone above them is occupied by the primordial tooth germ tissue or anlage.[7]

# Clinical Signs of Sinus Disease and Diagnostic Techniques

History and diagnostic methods for sinus disease are similar to those for diseases of the nasal passages and are covered in Chapter 17. The following are additional points that apply to the sinuses.

Most sinus diseases cause a unilateral mucopurulent nasal discharge unless inflammation occludes the nasomaxillary opening so that fluid is retained in the sinuses. A bilateral discharge[8–11] is rare because the source of fluid is usually rostral to the most caudal end of the nasal septum. This feature can help distinguish between diseases of the sinuses and guttural pouches. Blood-stained nasal discharge may be evident in horses with tumors or fungal infections. In long-standing cases, unilateral facial swelling is evident in the maxilla and is usually more severe in young horses (Fig. 18–4). Exophthalmos may be seen with a fungal granuloma and epiphora can be seen in some diseases due to compression of the osseous nasolacrimal duct. The latter is not always associated with facial distortion.[8,11]

Percussion can be useful in detecting fluid or space-occupying masses within the sinuses but is not always reliable and may be resented in inflammatory conditions. To percuss the sinuses, the fingers of one hand are tapped sharply against the overlying bones and the corresponding area on the normal side is percussed immediately afterwards for comparison. If the mouth is held open simultaneously, resonance will increase and abnormalities will be easier to detect. An oral examination should be performed to detect dental abnormalities, but these can be difficult to recognize. An infundibulum pick can be used to detect a patent infundibulum or fracture.[12]

Changes in peripheral blood samples are uncommon, except that the packed cell volume may be decreased in horses with chronic infections or neoplasia. Samples of the nasal discharge can be submitted for culture and sensitivity, but the results must always be interpreted with caution because commensal organisms reside in the nasal passages.

## *Endoscopy*

Endoscopy is used to detect abnormalities extending from sinuses into the nasal passages and to rule out other diseases of the upper respiratory tract and guttural pouches that can present with similar clinical signs. Endoscopic examination may not reveal any abnormality if the lesion has not extended or

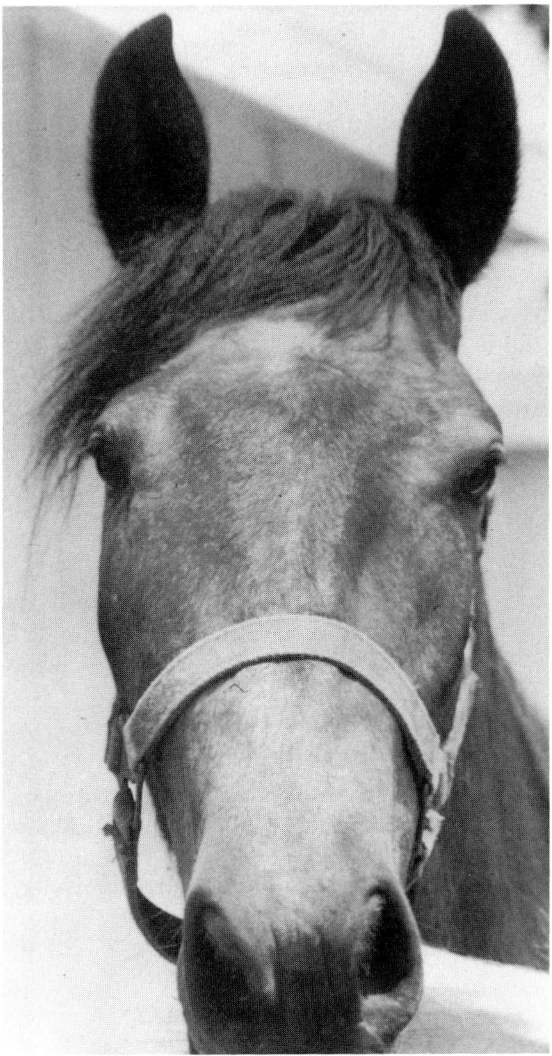

**FIG. 18–4.** Horse with bony enlargement of the right maxillary sinus and epiphora caused by a cementoma (see also Figures 18–13, 18–14, 18–16, which are from the same horse). This horse did not have nasal discharge, presumably because the lesion had obstructed drainage openings from the sinuses. The mild upper lip deviation was caused by voluntary lip movements and not by a disease process.

drained into the nasal passage. The method of performing endoscopic examination has been described in Chapter 17. However, special attention must be paid to the ethmoturbinates and the caudal end of the middle meatus because blood, pus, and masses can be seen at these sites in horses with sinus diseases.

## *Radiology*

Although radiographs are invaluable in diagnosis of sinus and dental diseases, they can be difficult to interpret.[13] Air in the sinuses provides a natural negative contrast medium for the surrounding bone and teeth and for soft tissue densities and fluid. However, angles of projection and exposure factors must be selected carefully because structures in the sinuses span a wide range of radiodensities from thin plates of bone to dense enamel.[7,14]

Interpretation of dental lesions requires an understanding of normal radiographic anatomy of the tooth root. In young horses, the root apices are smooth and round, but in older horses they become narrower and more pointed.[14] The anlages of permanent teeth are evident in radiographs to about 4 years of age, when the 6th cheek tooth erupts.[7] Eruption of a tooth is accompanied by an increase in vascularity of the tooth pulp and this can be seen on radiographs as a cystic distention of the lamina dura.[7] This change can be distinguished from an abscess by its smooth regular outline and association with an erupting tooth.[14] The lamina dura is a radiographic white line that represents the alveolar bone and periodontal ligament interface[7] and the latter appears as a radiolucent line around the tooth root.[7,14]

A lateral view is best to demonstrate fluid and soft tissue but fine detail in tooth roots may be obscured by fluid lines, trabecular patterns, and overlapping normal soft tissue densities.[15] If the head is extended, fluid lines will be obscured beneath tooth roots but, when the head is lowered, as under the influence of a sedative, fluid lines become more obvious.[16,17] A Mitchell marker should be used to demonstrate the orientation of fluid lines and help to distinguish them from other soft tissue densities.[17] Occasionally, removal of fluid from sinuses allows more complete assessment of lesions obscured by fluid lines.[17] The procedure for lateral radiographs in the standing horse has been described in Chapter 17.

In lateral radiographs, the side close to the beam will be magnified and superimposed on areas of interest. Therefore, to improve views of tooth roots, the cassette can be held at a 30° to 40° angle beneath the jaw on the affected side and the beam can be directed obliquely in a dorsal to ventral direction.[7,15,17] Powerful equipment, rare earth screens, and film combinations are required for these projections.[15] Greater detail of cheek teeth can be obtained by intraoral films,[7] but these are difficult to use in the back of the mouth.[16] Sinus cavities are difficult to evaluate on dorsoventral views because the upper and lower cheek teeth and the overlying masseter muscles obscure much of the field.[17]

## Centesis

This procedure is used to sample fluid or to flush the sinuses and can be performed with the horse standing and mildly sedated. The site for centesis is determined by clinical and radiographic findings but, if a generalized sinus problem is suspected, it is 2.5 to 3 cm dorsal to the facial crest and the same distance rostral to the orbit (Fig. 18–5).[18] If only the rostral maxillary sinus is involved, the area chosen for centesis is 3 cm dorsal to the facial crest and approximately 3 cm caudal to the infraorbital foramen (Fig. 18–5).

The site is prepared for aseptic surgery and infiltrated with local anesthetic. A 1-cm-long incision is then made through the skin and subcutaneous tissues and a 2-mm diameter Steinmann pin attached to a Jacob's chuck is used to drill a hole through the bone. In some horses, a 16-gauge needle alone can be used to penetrate the bone, without the need to drill a hole beforehand. Fluid within the sinus is aspirated and submitted for Gram stain, cytologic examination, culture, and sensitivity testing. If the fluid is inaccessible or too viscous to aspirate, a small quantity of sterile saline, free of bacteriostatic agents, is injected into the sinus cavity to mix with fluid contents and the mixture is then aspirated. A large volume of fluid is then delivered by gravity into the sinus cavity and, if the nasomaxillary opening is patent, fluid and exudate should flow freely from the nasal passage. Complications of centesis are rare, but purulent material within the sinus can escape through the bone hole and induce local cellulitis.

## Examination Through the Arthroscope

The sinuses can be examined through the arthroscope with the horse standing and sedated.[19] A site midway between the midline and medial canthus is prepared for aseptic surgery and infiltrated with local anesthetic. The skin and underlying soft tissues are incised and a hole is drilled in the bone with a

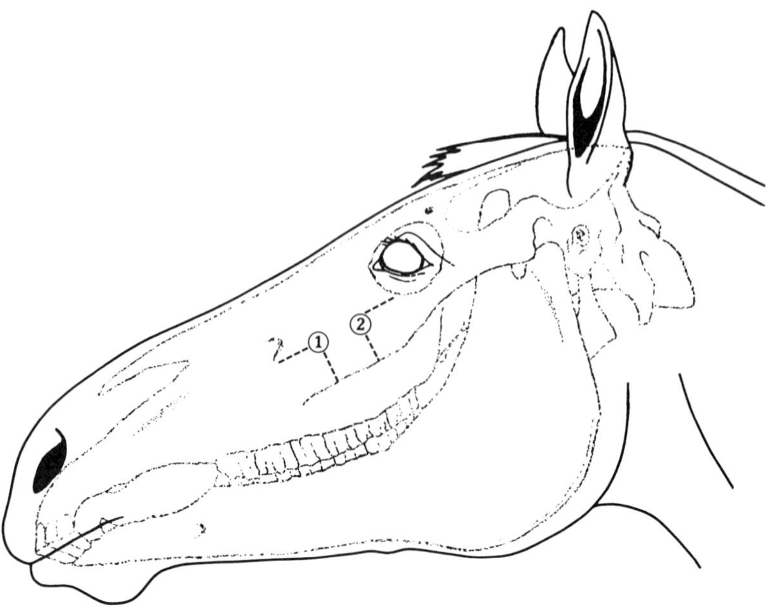


**FIG. 18–5.** Sites for centesis of the rostral (1) and caudal maxillary (2) sinuses. Broken lines represent distances of 2.5 to 3.0 cm from landmarks (see text).

¼-inch Steinmann pin held in a Jacob's chuck.[19] The arthroscope is inserted through the hole to obtain a bloodless view of the frontoconchal sinus and, through the frontomaxillary opening, of the caudal maxillary sinus.[19] A sample of abnormal tissue can be removed by inserting a biopsy instrument through a second hole that is placed close to the lesion and in view through the scope.[19] The arthroscope can be inserted through the caudal maxillary sinus at the site used for centesis (Fig. 18–5) but this approach may not allow adequate inspection of the conchofrontal sinus.[20]

## Diseases of the Paranasal Sinuses

### *Primary Sinusitis*

Primary sinusitis usually is caused by an upper respiratory tract infection that has extended into the paranasal sinuses, whereas secondary sinusitis is caused by a tooth infection. In recent retrospective studies, the ratios of primary sinusitis to secondary sinusitis in total numbers are 29 to 18,[21] 7 to 9,[1] 14 to 14[8] and 5 to 8.[17] Primary sinusitis can be seen in horses over a wide age range,[21,22] whereas dental disease is less common in horses before 4 years of age.[8,13,21] Primary sinusitis usually involves all sinus cavities but can be confined to the ventral conchal sinus[22,23] (Fig. 18–3). Persistent infections in this site can be attributed to occlusion of the conchomaxillary opening by mucosal swelling and granulation tissue.

***Cause.*** The organisms most commonly involved are Streptococcus equi and Streptococcus zooepidemicus.[11,18,22,23] A rare cause is staphylococcal granuloma (botryomycosis).[24] Inflammation and swelling in the nasal mucosa from a viral infection can occlude the nasomaxillary opening, obstruct drainage, and thereby predispose to secondary bacterial infection.[25]

***Clinical Signs.*** The most common clinical sign of primary sinusitis is a unilateral, mucopurulent nasal discharge.[25] Bilateral nasal discharge is rare[8] and could indicate bilateral sinusitis.[11] Nasal discharge usually increases during exercise[25,26] and stertorous breathing may be evident during work or at rest.

Facial distortion is unusual with primary sinusitis[21] but can develop in the more chronic stages of the disease, especially in young horses.[25] Epiphora may be evident with or without facial distortion.[8,11] Less common signs are submandibular lymph node enlargement,[23] depression, anorexia, and fever. In advanced cases, the overlying bone may be thin and pliable and hair may be sparse and erect.[12]

Neurologic signs are rare but can be seen with severe and chronic cases in which the infection has extended from the frontal sinus through the cribriform plate and caused purulent meningoencephalitis.[25] Severe infections of the sphenopalatine sinus, associated with considerable soft tissue and bony destruction, can cause blindness, exophthalmos, strabismus and meningitis; however, these complications are rare.[25]

***Diagnosis.*** Sinusitis may be suspected in a horse with the preceding clinical signs and dullness on percussion of the involved sinuses. On endoscopic examination, pus may be seen draining from the nasomaxillary opening into the middle meatus. On radiographs, fluid lines should be evident (Fig. 18–6), and in more severe cases, contents appear mineralized.[13] In one review, opacification of the sinuses served as a reliable differential feature between primary and secondary sinusitis.[13]

If infection is confined to the ventral conchal sinus, radiographs may demonstrate a soft tissue density dorsal to the third to fifth cheek teeth[22] and confined to the ventral conchal sinus on dorsoventral projections.[23] An intraoral examination and radiographs of tooth roots should be used to rule out secondary sinusitis.

***Treatment.*** Failure to institute appropriate treatment during the early stages of primary sinusitis will allow it to progress to a chronic problem with osteitis, advanced necrosis and destruction of soft tissue and bone, and formation of deep seated abscesses. Response to systemic antibiotic therapy can be favorable, especially if the choice of antibiotics is based

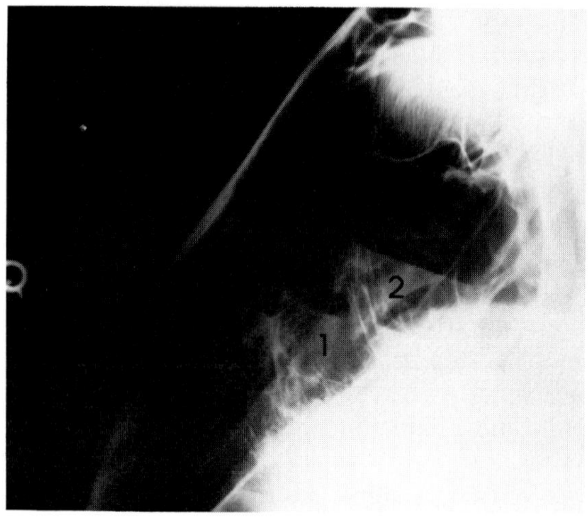


**FIG. 18–6.** Fluid lines on lateral views of the sinuses. 1 = Fluid line in the rostral maxillary sinus; 2 = fluid line in the caudal maxillary sinus. Note the Mitchell marker to the left side of the radiograph, which provides an accurate orientation of the fluid line.

upon culture and sensitivity testing of aspirates collected by centesis. Empirical use of antibiotics in racehorses may be palliative and allow training to continue but infection can recur after antibiotic therapy ceases.

Antibiotic therapy can be combined with daily lavage of the sinus with large volumes of warm, sterile physiologic saline solution delivered by gravity flow through polyethylene tubing. Tubing can be inserted through a hole, placed as for centesis (Fig. 18–5), and secured by "butterflies" of adhesive tape sutured to the adjacent skin. Irrigation removes debris and bacteria from the sinus and thereby enhances the effects of antibiotics. It has been claimed that enzymes, such as trypsin,[8,25] streptokinase, and streptodornase, can liquefy inspissated pus in the sinuses,[18] but they have not been critically evaluated for this purpose. Dilute solutions of antiseptics, such as 0.1% potassium permanganate,[18] 1% povidine iodine or 1% chlorhexidine, can be infused, but concentrated antiseptic solutions may exacerbate inflammation.[11] Antibiotics can be infused but combinations of antibiotics and other drugs should be avoided and many antibiotics will be rendered ineffective by organic material and by the acid pH in infected sinuses.[27] It has been suggested that exercise is of benefit because it may induce vasoconstriction and improve drainage by enlarging the nasomaxillary openings.[25,28] Nonsteroidal anti-inflammatory drugs, such as phenylbutazone and flunixin meglumine, can be administered to reduce inflammation and swelling around the drainage openings. At least 14 days of medical treatment may be needed before improvement is seen.

Long-standing cases of persistent sinusitis can be treated successfully by surgical debridement and curettage through a bone flap. The postoperative course is often protracted if the infection has become deep-seated and extensive bony necrosis, osteitis, and associated facial swelling have developed.[8] Surgical treatment is advised for horses with inspissated pus in the ventral conchal sinus and is usually successful.[22,23]

## Secondary Sinusitis

The most common causes of secondary sinusitis are diseases of cheek teeth, such as fractures, patent infundibulum, displaced teeth, dental malposition, and crown defects.[6–8,25,26,29] The teeth involved in decreasing order of frequency are the 1st molar, 4th premolar, and 3rd premolar.[13,21] In some horses, two or more adjacent teeth may be involved.[13,21] Open wounds and any destructive disease of the sinuses also can cause secondary sinusitis.

The most severe form of maxillary dental disease in the horse is pulpitis secondary to infection along a fractured tooth or from cement necrosis.[7] This condition causes inflammation in the alveolar bone, periodontal membrane, cementum and sinus mucous membrane.[7] This is followed by osteolysis and localized osteitis, accompanied by new bone and new cement formation as localized attempts to confine the infection.[7] The result is an apical granuloma on the involved tooth root or diffuse alveolar periostitis if the process spreads.[7] If the infection extends into the maxillary sinus, sinusitis develops.

***Clinical Signs.*** Clinical signs of secondary sinusitis closely resemble those of primary sinusitis, but the nasal discharge may be fetid and sinus tracts from rostral cheek teeth may drain onto the skin.[21] Horses with dental disease rarely have difficulties in masticating.

***Diagnosis.*** A tentative diagnosis can be made on the basis of clinical signs. Inflammation around the mucosa, fractures of teeth, patent infundibulum or malocclusion, may be seen on oral examination; however, the absence of dental lesions does not rule out the diagnosis of apical granuloma.[8] On radiographs, an apical granuloma can be recognized by disruption of the lamina dura, loss of normal root outline over the apex, and osteolysis over the affected root.[7,8,14,16] The zone of osteolysis is usually surrounded by sclerotic bone and cement deposition ("clubbing").[7,14] Interpretation of more subtle radiographic abnormalities is difficult.[13]

***Treatment.*** Treatment of secondary sinusitis involves removal of the diseased tooth or other primary problem and treatment of infection by surgical removal of abnormal mucosa, irrigation of the sinus cavity, and systemic antibiotics. Postoperative care is tedious (see section on surgery) and the prognosis is only fair in advanced cases.[8] Unsuccessful treatment can be attributed to persistent osteitis, abscesses, and failure to remove all the involved root and infected bone. Recent evidence that obligate anaerobes can be involved in dental abscesses in horses may explain the poor clinical response to postoperative antibiotics.[23,30] Although systemic (oral) medication is most frequent, topical treatment with metronidazole (0.5% solution) has also been used.[30] Special sample handling and isolation techniques should be used for culturing anaerobes.

## *Ethmoid Hematoma*

Ethmoid hematoma is a progressive and locally destructive mass of unknown cause in the paranasal sinuses that closely resembles a tumor in appearance and development, but it is not neoplastic (Fig. 18–7).[31] Diseases that can be confused with ethmoid hematomas include ulcerative or mycotic rhinitis, nasal polyps, neoplasia, fungal granuloma, botryomycosis, and trauma to the nasal passages and sinuses.

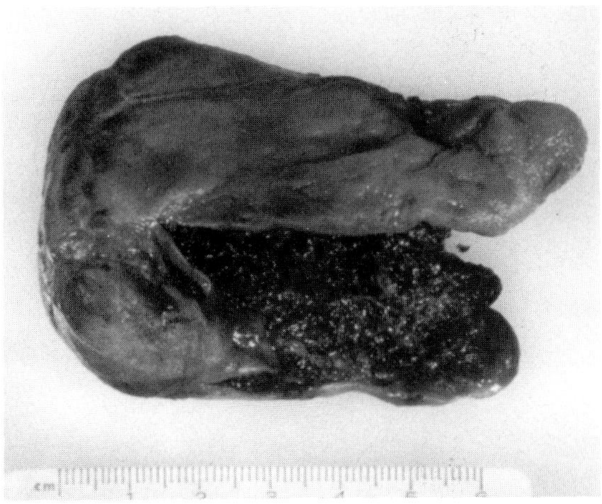

**FIG. 18–7.** Typical appearance of an ethmoid hematoma. The rounded surface to the left extended into the nasal passages. The capsule has been incised to demonstrate the dark hemorrhagic contents.

The largest hematomas arise from the ethmoidal labyrinth, whereas smaller ones originate from the floor and walls of the maxillary and frontal sinuses.[31,32] These smaller, less common lesions arise by a stalk from the mucoperiosteum of the sinus and rarely invade the nasal passages.[31] As an ethmoid hematoma expands, the surface of its capsule ulcerates, and this is responsible for epistaxis. The expanding hematoma also causes pressure necrosis of surrounding bone[31,32] and spreads into the frontal sinus, the sphenopalatine sinus,[31] nasal passages, and nasopharynx.[31]

On histologic examination, the smooth-walled hemorrhagic mass is highly vascular with changes that suggest repeated local hemorrhage, breakdown of hemoglobin, and organization.[33] The capsule is composed largely of respiratory epithelium and fibrous tissue, and the stroma contains blood, fibrous tissue, macrophages, multinucleated giant cells, and deposits of hemosiderin.[33] The degree of changes can vary within the same specimen.[33]

***Clinical Signs.*** Ethmoid hematomas are seen usually in horses older than 4 years but most often at 10 to 12 years of age.[31] The most consistent clinical sign is mild, spontaneous, intermittent unilateral epistaxis that may be present for months to years.[31] It is milder than hemorrhage from guttural pouch mycosis.

A stertorous respiratory noise may be heard

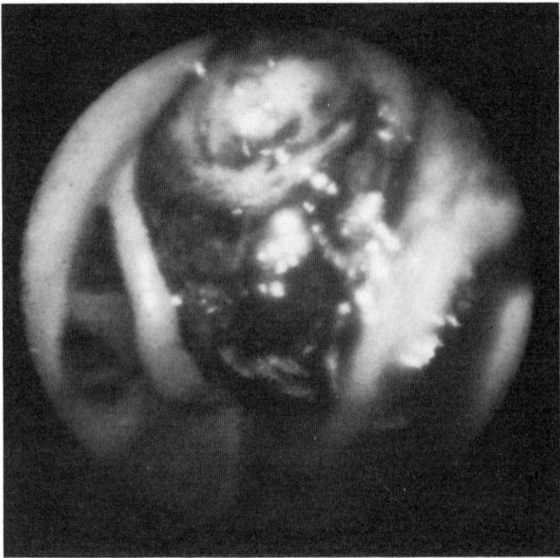

**FIG. 18–8.** View through endoscope of an ethmoid hematoma extending from the right ethmoturbinate region into the nasal passage. There is evidence of old (dark area) and fresh hemorrhage on the surface of the lesion, and some fresh blood can be seen on the nasal septum to the right of this view.

at rest, but is more pronounced during exercise and air flow may be reduced through the nostril on the affected side. The sinuses are usually normal on percussion and facial distortion is rare. Some horses have a mild mucopurulent discharge in conjunction with epistaxis and rarer signs are coughing, malodorous breath, and head shaking.[31] Extremely large hematomas can extend far enough to impinge on the soft palate and cause dysphagia.[34] Bilateral cases are unusual.[31]

***Diagnosis.*** A history of mild, spontaneous epistaxis, especially in an aged horse, is highly suggestive of ethmoid hematoma. On endoscopic examination, a smooth-walled green, black, and red mass with some ulceration can be seen extending from the ethmoid region (Fig. 18–8). Small amounts of blood can be seen on the surface of the lesion and in the nasal passage (Fig. 18–8). The absence of a mass in the nasal passage does not rule out a diagnosis of ethmoid hematoma because small lesions can remain within the sinuses.[32] When the mass is large, its caudal edge can be seen through an endoscope inserted in the contralateral nasal passage.

The hematoma can be seen on radiographs as a smooth-walled, well-circumscribed density that contrasts well with air in the sinus cavity (Figs. 18–9 and 18–10). Fluid lines can be attributed to secondary infection. On a dorsoventral projection of the head, the mass may be seen in the nasal passages where it impinges on, but rarely displaces, the nasal septum[13] (Fig. 18–10).

***Treatment.*** Treatment is surgical removal of the entire lesion through a frontonasal flap sinusotomy.[35] Its origin must be removed but may be difficult to approach within the ethmoidal labyrinth or sphenopalatine sinuses[26] or it may be obscured by copious hemorrhage during surgery. Cryosurgery through a bone flap reduces intraoperative hemorrhage and obviates the need for sinus packing.[31,35] The base of the lesion is frozen and left to slough and the remainder is removed.[36] Disadvantages are risk of damage to the infraorbital nerve and cribriform plate[31] and the copious mucopurulent discharge that may persist for months after surgery, while frozen tissues slough.[31,36] An ethmoid hematoma has been removed successfully by a wire snare,[1] but recurrence is likely after this procedure because it does not remove the lesion completely.[34]

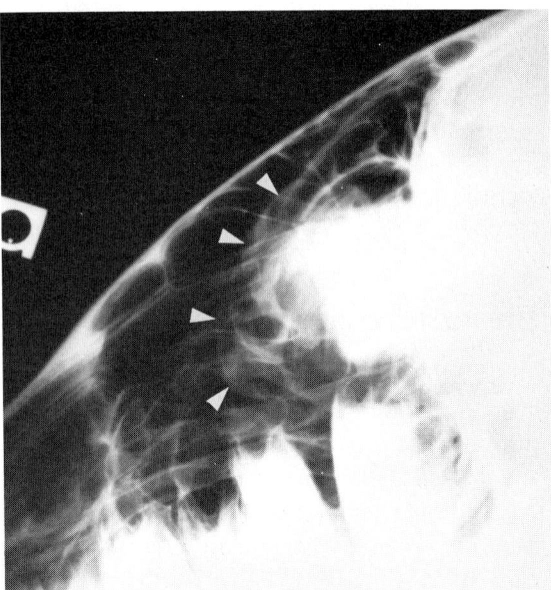

**FIG. 18–9.** Lateral view of an ethmoid hematoma (arrowheads) in the paranasal sinuses. This is the typical location of the lesion, rostral to the ethmoid labyrinth.

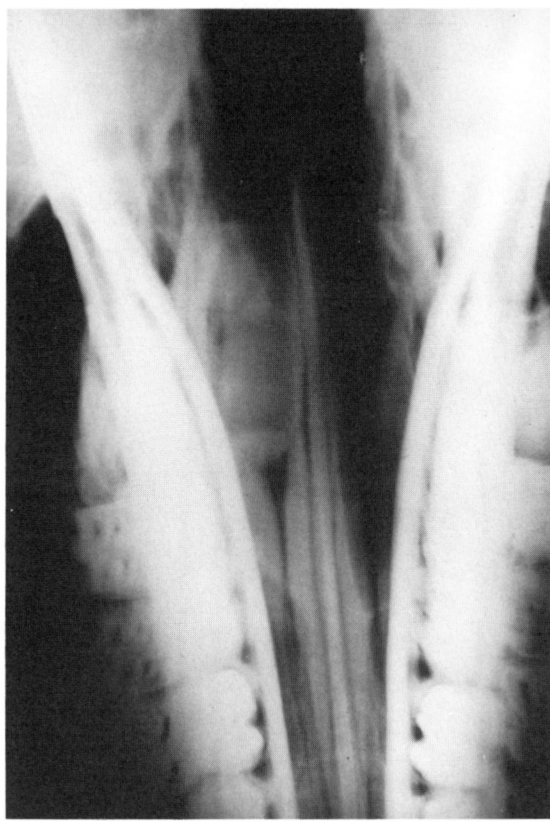

**FIG. 18–10.** Dorsoventral radiograph of a horse with an ethmoid hematoma extending into the right nasal passage. Although the hematoma is impinging on the nasal septum, it is not displacing it.

The recurrence rate after surgical removal of ethmoid hematomas through a sinus flap has been estimated at 42%[31] but may be less after cryosurgery.[1,31,35] Recurrence may be recognized within the first 12 months after surgery. Selective occlusion of vessels to the lesion might prevent recurrence, but it has not been possible to identify any associated vascular abnormalities by angiography to date.[21]

## Sinus Cysts

Sinus cysts are single or loculated fluid-filled cavities with an epithelial lining that develop principally in the maxillary sinuses but can extend into the frontal sinus. Some appear to develop as expanded turbinate structures that fill adjacent sinus cavities.[37] Congenital cysts have been reported in foals that had facial swelling and dyspnea since birth,[38] but a congenital cause would seem unlikely in older horses.[37] The condition has been attributed to a tooth root abnormality,[39–42] but cysts can develop without dental attachments.[38]

***Pathologic Findings.*** Sinus cysts can destroy, distort, or replace bone[39] and displace and deform teeth, but they rarely extend into the nasal cavity.[37] On gross inspection, the cysts appear to be formed of a thick and spongy mucous membrane containing incomplete plates of bone and large cavities filled with a yellow, acellular fluid.[37,40] The fluid can be turbid and viscous if the cyst occludes drainage openings and causes secondary infection.[37,41]

Lane et al proposed that paranasal sinus cysts have the same underlying pathogenesis as ethmoid hematomas.[37] In spite of the gross and histopathologic differences between the two lesions, they also share features such as recent and old partly organized hemorrhage beneath an ulcerated and inflamed respiratory epithelium.[37]

***Clinical Signs.*** Sinus cysts can be found mainly in two age groups, one composed of horses of 1 year and younger and the other of horses older than 9 years.[37] The major clinical signs are mild facial swelling, nasal discharge, and partial airway obstruction.[37] The nasal discharge is rarely malodorous or bloody.[37]

***Diagnosis.*** On endoscopic examination of the nasal passage, the ventral concha can appear enlarged and, in rare cases, a mass can be seen extending into the nasal passage.[37] On radiographs, multiloculated densities (Fig. 18–11) and fluid lines can be seen in the sinuses, but single fluid-filled cavities are found in some horses (Fig. 18–12). The surrounding bone may be thickened and other radiographic findings are dental distortion and displacement (Fig. 18–11), flattening of tooth roots, and soft tissue mineralization.[37] On dorsoventral projections, considerable deviation of the nasal septum and vomer bones can be seen (Fig. 18–11). Fluid samples collected by centesis are usually vivid amber-yellow color[37] and acellular,[40] unlike the thick, cloudy exudate of sinusitis.

***Treatment.*** Sinus cysts are approached

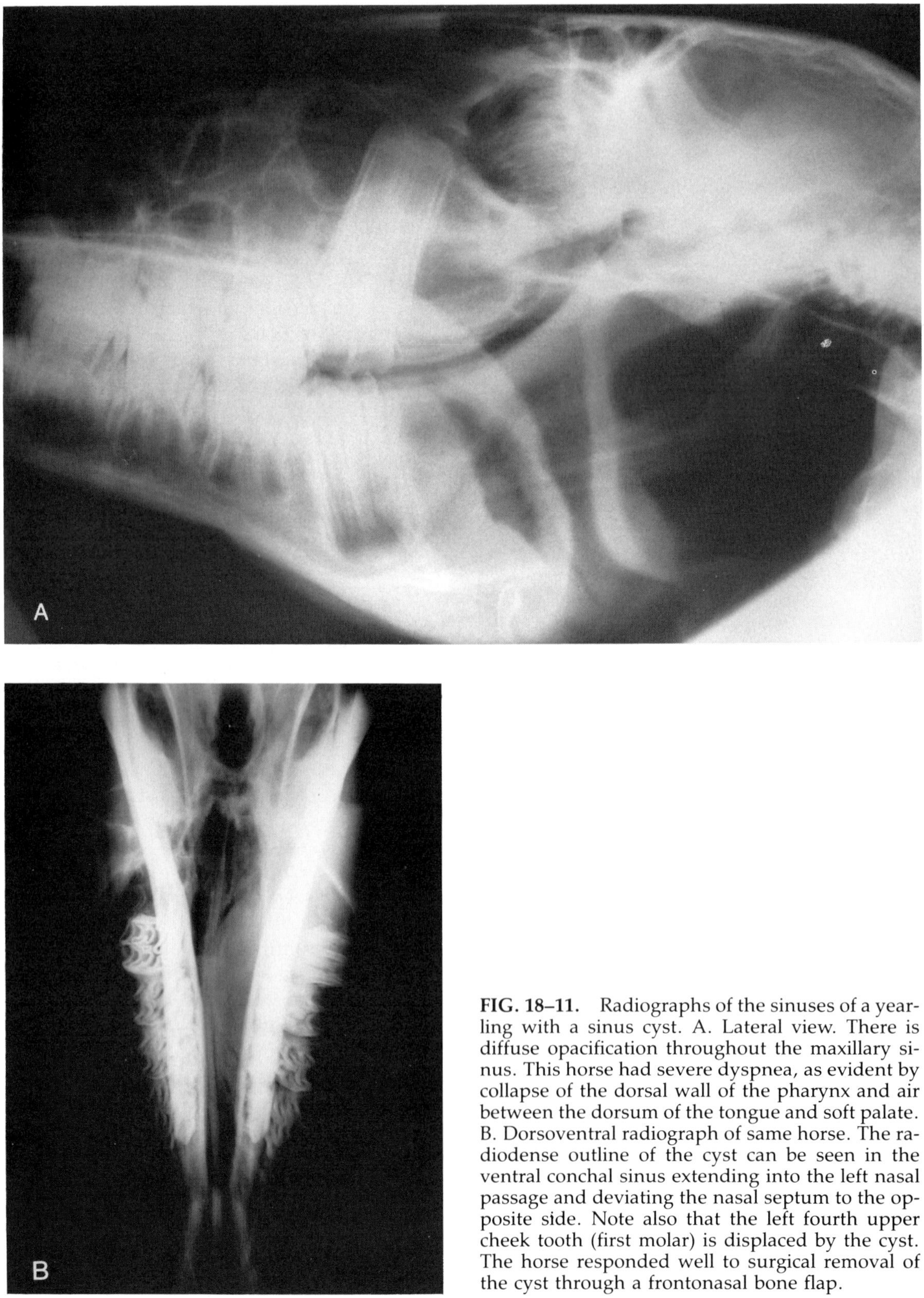

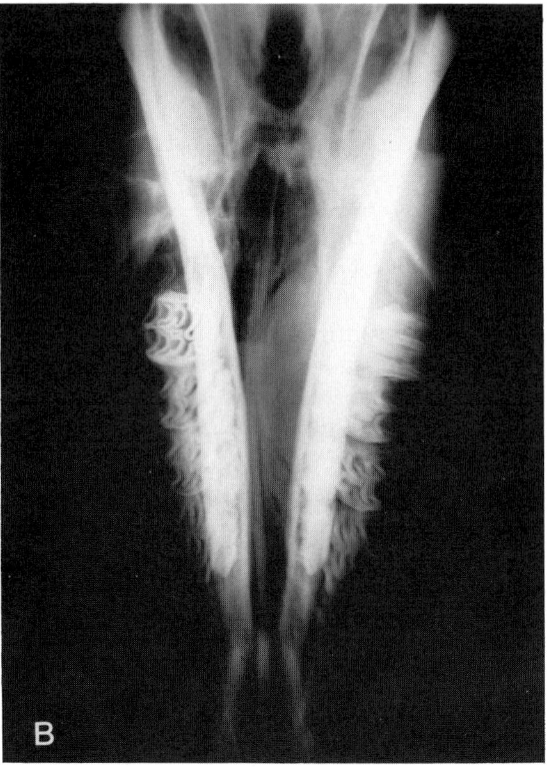


**FIG. 18–11.** Radiographs of the sinuses of a yearling with a sinus cyst. A. Lateral view. There is diffuse opacification throughout the maxillary sinus. This horse had severe dyspnea, as evident by collapse of the dorsal wall of the pharynx and air between the dorsum of the tongue and soft palate. B. Dorsoventral radiograph of same horse. The radiodense outline of the cyst can be seen in the ventral conchal sinus extending into the left nasal passage and deviating the nasal septum to the opposite side. Note also that the left fourth upper cheek tooth (first molar) is displaced by the cyst. The horse responded well to surgical removal of the cyst through a frontonasal bone flap.

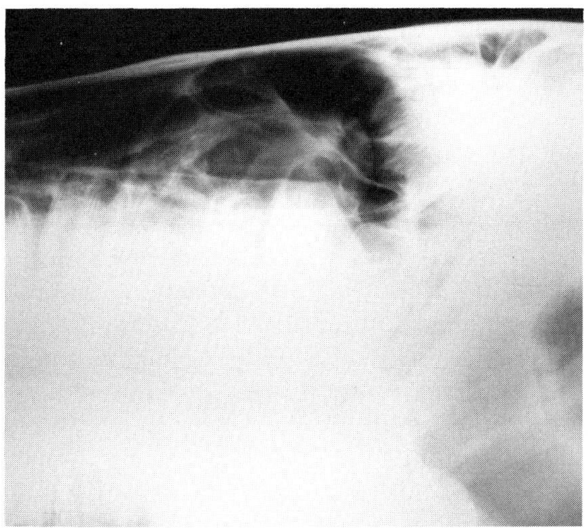

**FIG. 18–12.** Lateral view of a sinus cyst in a 3-year-old Standardbred colt. The cyst has a smooth border projecting into the frontal sinus. Free fluid in the frontal sinus was from a secondary infection.

through a frontal or maxillary bone flap and the entire cyst can be separated from surrounding structures by digital dissection.[37] Some recommend removal of an involved tooth[42,43] but this is of questionable value because it is not evident that sinus cysts arise from tooth roots. Removal can be followed by hemorrhage, especially from attachments to the ventral concha. The normal sinus boundaries are frequently disrupted by the cyst so that a large communication is established between the sinuses and nasal passage.

***Prognosis.*** The prognosis is good after surgical treatment and the recurrence rate is low.[37] Most of the facial distortion resolves after surgery so that facial contour returns to normal over time,[37] especially in young horses. Some horses have a permanent, mild, mucous discharge from the nostril after surgery but this does not appear to be associated with any problems.

## Mucocele

A mucocele is a secreting cyst lined by sinus membrane.[44,45] Although the cause and the pathogenesis of the condition are unknown, it appears to be caused by a congenital absence of the normal nasomaxillary opening.[44] In this way, it may differ from a sinus cyst, although the distinction may not be as simple. It is usually seen in horses under 2 years of age.[44,45]

***Clinical Signs and Diagnosis.*** The predominant clinical features of this disease are bulging of the maxilla and respiratory obstruction, without nasal discharge.[44] Clear, straw-colored, acellular, sterile fluid can be aspirated from the sinus,[45] but the fluid may be thick and mucoid also.[44] On radiographs, the affected sinus is filled with homogeneous fluid.[44]

***Treatment.*** This involves creation of a drainage opening from the sinuses into the nasal passages and is described in the section on surgery.

***Prognosis.*** The response to surgical treatment is good and the newly created drainage hole functions effectively.[44] Shortly after surgery, the facial deformity regresses and the head returns to a normal shape and contour. If the condition is not treated, a secondary infection can develop.[44,45]

## Wounds and Fractures

Blunt injuries to the frontal and nasal bones usually are caused by kicks from other horses or collisions with fixed objects.[1] They can be open or closed.

***Clinical Signs.*** A closed fracture over the sinuses is usually evident as a painful swelling or depression. It can go unnoticed for some time because the fracture fragments are forced into the sinus cavity and the space between them and overlying skin fills with blood so that facial contour is close to normal. As healing progresses, a depression forms along the fracture line. If fracture fragments are not depressed, organization of the hematoma and fracture callous produce a firm, subcutaneous swelling.

Epistaxis and subcutaneous emphysema are common clinical signs of sinus trauma and less common signs are dyspnea and epiphora. In acute cases, it may be possible to feel a hematoma and fracture fragments.[1] Severe trauma to the head and sinuses can cause ocular and central nervous system abnormalities.[46]

***Diagnosis.*** Diagnosis of a depression fracture or sinus trauma can be made on history, clinical signs, and by radiography. History of direct trauma to the head is rarely available but can be suspected, especially if the horse is kept outside with others. On radiographs, fracture fragments and fluid lines from blood can be seen within the involved sinuses, but several oblique views may be required to demonstrate most fragments. In many cases, the fracture is more extensive than the external soft tissue injury and radiographic findings would suggest.[47]

Different forms of nonpainful swellings should not be confused with traumatic injuries. It is not unusual for the reserve tooth crowns of young Welsh ponies and crosses to project a considerable distance into the sinus cavities to cause firm, painless, bilateral swellings in the nasal bones and maxilla. Similar bony lumps may be evident along the mandible and they correspond on radiographs to prominent dental sacs.[21] Facial lumps or "horns" can be seen in horses as symmetrical, painless prominences of the nasal and frontal bones and can be attributed tentatively to an embryologic fault.[44]

***Treatment.*** If the injury is recent, several days or a week can be allowed before surgical treatment and during that time, the horse is treated with nonsteroidal anti-inflammatory drugs, antibiotics and local cold compresses to reduce edema.[46] If the skin is intact, the fracture fragments can be exposed through a large curvilinear skin flap that can provide adequate soft tissue coverage of the repaired bone and implants.[46,47] After the fracture fragments have been exposed, blood clots are removed and the sinus cavity is flushed liberally with saline solution.[46] To facilitate elevation of the fracture fragments, small holes can be drilled in adjacent bone and a periosteal elevator or Langenbeck retractors can be passed through these to pry up depressed fragments.[46,47] If the fragments wedge firmly together in their normal position and form a stable union, it may be unnecessary to wire them.[46,47] If small pieces of bone have been lost or have to be removed, remaining fragments may have to be wired into position. All small fragments without periosteal attachments should be removed.[47] In horses with long-standing, healed depression fractures, fluorocarbon polymer and carbon fiber can be used to restore facial contour.[48] Alternatively, the healed fracture fragments can be cut with a saw and elevated into position. However, a better cosmetic appearance can be obtained by primary open reduction shortly after injury rather than facial reconstruction later.[47]

Untreated, open wounds can form chronic sinus or nasal fistulas. These can be repaired with single or double periosteal flaps reflected from adjacent normal bone so that the osteogenic (inner) layer faces externally.[49] Bone grafts can be applied to periosteal flaps but they are not essential and could retard facial growth in young horses.[49,50] Sinus fistulas can be repaired also by a temporalis muscle flap and a split-thickness skin graft.[51] Postoperative care with all techniques involves systemic antibiotics and a firm pressure bandage to decrease edema and subcutaneous emphysema.[47] If sinusitis develops, daily irrigations may be indicated.[46] Large defects that are not repaired can heal gradually over several months and, during that time, the advancing skin edges should be elevated frequently to prevent them from curling inward.[43,52]

***Prognosis.*** Many fractures into sinuses heal spontaneously and surgery is unnecessary when the injury is minor or cosmetic repair is not essential. If severe cases are not treated, complications such as sinusitis, sequestra formation, deformity, and even nasal obstruction can be expected.[47] After repair of acute wounds, healing is usually excellent and cosmetically acceptable. It can be difficult to mobilize skin over long-standing fistulas and dehiscence can be expected if flaps are not provided with adequate soft tissue or bony support.[49,51] Severe injury to sinuses or nasal passages of young horses can interfere with bone growth and cause facial deformities.[12]

## *Neoplasia and Neoplasia-Like Lesions*

General comments about sinus tumors in horses can be found in Chapter 17. The most common type of neoplasm of the paranasal sinuses of the horse is squamous cell carcinoma.[53–56] Squamous cell carcinomas in the sinuses may arise from squamous metaplasia

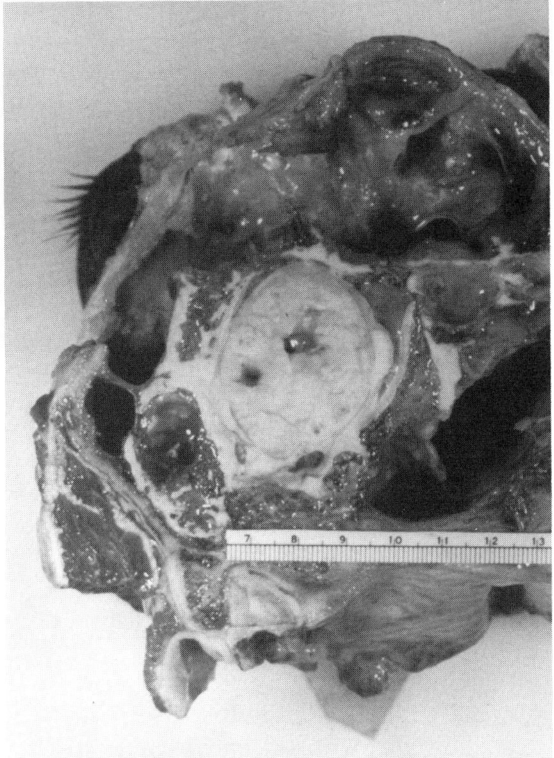


**FIG. 18–13.** Transverse section of the head of a horse with a cementoma of the third cheek tooth (fourth premolar) in the right maxillary sinus (this is the same horse as shown in Figure 18–4). There is marked destruction of the sinus architecture and compression of the ipsilateral nasal passage. Sinuses were filled with a thick brown fluid.

of the mucosal epithelium or could originate in the buccal mucosa; however, they are usually found in the sinuses without any lesions in the oral cavity.[54,57]

Other tumors of the paranasal sinuses are adenocarcinoma,[53,54,58] spindle cell sarcoma,[59] osteosarcoma,[14,39,54,60] fibrosarcoma,[53,61] fibroma,[53] round cell sarcoma,[54] ethmoid carcinoma,[62] neurofibroma,[1] mast cell tumor,[1] myxoma,[10,53] lymphosarcoma,[23] and chondrosarcoma.[17] Adamantinomas are seen usually in young horses but are more common in the mandible than in the upper jaw.[54] Complex odontomas originate from dental follicles and have been described in the horse.[63] An odontoma is not a true neoplasm but a tumor-like malformation or hamartoma, composed of dentin, enamel, and cementum.[55]

Cementomas are rare, irritative, hyperplastic lesions of cementum of the root apex[17,64,65] (Figs. 18–13 and 18–14). Fibrous dysplasia, which is a dysplastic focal proliferation of stroma and bone, different from osteodystrophia fibrosa, has been described in the maxillary sinus of a horse.[66]

Although tumors of the paranasal sinuses are more likely to be seen in older horses,[53,54] they have been reported also in young horses. These include osteoma in horses ranging from 6 weeks[13] to 2 years old,[44,67–70] osteosarcoma in a 2-year-old Thoroughbred colt,[39] fibrosarcoma in an 11-month-old Arabian filly,[61] angiosarcoma in a 4 year old,[9] and lymphosarcoma in an 18-month-old Thoroughbred filly.[71] Sinus osteomas in horses have been reported only in males.[44,67–69] Congenital tumors in the maxillary sinuses of horses are rare and include an ethmoid carcinoma,[62] fibrosarcoma, and a possible spindle cell sarcoma.[61] Congenital ameloblastic odontomas have been described in the maxillary sinus of foals.[72,73]

***Gross Pathologic Changes.*** Severe clinical

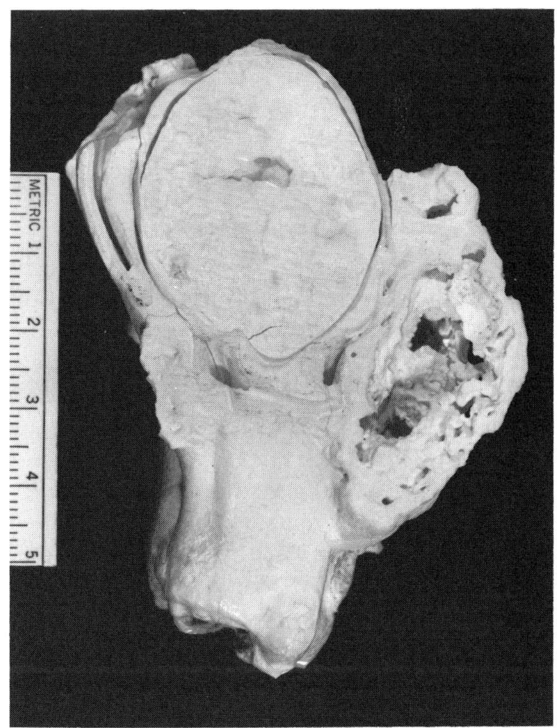


**FIG. 18–14.** Section of affected tooth with cementoma after soft tissues have been removed by boiling. The large ovoid mass that constitutes the cementoma incorporates the root of the third cheek tooth.

signs in horses with neoplasia or neoplasia-like masses in the paranasal sinuses can be attributed to the extent and severity of tissue damage by the time diagnosis is made (Fig. 18–13). Tumors can spread rapidly from the sinuses into the nasopharynx and nasal passages and also in the opposite direction.[74] Local destruction can expose the infraorbital nerve, loosen tooth roots, damage large arteries,[73] and extend to the hard palate[75] and cranial cavity.[54,56,58] Secondary infection usually develops in association with aggressive sinus tumors and contributes to the local destruction. Metastasis is not common and may be limited to adjacent lymph nodes.

***Clinical Signs.*** Clinical signs of sinus neoplasia resemble those of secondary sinusitis but are usually more severe. Bone destruction and facial distortion are more pronounced and the mucopurulent nasal discharge is fetid and usually bloodstained. Bone over the sinuses may become thin and soft and sometimes be completely destroyed. Neurologic signs and blindness are evidence that the tumor has involved the cranial cavity and caused brain damage.[58] Other signs that can be seen are enlarged local lymph nodes,[59,71] anorexia, weight loss,[58] head shaking,[70] and torticollis.[68]

***Diagnosis.*** Clinical signs, history, endoscopic and radiographic examinations may not be sufficient to distinguish sinus neoplasia from primary or secondary sinusitis, fungal granulomas, chronic inflammatory polyps, amyloid degeneration in the nasal passages, or osteodystrophy.[54] On oral examination, it may be possible to see a mucosal defect on the hard palate or retraction of the hard palate mucosa from the molars in horses with squamous cell carcinoma.[76,77] On radiographs, diffuse changes may be evident, such as severe osteolysis, distortion, proliferation, and opacification.[17] An osteoma can vary in density from soft tissue to compact bone[13,14,44,67,69,70] (Fig. 18–15) and an odontoma may appear as a radiopaque mass, composed of mineralized tissues and dentricles within a soft tissue stroma.[72,73] A cementoma is usually dense and can be seen above and incorporating a tooth root (Fig. 18–16).

Definitive diagnosis is made by histopathologic examination of biopsy specimens. Samples of tumor can be removed through a trephine hole with the horse standing, but more representative samples can be obtained through a bone flap with the horse under general anesthesia.

***Treatment and Prognosis.*** Surgical treatment is generally unsuccessful because the tumor is usually too extensive and tissue destruction too great by the time diagnosis is made. In addition, the advanced state of the disease warrants aggressive therapy in an area where anatomy is complex and the risks of iatrogenic injuries are considerable. Many sinus tumors, especially carcinomas, are locally invasive and likely to recur.[62] Radiation therapy[75,78] could be considered for discrete lesions and cryotherapy for lesions[63] that do not involve tooth roots, the infraorbital canal, or the cribriform plate.

Successful surgical treatment without recurrence has been described for a squamous cell carcinoma with 2 years' follow-up,[1] fibrosarcoma with 10 months follow-up[79] and ossified fibromas with unspecified follow-up.[26] Radiographic examination of the sinuses at 2- to 3-month intervals is recommended to detect early signs of recurrence.[79]

An osteoma is usually amenable to treatment because it is benign, grows slowly, has pedunculated or sessile attachments over a small base, and tends to form a well-circumscribed mass (Fig. 18–15) rather than to infiltrate.[68] The tumor may have to be divided and removed in piecemeal fashion[67] and two bone flaps may be required,[68] but tooth removal[70] is rarely indicated. It is usually difficult to identify points of attachment and the site of origin[68,69] of an osteoma and failure to remove all the tumor could lead to recurrence.[68]

## Fungal Diseases

Fungal infections of the sinuses are rare and sporadic and difficult to treat, and generally carry a guarded prognosis. Many of the organisms involved are saprophytes that can be found in barnyard soil and manure and some of them may be endemic in parts of the southwestern United States.[80] Granulomas caused by Cryptococcus neoformans,[24,81–86] Coccidioides immitis,[52,87] Allescheria boydii (Mad-

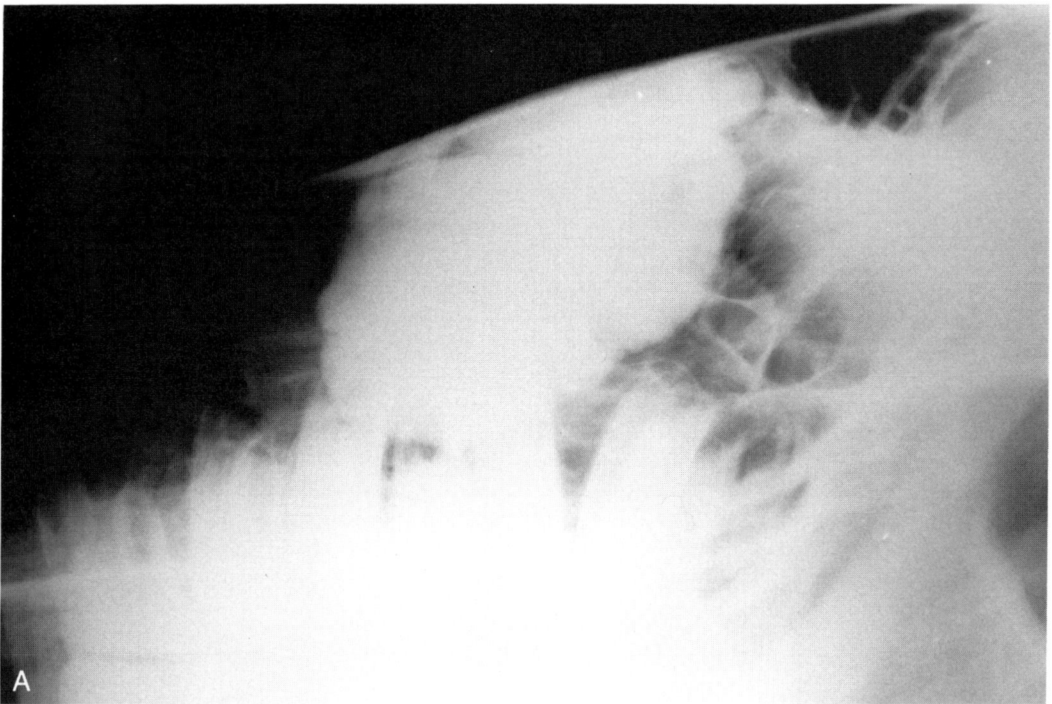


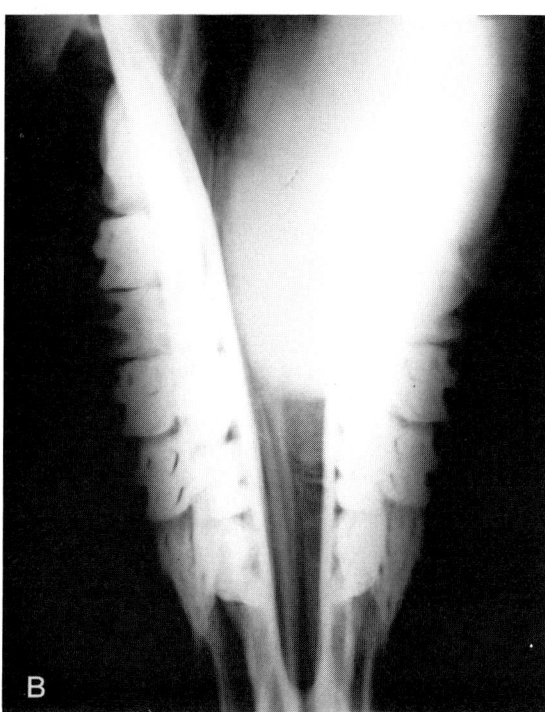


**FIG. 18–15.** Radiographs of the head of a horse with an osteoma. A. Lateral view of the sinuses showing the dense lesion within the maxillary and frontal sinuses. B. Dorsoventral view showing the smooth, well defined, and radiodense form of the osteoma impinging on the left nasal passage and deviating the nasal septum to the opposite site. This was removed successfully through a large frontonasal flap approach.

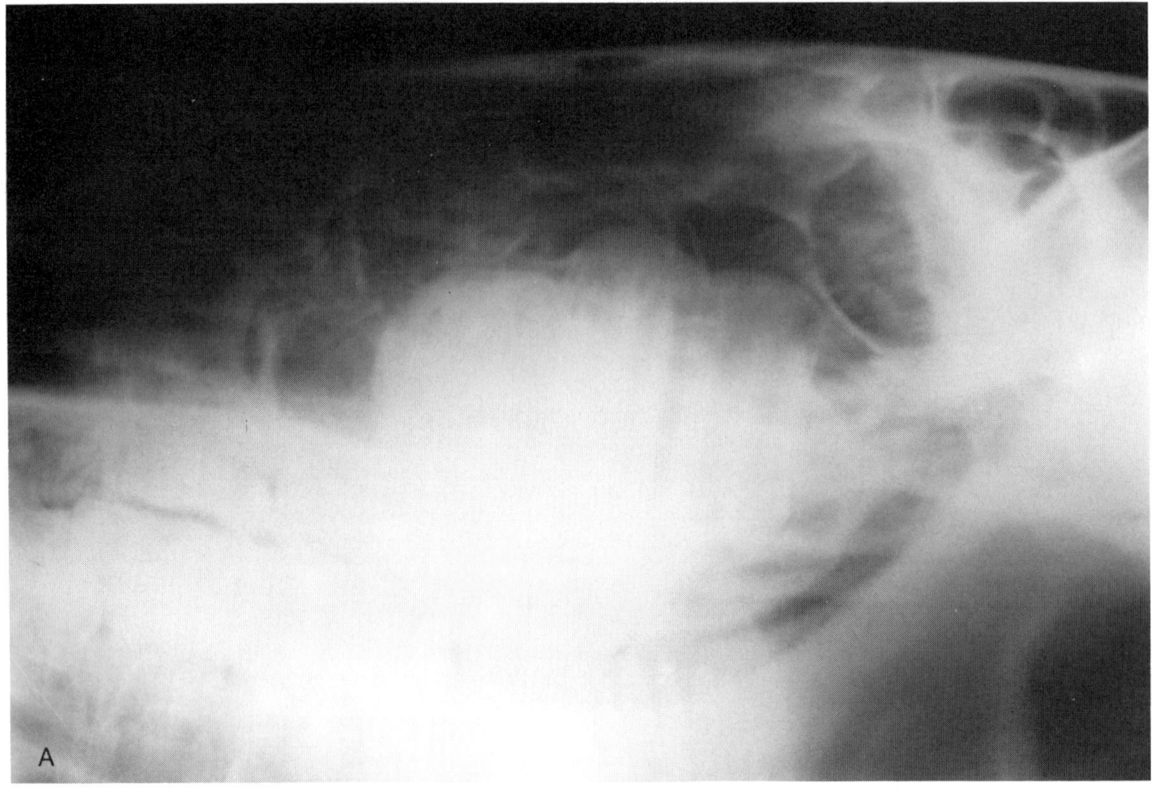


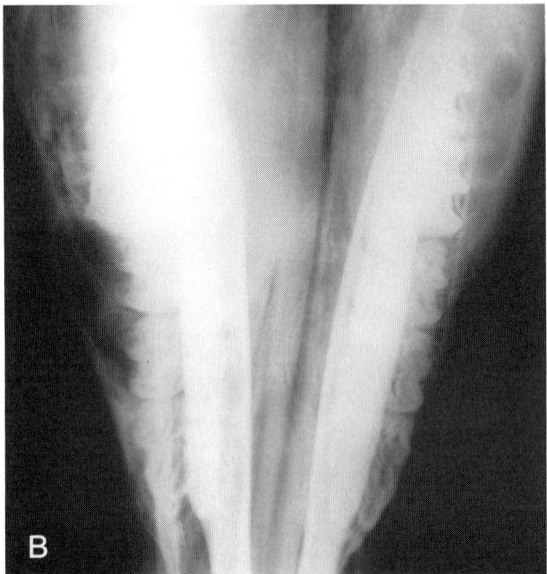


**FIG. 18–16.** Radiographs of horse with cementoma involving the third cheek tooth. This is the same horse as shown in Figures 18–4, 18–13, and 18–14. A. The radiodense outline of the cementoma can be seen involving and incorporating the root of the third cheek tooth on the lateral projection; opacification throughout the sinus cavities is evidence of fluid accumulation and associated reaction within the sinuses. B. Dorsoventral view of cementoma in the right maxillary sinus. The mass and associated sinus enlargement have completely occluded the right nasal passage and deviated the septum toward the opposite side.

uromycosis),[88] and Pseudallescheria boydii[20] have been reported in the nasal passages, frontal and maxillary sinuses, cribriform plate, nasopharynx, conchae, conchal sinuses, and sphenopalatine sinus of horses. Granulomas usually distort and destroy bone in a progressive fashion and can produce a retrobulbar mass and displace the cerebral hemisphere.[83,88] Spread to distant organs is unusual, but a horse with a long-standing cryptococcal granuloma developed lesions in the lungs and jejunum.[81] Discrete lesions caused by Aspergillus sp and a Penicillium sp can be confined to the involved sinus.[13] Predisposing causes are identified rarely.[88]

***Clinical Signs.*** Clinical signs closely resemble those of sinus neoplasia, and can include severe facial distortion, swollen periorbital region and exophthalmos,[81,83] blindness with postorbital lesions,[83] epistaxis,[24,84] and weight loss.[85]

***Diagnosis.*** Information about the horse's origin may be valuable in making a diagnosis because some infections, such as coccidioidomycosis, are considered to be endemic in arid parts of the United States.[52] On endoscopic examination, fungal granulomas are usually evident in the nasal passages as large, firm, lobulated or nonlobulated masses covered by intact, smooth, and glistening mucosa.[24,52,81] Parts of the mucosal surface may be ulcerated. On radiographs, fungal granulomas can be recognized as smooth-walled, well-demarcated soft tissue densities in the nasal passages and sinuses with fluid lines in the sinuses.[52,81,85] Small fungal lesions confined to the interior of the paranasal sinuses cannot be seen on radiographs.[13] The most definitive diagnosis can be made by biopsy of representative samples of tissue taken through the endoscope, with a uterine biopsy forceps or excised through a trephine opening or bone flap. It should be possible to identify the organisms by microscopic examination and fungal cultures. Immunologic techniques are used for presumptive diagnosis of systemic mycoses in other animals and human beings[89–91] and might be especially useful in the horse because deep granulomas are not readily accessible for other diagnostic methods.

***Treatment.*** It has been recommended that infected animals be destroyed for public health reasons,[83] but the condition can be treated by surgery through large bone flaps. Some horses that have responded to surgery in one site have subsequently developed similar lesions in the opposite nasal passages and sinuses.[24,87] Cryotherapy has been used successfully in a cryptococcal granuloma.[82] Humane destruction is recommended when the disease has become too extensive and irreversible damage has developed.

Amphotericin B, given IV daily for at least a month, is effective against many fungal granulomas but was not effective in 1 horse with cryptococcosis in the frontal and maxillary sinuses.[82] Ketoconazole has been used for treatment of fungal granulomas in other species.[89] Topical treatment with antifungal agents would appear to have little place in the treatment of large fungal granulomas but could be applied after the bulk of the lesion has been removed surgically.

## *Micronema deletrix Infection*

Micronema deletrix is a saprophytic nematode found in decaying humus[92] and infection with these organisms has been described in many countries, including the United States.[93,94] Infection produces a mass of gray, yellow fibrous tissue that obliterates the sinuses and their walls, loosens teeth and distorts sinus architecture.[92,93] Infection can be unilateral[92] or bilateral,[93] involve both the upper and lower jaws,[92] and spread to the kidneys and cerebellum.[92,94]

The predominant clinical signs are facial distortion with firm swellings in the maxilla, unilateral or bilateral nasal discharge, marked dyspnea and stridor, difficulty in eating, and weight loss.[93] The condition can be confused with squamous cell carcinoma but the female rhabditiform nematodes, their larvae and eggs, can be seen in clusters or scattered throughout a biopsy specimen.[92,93] Ivermectin can be used for treatment,[92] but the prognosis appears to be poor and there is a risk of spread to other organs.[92,94]

## *Miscellaneous*

Frontal sinus eversion has been described as a hard, slow-growing protuberance over the frontal sinus, probably of congenital origin, and in direct communication with the sinus cavity.[95] The bony protuberance can be removed through a large elliptical incision and the resulting defect in the frontal bone repaired with synthetic polypropylene mesh (Marlex) and skin.[95]

Osteodystrophia fibrosa or secondary nutritional hyperparathyroidism is rarely if ever seen under modern management conditions.[96] It can develop in horses on a diet high in foods containing phosphorus, such as bran, and can be attributed to calcium deficiency.[44] Early clinical signs are changes in gait and lameness and these are followed by bilateral enlargement of the mandible, maxilla, and conchae.[44,96] The condition can cause severe respiratory difficulty.[39]

A congenital lesion attributed to hemorrhage within a developing tooth and resembling a maxillary sinus cyst on radiographs was diagnosed as a dental cyst.[7] An oromaxillary fistula, possibly congenital, has been reported as a cause of sinusitis and dental displacement.[13]

# Surgery of the Paranasal Sinuses

The paranasal sinuses can be opened for exploration and removal of tumors, masses, diseased cheek teeth, abnormal and infected mucosa and to establish drainage into the nasal cavity. Although trephine openings can be used, they have been largely replaced by the more versatile bone flap techniques that allow greater access to the sinus cavities and more thorough debridement of abnormal tissues.

## *Frontonasal Flap Technique*

A frontonasal flap approach can be used to gain access to the conchofrontal and caudal maxillary sinuses and, by additional steps, to the rostral maxillary and ventral conchal sinuses. It can be used also for removal of 5th and 6th cheek teeth but access to the 4th cheek tooth is limited in some horses. The size and position of the flap can be designed to suit the lesion, but a large flap is generally recommended.

Before sinus surgery, a potential blood donor should be identified by cross-match with the patient and be made available. If severe blood loss is anticipated or the patient is already anemic, 8 L of whole blood should be collected shortly before surgery and be stored in citrate. Fluids are given intravenously during surgery.

### Surgical Landmarks

The caudal edge of the bone flap is on a line at right angles to the dorsal midline and midway between the supraorbital foramen and the medial canthus of the eye (Fig. 18–17). The lateral edge* is roughly parallel to the midline and 2 to 2.5 cm medial to the medial canthus of the eye (Fig. 18–17). It is approximately 9 to 10 cm long. The rostral edge is at right angles to the dorsal midline, two thirds the distance between the medial canthus of the eye and the infraorbital foramen (Fig. 18–17). A flap cut in this fashion has a base along the dorsal midline and lies ventral to the surgical field.

### Surgical Procedure

The skin is incised to overlap the bone incision by 5 mm and its corners are made slightly round. Few major vessels are encountered and bleeding is usually slight. The underlying periosteum is incised and the exposed bone is cut with an oscillating bone saw (Stryker) to create the three-sided rectangular flap. When the lateral bone incision is made, care should be taken to avoid the nasolacrimal duct immediately lateral to it (Fig. 18–17). The bone flap can be cut with a 45 degree angle to ensure a secure contact with the parent bone when repositioned,[24] but this is not necessary. The bone flap can be cut also with a #700 to #701-tapered fissured burr in a Hall

*For description of a nasofrontal bone flap, medial and lateral are used instead of dorsal and ventral because the frontal bone is flat and these margins are almost level on the most dorsal aspect of the head.

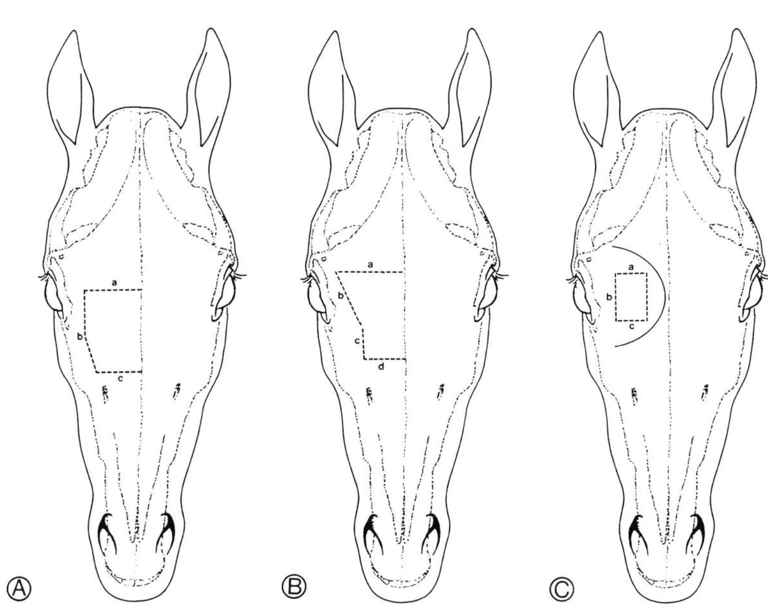


**FIG. 18–17.** A. Outline of frontonasal flap approach. a = Caudal, b = lateral, and c = rostral margins. The lateral margin angles medially to avoid the nasolacrimal duct. The duct follows a course from the medial canthus of the eye towards the nasoincisive notch (see Fig. 18–1B). B. Outline of triangulated flap approach for conchofrontal sinus.[24] a = Caudal margin (approximately 6 cm); b and c = lateral margin (angle between a and b = 60°); d = rostral margin (approximately 4.5 cm). Length of flap (a to d) is approximately 9 cm. C. Approach to frontal sinus through a curvilinear incision.[99,100] Key as in Figure 18–1A. The bone flap can be broken along a medial or lateral margin if it is retained. Alternatively, the entire bone flap can be removed and discarded.[26]

drill[97] or with an osteotome along lines that join drill holes at the corners of the flap.[98]

The small bony attachments or lamellae between the underside of the flap and floor of the frontal sinus are cut with a 9-mm osteotome, at the same time elevating the osteotome until the flap is completely freed. Wide periosteal elevators or osteotomes are placed under the rostral and caudal ends of the flap to pry it open and fracture it along the midline. When the flap is made in this fashion, the skin, fascia, and periosteum combine with incomplete points of fracture to form a solid hinge.

This approach allows direct access to the conchofrontal sinus and the caudal maxillary sinus. The bulla of the ventral conchal sinus and the rostral edge of the frontomaxillary opening can be broken down to allow access to the rostral maxillary sinus and ventral conchal sinus (Fig. 18–18). The lateral and ventral walls of the dorsal conchal sinus and the underlying ventral concha can then be disrupted to allow greater access to the rostral maxillary sinus and the ventral conchal sinus (Fig. 18–18). This step also establishes an opening from each conchal sinus into the nasal cavity and these can be enlarged if needed (Fig. 18–18). Disruption of conchal walls should be the last step in the procedure because it causes profuse hemorrhage that obscures the surgical field. Walls of the conchae should be opened with scissors or rongeurs. A hole can also be made by forcing a blunt instrument through the concha but this can produce small bone fragments that may obstruct the openings or form sequestra subsequently. The rigid septum that divides the maxillary sinus can be broken down completely to improve access to the rostral maxillary sinus; however, access to the most rostral end is limited.

To control the profuse hemorrhage that usually follows sinus surgery, the sinus cavity is packed with gauze soaked in 1:10,000 epinephrine[24,43] or saline alone. The major concern with epinephrine is the increased risk of cardiac arrhythmias in horses under halothane anesthesia.[24] The gauze packing should be folded in accordion fashion so that it will not become entangled during withdrawal. Its free end is drawn through the nasal passage and sutured to the roof of the false nostril. Alternatively, it can be brought out through

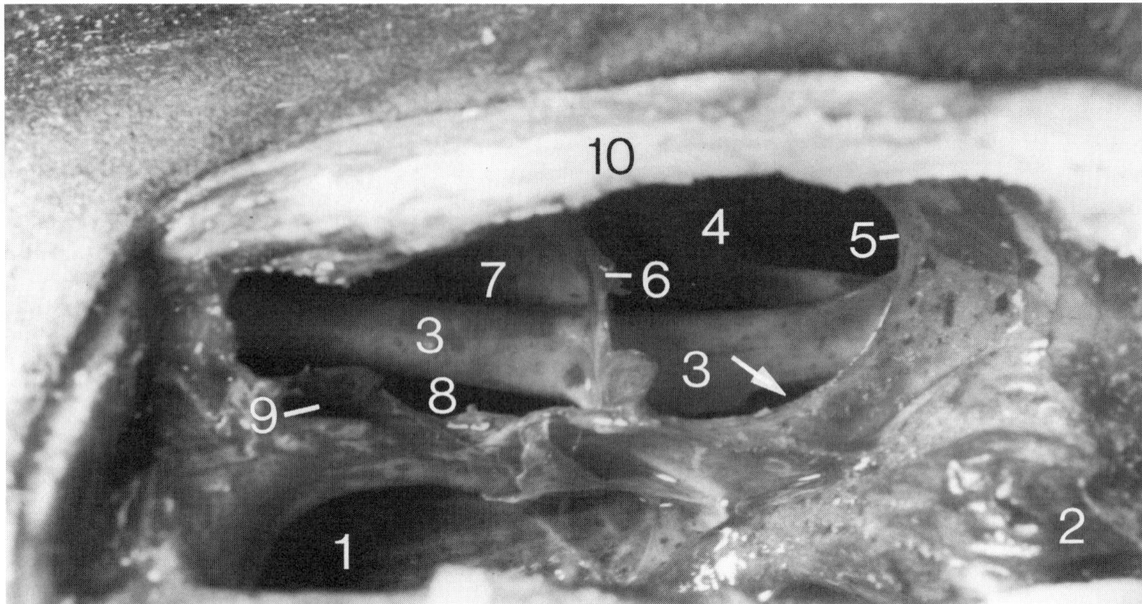


**FIG. 18–18.** View of sinus as through a right frontonasal bone flap (horse in left lateral recumbency and flap as in Figure 18–17A) after part of the floor of the frontal sinus, the dorsal and ventral conchae, and the conchal bulla have been removed to expose the rostral maxillary sinus and ventral conchal sinus (cadaver specimen). The rostral end of the head is to the left and the dorsal midline is along the bottom edge of the photograph. 1 = Dorsal conchal sinus (within dorsal concha); 2 = ethmoid labyrinth; 3 = infraorbital canal; 4 = caudal maxillary sinus; 5 = caudal edge of frontomaxillary opening; 6 = septum between rostral and caudal maxillary sinuses; 7 = rostral maxillary sinus; 8 = ventral conchal sinus (within ventral concha); 9 = opening into middle nasal meatus between cut edges of the conchae; 10 = lateral margin of opening (corresponds to b in Fig. 18–17A). Arrow points toward the sphenopalatine sinus, medial to the infraorbital canal and beneath the ethmoid labyrinth.

a small corner broken off the bone flap or through a trephine hole in adjacent intact bone.

The bone flap is repaired by drilling holes in the edges of the flap and at corresponding points in the parent bone with a 2-mm Steinmann pin. Simple interrupted sutures of #2 Vicryl or 25-gauge wire[98] are used to secure the bone in place and the subcutaneous fascia and skin are closed in routine fashion. The flap also can be repaired securely by suturing only the periosteum and fascia with absorbable material, without sutures in the bone itself.[24,97] Wire and other nonabsorbable sutures in bone can cause permanent subcutaneous nodules and any suture through the bone can be a nidus for infection from the sinuses.

## Aftercare

Packing is removed at 72 hours after surgery and removal is followed usually by mild to moderate hemorrhage for several minutes. Daily postoperative irrigation of the sinus is recommended for 10 to 14 days after surgery for septic or destructive lesions. The purpose is to remove necrotic tissue and blood and to promote drainage. The sinus can be flushed through a piece of tubing inserted through intact bone,[97] through a 24-F Foley balloon catheter inserted into the sinus through the nasal passages[26] or through a balloon catheter inserted through a separate trephine hole.[68] Antibiotics such as penicillin and gentamicin can be given on the morning of surgery and continued for 3 to 5 days afterwards.

## Alternative Procedures

The triangulated bone-flap technique is similar to the preceding except that the lateral bone incision follows the outline of the conchofrontal sinus more closely[24] (Fig. 18–17). This reduces rostral width of the flap and may thus limit lateral access to the ventral conchal sinus and rostral maxillary sinus (Fig. 18–17). An alternative approach to the conchofrontal sinus involves a curvilinear skin incision with its base approximately half-way between the midline and the medial canthus of the eye[99,100] (Fig. 18–17). The skin is reflected off the underlying tissues and a rectangular bone flap is then made within the confines of the skin incision[99,100] (Fig. 18–17). Consequently, the size of the sinus opening is smaller than in the preceding methods.

The combined skin and bone flap can be made with a lateral base, but it is difficult to fracture the bone cleanly along the medial canthus. Also, the flap must be retained out of the surgical field by stay sutures or clamps if it is fractured along the lateral margin. There is no evidence that blood supply to bone and attached soft tissues is jeopardized more with a flap attached medially than one attached laterally or vice versa.

The bone flap can be made after the skin has been separated off the underlying periosteum and reflected separately;[24,42,98,99] however, this appears to offer no particular advantage and could predispose to hematoma formation and cellulitis in the subcutaneous deadspace and necrosis of the bone flap. If a small flap is made, the bone can be discarded.[23,26,37]

## *Maxillary Sinus Flap*

The maxillary sinus flap approach is most suitable for lesions that are confined to the rostral maxillary sinus. The skin incision is curvilinear[99] or corresponds in shape with the rectangular bone flap and overlaps it by 5 mm. The caudal border of the bone flap* is at right angles to the facial crest and is 0.5 to 1 cm in front of the medial canthus of the eye (Fig. 18–19). The ventral border is 0.5 cm above and parallel with the facial crest and the rostral border is from the end of the facial crest and parallel with the caudal border (Fig. 18–19). Its dorsal limit is on a line from the nasoincisive notch to the medial canthus[101] (Fig. 18–19).

The bone flap is cut as for the nasofrontal flap technique.[97] The origins of the levator labii maxillaris and levator nasolabialis muscles must be elevated from the most rostral end of the flap and large branches from the angular artery of the eye and associated vein may have to be ligated and cut. Attachments of the flap to the septum that divides the maxillary sinus may have to be cut with an osteotome, unless it has been destroyed by the disease process.

The sagittal bony plate beneath the infraorbital canal can be broken down to remove inspissated pus from the ventral conchal sinus (Fig. 18–3). Pus in this site can also be removed through the empty alveolus if a tooth is repelled or through the narrow space over the infraorbital canal in young horses with prominent tooth roots.[22,23] In foals and young horses, the bone flap can be based along the facial crest to improve access over the cheek teeth.[36] An opening can be made into the nasal passage through the ventral concha to allow drainage from the ventral conchal sinus and this can be kept patent with gauze packing or a silastic tube sutured to the nostrils.[23]

The maxillary flap allows limited access to the sphenopalatine and frontal sinuses, but the flexible fiberoptic endoscope can be passed through the flap opening to inspect these areas.[101] For most purposes, the nasofrontal flap approach is superior to the maxillary approach because it allows greater access to most sinuses, is easier to make, and is associated with less hemorrhage. In general, any lesions medial and dorsal to the infraorbital canal are approached more easily through a nasofrontal flap.

### Healing

Healing of bone flaps is usually excellent, even in horses with extensive sinus infection. Draining tracts may develop along skin sutures, but these resolve rapidly if the involved sutures are removed and the tract is cleaned. Mucopurulent, fetid fluid may drain from the sinuses after surgery while old blood and devitalized tissue are sloughed but this ceases

*For descriptions of a maxillary bone flap, the terms dorsal and ventral are used where medial and lateral are more appropriate for the conchofrontal flap.

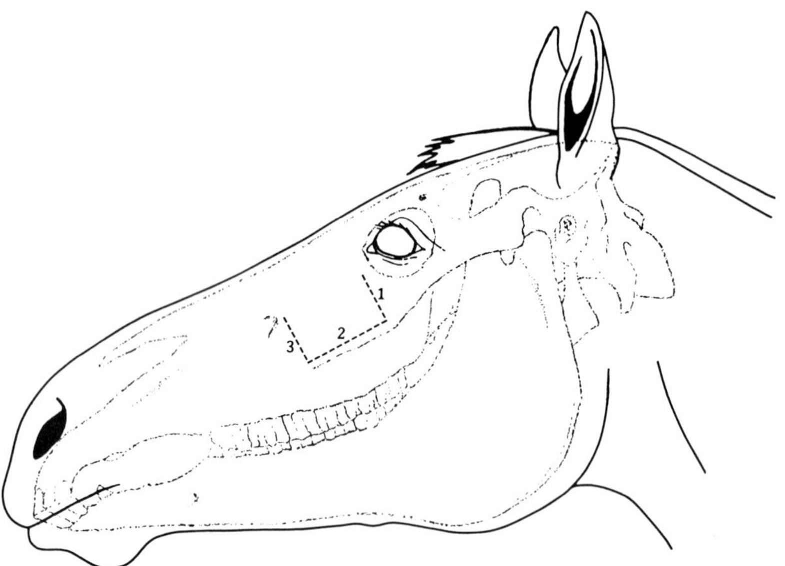


**FIG. 18–19.** Outline of maxillary sinus flap approach. 1 = Caudal, 2 = ventral, 3 = rostral margins.

after 10 to 14 days in uncomplicated cases. If the edge of the flap is severely traumatized during surgery or an underlying septic process invades it, bone and skin along the free edge may slough. To reduce this risk, remove any fragments of bone that break off the flap edge during surgery.

Many diseases of the sinuses destroy much of the sinus walls so that when abnormal tissue is removed, large communications are established between the sinuses and nasal passages, sometimes of sufficient size to convert them all to a single cavity. This may cause turbulence and an abnormal respiratory noise during fast work[67] but does not appear to affect performance. A large opening into the nasal cavity is recommended because it will become gradually smaller and a small hole could seal before drainage is complete. Sinus surgery in young horses can interfere with facial development and cause malocclusion if surgery produces massive callus bridging of sutures or results in extensive loss of bone and periosteum.[50,102,103]

## *Carotid Occlusion*

Temporary bilateral, carotid artery occlusion can be used to reduce intraoperative hemorrhage during sinus surgery so that exposure is improved without the need for constant suction or swabbing.[104] Both arteries can be approached through an 8-cm long incision in the uppermost jugular groove with blunt dissection over the trachea to expose the opposite artery. This is more convenient than exposing each artery through a separate incision[104] because it allows carotid dissection to start at the same time as sinus surgery, eliminates the need for turnover, and maintains surgery time as short as possible. After each artery is exposed, it is carefully separated from the vagosympathetic trunk and recurrent laryngeal nerve and a loop of ¼ inch-wide umbilical tape is secured snugly around it with a hemostat. Both carotid arteries have been occluded for up to 16 minutes without adverse effects,[104] but the effect on sinus hemorrhage appears to be variable.[37] Also, the risk of damage to the recurrent laryngeal nerve should be considered in athletic horses.

## *Trephination*

Trephination allows limited access to the sinuses but can be used as a simple and inexpensive field procedure in the sedated, standing horse for biopsy, aspiration, and irrigation. It can be used also for selective repulsion of diseased cheek teeth with the horse under general anesthesia but would be inadequate for the amount of debridement and curettage required in some cases.

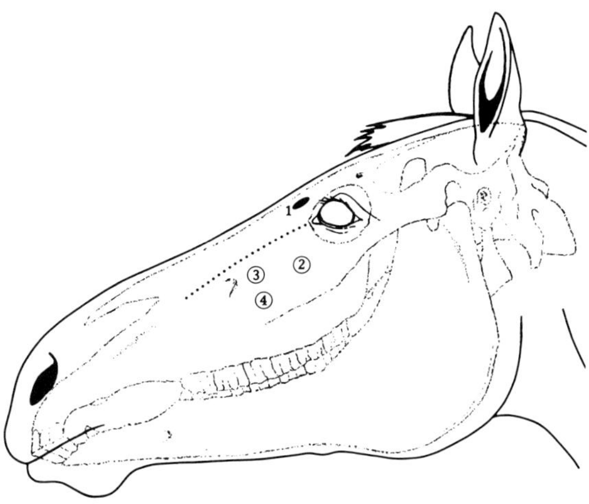


**FIG. 18–20.** Sites for trephine holes in the paranasal sinuses. 1 = Frontal sinus; 2 = caudal maxillary sinus; 3 = rostral maxillary sinus (young horse); 4 = site for rostral maxillary sinus that can be used in an older horse but is not recommended for young horses.

## Sites for Trephination

For generalized sinusitis, the site for trephination is on a point midway between the medial canthus of the eye and the dorsal midline of the skull (Fig. 18–20). The caudal maxillary sinus can be opened also through the site used for centesis (Figs. 18–5 and 18–20). A trephine opening into the rostral maxillary sinus requires careful placement. In young horses, an opening close to the floor of the sinus is against the cheek teeth and the intervening space fills rapidly with granulation tissue[28] (Fig. 18–20). An opening at the level of the infraorbital foramen and 1 to 2 cm caudal to the end of the facial crest avoids this problem and allows access to the ventral conchal sinus over the infraorbital canal[28] (Fig. 18–20). Care must be taken in this site to avoid the levator nasolabialis muscle and the nasolacrimal duct.[28] If the septum between the maxillary sinuses is broken down, a gauze seton can be placed through the opening in the rostral maxillary sinus and retrieved through an opening in the frontal sinus to be tied on the face. This can be replaced daily and used to keep the openings patent for flushing.

## Surgical Technique

The area is prepared for aseptic surgery and a circle of skin marked with the trephine is excised along with the underlying fascia and periosteum. The trocar point guide of the trephine is then advanced 1 cm beyond the teeth and used to make a small hole in the exposed bone. The trocar point is then used to stabilize the trephine and a rotary cutting motion is used to remove a plug of bone. If a number of trephine holes are placed close together to make a single large opening,[52] some of the overlying skin should be preserved to cover the defect and hasten healing. In horses with severe infection, the bone overlying the sinus may be eroded by sepsis and can be incised with a scalpel or scissors.

## Aftercare

Fluid can be infused through the trephine openings daily to remove exudate and necrotic material from the sinuses. Infusion of warm water through a hose at the maximum flow rate that the horse will tolerate is the method of choice, but dilute antiseptic solutions (1% povidone iodine) or normal saline solution can be used instead. The horse can be mildly sedated during infusion so that it lowers its head and allows drainage through the nasal passage. While fluid is being delivered through one trephine opening, others should be temporarily occluded to encourage fluid to distribute throughout the sinuses and to drain through the nasal passages.[25] Between irrigations, the trephine opening should be packed with a rolled wad of sterile gauze soaked with an antibiotic solution and this should be changed daily.

The trephine hole heals by granulation and usually closes after 21 to 30 days. The scar may be imperceptible or a small blemish may remain in the form of a depression, darkening of the skin, loss of hair,[8] or a patch of white hair.

# *Tooth Repulsion*

Diseased cheek teeth can be removed by extraction but repulsion is preferred, especially in young horses with long reserve crowns. The horse is placed under general anesthesia with the affected side uppermost and a trephine, or preferably a bone flap, is used. The upper limit of a trephine hole should be immediately below a line from the medial canthus of the eye to the nasoincisive notch to avoid damage to the osseous portion of the nasolacrimal duct. In older horses, the hole can be placed closer to the facial crest. To repel the 3rd molar, the trephine opening is placed midway between the dorsal midline and medial canthus of the eye and the punch is placed through the frontomaxillary opening.

For the first two cheek teeth (2nd and 3rd premolars), the trephine opening should be made directly above their table surfaces. For the 3rd to 6th cheek teeth, which have considerable caudal curvature in horses under 8 years of age, the opening should be on a vertical line from the caudal edge of the occlusal surface.[36] In horses over 8 years of age, the 4th cheek tooth tends to be more perpendicular from the occlusal surface.[36] Accurate placement of the trephine opening can be guided by radiographs. If the horse has a sinus tract from the affected tooth, radiographs taken with a metal probe through the tract will help identify the involved root.[36]

The infraorbital canal lies directly above the cheek teeth and a curved or offset dental punch should be used to avoid it. When the 6th cheek tooth is repelled, special care must be taken to avoid the nearby infraorbital, major palatine, and sphenopalatine arteries. The major palatine artery can be lacerated if the dental punch is driven through the palatine bone medial to any cheek tooth.

## Surgical Procedure

The dental punch is positioned over the tooth root and struck sharply and repeatedly with an orthopedic mallet or hammer. An assistant should place a finger against the occlusal surface of the affected tooth to confirm that each blow is transmitted through it. As the tooth is removed, it may be necessary to cut sections from it with molar cutters so that it can clear the space between the upper and lower teeth.

After removal, the tooth should be checked to confirm that it was abnormal, the alveolar socket should be palpated for fragments, and intraoperative radiographs should be taken to ensure that all fragments of teeth and bone have been removed. The alveolar socket is then packed with gauze or dental acrylic to prevent migration of food from the oral cavity into the maxillary sinus. Packing should not be placed too deep in the socket or it might interfere with healing.[43]

A gauze pack is made from a roll of 3 or 4 surgical sponges and tied with a doubled gauze strip to a second gauze spindle on the outside of the trephine opening. After the first 3 days, the pack is changed daily by pulling it through the mouth, after the outside spindle has been removed and a length of new gauze attached to that end of the old gauze strip.[105] At this point, the sinus cavity is liberally irrigated with warm water from a hose. A fresh spindle of gauze sponges is attached to the strip of gauze extending from the mouth and is drawn into the socket by pulling on the ends from the trephine opening. During the next 3 to 4 weeks, the alveolus fills with granulation tissue and all packing can be removed.[105] The horse should be muzzled and held off feed for 48 to 72 hours after pack removal to allow the socket to fill completely with granulation tissue.[105]

A plug of Optosil (Unitek Corporation, Monrovia, CA) or methyl methacrylate can be used instead of gauze and is easier to manage. The plug is molded around 18-gauge stainless steel wire and the wire is drawn through the sinus and secured to gauze sponges outside the trephine hole. The pack is removed after 3 to 4 weeks by cutting the wires at the trephine hole and pulling the plug from the mouth.[36] Dental acrylic without wire ties usually remains for a sufficient time for granulation tissue to fill the socket.

Cheek teeth can be removed through a buccotomy to preserve the alveolus and avoid establishing a communication between the oral cavity and sinuses.[106] This procedure is technically difficult and breakdown of a large tooth can be a protracted procedure.

## Complications

Removal of upper cheek teeth in the horse is fraught with numerous complications and aftercare is tedious. Failure to resolve sinusitis can be attributed to migration of oral contents into the sinus, removal of the wrong tooth, or fracture of the adjacent alveolar plate during surgery.[36] Recurrent sinusitis after tooth removal can be attributed to persistent foci of infection in isolated pockets and to sequestra and osteitis. The most common cause of recurrent problems after tooth removal, and hence the greatest need for reoperation, is failure to remove all pieces of bone and tooth fragments from the alveolus.[30,107] These fragments can be recognized on radiographs. Rarer complications include fracture of the maxilla or palatine bone.

## *Treatment of Mucocele*

Mucoceles are treated by creation of a new drainage opening into the nasal passage.[25] With the horse under general anesthesia, the conchofrontal sinus is opened by trephine immediately rostral to and on the midpoint of a line between the medial canthus of the eye and the dorsal midline of the face.[25] A metal probe or catheter is passed through the nasal passage into the middle meatus until it can be felt through the wall of the dorsal conchal sinus.[25] It is then thrust through this wall and a 4-foot length of gauze bandage material is tied to the catheter tip.[25] The catheter is then withdrawn so that the tape is pulled through the trephine opening and through the newly established hole in the floor of the dorsal conchal sinus.[25] The gauze is then drawn through the nostrils and the two ends are tied together on the outside of the face to form a seton.[25] This seton is changed every 2 to 3 days and the sinuses and nasal passages are irrigated daily through the trephine opening with warm water from a hose. After 2 weeks, a permanent opening should form between the dorsal conchal sinus and the middle meatus.

Mucoceles can also be treated through a nasofrontal bone flap, which allows more complete evaluation of the lesion and creation of a large opening into the nasal passage. This is the approach of choice if there is some doubt about the diagnosis.

# References


1. Boulton CH. Equine nasal cavity and paranasal sinus disease: A review of 85 cases. Equine Vet Sci, *5*:268, 1985.
2. Hillmann DJ. Skull. In: Sisson and Grossman's The Anatomy of the Domestic Animals. 5th Ed. R Getty (Ed). Philadelphia, WB Saunders Co, 1975, p 318.
3. Dyce KM, Sack WO, Wensing CJG. Textbook of Veterinary Anatomy. Philadelphia, WB Saunders Co, 1987, p 462.
4. Nickel R, Schummer A, Seiferle E, et al. The Viscera of the Domestic Mammals. New York, Springer-Verlag, 1977, p 273.
5. Hare WCD. Equine respiratory system. In: Sisson and Grossman's the Anatomy of the Domestic Animals. 5th Ed. R Getty (Ed). Philadelphia, WB Saunders Co, 1975, p 498.
6. Baker GJ. Some aspects of equine dental disease. Equine Vet J, *2*:105, 1970.
7. Baker GJ. Some aspects of equine dental radiology. Equine Vet J, *3*:46, 1971.
8. Mason BJE. Empyema of the equine paranasal sinuses. J Am Vet Med Assoc, *167*:727, 1975.
9. Chan CW, Collins EA. Case of angiosarcoma of the nasal passage of the horse—ultrastructure and differential diagnosis from progressive haematoma. Equine Vet J, *17*:214, 1985.
10. Rahko T, Alitalo I, Paatsama S. Myxoma in the nasal cavity of the Finnish-bred horse. Acta Vet Scand, *13*:131, 1972.
11. Coumbe KM, Jones RD, Kenward JH. Bilateral sinus empyema in a 6-year-old mare. Equine Vet J, *19*:559, 1987.
12. Goble DO, Geiser DR, Jones RD. Examination, diagnosis and treatment of equine upper respiratory disorders: part I. J Equine Med Surg, *3*:162, 1979.
13. Gibbs D, Lane JG. Radiographic examination of the facial, nasal and paranasal sinus regions of the horse. II. Radiological findings. Equine Vet J, *19*:474, 1987.
14. Wyn-Jones G. Interpreting radiographs 6: Radiology of the equine head (Part 2). Equine Vet J, *17*:417, 1985.
15. Wyn-Jones G. Interpreting radiographs 6: The head. Equine Vet J, *17*:274, 1985.
16. Gibbs C. The equine skull: Its radiologic investigation. J Am Vet Radiol Soc, *15*:70, 1974.
17. Finn ST, Park RD. Radiology of the nasal cavity and paranasal sinuses in the horse. Proc Am Assoc Equine Pract, *33*:383, 1987.
18. Kral F. Equine sinusitis—A new therapeutic approach. J Am Vet Med Assoc, *124*:373, 1954.
19. McIlwraith CW. Diagnostic and Surgical Arthroscopy in the Horse. Edwardsville, Veterinary Medicine Publishing Company, 1984, p 136.
20. Brearley JC, McCandlish IAP, Sullivan M, et al. Nasal granuloma caused by *Pseudallescheria boydii*. Equine Vet J, *18*:151, 1986.
21. Lane JG, Gibbs C, Meynink SE, et al. Radiographic examination of the facial, nasal and paranasal sinus

regions of the horse: I. indications and procedures in 235 cases. Equine Vet J, *19*:466, 1987.
22. Schumacher J, Honnas C, Smith B. Paranasal sinusitis complicated by inspissated exudate in the ventral conchal sinus. Vet Surg, *16*:373, 1987.
23. De Moor Von A, Verschooten F. Empyem und Nekrose der Nasenmuscheln beim Pferd (Empyema and necrosis of the nasal conchae in a horse). Dtsch tierarztl Wschr, *89*:275, 1982.
24. Blackford JT, Goble DO, Henry RW, et al. Triangulated flap technique for nasofrontal surgery: results in 5 horses. Vet Surg, *4*:287, 1985.
25. Cook WR. Sinusitis, paranasal; horse. Int Encyclopedia Vet Med, *5*:2689, 1966.
26. Greet TRC. The respiratory tract. In: Equine Surgery and Medicine. Vol. 1. J Hickman (ed). New York, Academic Press, 1985, p 247.
27. Aronson AL, Kirk RW. Antimicrobial drugs. In: Textbook of Veterinary Internal Medicine. Diseases of the Dog and Cat. 2nd Ed. SJ Ettinger (ed). Philadelphia, WB Saunders Co, 1983, p 338.
28. Cook WR. Clinical observations on the anatomy and physiology of the equine upper respiratory tract. Vet Rec, *79*:440, 1966.
29. Baker GJ. Some aspects of equine dental decay. Equine Vet J, *6*:127, 1974.
30. Mackintosh ME, Colles CM. Anaerobic bacteria associated with dental abscesses in the horse and donkey. Equine Vet J, *19*:360, 1987.
31. Cook WR, Littlewort MCG. Progressive haematoma of the ethmoid region in the horse. Equine Vet J, *6*:101, 1974.
32. Sullivan M, Burrell MH, McCandlish IAP. Progressive haematoma of the maxillary sinus in a horse. Vet Rec, *114*:191, 1984.
33. Platt H. Haemorrhagic nasal polyps of the horse. J Pathol, *115*:51, 1975.
34. Hanselka DV, Young MF. Ethmoidal hematoma in the horse. VM/SAC, *70*:1289, 1975.
35. Meagher DM. The elevation and surgical treatment of ethmoid hematomas in the horse (Abstr.). Vet Surg, *15*:128, 1986.
36. Pascoe JR. Specific aspects of equine dental surgery. In: Symposium on Surgery and Diseases of the Oral Cavity and Respiratory Tract. RJ Rose (ed). The Australian Equine Veterinary Association, 1981, p 20.
37. Lane JG, Longstaffe JA, Gibbs C. Equine paranasal sinus cysts: A report of 15 cases. Equine Vet J, *19*:537, 1987.
38. Sanders-Shamis M, Robertson JT. Congenital sinus cyst in a foal. J Am Vet Med Assoc, *190*:1011, 1987.
39. Leyland A, Baker JR. Lesions of the nasal and paranasal sinuses of the horse causing dyspnoea. Br Vet J, *131*:339, 1975.
40. Boles C. Abnormalities of the upper respiratory tract. Vet Clin N Am, *1*:89, 1979.
41. Cannon JH, Grant BD, Sande RD. Diagnosis and surgical treatment of cystlike lesions of the equine paranasal sinuses. J Am Vet Med Assoc, *169*:610, 1976.
42. Haynes PF. Surgery of the equine respiratory tract. In: The Practice of Large Animal Surgery. PB Jennings (ed). Philadelphia, WB Saunders Co, 1984, p 388.
43. Boles C. Treatment of upper airway abnormalities. Vet Clin North Am, *1*:127, 1979.
44. Cook WR. Skeletal radiology of the equine head. J Am Vet Rad Soc, *11*:35, 1970.
45. Hensley RM, Thomas EW. Mucocele sinusitis in a Thoroughbred filly. J Am Vet Med Assoc, *130*:133, 1957.
46. Levine SB. Depression fractures of the nasal and frontal bones of the horse. J Equine Med Surg, *3*:186, 1979.
47. Turner AS. Surgical management of depression fractures of the equine skull. Vet Surg, *8*:29, 1979.
48. Valdez H, Rook JS. Use of fluorocarbon polymer and carbon fiber for restoration of facial contour in a horse. J Am Vet Med Assoc, *178*:249, 1981.
49. Schumacher J, Auer JA, Shamis L. Repair of facial defects with periosteal flaps in two horses. Vet Surg, *14*:235, 1985.
50. Engdahl E. Bone regeneration in maxillary defects. An experimental investigation on the significance of the periosteum and various media (blood, surgical, bone marrow and bone grafts) on bone formation and maxillary growth. Scand J Plast Reconstr Surg, *8*[Suppl]:1, 1972.
51. Campbell ML, Peyton LC. Muscle flap closure of a frontocutaneous fistula in a horse. Vet Surg, *13*:185, 1984.
52. Reed SM, Boles CL, Dade AW, et al. Localized equine nasal coccidioidomycosis granuloma. J Equine Med Surg, *3*:119, 1979.
53. Madewell BR, Priester WA, Gillette EL, et al. Neoplasms of the nasal passages and paranasal sinuses in domesticated animals as reported by 13 veterinary colleges. Am J Vet Res, *37*:851, 1976.
54. Cotchin E. Spontaneous neoplasms of the upper respiratory tract in animals. In: Cancer of the Nasopharynx. Muir C, Shanmugaratnam K, eds. UICC Monograph Series, Vol. 1. Copenhagen, Monksgaard, 1967, p 203.
55. Moulton JE (ed). Tumors in Domestic Animals. Los Angeles, University of California Press, 1978, p 211.
56. Schuh JCL. Squamous cell carcinoma of the oral, pharyngeal and nasal mucosa of the horse. Vet Pathol, *23*:205, 1986.
57. Noack P. Die Geschwulste der oberen Atmungswege bei den Haussaugetieren (Teile I, II). Wiss Z Humboldt-Univ, *6*:293, 373, 1956 (cited in references 54 and 55).
58. Reynolds BL, Stedham MA, Lawrence JM, et al. Adenocarcinoma of the frontal sinus with extension to the brain in a horse. J Am Vet Med Assoc, *174*:734, 1979.
59. Mason BJE. Spindle-cell sarcoma of the equine paranasal sinuses and nasal chamber. Vet Rec, *96*:287, 1975.
60. Cotchin E. Tumors of farm animals: A survey of tumors at the Royal Veterinary College, London, during 1950–60. Vet Rec, *72*:816, 1960.
61. Hultgren BD, Watrous BJ, Wagner PC, et al. Nasal-maxillary fibrosarcoma in young horses: A light and electron microscopic study. Vet Pathol, *24*:194, 1987.
62. Acland HM, Orsini J, Elkins S, et al. Congenital ethmoid carcinoma in a foal. J Am Vet Med Assoc, *184*:979, 1984.

63. Dillehay DL, Schoeb TR. Complex odontoma in a horse. Vet Pathol, *23*:341, 1986.
64. Jubb KVF, Kennedy PC. Pathology of Domestic Animals. New York, Academic Press, 1970, p 40.
65. Jones TC, Hunt RD. Veterinary Pathology. 5th ed. Philadelphia, Lea & Febiger, 1983, p 1356.
66. Jacobson SA. Tumors of bone and cartilage. In: The Comparative Pathology of Tumors of Bone. Springfield, Charles C Thomas, 1971, p 355.
67. Peterson FB, Martens RJ, Montali RJ. Surgical treatment of an osteoma in the paranasal sinuses of a horse. J Equine Med Surg, *2*:279, 1978.
68. Schumacher J, Smith BL, Morgan SJ. Osteoma of paranasal sinuses of a horse. J Am Vet Med Assoc, *192*:1449, 1988.
69. Fisher AK. A compact osteoma in the skull of a horse. J Am Vet Med Assoc, *121*:42, 1952.
70. Kold SE, Ostblom LC. Headshaking caused by a maxillary osteoma in a horse. Equine Vet J, *14*:167, 1982.
71. Meschter CL, Allen D. Lymphosarcoma within the nasal cavities of an 18-month-old filly. Equine Vet J, *16*:475, 1984.
72. Roberts MC, Groenendyk S, Kelly WR. Ameloblastic odontoma in a foal. Equine Vet J, *10*:91, 1978.
73. Lingard DR, Crawford TB. Congenital ameloblastic odontoma in a foal. Am J Vet Res, *31*:801, 1970.
74. Traver DS, Coffman JR, Moore JN, et al. Non-invasive diagnosis of growths in the equine nasal passage. VM/SAC, *72*:848, 1977.
75. Koch DB. The oral cavity, oropharynx and salivary glands. In: Equine Medicine and Surgery. RA Mannsmann and ES McAllister (eds). Santa Barbara, American Veterinary Publications, 1982, p 469.
76. Leuthold A. Vorkommen und Diagnose des Kieferhöhlenkarzinoms beim Pferd. Wien Tierarztl Wochenschr, *25*:655, 1938.
77. Pascoe RR, Summers PM. Clinical survey of tumours and tumour-like lesions in horses in south east Queensland. Equine Vet J, *13*:235, 1981.
78. Reid CF. Proceedings of radiology panel, film interpretation session. Proc Am Assoc Equine Pract, 22, 1976.
79. Schmotzer WG, Watrous BJ, Hedstrom OR, et al. Nasomaxillary fibrosarcomas in three young horses. J Am Vet Med Assoc, *191*:437, 1987.
80. Bridges CH. Systemic myocoses. In: Equine Medicine and Surgery. 2nd Ed. EJ Catcott, JF Smithcors (eds). Wheaton, American Veterinary Publications, Inc, 1972, p 119.
81. Roberts MC, Sutton RH, Lovell DK. A protracted case of cryptococcal nasal granuloma in a stallion. Aust Vet J, *57*:287, 1981.
82. Joyce JR, McMullan WC, Burns SJ. The use of amphotericin B in late pregnancy in mares. J Equine Med Surg, *1*:256, 1977.
83. Scott EA, Duncan JR, McCormack JE. Cryptococcosis involving the postorbital area and frontal sinus in a horse. J Am Vet Med Assoc, *165*:626, 1974.
84. Watt DA. A case of cryptococcal granuloma in the nasal cavity of a horse. Aust Vet J, *46*:493, 1970.
85. Carrig CB. What is your diagnosis? J Am Vet Med Assoc, *153*:1206, 1968.
86. Corrier DE, Wilson SR, Scrutchfield WL. Equine cryptococcal rhinitis. Comp Cont Ed Pract Vet, *6*:S556, 1984.
87. Hodgin EC, Conaway DH, Ortenburger AI. Recurrence of coccidioidal granuloma in a horse. J Am Vet Med Assoc, *184*:339, 1984.
88. Johnson GR, Schiefer B, Pentekoek JFCA. Maduromycosis in a horse in western Canada. Can Vet J, *16*:341, 1975.
89. Pentlarge VW, Martin RA. Treatment of cryptococcosis in three cats, using ketoconazole. J Am Vet Med Assoc, *188*:536, 1986.
90. Jackson JA. Immunodiagnosis of systemic mycoses in animals: A review. J Am Vet Med Assoc, *188*:702, 1986.
91. Penn RL, Lambert RS, Goerge RB. Invasive fungal infections. The use of serologic tests in diagnosis and management. Arch Intern Med, *143*:1215, 1983.
92. Keg PR, Mirck MH, Dik KJ, et al. *Micronema deletrix* infection in a Shetland pony stallion. Equine Vet J, *16*:471, 1984.
93. Johnson KH, Johnson DW. Granulomas associated with *Micronema deletrix* in the maxillae of a horse. J Am Vet Med Assoc, *149*:155, 1966.
94. Rubin HC, Woodard JC. Equine infections with *Micronema deletrix*. J Am Vet Med Assoc, *165*:256, 1974.
95. Martin GS, McIlwraith CW. Repair of a frontal sinus eversion in a horse. Vet Surg, *10*:149, 1981.
96. Rubarth S, Krook L. Etiology and pathogenesis of so-called mucoid degeneration of the nasal conchae in the horse. Acta Vet Scand, *9*:253, 1968.
97. Wheat JD. Sinus drainage and tooth repulsion in the horse. Proc Am Assoc Equine Pract, *19*:171, 1973.
98. McIlwraith CW, Turner AS. Equine Surgery Advanced Techniques. Philadelphia, Lea & Febiger, 1987, p 244.
99. Milne DW, Turner AS. An Atlas of Surgical Approaches to the Bones of the Horse. Philadelphia, WB Saunders Co, 1979, p 178.
100. Shappell KK, Baker GJ. Diagnosis and surgical treatment of a frontal-maxillary sinus cyst in a horse. Comp Cont Ed Pract Vet, *9*:1226, 1987.
101. Barclay WP, Phillips TN, Foerner JJ, et al. Sinusotomy for paranasal sinus drainage in the horse. Mod Vet Pract, *68*:169, 1987.
102. Goring RL, Campbell M, Hillidge CJ. Surgical correction of congenital bilateral choanal atresia in a foal. Vet Surg, *13*:211, 1984.
103. Hellquist R. Facial skeleton growth after periosteal resection. An osteometric, roentgenographic and histologic study in the rabbit and guinea pig. Scand J Plast Reconstr Surg, *10*[Suppl]:1, 1972.
104. Wyn-Jones G, Jones RS, Church S. Temporary bilateral carotid artery occlusion as an aid to nasal surgery in the horse. Eq Vet J *18*:125, 1986.
105. Raker CW. Diseases of the nostrils, nasal septum, and cranial sinuses. Lecture notes. University of Pennsylvania, 1980.
106. Evans LH, Tate LP, LaDow CS. Extraction of the equine 4th upper premolar and 1st and 2nd upper molars through a lateral buccotomy. Proc Am Assoc Equine Pract, *27*:249, 1982.
107. Scott EA, Gallagher K, Boles CC, et al. Dental disease in the horse: 5 case reports. J Equine Med Surg, *1*:301, 1977.

# CHAPTER 19

# GUTTURAL POUCHES

*DAVID E. FREEMAN*

Diseases of the guttural pouch are rare but must be considered in a list of differential diagnoses when a horse has spontaneous epistaxis, cranial nerve damage, parotid distention, and signs of upper respiratory disease. Because of their complex anatomy, direct examination of the guttural pouches is difficult and some forms of treatment carry a high risk of iatrogenic injuries.

## Anatomy

The guttural pouches are diverticula of the eustachian tubes and each has a capacity of approximately 300 ml.[1] The right and left guttural pouches are separated caudally by the rectus capitis ventralis and longus capitis muscles and rostrally by a thin median septum, formed by apposition of their mucosal linings. Each guttural pouch is divided ventrally and caudally into medial and lateral compartments by the stylohyoid bone (Figs. 19–1 and 19–2) and the medial compartment accounts for two-thirds of the total capacity.[1] It extends rostrally from the base of the sphenoid and occipital bones to the pharyngeal orifice of the auditory (eustachian) tube and ventrally to the pharynx and esophagus. The caudal extent approaches the level of the atlantoaxial articulation, ventral to the atlantal attachment of the longus colli muscle. However, its exact size, shape, and position are variable.[1]

Each guttural pouch communicates with the pharynx through the pharyngeal orifice of the eustachian tube. This is a slit-like opening situated rostral and ventral to the pharyngeal recess and bounded medially by the medial lamina of the eustachian tube. This lamina is fibrocartilaginous and its free edge slopes caudally and ventrally along the wall of the pharynx. The pharyngeal orifice of the guttural pouch is a funnel-shaped vestibule that is wider rostrally than caudally. The caudal narrowing is due to a transverse fold of mucous membrane (plica salpingopharyngea) on the floor of the opening that connects the medial lamina of the eustachian tube to the lateral wall of the pharynx.[1]

The internal carotid artery, the cranial cervical ganglion, the cervical sympathetic trunk, and the vagus, glossopharyngeal, hypoglossal, and spinal accessory nerves are all contained in a fold of mucous membrane that extends from the roof of the guttural pouch and traverses the caudal wall of the medial compartment[1] (Fig. 19–1). The pharyngeal branch of the vagus nerve, the cranial laryngeal nerve, and the retropharyngeal lymph nodes lie beneath the mucosa on the floor of the medial compartment[1] (Figs. 19–1 and 19–2).

The external carotid artery passes rostrally along the ventral surface of the lateral compartment of the guttural pouch, where it is accompanied in part of its course by the glossopharyngeal and hypoglossal nerves[1] (Fig. 19–1). It turns dorsally to continue as the maxillary artery along the lateral and dorsal walls of the lateral compartment, caudal to the maxillary vein, and is crossed by the chorda tympani nerve and branches of the mandibular

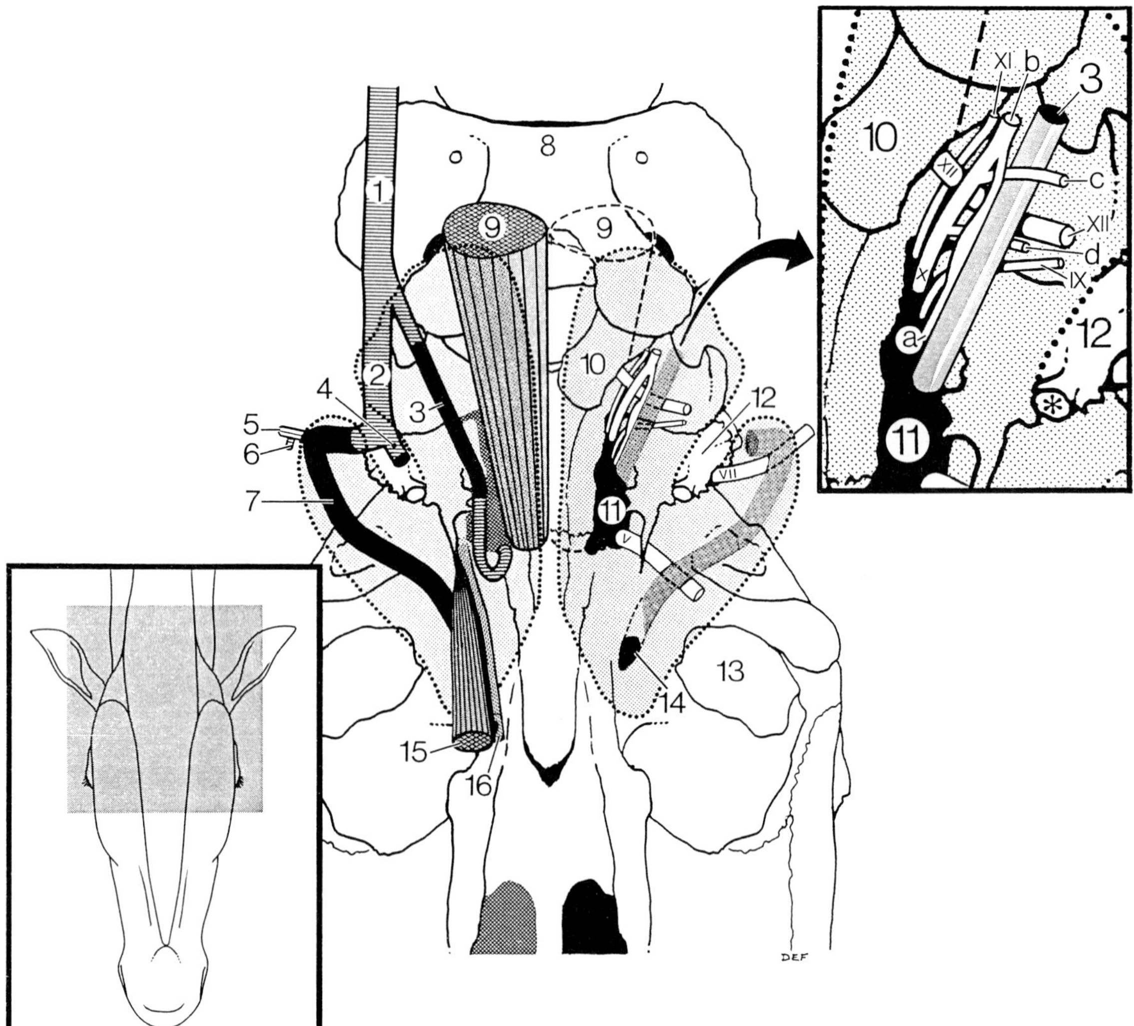


**FIG. 19–1.** Anatomy of the guttural pouches from a ventral view. Lower Inset: Shaded area is the area of interest, shown in detail from the ventral aspect. Upper Inset: Detail of that part of the roof from which the arrow is directed. The lightly shaded area with the dotted outline is the guttural pouch, as determined by radiographs and dissections. The black segments of arteries are those parts that lie beneath the guttural pouch mucosa. Corresponding segments on the right side are shaded. Arteries: 1 = common carotid artery; 2 = external carotid artery; 3 = internal carotid artery; 4 = linguofacial trunk; 5 = superficial temporal artery; 6 = transverse facial artery; 7 = maxillary artery. Other land marks: 8 = atlas; 9 = longus capitis and rectus capitis ventralis muscles (ventral straight muscles of the head; the muscles on the right are outlined by a broken line); 10 = occipital condyle; 11 = foramen lacerum; 12 = temporal bone; 13 = orbit; 14 = caudal alar foramen; 15 = tensor veli palatini muscle; 16 = medial lamina of auditory tube; V = mandibular nerve, branch of the trigeminal nerve; VII = facial nerve. Key for upper right hand inset: IX = glossopharyngeal nerve; X = vagus nerve; XI = accessory nerve; XII = hypoglossal nerve; a = internal carotid nerve, arising from the cranial cervical ganglion (stippled fusiform dilatation); b = vagosympathetic trunk, formed by the vagus nerve and cervical sympathetic trunk; c = pharyngeal branch of the vagus nerve (X); d = cranial laryngeal nerve; * = styloid process of petrous part of the temporal bone.

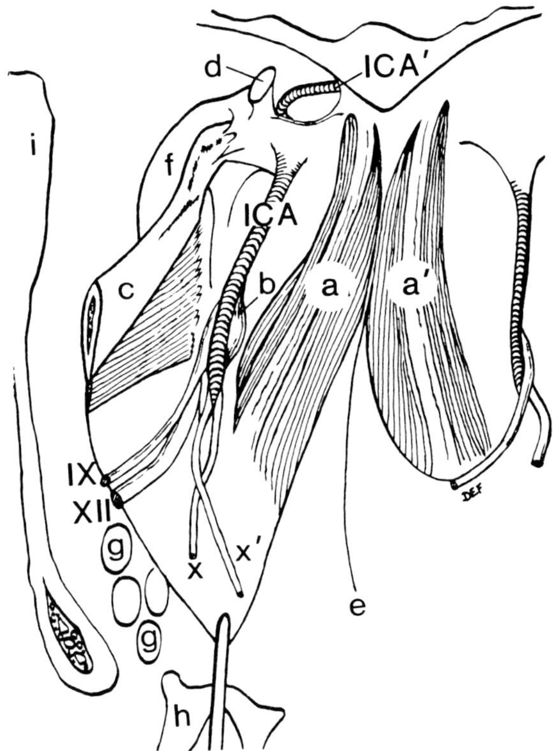


**FIG. 19–2.** View of the interior of the right guttural pouch from the rostral aspect. The specimen is cut transversely and the view is slightly oblique. ICA = Internal carotid artery; ICA' = internal carotid artery within the venous sinuses where it forms a sigmoid flexure; a a' = ventral straight muscles of the head; b = cranial cervical ganglion; c = stylohyoid bone; d = medial lamina of eustachian tube; e = median septum; f = lateral compartment; g = retropharyngeal lymph nodes; h = arytenoid cartilage; i = mandible; IX = glossopharyngeal nerve; XII = hypoglossal nerve; x = cranial laryngeal nerve; x' = pharyngeal branch of the vagus nerve. (From Freeman DE. Diagnosis and treatment of diseases of the guttural pouch (Part I). Compendium of Continuing Education for the Practicing Veterinarian, 2:S3, 1980.)

nerve.[1] At the end of its course in the guttural pouch, the maxillary artery passes above the tensor veli palatine muscle and enters the caudal alar foramen.

The facial nerve emerges through the stylomastoid foramen and courses for 3 to 4 cm over the caudal dorsal aspect of the lateral compartment[1] (Fig. 19–1). It then passes between the mandible and the parotid gland. The mandibular nerve emerges from the foramen lacerum, passes above the muscular process of the petrous part of the temporal bone and continues rostrally along the roof of the lateral compartment (Fig. 19–1).

The epithelial lining of the guttural pouch is ciliated and pseudostratified, and contains goblet cells.[1] Mucous glands are found beneath the epithelium and numerous lymph nodules are present in the young horse.[1]

The function of the guttural pouches is unknown, although the eustachian tube probably serves to equalize air pressure on both sides of the tympanic membrane. The guttural pouches are thought to fill with warm air during expiration, part of which is exchanged for cold air during the expiratory pause;[2] however, there is no evidence to support this theory. Cinefluoroscopic studies have shown that, during swallowing, the pharyngeal orifices open and the soft palate contacts the pharyngeal roof caudal to the openings.[3] The medial laminae do not meet on the midline and therefore do not appear to contribute to the nasopharyngeal sphincter mechanism, as was once proposed.[4]

## Endoscopic Examination

Some evidence of guttural pouch disease may be found on endoscopic examination of the pharynx. Examples are dorsal displacement of the soft palate, collapse of the roof of the pharynx from compression by a distended pouch, laryngeal hemiplegia, and blood or pus draining from the pharyngeal orifice. However, many of these are nonspecific findings and blood or pus from other sources can be aspirated into the guttural pouch opening, thereby appearing to drain from there. Direct endoscopic examination of the guttural pouches can be performed with a flexible fiberoptic endoscope. General anesthesia or a sedative/narcotic combination may have to be used on fractious horses, but most can be examined with mild sedation. The fiberoptic endoscope is difficult to insert into guttural pouches because it has a blunt, wide, and flexible end. However, if the biopsy attachment is introduced into the guttural pouch under endoscopic control, it can serve as a guide wire, over which the endoscope can be threaded (Fig. 19–3). Once the

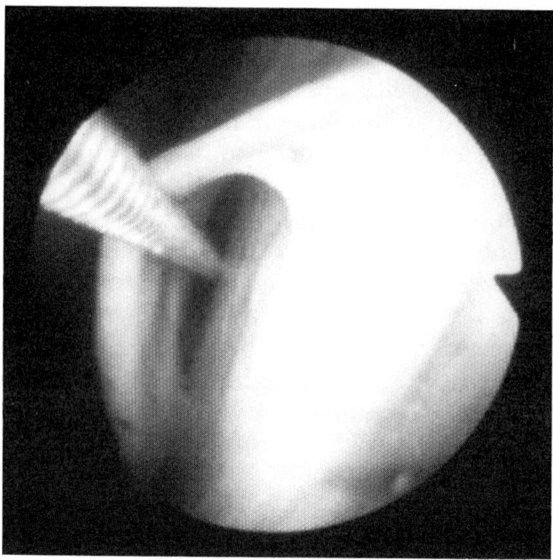

**FIG. 19–3.** Method of inserting the endoscope into the guttural pouch using the biopsy instrument to prop the medial lamina into an open position. Note that the biopsy instrument is closer to the lumen of the nasopharynx than the viewing objective of the endoscope.

biopsy instrument is through the guttural pouch opening, the endoscope is carefully rotated, without twisting it or its connections, until the biopsy instrument is toward the pharyngeal lumen and away from the wall of the pharynx. This maneuver props the cartilaginous flap into an open position (Fig. 19–3) and the endoscope can be introduced under visual guidance. Alternatively, a stiff metal or plastic catheter can be inserted into the guttural pouch under endoscopic guidance and used to prop open the medial lamina. Insertion by any method is difficult if the endoscope is not kept along the floor of the ventral meatus. Insertion under anesthesia is difficult because the soft palate is elevated dorsally by the endotracheal tube and this prevents an approach to the pharyngeal orifice from a ventral position. Both guttural pouches should be examined to determine if a disease is bilateral. On endoscopic examination, the normal guttural pouch has a translucent, glistening mucosa that is thin enough to permit recognition of all underlying structures. A small volume of mucus draining from the guttural pouch openings, especially after exercise, is not an abnormal finding.

## Catheterization

The guttural pouches can be catheterized to collect samples for culture and sensitivity testing and for treatment. If the catheter is to be placed blindly, it should be marked at a distance from its tip that corresponds to the distance from the lateral canthus of the eye to the nostril. The mark should be placed on the side to which the tip is bent. The catheter is inserted into the ventral meatus until its tip is felt to contact the wall of the pharynx, at which point the mark should be at the nostril. If the horse swallows, the pharyngeal orifice will open and the tip can be passed into the guttural pouch. If the horse does not swallow, the curved tip of the catheter should be directed laterally and the end outside the nostrils should be pressed toward the midline. This directs the tip beneath the flap of the medial lamina. The tip should then be rotated to free it of the plica salpingopharyngea and advanced into the guttural pouch. Successful passage into the pouch is indicated by lack of resistance as the catheter is inserted deeper than if it were in the pharynx. The catheter can be inserted easily if the endoscope is placed in the opposite nasal passage so that the catheter tip can be guided into the pharyngeal orifice under direct view.

For brief and temporary catheterization, a Chamber's mare catheter can be used.[5] Rubber or plastic catheters with self-retaining devices are used for indwelling systems for repeated infusions. A 27F balloon catheter (Foley) can be inserted over a wire stylet and retained in place by inflating the balloon with saline.[6] Another method is a self-retaining intrauterine catheter with a ram's horn on its distal tip (Fig. 19–4). This is inserted through its introducer, which has been bent 2 cm from its tip, and guided into the guttural pouch under endoscopic observation. When the coiled ram's horn of the catheter is advanced into the pouch, the introducer is removed, and a butterfly bandage of adhesive tape is applied to the catheter shaft and sutured to the nostril. The disadvantage of this catheter is that the plastic ram's horn (Fig. 19–4) can become adhered to the inflamed mucosa with time and detach when the catheter is re-

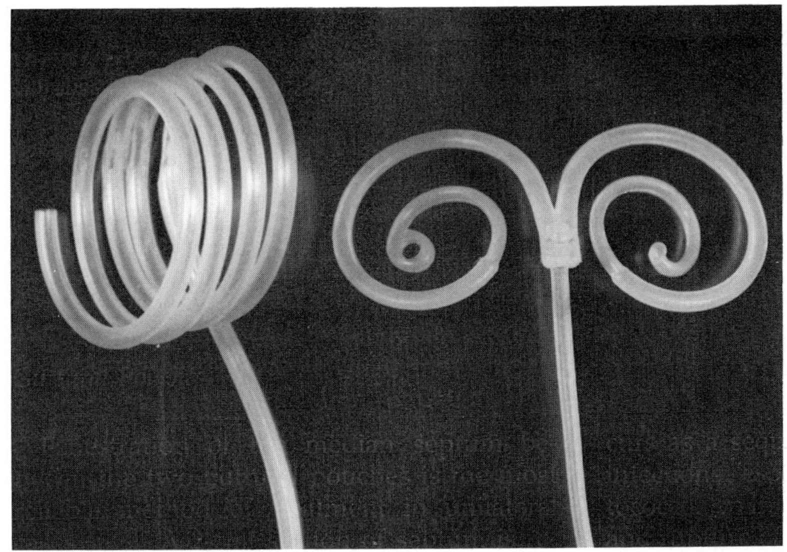

**FIG. 19–4.** Distal tips of two types of indwelling irrigation catheters for the guttural pouch. On the right is the commercially available intrauterine catheter with a ram's horn grapple on the distal tip. On the left is the distal tip of a catheter constructed from PE 240 tubing (see text for description of catheter construction).

moved. A more satisfactory indwelling catheter can be made from a length of PE 240 polyethylene tubing that is coiled at one end by heating it with hot water and wrapping it around the barrel of a 50-ml syringe (Fig. 19–4). The coils are then fixed by immersion in cold water. This tubing can also be inserted through the introducer of the intrauterine catheter and is advanced until all its coils lie within the cavity of the guttural pouch. A similar type catheter can be made from an 8 F male-dog polypropylene urinary catheter and inserted into the guttural pouch over a wire stylet with a 30° bend at its tip.[7–10] All indwelling catheters can cause superficial necrosis of the medial lamina of the auditory tube.[10]

The guttural pouch can also be catheterized at Viborg's triangle with a 5¼-inch, 14-gauge intravenous catheter or with a length of PE 240 polyethylene tubing inserted percutaneously through a large-bore needle.[11] A disadvantage of this method is that the percutaneous catheter provides a tract that allows infection to spread into tissue outside the guttural pouch.

## Radiology

Radiographic examination may be particularly rewarding in those cases in which the abnormality prevents a clear view of the guttural pouch interior through the endoscope.[12,13] It is useful to determine the presence of fluid lines, fractures and exostosis of the stylohyoid bone, radiopaque foreign bodies, and space occupying masses.[12,13]

The guttural pouches can be radiographed with portable x-ray units because they are air-filled cavities with little overlying bone and soft tissue (Fig. 19–5). Longer exposure times may be needed with large horses but can be reduced by use of high-speed films and screens.[13] Tranquilization can be used to reduce patient movement.

Arteriography can be used to identify the affected vessel in horses with guttural pouch mycosis.[14] Arteriograms of the common carotid artery can be obtained by injection of radiopaque dye into the artery or directly into selected branches with the horse under general anesthesia[14] (Fig. 19–6). An 8 French polyethylene or similar catheter is placed in the common carotid artery, and 20 to 30 ml of warmed contrast agent (iothalamate meglumine) is injected rapidly as a single bolus. An automatic rapid changer can be used to determine the order in which vessels fill.

## Diseases of the Guttural Pouch

### *Tympany*

The cause of guttural pouch tympany is not known although a number of mechanisms

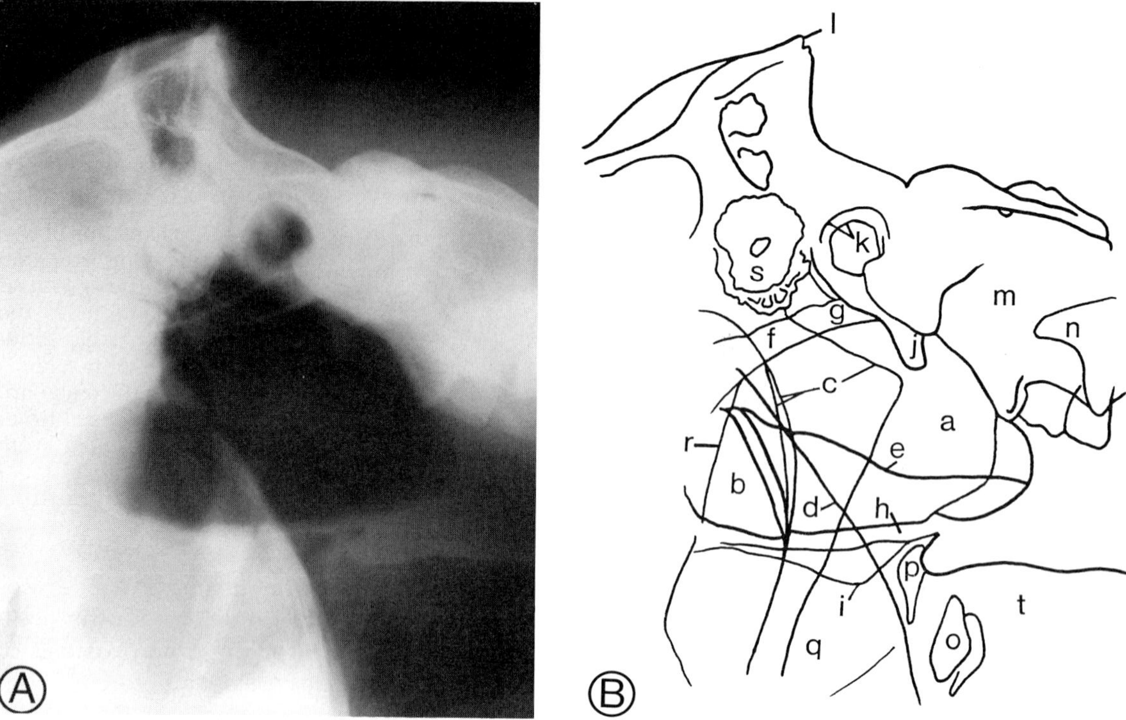


**FIG. 19–5.** A. Radiograph of normal guttural pouch. B. The line drawing from this radiograph, a = medial compartment; b = lateral compartment; c = right and left stylohyoid bones; d = mandible; e = edge of ventral straight muscles of the head; f = body of basisphenoid; g = basilar part of the occipital bone; h = dorsal wall of the pharynx; i = floor of medial compartment of the guttural pouch; j = jugular process; k = condyloid fossa; l = nuchal crest; m = atlas; n = dens of axis; o = ventricles of the larynx; p = arytenoid cartilage; q = pharynx; r = medial lamina of eustachian tube; s = petrous part of the temporal bone; t = larynx. (From Freeman DE. Diagnosis and treatment of diseases of the guttural pouch (Part II). Compendium of Continuing Education for the Practicing Veterinarian, 2:S25, 1980.)

have been postulated. It has been suggested that air that normally enters the pouch during expiration cannot leave because the plica salpingopharyngea acts as a one-way valve and collapses across the pharyngeal orifice as air is expelled.[2,15] Redundant tissue in this fold may be a congenital defect or it may be enlarged as a result of inflammation from an upper airway infection.[16,17] In most cases, no abnormality can be detected on endoscopic or intraoperative visual and digital examinations of the guttural pouch opening during surgery, evidence that a functional rather than anatomic defect is involved.[18] Excessive coughing[18,19] and muscle paralysis[20] have been considered as possible causes.

There is a marked preponderance of fillies affected with this condition (9 out of 11 cases in the veterinary literature,[15,17,21-25] and 11 of 14 cases seen at the University of Pennsylvania over a 9-year period). The condition is usually unilateral.[2]

## Clinical Signs and Diagnosis

Tympany of the guttural pouch develops in foals shortly after birth and up to 1 year of age.[2,17-19] The affected guttural pouch becomes distended with air and forms a characteristic nonpainful and elastic swelling in the parotid region (Fig. 19–7). The degree of tympanitic swelling is variable. Some foals develop stertorous breathing and even severe dyspnea as the distended guttural pouch collapses the dorsal wall of the pharynx. Although the swelling is most prominent on the affected side, it can extend across the neck and displace the opposite guttural pouch, the trachea, and hyoid bone (Fig. 19–8).[15] This distribution of swelling gives the impression

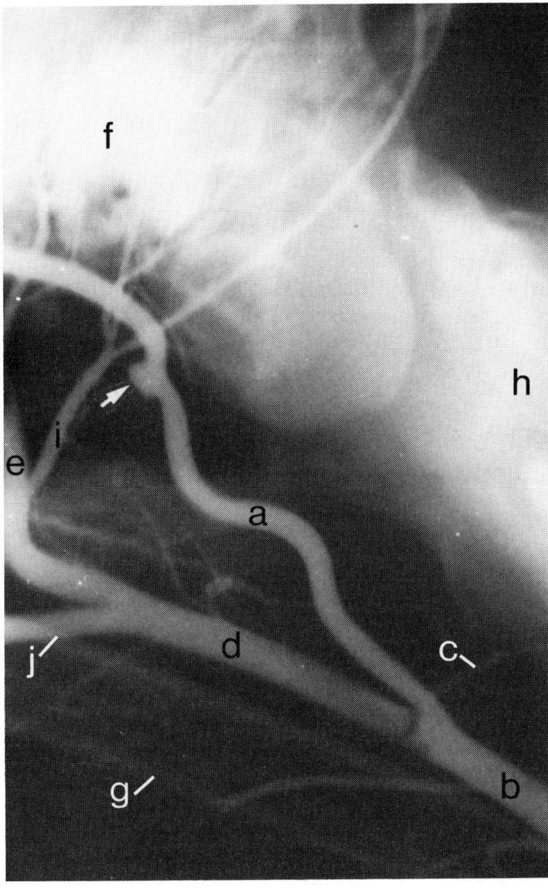


**FIG. 19–6.** Carotid arteriogram from a foal with a defect (arrow) on the internal carotid artery (a) caused by guttural pouch mycosis. b = Common carotid artery; c = occipital artery; d = external carotid artery; e = maxillary artery; f = petrous part of the temporal bone; g = endotracheal tube; h = atlas; i = superficial temporal artery; j = linguofacial trunk. (Radiograph courtesy of Dr. Jeff Witwer, Delaware Equine Center, Cochranville, PA. From Freeman DE. Diagnosis and treatment of diseases of the guttural pouch (Part II). Compendium of Continuing Education for the Practicing Veterinarian, 2:S25, 1980.)

of bilateral involvement when the condition is unilateral.[2,15] Dorsoventral radiographs will help determine if one or both guttural pouches are involved.[26] Also, if guttural pouch tympany is unilateral, aspiration of air from the distended guttural pouch causes much improvement in size and contour of the parotid region. However, if the condition is bilateral, much of the tympanitic swelling remains following removal of air from one guttural pouch. In unusual cases, tympany can also collapse the opposite guttural pouch, compress the pharynx, and cause dyspnea without causing any external swelling.

In many foals, severe distention of the guttural pouch is well tolerated and does not interfere with growth and development. In severe cases, the foal has dysphagia and may aspirate milk and develop inhalation pneumonia. A secondary infection may develop in the affected guttural pouch and is recognized as fluid lines on lateral radiographs (Fig. 19–8). On endoscopic examination, the pharyngeal openings to the guttural pouches usually appear normal, but the roof of the pharynx may be collapsed. Radiographic diagnosis of tympany is straightforward in severe cases (Fig. 19–8); however, on radiographic examination, it should be remembered that the guttural pouch outline can extend farther caudally than the ventral tubercle of the atlas in normal horses.[13]

## Treatment

Temporary alleviation of guttural pouch tympany can be achieved by aspiration of air from the affected pouch through a needle inserted at the point of greatest distention or through a catheter introduced through the pharyngeal orifice of the eustachian tube. The catheter can be sutured to the nostril and left in place to allow continuous removal of air. In some foals, air can be expressed from the affected pouch by applying digital pressure to the point of greatest distention.[18] However, the guttural pouch rapidly refills when these measures are discontinued.[18]

Surgery provides the most satisfactory method of treatment. The affected guttural pouch is usually entered through Viborg's triangle (vide infra), where the mucosal lining has been expanded to a subcutaneous position or through a modified Whitehouse approach (vide infra). A small segment (1.5 × 2.5 cm) of the medial lamina is excised within the guttural pouch orifice to create a larger opening into the pharynx.[2,27] Some foals have also been treated successfully by excising the excess plica salpingopharyngea with scissors or by splitting it with a bistoury.[21] However, swelling and inflammation along the cut edge of the fold can close the pharyngeal orifice and cause empyema.[22]

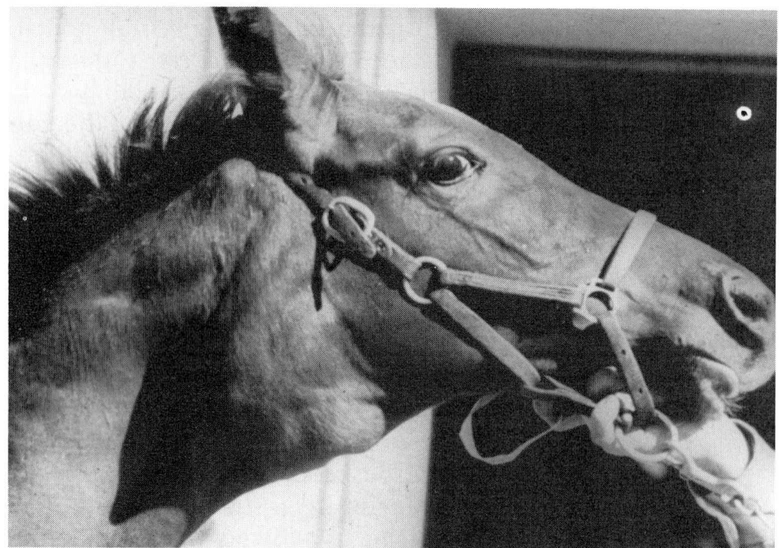

**FIG. 19–7.** Foal with tympany of the guttural pouch. The parotid region is distended. (From Freeman DE. Diagnosis and treatment of diseases of the guttural pouch (Part I). Compendium of Continuing Education for the Practicing Veterinarian, 2:S3, 1980.)

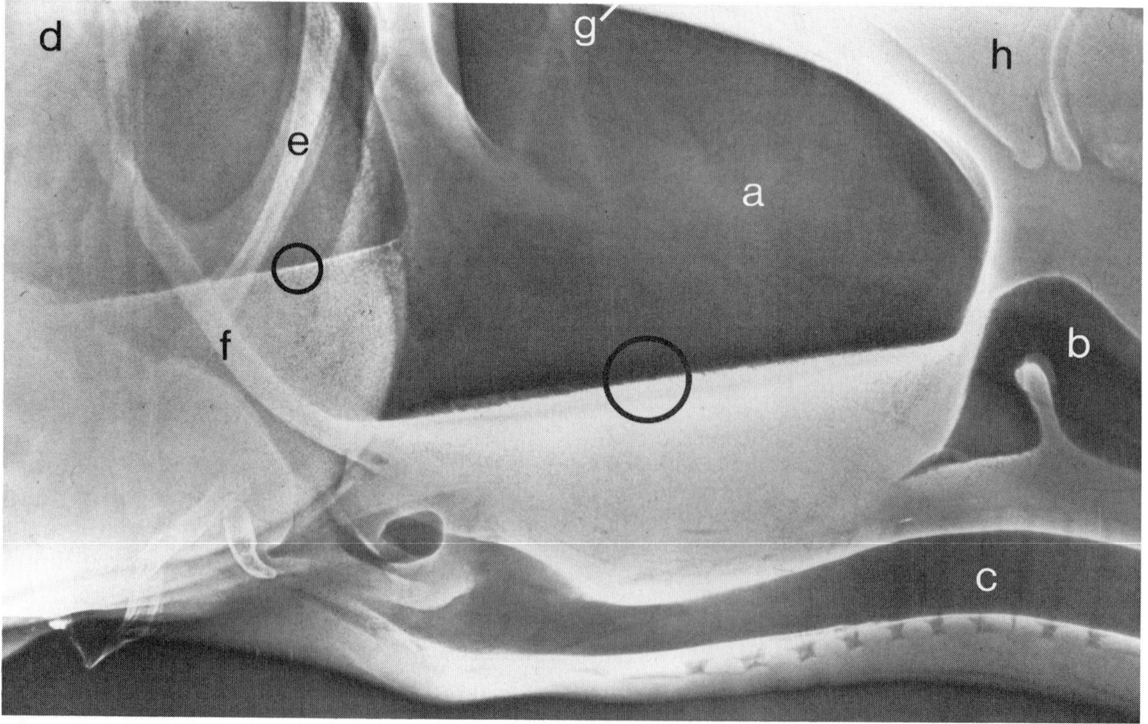


**FIG. 19–8.** Lateral xeroradiograph of head and neck of the foal in Figure 19–7 with tympany of the right guttural pouch. a = Cavity of the medial compartment of the right guttural pouch; b = esophagus; c = trachea; d = basilar part of the occipital bone; e = stylohyoid bone; f = roof of the pharynx; g = atlas; h = axis. The large circle indicates a fluid line in the medial compartment of the guttural pouch and the small circle indicates a fluid line in the lateral compartment. Note that the trachea and larynx are compressed ventrally and the esophagus is buckled. This foal did not have dysphagia or dyspnea at rest in spite of these changes. (From Freeman DE. Diagnosis and treatment of diseases of the guttural pouch (Part I). Compendium of Continuing Education for the Practicing Veterinarian, 2:S3, 1980.)

Fenestration of the median septum between the two guttural pouches is the most reliable method of treatment in unilateral cases.[2,4,17,18] A 2-cm$^2$ section of septum is removed so that the pharyngeal orifice of the unaffected guttural pouch can allow egress of trapped air from the tympanitic pouch. Intraoperative identification of the median septum can be difficult as it is often collapsed towards the opposite guttural pouch. To obviate this problem, a Chamber's mare catheter or a lighted fiberoptic endoscope can be inserted into the healthy pouch to elevate the septum towards the incision.[22] The mucosa on the septum from both guttural pouches must be trimmed so that the openings in them are not staggered or the fenestration will seal. Any purulent material is lavaged from the guttural pouch with physiologic saline solution and the surgical incision can be closed or left open, depending on the severity of any secondary infections. The foal can be allowed to nurse immediately after the surgical procedure.

Fenestration can be performed also by diathermy through a fiberoptic endoscope introduced through the ventral meatus and used to guide the cautery instrument within the guttural pouch.[17] Transendoscopic diathermy has been used successfully to treat tympany by creating a fistula between the guttural pouch and pharynx, close to the pharyngeal recess.[17] The laser instrument may prove to be more suitable for these procedures.

The fenestration procedure will fail if the opening seals or the condition is bilateral. If bilateral, one or both pharyngeal openings will have to be enlarged and trimmed in combination with fenestration of the median septum. The prognosis for complete recovery is favorable and complications are rare.[2] Secondary infections in the pouch usually resolve spontaneously after successful treatment of the tympany. However, the prognosis is guarded for foals that have developed aspiration pneumonia and intensive antibiotic therapy is required to treat this complication.

## *Empyema*

Empyema of the guttural pouches can affect horses of any age. The condition usually occurs as a sequela to upper respiratory tract infections, especially those caused by Streptococcus sp in young animals.[28] Abscessation and rupture of retropharyngeal lymph nodes into the guttural pouch produce exudate but there may be little inflammation deep to the mucosal surface.[29] Empyema can develop as a complication of local treatment with irritant drugs or as a sequela to other guttural pouch diseases.[17] In one report, the highest incidence of classical guttural pouch empyema was in small, mature ponies, in which congenital stenosis of the pharyngeal orifice was a possible cause.[17] In chronic cases of guttural pouch empyema, the purulent material in the pouch becomes inspissated and forms ovoid masses, called chondroids.

### Clinical Signs

Clinical signs of guttural pouch empyema include intermittent nasal discharge, swelling of adjacent lymph nodes, parotid swelling and pain, extended head carriage, and difficulties in swallowing and breathing. The nasal discharge is usually nonodorous, white, and opaque, and contains yellowish-white floccules of variable size. The discharge is usually unilateral when only one pouch is affected but can be bilateral. The discharge is food-stained in horses that develop dysphagia.[8]

Bilateral guttural pouch empyema can cause neurologic problems such as soft palate displacement, pharyngeal paresis, and laryngeal muscle paresis.[8] These are rare and usually transient; however, the dysphagia can be severe enough to cause aspiration pneumonia.[8] Empyema rarely causes epistaxis and then the quantity of blood is only sufficient to stain the mucopurulent discharge.[30] Blood may originate from the site of retropharyngeal lymph node rupture or from granulating surfaces on the floor of the pouch, but not from erosion of large blood vessels.[30]

### Diagnosis

Exudate from the lungs or from an infected sinus can resemble the discharge of guttural pouch empyema[17] so that additional diagnostic steps are required. On endoscopic examination of the pharynx, a purulent discharge

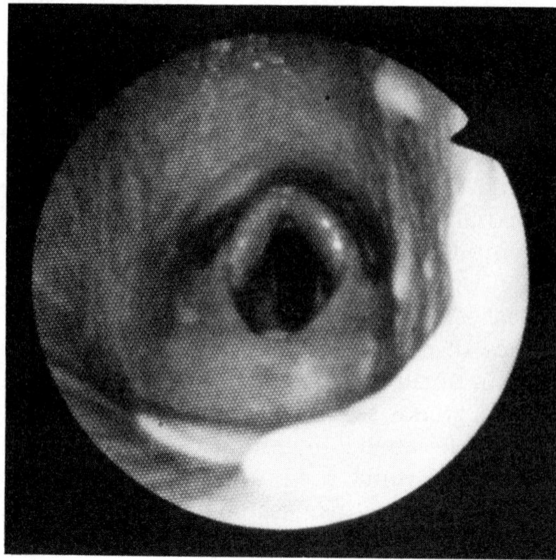

**FIG. 19–9.** Endoscopic view of the pharynx of a horse with empyema. Thick white exudate can be seen draining from the pharyngeal orifice of the guttural pouch and lying on the floor of the soft palate. This horse has cranial nerve damage, which explains the persistent dorsal displacement of the soft palate.

can be seen at the orifice of the affected guttural pouch (Fig. 19–9). An accumulation of exudate within the guttural pouch can be seen on standing lateral radiographs.

To obtain fluid from the affected guttural pouch for diagnostic purposes, a sterile saline solution that does not contain a bacteriostat should be injected through a catheter and aspirated. Bacterial cultures and sensitivity testing of fluid aspirates or saline washings should be interpreted in the light of clinical findings because bacteria and fungi can be retrieved from normal guttural pouches and other parts of the horse's upper respiratory tract.

## Treatment

Treatment of guttural pouch empyema is complicated by poor drainage from the affected pouch. In normal horses, the pharyngeal orifice of the eustachian tube is dorsal to the floor of the guttural pouch and distention may expand the floor further ventrally. In addition, inflammation of mucosa around the pharyngeal orifice can occlude the normal drainage point. Nonsteroidal anti-inflammatory drugs should be given to combat this problem. If the horse is severely dyspneic from guttural pouch distention, a tracheotomy should be done.

In the early stages of this disease, the pouch may respond to daily irrigations with physiologic saline solutions. The purpose of topical infusions is to dislodge and remove dead cells, debris, and mediators of the inflammatory response from the guttural pouch. Infusions should be repeated once or twice daily until the infection has resolved, and the horse should be sedated for the first infusion so that it lowers its head and fluid can drain without risk of aspiration. The horse should be fed from the ground to allow drainage of exudate and infusion solutions. After 7 to 10 days, topical treatment should be interrupted briefly to assess the response.

Irritating solutions such as hydrogen peroxide or concentrated antiseptics should not be infused because they can induce neuritis of the cranial nerves in the guttural pouch, resulting in coughing and dysphagia. They can also modify the nature of and increase the amount of nasal discharge,[10] thereby masking the outward signs of response to treatment. If an antibiotic is given topically, it should not be combined with other antibiotics or other drugs unless there is synergism or the combination is known to have no adverse effects or interactions. The pH and ionic composition of the infusion solution should also be close to optimal. Topical antibiotics are rarely effective in guttural pouch empyema because they are unable to penetrate tissues or kill organisms within the brief contact period achieved, and many are inactivated by the products of inflammation.[31]

The most popular antiseptic for guttural pouch infusion is a 10% (v/v) solution of povidone-iodine in physiologic saline or in water. The free iodine liberated from this solution accounts for its low to intermediate germicidal properties.[32] However, iodine may be neutralized in the presence of exudates[32] and a 10% solution can be irritating to the guttural pouch mucosa.[10] Dilute solutions of povidone-iodine, such as 1%, can be more effective than concentrated solutions because free iodine dissociates more readily from the organic carrier at low concentrations.[32]

Systemic treatment of guttural pouch empyema is rarely indicated unless there is evidence that the infection is spreading and involving other tissues. In these cases, penicillin is often the drug of choice because streptococci, the most common causes of guttural pouch and upper respiratory tract infections in the horse, are usually sensitive to it.[31] Penicillin is less effective against bacteria that are not actively growing and multiplying, as in the late stages of infection or in suppurative processes contained in cavities[31] like the guttural pouch. This underscores the need for drainage, preferably by local irrigation, rather than total reliance on systemic antibiotics.

In many cases, treatment for 1 week with a combination of saline irrigations and systemic antibiotics is successful. If the response to this treatment is poor, or if the purulent material becomes inspissated, surgical drainage of the guttural pouch will have to be considered. If the inspissated pus forms dense, tightly adherent plaques on the mucosal surface, they can be difficult or impossible to remove. A hyovertebrotomy incision combined with ventral drainage through Viborg's triangle or a modified Whitehouse incision are the approaches of choice.

## Guttural Pouch Mycosis

Guttural pouch mycosis affects the roof of the medial compartment of the guttural pouch, caudal and medial to the articulation of the stylohyoid bone with the petrous part of the temporal bone.[33] In this area, it can damage a number of structures and cause a variety of clinical signs. There is no age, sex, breed, or geographic predisposition to this disease, although it seems to occur more frequently in stabled horses during the warmer months of the year.[34] It appears also to be more common in the United Kingdom[6,35] than the United States and in the northern hemisphere than in the south.

### Pathologic Changes

The lesion caused by guttural pouch mycosis is a diphtheritic membrane (Fig. 19–10) that is closely attached to the underlying tissues and has an irregular surface.[33] This membrane is usually composed of necrotic tissue and debris and has a variety of bacteria on its surface.[33] It may be brown, yellow, or black and white and can vary from a discrete nodule to an extensive covering on the roof of the medial and lateral compartments.[33]

On histopathologic examination, fungal mycelia can be found throughout the depth of the diphtheritic membrane and also invading the underlying tissues, nerve fibers, and arteries.[33] Erosion of the wall of the internal carotid artery results in aneurysmal dilatation and eventual rupture.[14,33] An aneurysm may not form in every case but instead, a segment of necrotic arterial wall can form a full-thickness defect without any change in arterial diameter. There is usually a partial thrombosis in the wall of the artery[30,36] but this does not occlude the lumen or appear to prevent hemorrhage. Active inflammation can extend to the underlying bone and cause profuse exostoses.[17,33] In one horse, fungal infection eroded tendons of insertion of the ventral straight muscles of the head and predisposed to their rupture.[37] The infection can cause a fistula between the pharyngeal recess and guttural pouch, or erode the septum and invade the opposite guttural pouch.[6,7,33] If the fistula is in the caudal part of the pharynx or the horse has dysphagia, food can enter the guttural pouch through it.[34] As the mycotic lesion heals, submucosal scarring and fibrosis develop at the site of infection.[33]

The cause of guttural pouch mycosis is not known and, although a number of fungi, especially Aspergillus nidulans and Aspergillus fumigatus, have been identified in the lesion, these organisms are unlikely to be the primary pathogens.[33,38] They are ubiquitous and can be recovered in saline washings from healthy guttural pouches, as well as from other parts of the upper respiratory tract.[33] In one case of guttural pouch mycosis, an aberrant parasitic infection appeared to be involved.[11]

### Clinical Signs

The most common clinical sign of guttural pouch mycosis is epistaxis, which is caused by fungal erosion of the wall of the internal

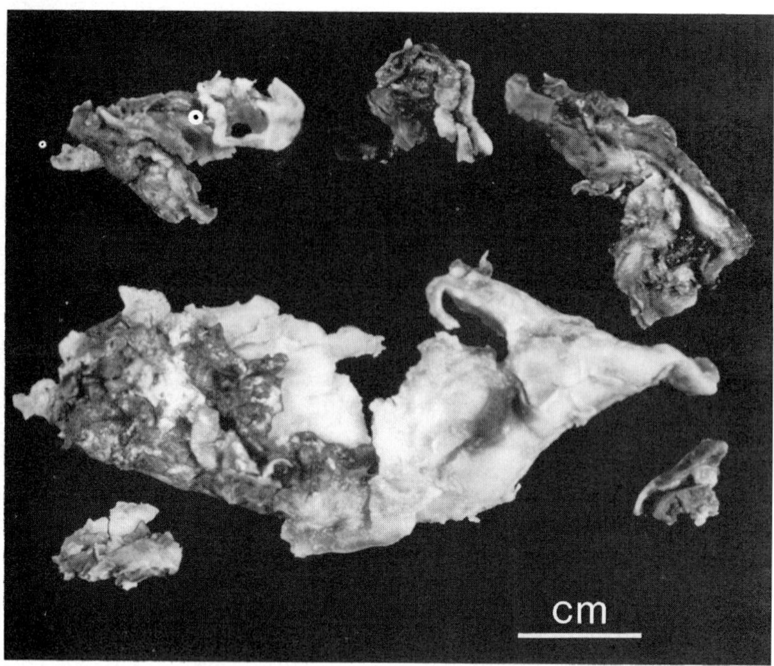


**FIG. 19–10.** Several plaques of diphtheritic membrane removed surgically from the roof of the guttural pouch from a horse with guttural pouch mycosis.

carotid artery in most cases[6,33–35] and the external carotid and maxillary arteries in some.[30,39,40] Epistaxis can be preceded by a mild, mucoid discharge on the nostril of the affected side.[34] In most cases, epistaxis is severe and usually there are several bouts over a period of weeks preceding a fatal hemorrhage.[34] Approximately 50% of horses with hemorrhage die from this complication.[33,34,39,41]

Guttural pouch mycosis is usually unilateral but bilateral cases have been reported.[34,35] Epistaxis is usually bilateral in a horse with one affected guttural pouch but is considerably more severe on the affected side. During hemorrhage, the blood is bright red and free-flowing, but mucus and dark blood continue to drain from the nostril on the affected side for approximately 1 week after hemorrhage ceases. This can be attributed to retention of blood in the guttural pouches over that time with slow drainage through the pharyngeal orifice. By contrast, epistaxis ceases more rapidly in horses with exercise induced pulmonary hemorrhage or nasal trauma and is usually considerably milder in horses with an ethmoid hematoma.

The second most common clinical sign of guttural pouch mycosis is dysphagia.[34] This is manifested in its severe form as masticated food in the nasal discharge, coughing and sneezing, and water flowing freely from the nostrils as the horse drinks. A horse with dysphagia will spend several hours trying to drink in response to severe dehydration. Dysphagia can develop suddenly or slowly and can be explained by involvement of the pharyngeal branches of the vagus and glossopharyngeal nerves.[34] The vulnerability of the glossopharyngeal nerve to damage has been explained by its prominent position in the fold of mucous membrane that contains the other cranial nerves and internal carotid artery (Fig. 19–1). The cranial laryngeal nerve of the vagus is an important component of the reflex arc of deglutition and its destruction could also cause dysphagia.

Other signs of guttural pouch mycosis are parotid pain, nasal discharge, abnormal head posture, head shyness, abnormal respiratory noise, sweating and shivering, Horner's syndrome (Fig. 19–11), corneal ulcers, colic, and facial nerve paralysis.[34,39,42] Parotid pain can be demonstrated by digital pressure to the conchal cartilage on the side of the affected guttural pouch.[34] This region is especially sensitive during the acute stages of the disease or in those horses in which the mycotic infection and hemorrhage have extended into the tissues surrounding the caudal wall of the

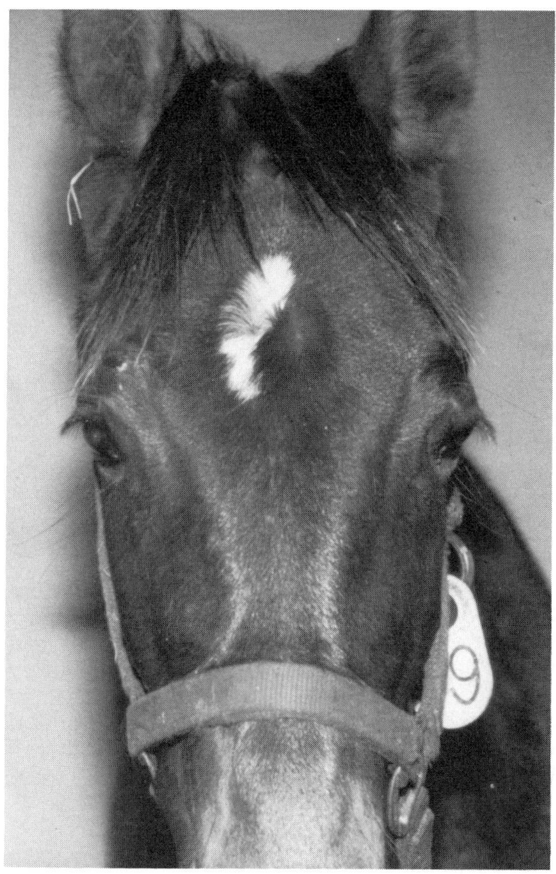


**FIG. 19–11.** A horse with ptosis caused by guttural pouch mycosis. Note that the eyelid on the left (affected) side is drooped and the palpebral fissure is narrow. This horse did not have any other signs of Horner's syndrome. Figure 19–13 is an endoscopic view of the lesion in its guttural pouch.

guttural pouch.[34] Hemorrhage into the retropharyngeal space can be severe enough to cause marked dyspnea[35] and mycosis in the lateral compartment can cause abscessation.[17] The nasal discharge that occurs in cases of guttural pouch mycosis is usually scanty, unilateral and mucoid. The abnormal respiratory noise may be attributed to soft palate paresis and pharyngeal paralysis. Laryngeal hemiplegia can also be caused by guttural pouch mycosis and can be attributed to involvement of the recurrent laryngeal nerve within the vagus.

Horner's syndrome can be explained by damage to the cranial cervical ganglion and postganglionic sympathetic fibers and can be permanent or temporary.[34] Any lesion that involves the internal carotid artery can easily damage the sympathetic nerve trunk and ganglion (Figs. 19–1 and 19–2). The most consistent clinical sign of Horner's syndrome is ptosis, which can be recognized by narrowing of the palpebral fissure and ventral deviation of the upper eyelid (Fig. 19–11). Other ocular signs are miosis, enophthalmos (retraction of the eyeball) and protrusion of the nictitating membrane. These are difficult to detect and may not be evident in many cases.[43–45] The nasal mucosa may become congested for the first few days after sympathetic nerve damage but this finding is also inconsistent, even after a complete neurectomy.[44] Another sign of Horner's syndrome is increased skin temperature and localized sweating, which is usually patchy and confined to the base of the ears, under the halter, and around the eyes.[45,46]

Facial nerve damage can be from direct injury to the nerve or from infection in the temporal bone.[12,13,17,47] Facial nerve paralysis could also cause ptosis because this nerve is distributed to the levator anguli oculi medialis muscle.[47] In this case, the horse will not have miosis, but may have keratitis sicca.[47] The latter can be explained by reduced blinking and lacrimation and can predispose to corneal opacity and ulceration, epiphora, photophobia, and conjunctivitis.[34,47]

Abnormal head posture can be due to parotid pain or to sternocephalicus muscle atrophy from damage to the accessory nerve.[34] Extended head carriage, stiffness, and pain on manipulation of the head and neck are signs that the infection has invaded the atlanto-occipital joint and caused septic arthritis.[43,48] Paralysis of the tongue is a rare consequence of guttural pouch mycosis[6] and can be attributed to damage to the hypoglossal nerve. Blindness and locomotor disturbances are rare and can be caused by a spread of inflammation to the brain[49] or by embolic fungal encephalitis.[50,51]

## Diagnosis

Diagnosis of guttural pouch mycosis can be made on the basis of clinical signs, history, and endoscopic examination. On endoscopic examination, blood and occasionally mucus can be seen draining from the pharyngeal orifice if the horse bled within the previous 3

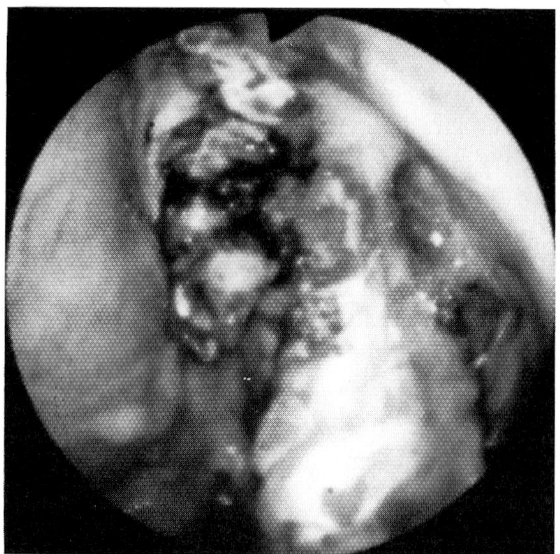

FIG. 19–12. Endoscopic view of the caudal and medial aspect of the guttural pouch from a horse with a history of hemorrhage from the internal carotid artery. The mycotic plaque is located on the roof of the medial compartment and much of the lesion extends along the shaft of the stylohyoid bone.

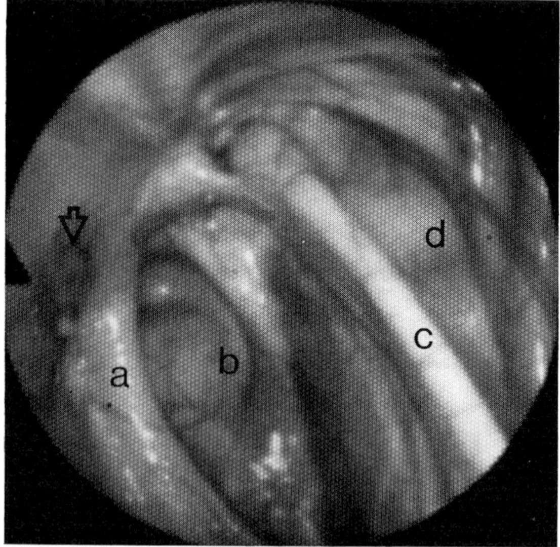


FIG. 19–13. Endoscopic view of the left guttural pouch of a horse with a small lesion caused by guttural pouch mycosis (arrow). This horse had severe hemorrhage from the internal carotid artery and also had signs of Horner's syndrome (same horse as Figure 19–11). a = Internal carotid artery; b = medial compartment; c = stylohyoid bone; d = lateral compartment.

to 5 days. Because blood from other parts of the respiratory tract may be seen on the pharyngeal wall beneath the pharyngeal opening, the guttural pouch interior must be examined to determine if it is the source. In horses with dysphagia, food material can be seen in the nasopharynx and the roof of the pharynx may be collapsed and the soft palate displaced dorsally. In these horses, a barium swallow can be used to assess the severity of pharyngeal paralysis.[6]

When the pouch is examined with the endoscope, the mycotic lesion can be seen on its roof (Figs. 19–12 and 19–13) but may be obscured by clotted blood if hemorrhage was recent. If an eroded artery is to be occluded surgically to prevent epistaxis, an attempt should be made to determine if the lesion is on the internal carotid artery (Figs. 19–12 and 19–13) or on the maxillary artery (Figs. 19–14 and 19–15). The mycelium stimulates an intense inflammatory response in the surrounding mucosa which subsequently thickens and acquires a dull, brick-red color. The size of the lesion bears no relationship to the severity of clinical signs (Fig. 19–13).

It is sometimes possible to see the mycotic

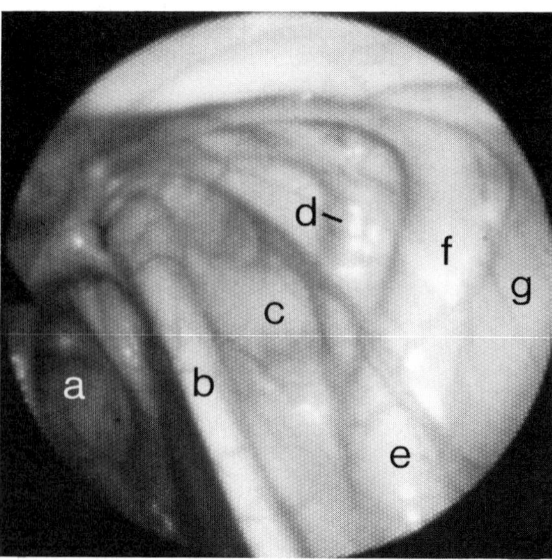


FIG. 19–14. Endoscopic view of the normal lateral compartment of the left guttural pouch. a = Medial compartment; b = stylohyoid bone; c = lateral compartment; d = superficial temporal artery; e = external carotid artery; f = maxillary artery; g = maxillary vein.

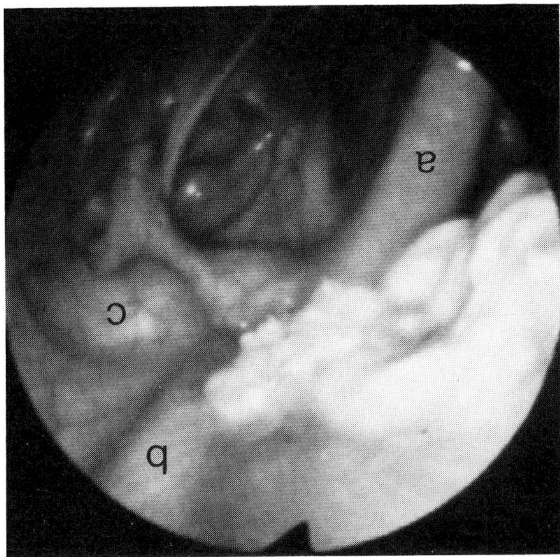


**FIG. 19–15.** Endoscopic view of the right guttural pouch of a horse with guttural pouch mycosis along the maxillary artery. a = Stylohyoid bone; b = the tensor veli palatini muscle; c = internal carotid artery in the medial compartment.

plaque on lateral radiographs of the guttural pouch and also any exostosis or lysis on the stylohyoid bone. However, radiographs may fail to detect changes of septic arthritis in the atlanto-occipital joint.[43,48] Serologic tests for precipitating antibody have been used in horses with suspected Aspergillus infections[52,53] and with some success in a horse with guttural pouch mycosis.[43] Antibodies may be present in a small number of normal horses.[53]

In some horses, the signs of Horner's syndrome may be too subtle to detect and the only evidence of cervical sympathetic damage may be slight ptosis. Some signs of Horner's syndrome can disappear 24 to 48 hours after damage to the sympathetic nerve, even after total neurectomy.[46] However, the denervated area of the face and neck remains highly responsive to sudorific drugs and to exercise.[46] Epinephrine, intravenous xylazine, excitement, and direct radiant heat from an electric heater, can all induce sweating in the horse, but, if Horner's syndrome is present, the sweating will be more obvious on the affected side of the face with a clear line of demarcation on the dorsal midline.[44–46] Therefore, the administration of xylazine or epinephrine can be a useful diagnostic step in horses suspected of having guttural pouch mycosis. There is little evidence of sympathetic innervation to sweat glands in horses;[46] however, epinephrine-induced sweating of Horner's syndrome can be attributed to cutaneous vasodilatation and increased delivery of epinephrine to the sweat glands[46] with subsequent stimulation of their $\beta_2$ adrenoreceptors.[54]

## Topical Treatment

Guttural pouch mycosis can be treated by topical infusions using the same principles and methods described for topical treatment of empyema. Infusions should be daily for 4 to 6 weeks, but the response is slow.[6] It is difficult to apply medication directly to the infection site because it is usually confined to the roof of the guttural pouch and the organisms are well protected within a superficial layer of necrotic tissue and fibrin. This problem can be circumvented by nebulizing fungicidal and fungistatic agents through a catheter placed in the guttural pouch, or the horse can be anesthetized and placed in dorsal recumbency so that infusion solutions can bathe the roof of the medial compartment.[17] However, these methods are cumbersome and a simpler method is controlled delivery of medication through polyethylene tubing in the biopsy channel of the endoscope in the standing, sedated horse. With this approach, solutions can be infused directly beneath the diphtheritic membrane and against the infected mucosal surface every day or every other day. Vigorous flushing of the lesion can macerate, undermine, and detach the necrotic debris and fungal mat. Parts of the lesion can be debrided before flushing by abrading the fungal mat with a cytology brush inserted through the endoscope. This can be repeated on a daily basis until the entire plaque is removed but debridement should be done only after an eroded artery has been occluded.

The inciting cause of guttural pouch mycosis is often unknown, so topical treatment must often be directed against a presumptive pathogen such as Aspergillus sp. A dilute solution of povidone-iodine is both fungicidal and fungistatic[32] but limitations of this form of treatment have been outlined in the section on empyema. Daily infusions of 1% gentian violet have been used,[55] but this dye is only effective against Candida sp, an organism that is rarely involved. A 4% solution of formaldehyde has been used also[17] but this agent is slow-acting, inactivated by organic matter, and irritating to mucosal surfaces when applied in effective concentrations.[32] Thiabendazole (10 to 20%) has been infused[7,40,48] on the basis that this drug is fungicidal and fungistatic.[56,57]

Antifungal drugs such as amphotericin B, nystatin, and natamycin have been used for topical treatment of guttural pouch mycosis. Amphotericin B is unstable, especially in an acid environment, and binding to tissue constituents may limit its diffusion to the infected areas.[58]

Natamycin,[6,59] nystatin,[35] and miconazole have been used in horses with guttural pouch mycosis; however, in vitro sensitivity testing with natamycin and miconazole has shown considerable variation among different species of Aspergillus.[60,61] Miconazole has been used topically at a concentration of 1 mg per ml. Enilconazole has been claimed to be effective against Aspergillus sp[65] and has shown some efficacy in topical treatment of nasal aspergillosis in dogs.[66] The efficacy of ketoconazole against Aspergillus sp is controversial.[61,65] Topical ketoconazole (1 to 5%) has been effective in treatment of keratomycosis.[62,63] In vitro, clotrimazole has broad antifungal activity and is effective against Aspergillus sp; however, to my knowledge its use in guttural pouch mycosis has not been reported and safety and efficacy are unknown. There is some evidence that delivery of antibiotic in powder form may be of benefit because the powder coats the mycotic plaque and thus contact is prolonged.[35] Topical treatment with griseofulvin is not justified because this drug is ineffective against the types of fungi involved in guttural pouch mycosis.[58,60] Topical silver sulphadiazine has been effective for treatment of human keratomycosis caused by Aspergillus sp and Fusarium sp and also has antibacterial activity;[64] its use in the guttural pouch has not, to my knowledge, been reported.

Enzymes have been applied topically to the diphtheritic membrane in an attempt to remove clotted blood, mucous, and fibrinous and purulent exudate.[17] The value of this treatment is questionable because enzymes have specific pH requirements and must have prolonged and intimate contact with their substrates.[67] They can also induce a local inflammatory response, remove tissue barriers that limit spread of infection, and interfere with blood clotting.[67] Dimethylsulfoxide has been used as a vehicle to enhance drug penetration to infected tissues but is too irritating to infuse into the guttural pouch over a prolonged period.

## Systemic and Oral Treatment

Many antifungal agents, such as griseofulvin, are only active against dermatophytes[60] and have no place in the treatment of guttural pouch mycosis. The imidazoles, miconazole and ketoconazole, are effective against many systemic mycoses but, as previously mentioned, Aspergillus sp. may be resistant to them.[61,65,68,69] Although there are no reports on the use of amphotericin B intravenously in the treatment of guttural pouch mycosis, it has been used systemically and topically for the treatment of other fungal infections in the horse.[70] Horses appear to tolerate amphotericin B, although it can cause phlebitis, depression, nephrotoxicity, fever, hypokalemia, and weight loss.[65,70] Prolonged therapy can also cause anemia, which, although usually mild,[65,70] could be a grave complication in a horse prone to hemorrhage. Potassium iodide has been given orally (10 g per os daily) and sodium iodide (15 ml of 20% solution twice daily) intravenously to treat guttural pouch mycosis,[36] but there is little critical assessment of these forms of treatment and no evidence that these drugs are effective against infections with Aspergillus sp.[65]

Corticosteroids or phenylbutazone may be administered to alleviate the inflammatory response to mycotic infections and to reduce neuritis and fibrosis in infected tissues. However, prolonged corticosteroid therapy can exacerbate the mycotic invasion by reducing local tissue defenses.

Oral thiabendazole, at a dose rate of 10 mg/kg twice daily or 50 mg/kg daily for 4 to 6 weeks, has been used in horses with guttural pouch mycosis,[7] but the number of horses treated is insufficient to allow critical assessment of its efficacy. Initial results suggested that thiabendazole might be effective in treatment of nasal aspergillosis in dogs,[7] but later it was shown in a large survey to be of little value.[72] It is a potent, broad-spectrum fungicidal and fungistatic agent in vitro at concentrations that can be achieved in serum of dogs after oral administration.[57] Although oral thiabendazole is readily absorbed, a large part of the absorbed drug is converted into metabolic products that are less fungicidal than the parent compound.[57]

Whole blood should be administered to horses that have suffered acute and massive hemorrhage, and polyionic solutions should be given to supplement blood transfusions or as the sole means of fluid replacement if blood is not available. Tranquilizers, such as acepromazine, should not be given to drop blood pressure and reduce severity of hemorrhage because hypotensive agents can exacerbate hemorrhagic shock. Horses with dysphagia should be given intravenous fluids and nutritional support by nasogastric tube or through an esophagostomy if necessary.

In summary, few treatments are available for guttural pouch mycosis and none has been critically evaluated in a large number of cases. Even under optimal conditions, the response to medical treatment is too slow to reduce the risk of complications such as fatal hemorrhage. Some cases resolve spontaneously, and this must be considered when evaluating a treatment method. In addition, there are few if any outward signs that can be used to monitor the response to treatment, although serologic tests for antibody to Aspergillus sp. or for Aspergillus antigen could be considered for this purpose.[73,74]

## Surgical Treatment

Surgical removal of the diphtheritic membrane can cause severe hemorrhage and cranial nerve deficits[38,75] and should only be done after the involved vessels are occluded. The best approach is through a modified Whitehouse incision and the plaques can be detached by a combination of gentle swabbing with saline-soaked gauze sponges and by peeling them off with sponge forceps. Then the guttural pouch cavity is irrigated with copious amounts of sterile saline and topical antifungal agents. Surgical removal of the lesion can eliminate the infection completely and recurrence is highly unlikely. However, it does not ensure against the risk of hemorrhage from an eroded artery and it also fails to retard progression of neurologic signs. When its inherent risks are considered, surgical debridement offers few advantages in the treatment of guttural pouch mycosis.

Surgical treatment of guttural pouch mycosis should be directed at occlusion of the affected artery in horses that have had hemorrhage. Endoscopy alone is adequate for identification of the affected artery and I do not use arteriography[14] because it requires additional anesthesia time that may not be tolerated well in horses with blood loss. If the lesion is discrete and situated on one artery only, attempts are made to occlude that vessel. If the lesion is extensive and overlies both the internal and the external carotid arteries and branches of the latter, then both vessels are occluded. The artery most frequently eroded in guttural pouch mycosis is the internal carotid artery. In bilateral infections, both internal carotid arteries can be ligated simultaneously without any adverse effects.[27,35] The site for ligation of the internal carotid artery is immediately distal to its origin from the common carotid artery, outside the guttural pouch. The approach is similar to that for a hyovertebrotomy but is placed more ventrally. The internal carotid originates on the cardiac side of the occipital artery and travels deep to that vessel and in a more rostral direction. It may be difficult to distinguish between these vessels in some horses, especially those in which both arteries arise as a single trunk and bifurcate at a variable distance from the common carotid artery. If there is any doubt about identification, both the internal carotid and occipital arteries can be ligated safely.[27,35]

It has been shown that a single ligature on the internal carotid artery, close to its origin, is sufficient to prevent fatal hemorrhage in most cases.[6,35] The high success rate achieved with single ligation has been attributed to thrombosis of the vessel during the week following surgery.[18,27] Thrombosis is favored after ligation because the column of blood distal to the ligature becomes stagnant. Fatal or severe hemorrhage after proximal ligation has been reported and can be attributed to aberrant vasculature with occlusion of the wrong vessel or to retrograde flow from the cerebral arterial circle.[6,11,27,35]

To prevent hemorrhage caused by backflow from the cerebral arterial circle (circle of Willis), an additional ligature has been placed distal to the mycotic infection.[11,36,75] However, this is difficult because the artery must be ligated close to the point where it enters the venous sinuses and the involved segment can be obscured by the diphtheritic membrane. Consequently, the ligature has to be placed blindly and may fail to include the vessel[75] or may incorporate the sympathetic trunk and cause Horner's syndrome.[11]

## Balloon-Catheter Occlusion of the Internal Carotid Artery

We have shown that ligation does not drop blood pressure in the internal carotid artery distal to a ligature so that this procedure may not be immediately effective. A balloon catheter technique* has been devised to allow immediate intravascular occlusion of the artery beneath the guttural pouch mucosa and to prevent retrograde flow from the cerebral arterial circle through the vascular defect.[55,76] The internal carotid artery is isolated close to its origin from the common carotid artery and freed from surrounding fascia. It is then ligated and a small arteriotomy is made in its wall distal to the ligature. A 4- to 8-F balloon-tipped silicone rubber catheter, constructed especially,[76] or a venous thrombectomy catheter (Fogarty-Edwards Laboratories) is inserted through the arteriotomy for a distance of approximately 13 cm.[55,76] This distance usually places the balloon tip of the catheter at the second flexure of the sigmoid, within the venous sinuses on the roof of the guttural pouch and therefore distant to the site of infection (Figs. 19–16 and 19–17). Fluoroscopy is not required to confirm this because when the catheter tip reaches the second flexure of the sigmoid, it becomes difficult to advance. The catheter is inflated with sterile saline and secured in position by a ligature applied distal to the site of insertion. The redundant portion of the catheter is buried in the deeper tissues and the incision is closed in routine fashion. Catheter insertion to the required point may be difficult if the diseased segment has undergone thrombosis,[59] but this is unusual.

Complications associated with this procedure are rare and the most common is infection in the surgical site.[55,59] This problem can be resolved easily by removal of the catheter and establishing drainage and prevented by inflating the balloon to a sufficient diameter (at least 8 mm) to prevent blood pressure from forcing it back into the original infected segment. It is unnecessary to treat the fungal lesion afterwards or to remove the catheter after surgery, unless infection tracks along it and invades the surgical incision. The horse can resume normal activity when wound healing is complete and its PCV has returned to normal. The balloon catheter technique has been found to be a successful, safe and easy technique for preventing hemorrhage from guttural pouch mycosis.[59]

## Ligation of the External Carotid Artery

The external carotid artery can be approached through a similar incision to that for internal carotid artery ligation and ligated distal to the origin of the linguofacial trunk[40] (Fig. 19–18). However, this procedure is generally unsuccessful because the external carotid artery has numerous collateral channels that allow retrograde flow to the infected segment.[40]

After the external carotid artery continues as the maxillary artery (Figs. 19–1 and 19–18), it gives off several large branches that can provide retrograde flow to the lesion. The most likely source of retrograde flow, based on size alone, is the major palatine artery. This joins the contralateral major palatine artery behind the upper row of incisor teeth to form a large arterial loop around the upper jaw (Fig. 19–17).

*The procedure was also described in: Mongeon R. Un cas de mycose des poches gutturales chez un cheval de competition. MV Quebec, 7:28, 1977. However, this report described case 1 from reference 55.

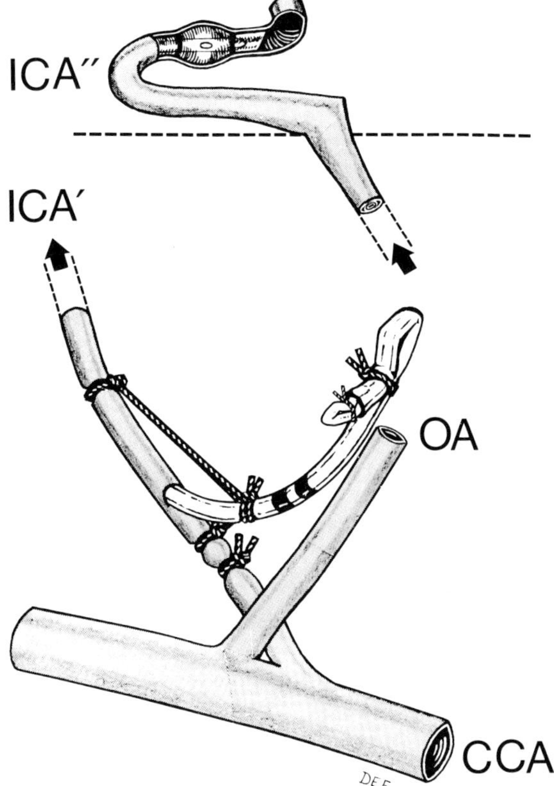


**FIG. 19–16.** Method of placing a balloon catheter in the internal carotid artery. The final position of the balloon is midway between the two flexures of the sigmoid of the internal carotid artery. The catheter is secured to the artery so that it does not become dislodged and so that the balloon remains inflated. The arrows and broken lines continuous with the artery indicate continuity between the two parts of the diagram. OA = Occipital artery; CCA = common carotid artery; ICA′ = internal carotid artery in the guttural pouch; ICA″ = internal carotid artery in the venous sinuses. The heavy broken line represents the roof of the guttural pouch. Note that the sigmoid flexure of the internal carotid artery is within the venous sinuses and therefore cannot be seen from the guttural pouch. Freeman DE, Donawick WJ. Occlusion of internal carotid artery in the horse by means of a balloon-tipped catheter: Clinical use of a method to prevent epistaxis caused by guttural pouch mycosis. (Reproduced with permission from JAVMA, *176*:236, 1980.)

## Balloon-Catheter Occlusion of the External Carotid Artery and Its Branches

Attempts to occlude the external carotid artery by a single balloon-tipped catheter have proven unsatisfactory because it is impossible to control the direction of the catheter tip in distal branches and it can readily enter the superficial temporal artery rather than the maxillary artery (Fig. 19–18). In this event, the catheter accomplishes little more than single ligation because the most common site of infection is farther distally on the maxillary artery (Fig. 19–18). To overcome this problem, the external carotid artery is ligated at its origin and a 6-F Fogarty venous thrombectomy catheter is inserted into the major palatine artery, 3 cm caudal to the corner incisor tooth (Fig. 19–17). This catheter is placed so that its balloon can occlude the maxillary artery, caudal to the caudal alar foramen and thus prevent retrograde flow to this segment (Fig. 19–17). The catheter is inserted for approximately 2 to 3 cm beyond the shortest distance from the arteriotomy to the articular tubercle of the temporal bone and the balloon is partly inflated. The catheter is gently retracted until some resistance is encountered, at which point it is assumed that the balloon is at the caudal alar foramen (Fig. 19–17). It is then fully inflated with sterile saline.

As an alternative to ligation distal to the origin of the linguofacial trunk, which involves deep dissection, the external carotid artery can also be occluded by inserting a catheter through the transverse facial artery beneath the articular tubercle of the temporal bone (Figs. 19–17 and 19–18). This catheter is advanced in retrograde fashion so that its tip is approximately 12 cm from the arteriotomy and then it is inflated with saline. It has been shown by measurement in cadavers that the balloon at this distance is in the external carotid artery (Fig. 19–17). The redundant ends of the catheters in the transverse facial and major palatine arteries are secured with tape and incorporated into a stockinet hood.

There are several branches from the maxillary artery in the segment intervening between the points of balloon inflation and it is possible that these may still provide some ret-

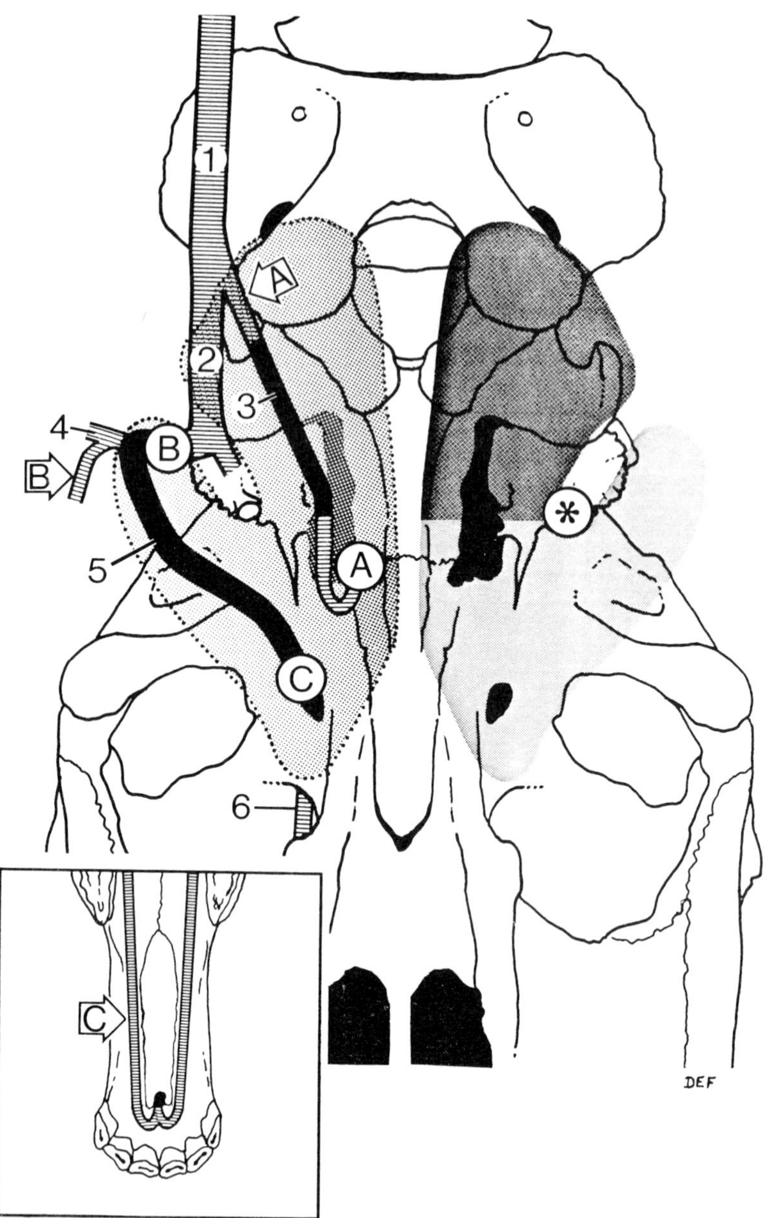


**FIG. 19–17.** Sites of insertion (lettered arrows) and sites of balloon inflation (lettered circles) to treat horses with hemorrhage from branches of the common carotid artery within the guttural pouch. 1 = Common carotid artery; 2 = external carotid artery; 3 = internal carotid artery; 4 = superficial temporal artery; 5 = maxillary artery; 6 = descending palatine artery. The black segments of arteries are those parts that are contained beneath the mucosa of the guttural pouch and are thus vulnerable to damage from guttural pouch mycosis. A = Sites for insertion and balloon inflation in the internal carotid artery; B (arrow) = site of insertion of balloon catheter in the transverse facial artery; B (circled) = site of balloon inflation for that catheter in the external carotid artery; C (arrow in inset) = site of catheter insertion in major palatine artery; and C (circled) = site of balloon inflation of that catheter in the maxillary artery, caudal to the caudal alar foramen. The system for determining the artery most likely affected is shown in the shaded outline of the guttural pouch on the right side. If the mycotic infection is located on endoscopic examination in the area identified by the dark shading, the internal carotid artery is most likely involved. If the segment indicated by the lighter shading contains the mycotic lesion, then the external carotid and maxillary arteries are probably involved. The asterisk marks the temporohyoid joint which serves as a useful landmark for the border between these two areas of the guttural pouch.

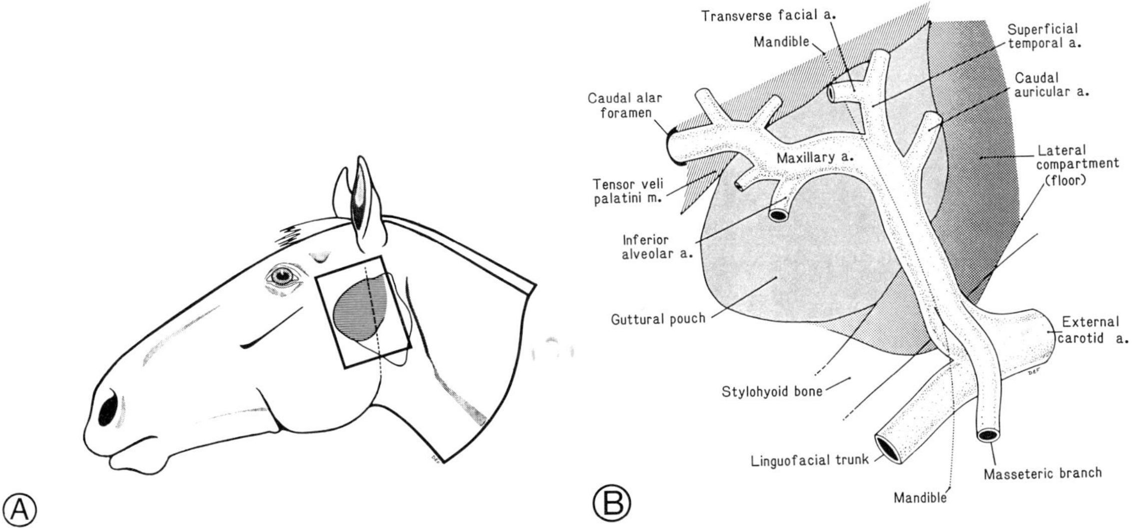


**FIG. 19–18.** Relationship of the maxillary artery to the guttural pouch. A. The rectangle encloses the segment of guttural pouch illustrated in Figure 19–18B. The shaded segment within the guttural pouch outline is the most rostral part, including the lateral compartment shown in Figure 19–18B. B. Lateral aspect of the left guttural pouch, illustrating the course of the external carotid artery and its branches along the wall and roof of the lateral compartment. a = Artery; m = muscle. Freeman DE, Ross MW, Donawick WJ, et al. Occlusion of the external carotid and maxillary arteries in the horse to prevent hemorrhage from guttural pouch mycosis. (Reproduced with permission from Veterinary Surgery, *18*:39, 1989.)

rograde flow to the infected segment (Fig. 19–18). However, this procedure has been effective in a small number of horses to date. All these catheters are removed after 7 to 10 days and removal does not require sedation or local anesthesia.

The major potential complication of external carotid occlusion is blindness,[40] although this has not been observed in the small number of horses treated by the above procedure, regardless of whether it was done alone or combined with occlusion of the internal carotid artery. However, the owner should be advised of this risk and the affects of unilateral blindness on the horse's future should be considered before proceeding with the surgery.

## Prognosis

The risk of fatal hemorrhage from guttural pouch mycosis is at least 50%; however, balloon occlusion of the involved vessel can abolish this risk if the internal carotid artery is eroded and reduces it considerably if the external carotid or maxillary arteries are affected. Laryngeal hemiplegia is usually permanent,[18] but a rare recovery has been reported.[6] Some horses that develop dysphagia may eventually recover,[18,48,77] but this may take at least 6 to 18 months.[6] Recovery from dysphagia may not be complete but, instead, the horse may learn to compensate for a mild paresis of the pharyngeal musculature.[18] The prognosis is poor in horses that are unable to maintain themselves throughout the recovery period.[6] Horses can recover from Horner's syndrome and facial nerve paralysis. Pharyngeal fistulas can heal spontaneously.[7]

## *Neoplasia*

Neoplasia of the guttural pouches is rare but tumors reported include a squamous cell carcinoma,[78,79] a round cell sarcoma,[13] a fibroma,[80] hemangioma,[81] hemangiosarcoma,[82] and a melanoma of the parotid region that involved the lateral wall of the guttural pouch and the retropharyngeal lymph nodes.[17] Tumors of the guttural pouches can cause epistaxis[82] and signs of cranial nerve damage.[81] Radiography and biopsy are useful in making the diagnosis.[13,17] Surgical removal is difficult because the lesion is usually extensive and adjacent vital structures may be involved.[79]

## Fractures

Fracture of the stylohyoid bone, close to its articulation with the petrous part of the temporal bone, can cause signs of guttural pouch disease or may be an incidental finding at necropsy.[12] Fractures of this bone may be secondary to guttural pouch mycosis[34] or may be caused by the horse falling over backwards or by excess traction to the tongue during oral examination.[12,13] Bone necrosis can follow and clinical signs include dysphagia, pharyngeal swelling, and empyema.[12,34] Fracture of the jugular process from falling over backwards can cause copious hemorrhage from the guttural pouch.[12]

## Foreign Bodies

Segments of drainage catheters have been found in the guttural pouch[13] and wire impacted in the retropharyngeal space can lacerate an artery in the guttural pouch and cause epistaxis.[83]

## Otitis

Otitis media, ruptured tympanic membrane, and otitis externa have occurred in association with empyema of the guttural pouches[17] and otitis media in association with guttural pouch mycosis.[17,39,43] A syndrome of vestibulocochlear and facial nerve dysfunction with chronic periosteal bony proliferation of the tympanic bulla, petrous part of the temporal bone, and stylohyoid bone, fusion of the temporohyoid joint and the petrous part of the temporal bone may be secondary to otitis media-interna in horses.[84,85] Horses over a wide age range are affected with this syndrome,[85] but it is more common in horses over 11 years.[47,84] Clinical signs include peripheral vestibular ataxia, transitory dysphagia, facial nerve paralysis, and keratitis due to paralysis of the eyelids.[85] The bony lesions can be demonstrated most readily on dorsoventral projections[84,85] and prominent, smooth exostoses can be seen along the shaft of the stylohyoid bone on endoscopic examination of the guttural pouch. Clinical signs are ameliorated by treatment with antibiotics and antiinflammatory drugs.[84,85]

Although these horses do not have guttural pouch infections, the bony lesions involve parts of the skull that contribute to formation of the guttural pouch or are contained directly beneath its mucosal lining. In rare cases, there can be hyperemia and edema in the guttural pouch lining.[84] Because many clinical signs of this syndrome can be seen in horses with guttural pouch mycosis,[12,13] endoscopic examination of the guttural pouch should be used to distinguish between them.

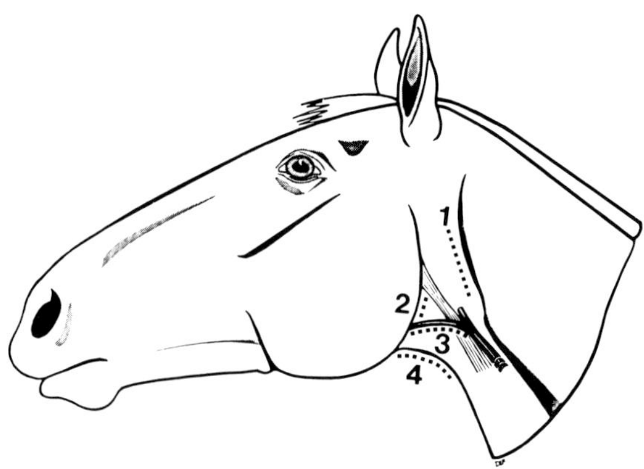

**FIG. 19–19.** Surgical approaches to the guttural pouch. 1 = Hyovertebrotomy; 2 = Viborg's triangle. This incision can be made horizontally or vertically in the triangle defined by the tendon of the sternocephalicus muscle, the linguofacial vein, and the ramus of the mandible. 3 = Modified Whitehouse approach; 4 = Whitehouse approach. (From Freeman DE. Diagnosis and treatment of diseases of the guttural pouch (Part II). Compendium of Continuing Education for the Veterinary Practitioner, 2:S25, 1980.)

# Surgery

The following surgical approaches are those most commonly used to enter the guttural pouch for removal of pus, mycotic plaques and foreign bodies, and to establish drainage (Fig. 19–19).

## Hyovertebrotomy

This approach involves a 10-cm long incision 2 cm cranial to and parallel with the wing of the atlas (Fig. 19–19). The dense fascia around the parotid gland is incised, and this gland and the overlying parotidoauricularis muscle are reflected cranially and the fascia and second cervical nerve are reflected caudally. The areolar tissue beneath the parotid gland is broken down by blunt dissection and the mandibular salivary gland is reflected cranially. The guttural pouch lining is grasped with rat teeth or Allis tissue forceps and is punctured with the closed tips of scissors or a hemostat. This opening is close to the internal carotid artery, the hypoglossal and glossopharyngeal nerves, and the cranial laryngeal and pharyngeal branches of the vagus nerve so that special care must be exercised. The incision is enlarged by spreading its edges with jaws of a hemostat or with fingers. This approach is often combined with an opening through Viborg's triangle to establish ventral drainage because drainage from the hyovertebrotomy alone is poor. In order to open the pouch through Viborg's triangle, a metal sound is passed through the hyovertebrotomy incision and directed ventrally so that its tip can be palpated at the proposed incision site (Fig. 19–19). The inspissated pus and chondroids are removed by a combination of lavage and swabbing the mucosal surface with saline-soaked sponges. A soft rubber drain or packing can then be placed in the pouch so that its tip exits at the ventral incision. The hyovertebrotomy can be closed in routine fashion or left partly open to provide ingress and egress for irrigating solutions. For this purpose, a soft rubber seton can be placed through both incisions to keep them patent.

## Viborg's Triangle

Viborg's triangle is an area defined by the tendon of the sternocephalicus muscle, the linguofacial vein, and the vertical ramus of the mandible (Fig. 19–19). The incision can be vertical or horizontal and care must be taken to avoid the parotid duct and the branches of the vagus nerve along the floor of the guttural pouch. This incision is usually allowed to heal by second intention and can be kept open with packing or with a soft rubber drain. The major problem with this approach is that it is confined, except in foals with tympany when the triangle is expanded (Fig. 19–7).

## Whitehouse

The horse is placed in dorsal recumbency and the incision is made on the ventral midline through the skin overlying the larynx (Fig. 19–19). Dissection is continued through the sternohyoideus and omohyoideus muscles and along the larynx to the side of the affected guttural pouch. The guttural pouch is opened medial to the stylohyoid bone, the external carotid artery, the glossopharyngeal nerve, and the hypoglossal nerve. The pharyngeal branch of the vagus nerve and the cranial laryngeal nerve are close to the incision and must be avoided. An opening can be made through the median septum to the opposite guttural pouch if needed.

## Modified Whitehouse Approach

The Whitehouse approach can be modified by placing the skin incision along the ventral edge of the linguofacial vein and extending it rostrally for 12 cm from the jugular vein (Fig. 19–19). The underlying fascia is incised and the lateral aspect of the larynx exposed. The incision is then continued as in the preceding until the guttural pouch cavity has been entered. The major advantage of this approach is that the incision through the sternohyoideus and omohyoideus muscles is avoided and dissection is through a natural fascial plane.

Advantages of both Whitehouse approaches are that they allow direct access to the roof of the guttural pouch, digital exploration of the lateral compartment, excellent ventral drainage, and simultaneous access to both pouches. However, both approaches involve deep dissection. It has been stated that the Whitehouse approaches have a high rate of complications, such as dysphagia, in horses with empyema.[86] However, these concerns apply equally to other approaches and the advantages of the Whitehouse methods are considerable.

## *Aftercare*

Open incisions in the guttural pouch are cleaned daily with gauze sponges soaked with warm water and dilute antiseptic solutions. The guttural pouch cavity should be flushed through the open incision daily with a nonirritating solution or saline solution in order to remove any accumulated purulent material. The incisions will close spontaneously within 14 days, by which time the infection should be resolved. The horse can be put on a course of postoperative antibiotics if desired, especially when dealing with a severe infection.

## *General Comments*

Surgery of the guttural pouch should be regarded as a last resort because it is fraught with the risk of iatrogenic nerve damage, regardless of the approach used. All incisions are directed internally toward the floor and caudal aspect of the medial compartment of the guttural pouch where the internal carotid artery and cranial nerves lie beneath a fold of guttural pouch mucosa. The positions of these nerves are not constant.[86]

Identification of the guttural pouch lining is extremely difficult and may be facilitated by prior insertion of a lighted endoscope into the medial compartment. Because the mucosa tends to collapse away from the plane of dissection, a fixed structure within the guttural pouch, such as the stylohyoid bone, should be identified by palpation and used as a guide. If the guttural pouch lining is thickened and inflamed, identification of fine nerve branches may be facilitated by illuminating the mucosa with the endoscope. The mucosa should not be incised with a scalpel or scissors because of the risk of severing important nerves. Retraction of incision edges can damage nerves and should be applied with care.

## References

1. Sisson S. The Ear. In: Sisson and Grossman's The Anatomy of the Domestic Animals. 5th Ed. Getty R (ed): Philadelphia, WB Saunders Co, 1975, p 723.
2. Raker CW. Diseases of the guttural pouch. Mod Vet Pract, *57*:549, 1976.
3. Heffron CJ, Baker JG. Endoscopic observations on the deglutition reflex in the horse. Equine Vet J, *11*:137, 1979.
4. Cook WR. Clinical observations on the anatomy and physiology of the equine upper respiratory tract. Vet Rec, *79*:440, 1966.
5. Tritschler LG, Morrow LL. Guttural pouch catheterization. VM/SAC, *67*:534, 1972.
6. Greet TRC. Outcome of treatment in 35 cases of guttural pouch mycosis. Equine Vet J, *19*:483, 1987.
7. Jacobs KA, Fretz PB. Fistula between the guttural pouches and the dorsal pharyngeal recess as a sequela to guttural pouch mycosis in the horse. Can Vet J, *23*:117, 1982.
8. Modransky PD, Reed SM, Barbee DD. Dysphagia associated with guttural pouch empyema and dorsal displacement of the soft palate. Equine Pract, *4*:34, 1982.
9. White SL, Williamson L. How to make a retention catheter to treat guttural pouch empyema. Vet Med, *82*:76, 1987.
10. Wilson J. Effects of indwelling catheters and povidone iodine flushes on the guttural pouches of the horse. Equine Vet J, *17*:242, 1985.
11. Owen R ap R. Epistaxis prevented by ligation of the internal carotid artery in the guttural pouch. Equine Vet J, *6*:143, 1974.
12. Cook WR. Skeletal radiology of the equine head. J Am Vet Radiol Soc, *11*:35, 1970.
13. Cook WR. The auditory tube diverticulum (guttural pouch) in the horse: Its radiographic examination. J Am Vet Radiol Soc, *14*:51, 1973.
14. Colles CM, Cook WR. Carotid and cerebral angiography in the horse. Vet Rec, *113*:483, 1983.
15. Wheat JD. Tympanites of the guttural pouch of the horse. J Am Vet Med Assoc, *140*:453, 1962.
16. Holmes RA. The guttural pouches of the horse. Mod Vet Pract, *43*:45, 1962.
17. Cook WR. Diseases of the ear, nose and throat in the horse. Part 1: The Ear. In: The Veterinary Annual. Grunsell CSG (ed). Bristol, John Wright and Sons, Ltd, 1971, p 12.
18. Cook WR. Diseases of the auditive tube diverticulum (guttural pouch). In: Current Therapy in Equine Medicine. 2nd Ed. NE Robinson (ed). Philadelphia, WB Saunders Co, 1987, p 612.
19. Wirstad HF. Luftposetympanitt hos foll. Nord Vet Med, *3*:87, 1951.
20. Hutyra F, Marek J, Manninger R. Special Pathology

and Therapeutics of Domestic Animals, Vol. 3. London, Bailliere, Tindall and Cox, 1946, p 626.
21. Mason TA. Tympany of the eustachian tube diverticulum (guttural pouch) in a foal. Equine Vet J, *4*:153, 1972.
22. Milne DW, and Fessler JR. Tympanites of the guttural pouch in a foal. J Am Vet Med Assoc, *161*:61, 1972.
23. O'Connor JR. A case of tympany of the guttural pouch. Ir Vet J, *25*:11, 1971.
24. Lokai MD, Hardenbrook HJ, Benson GH. Guttural pouch tympanites in a foal. VM/SAC, *71*:1625, 1976.
25. Forbes JRS, Bennel DG. Tympany of the guttural pouch in a foal. Aust Vet J, *51*:164, 1975.
26. Lattimer JC. Equine nasal passages, sinuses and guttural pouches. In: Textbook of Veterinary Diagnostic Radiology. DE Thrall (ed). Philadelphia, WB Saunders Co, 1986, p 64.
27. McIlwraith CW, Turner AS. Equine Surgery Advanced Techniques. Philadelphia, Lea & Febiger, 1987, p 228.
28. Sweeney CR, Whitlock RH, Meirs DA, et al. Complications associated with *Streptococcus equi* infection on a horse farm. J Am Vet Med Assoc, *191*:1446, 1987.
29. Knight AP, Voss JL, McChesney AE, et al. Experimentally-induced Streptococcus equi infection in horses with resultant guttural pouch empyema. VM/SAC, *70*:1194, 1975.
30. Nation PN. Epistaxis of guttural pouch origin in horses: pathology of three cases. Can Vet J, *19*:194. 1978.
31. Aronson AL, Kirk RW. Antimicrobial drugs. In: Textbook of Veterinary Internal Medicine. Diseases of the Dog and Cat. 2nd Ed. SJ Ettinger (ed). Philadelphia, WB Saunders Co, 1983, p 338.
32. Harvey SC. Antiseptics and disinfectants; fungicides; ectoparasiticides. In: Goodman and Gilman's The Pharmacological Basis of Therapeutics. 7th Ed. A Gilman, LS Goodman, TW Rall, and F Murad (eds). New York, MacMillan Publishing Co, 1985, p 959.
33. Cook WR, Campbell RSF, Dawson C. The pathology and aetiology of guttural pouch mycosis in the horse. Vet Rec, *83*:422, 1968.
34. Cook WR. The clinical features of guttural pouch mycosis in the horse. Vet Rec, *83*:336, 1968.
35. Church S, Wyn-Jones G, Park AH, et al. Treatment of guttural pouch mycosis. Equine Vet J, *18*:362, 1986.
36. Owen RR, McKelvey WAC. Ligation of the internal carotid artery to prevent epistaxis due to guttural pouch mycosis. Vet Rec, *104*:100, 1979.
37. Knight AP. Dysphagia resulting from unilateral rupture of the rectus capitis ventralis muscles in a horse. J Am Vet Med Assoc, *170*:735, 1977.
38. Johnson JH, Merriam JG, Attleberger M. A case of guttural pouch mycosis caused by *Aspergillus nidulans*. VM/SAC, *68*:771, 1973.
39. Bjorklund NE, Palsson G. Guttural pouch mycosis in the horse. A survey of 7 cases and a case report. Nord Vet Med, *22*:65, 1970.
40. Smith DM, Barber SM. Guttural pouch hemorrhage associated with lesions of the maxillary artery in two horses. Can Vet J, *25*:239, 1984.
41. Cook WR. Observations on the aetiology of epistaxis and cranial nerve paralysis in the horse. Vet Rec, *78*:396, 1966.
42. Hilbert BJ, Huxtable CR, Brighton AJ. Erosion of the internal carotid artery and cranial nerve damage caused by guttural pouch mycosis in a horse. Aust Vet J, *57*:346, 1981.
43. Dixon PM, Rowlands AC. Atlanto-occipital joint infection associated with guttural pouch mycosis in a horse. Equine Vet J, *13*:260, 1981.
44. Firth EC. Horner's syndrome in the horse: experimental induction and a case report. Equine Vet J, *10*:9, 1978.
45. Smith JS, Mayhew IG. Horner's syndrome in large animals. Cornell Vet, *67*:529, 1977.
46. Usenik EA. Sympathetic innervation of the head and neck of the horse; neuropharmacological studies of sweating in the horse. PhD Thesis, University of Minnesota, 1957.
47. Habel RE, King JM. Clinical anatomy of the guttural pouch. In: Proceedings. 20th World Veterinary Congress, *1*:113, 1975.
48. Walmsley JP. A case of atlantooccipital arthropathy following guttural pouch mycosis in a horse. The use of radioisotope bone scanning as an aid to diagnosis. Equine Vet J, *20*:219, 1988.
49. Hatziolos BC, Sass B, Albert TF, et al. Ocular changes in a horse with gutturomycosis. J Am Vet Med Assoc, *167*:51, 1975.
50. McLaughlin BG, O'Brien JL. Guttural pouch mycosis and mycotic encephalitis in a horse. Can Vet J, *27*:109, 1986.
51. Wagner PC, Miller RA, Gallina AM, et al. Mycotic encephalitis associated with a guttural pouch mycosis. J Equine Med Surg, *2*:355, 1978.
52. Greet TRC. Nasal aspergillosis in three horses. Vet Rec, *109*:487, 1981.
53. Lawson GHK, McPherson SA, Murphy JR, et al. The presence of precipitating antibodies in the sera of horses with chronic obstructive pulmonary disease. Equine Vet J, *11*:172, 1979.
54. Snow DH. Identification of the receptor involved in adrenaline mediated sweating in the horse. Res Vet Sci, *23*:246, 1977.
55. Freeman DE, Donawick WJ. Occlusion of internal carotid artery in the horse by means of a balloon-tipped catheter: clinical use of a method to prevent epistaxis caused by guttural pouch mycosis. J Am Vet Med Assoc, *176*:236, 1980.
56. Allen PM, Gottlieb D. Mechanism of action of the fungicide thiabendazole, 2-(4'-thiazolyl) benzimidazole. Appl Microbiol, *20*:919, 1970.
57. Robinson HJ, Phares HF, Graessle OE. Antimycotic properties of thiabendazole. J Invest Dermatol, *42*:479, 1964.
58. Sande MA, Mandell GL. Antifungal and antiviral agents. In: Goodman and Gilman's The Pharmacological Basis of Therapeutics. 7th Ed. A Gilman LS Goodman, TW Rall, and F Murad (eds): New York, MacMillan Publishing Co, 1985, p 1219.
59. Caron JP, Fretz PD, Bailey JV, et al. Balloon-tipped catheter arterial occlusion for prevention of hemor-

rhage caused by guttural pouch mycosis: 13 cases (1982–1985). J Am Vet Med Assoc, *191*:345, 1987.
60. Reynolds JEF (ed). Martindale the Extra Pharmacopoeia. 28th Ed. London, The Pharmaceutical Press, 1982, p 728.
61. Coad CT, Robinson NM, Wilhelmus KR. Antifungal sensitivity testing for equine keratomycosis. Am J Vet Res, *46*:676, 1985.
62. O'Day DM. Selection of appropriate antifungal therapy. Cornea, *6*:238, 1987.
63. Johns KJ, O'Day DM. Pharmacologic management of keratomycoses. Surv Ophthalmol, *33*:178, 1989.
64. Mohan M, Gupta SK, Kaha UK, et al. Topical silver sulphadiazine—A new drug for ocular keratomycosis. Br J Ophthalmol, *72*:192, 1988.
65. Utz JP. Chemotherapy of the systemic mycoses. Med Clin North Am, *66*:221, 1982.
66. Sharp NJH, Sullivan M. Treatment of canine nasal aspergillosis with systemic ketoconazole and topical enilconazole. Vet Rec, *118*:560, 1986.
67. Swinyard EA, Pathak MA. Surface-acting drugs. In: Goodman and Gilman's the Pharmacological Basis of Therapeutics. 7th Ed. A Gilman, LS Goodman, TW Rall, and F Murad (eds). New York, MacMillan Publishing Co, 1985, p 946.
68. Gabal MA. Antifungal activity of ketoconazole with emphasis on zoophilic fungal pathogens. Am J Vet Res, *47*:1229, 1986.
69. Stamm AM, Dismukes WE. Current therapy of pulmonary and disseminated fungal diseases. Chest, *83*:911, 1983.
70. McMullan WC, Joyce RJ, Hanselka DV, et al. Amphotericin B for the treatment of localized subcutaneous phycomycosis in the horse. J Am Vet Med Assoc, *170*:1293, 1977.
71. Lane JG, Clayton-Jones DG, Thoday KL, et al. The diagnosis and successful treatment of *Aspergillus fumigatus* infection of the frontal sinuses and nasal chambers of the dog. J Sm Anim Pract, *15*:79, 1974.
72. Harvey CE. Nasal aspergillosis and penicilliosis in dogs: results of treatment with thiabendazole. J Am Vet Med Assoc, *184*:48, 1984.
73. Glimp RA, Bayer AS. Pulmonary aspergilloma. Diagnostic and therapeutic considerations. Arch Intern Med, *143*:303, 1983.
74. Penn RL, Lambert RS, George RB. Invasive fungal infections: the use of serologic tests in diagnosis and management. Arch Intern Med, *143*:1215, 1983.
75. McIlwraith CW. Surgical treatment of acute epistaxis associated with guttural pouch mycosis. VM/SAC, *73*:67, 1978.
76. Freeman DE, Donawick WJ. Occlusion of internal carotid artery in the horse by means of a balloon-tipped catheter: Evaluation of a method designed to prevent epistaxis caused by guttural pouch mycosis. J Am Vet Med Assoc, *176*:232, 1980.
77. Rawlinson RJ, Jones RT. Guttural pouch mycosis in two horses. Aust Vet J, *54*:135, 1978.
78. Moulton JE (ed). Tumors in Domestic Animals. Los Angeles, University of California Press, 1978, p 211.
79. Trigo FJ, Nickels FA. Squamous cell carcinoma of a horse's guttural pouch. Mod Vet Pract, *62*:456, 1981.
80. Merriam JG. Guttural pouch fibroma in a mare. J Am Vet Med Assoc, *161*:487, 1972.
81. Greene HJ, O'Connor JP. Hemangioma of the guttural pouch of a 16-year-old Thoroughbred mare: Clinical and pathological findings. Vet Rec, *118*:445, 1986.
82. Raker CW. The nasopharynx. In: Equine Medicine and Surgery. 3rd Ed. RA Mannsmann, ES McAllister (eds). Santa Barbara, American Veterinary Publications, 1982, p 756.
83. Bayly WM, Robertson JT. Epistaxis caused by foreign body penetration of a guttural pouch. J Am Vet Med Assoc, *180*:1232, 1982.
84. Blythe LL, Watrous BJ, Schmitz JA, et al. Vestibular syndrome associated with temporohyoid joint fusion and temporal bone fracture in three horses. J Am Vet Med Assoc, *185*:775, 1984.
85. Power HT, Watrous BJ, deLahunta A. Facial and vestibulocochlear nerve disease in six horses. J Am Vet Med Assoc, *183*:1076, 1983.
86. Turner AS, McIlwraith CW. Techniques in Large Animal Surgery. Philadelphia, Lea & Febiger, 1982, p 194.

# CHAPTER 20

# PHARYNX AND LARYNX

*JAMES T. ROBERTSON*

## Dorsal Displacement of the Soft Palate

The soft palate is a musculomembranous sheet of tissue that extends from the hard palate to the entrance of the esophageal pharynx and serves to separate the oral cavity from the nasopharynx. Caudally, it has an opening, the ostium intrapharyngium, through which the epiglottis and the corniculate processes of the arytenoid project.[1,2] The boundaries of this opening are formed by the visible free border of the soft palate rostrally, the pillars of the soft palate laterally, and the palatopharyngeal arch caudodorsally. The muscles that control the soft palate are the palatine, the levator, and the tensor, which serve to shorten, raise, and tense the soft palate, respectively. Their innervation is derived from the trigeminal, vagus and glossopharyngeal nerves.[2]

The larynx articulates with the ostium intrapharyngium like a button in a button hole and, except during swallowing or coughing, the free border of the soft palate should remain beneath the epiglottis[1] (Fig. 20–1). It is important that the ostium intrapharyngeum is tightly fitted around the larynx and maintains an airtight seal when the horse is breathing. During inspiration, the corniculate processes dilate maximally, reinforcing this seal. The sternothyrohyoideus and omohyoideus muscles are accessory muscles of respiration that cause caudal retraction of the larynx, longitudinal stretching of the nasopharynx and a tilting of the glottis during inspiration.[1,3] Under normal circumstances, the effects of this muscular activity are beneficial, helping to reinforce the airtight seal between the dilated larynx and the ostium intrapharyngium and produce a straighter, more streamlined airway that is more resistant to collapse.[3]

Subluxation of the nasopharyngeal and laryngeal airways results in a displacement of the caudal free border of the soft palate to a position above the epiglottis (Figs. 20–2 and 20–3). Dorsal displacement of the soft palate (DDSP) causes a narrowing of the nasopharyngeal airway and creates air turbulence on inspiration and expiration. During expiration, air is expelled into both the nasopharynx and the oral cavity. DDSP may be intermittent or persistent and in some horses it may be a permanent condition. The condition is most frequently encountered in racehorses as an intermittent event that causes temporary obstruction and asphyxia at high speed.

Terms other than DDSP that have been used to describe this condition include soft palate paralysis or paresis and elongation of the soft palate. To date there is no evidence that there is a neurogenic etiology for the DDSP that is a common cause of temporary asphyxia in racehorses.[1,3] Histopathologic examinations of sections of the soft palate of horses that had intermittent DDSP show no evidence of a neuropathy or neurogenic atrophy of the palate musculature.[1] Horses that have damage to cranial nerves IX and X, as seen with a guttural pouch mycosis, or have a generalized neuromuscular disease such as botulism, have a true pharyngeal and soft palate paralysis that results in dysphagia. Dys-

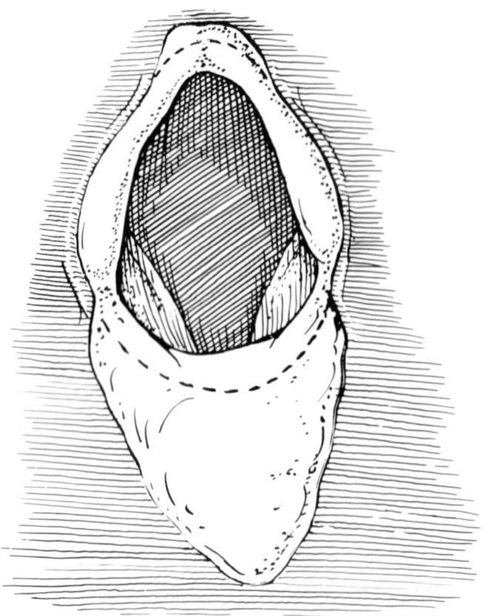

**FIG. 20–1.** In this sketch of an endoscopic view of the larynx, the epiglottis is visible and situated above the free border of the soft palate. The ostium intrapharyngium is denoted by the dotted lines.

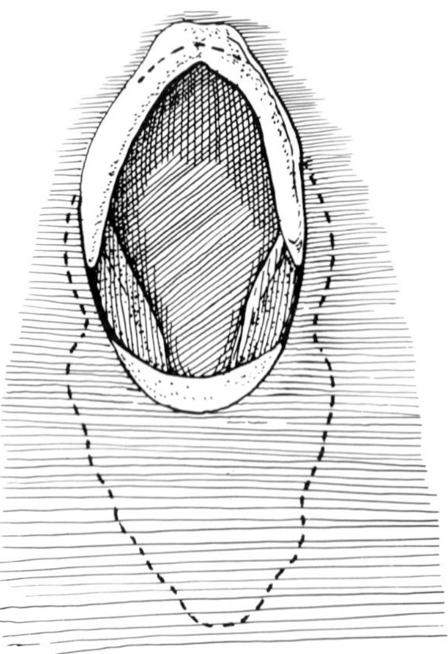

**FIG. 20–2.** This sketch shows a dorsal displacement of the soft palate. The rostral and lateral margins of the ostium intrapharyngium are visible, but the epiglottis (dotted outline) is not visible. The dotted line over the dorsum of the larynx represents the caudal margin of the ostium intrapharyngium, which is situated behind the apices of the corniculate processes.

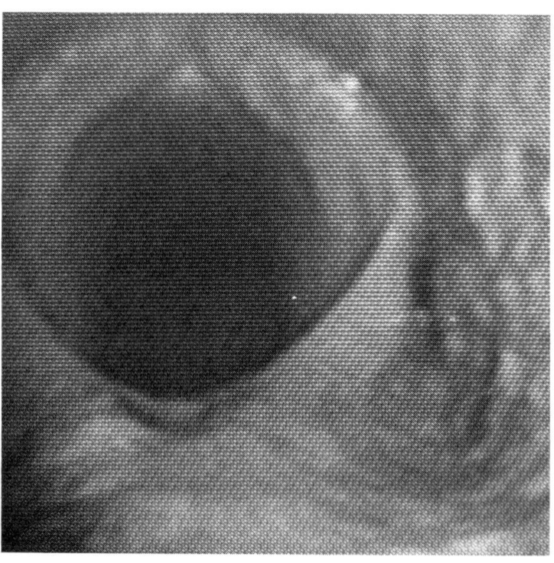

**FIG. 20–3.** Endoscopic view of a dorsal displacement of the soft palate.

phagia is not usually observed in horses with intermittent DDSP. The term "elongation of the soft palate" would also appear to be descriptively inaccurate. Although it is true that intermittent DDSP can be corrected in some horses by trimming the caudal margin of the soft palate, there is no evidence that there is an overabundance of palate tissue.

Cook has postulated that the DDSP responsible for temporary asphyxia in racehorses is a functional pharyngeal obstruction that results when mechanical and physical forces interact on the nasopharynx to produce a laryngopalatal subluxation.[1,3] Forces that produce either an elevation of the soft palate or a caudal retraction of the larynx threaten the stability of the laryngopalatal relationship.[1] Functional pharyngeal obstruction may be considered as a primary problem when it is not associated with other upper respiratory tract abnormalities. Numerous factors can contribute to a primary DDSP. One of the most common is retraction of the tongue which causes both an elevation of the soft palate by the base of the tongue and a caudal retraction of the larynx. Opening the mouth or swallowing during exercise may result in laryngopalatal dislocation. Flexion of the head causes a loss of the longitudinal stretching in the nasopharynx that is important for resisting dynamic collapse and maintaining a tight laryngopalatal seal, and produces a narrowing of the nasopharynx that creates an obstruction to airflow that results in greater negative intrapharyngeal air pressure.[1,3] It is possible to literally "choke" a horse during a race if the head is flexed excessively. It has been postulated that horses that have a great deal of nervous excitement are more likely to develop DDSP, likely because of overactivity or spasm of the sternothyrohyoid muscles.[1] Under normal circumstances, the action of these muscles is desirable, however, excessive activity can produce excessive caudal retraction of the larynx. Exaggerated activity of these muscles has been postulated to occur during periods of labored breathing, particularly near the end of a race, in response to overwork and hypoxia.[1,3]

Dorsal displacement of the soft palate may be related to a disease or a structural abnormality of the respiratory tract and be a secondary problem. Pharyngeal inflammation, abnormal narrowing of the nasopharynx, hypoplasia of the epiglottis, entrapment of the epiglottis, left laryngeal hemiplegia, arytenoid chondritis, and malformation of the laryngeal cartilages can all predispose to DDSP. Dorsal displacement of the soft palate is also seen as a complication following surgical resection of the arytenoepiglottic folds, likely as a result of subepiglottic scarring.[4] It is my opinion, as well as that of others, that it is also quite likely that chronic obstructive lung disease predisposes to intermittent DDSP in racehorses.[3]

Under normal conditions when a horse is examined endoscopically, the epiglottis should be clearly visible above the soft palate, with its serrated edges and distinct surface vasculature. If the soft palate is displaced dorsally, the epiglottis cannot be seen and the rostral and lateral margins of the ostium intrapharyngeum are visible. In some cases of DDSP, one may see a bulging under the caudal portion of the soft palate as a result of pressure from the epiglottis pushing up from beneath.

The diagnosis of intermittent DDSP is based on an evaluation of the horse's performance record, first hand observation of the horse performing or racing and an endoscopic examination. An endoscopic evaluation is best performed immediately after training or racing or during exercise on a high speed treadmill. Most racehorses or performance horses with exercise induced DDSP will appear normal at rest. The diagnosis is often made after all other potential causes of upper respiratory tract obstruction have been ruled out. The horse should be examined without tranquilization and with minimal restraint.

A horse that displaces its soft palate during a race will "choke" and make a loud gurgling or fluttering noise that is heard on both inspiration and expiration. This usually occurs in the last half of the race or it may be triggered by a rider or a driver having to take a strong "hold" of the horse to control its speed or alter course. Nervous and tense horses seem to be predisposed to DDSP. As an example, I have encountered some Standardbreds that will train at racing speed without a problem but in a race will displace their soft palate before they leave the starting gate.

As a result of the functional obstruction produced by DDSP, the horse is temporarily suffocated and speed slows dramatically. In severe cases of prolonged obstruction, the horse may become weak and ataxic from a lack of oxygen, and attempt to mouth breathe. The horse may swallow and return the palate to the normal breathing position shortly after it displaces, or the palate may remain displaced for the remainder of the race and even following the race. Usually, by the time the horse has returned to the paddock the noise has stopped and the palate is in a normal position. An endoscopic examination at this time may show intermittent dorsal displacement of the soft palate. If the palate is in a normal position, the horse can be made to swallow by spraying water from the endoscope into the pharynx in an attempt to produce a displacement. Once displaced, the palate should return to a normal position with the next swallow but if repeated swallowing efforts are required to replace it to its subepiglottic position, soft palate dysfunction should be suspected. Many horses with DDSP also have a small ulceration on the caudal free border of the palate, the rostral margin of the ostium intrapharyngeum, which may be secondary to the repeated trauma of laryngopalatal dislocation particularly if the

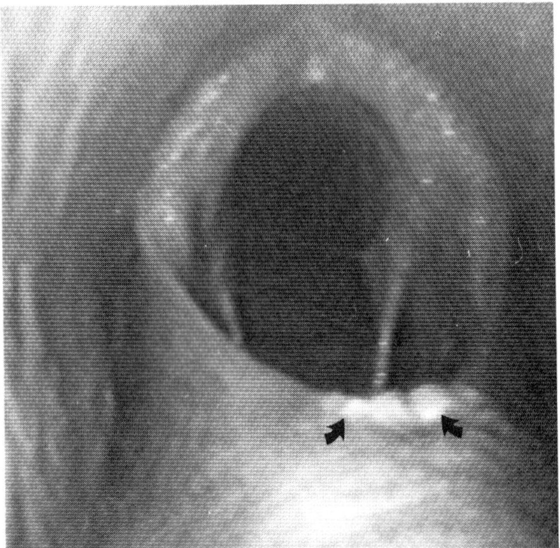

**FIG. 20–4.** Ulceration of the caudal free border of the soft palate (arrows) in a horse with intermittent dorsal displacement.

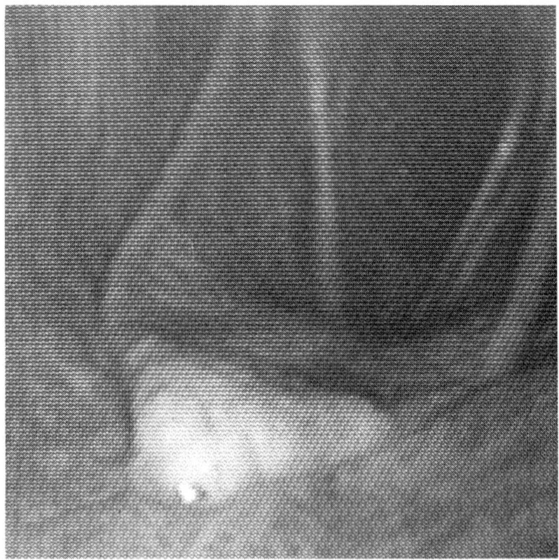

**FIG. 20–5.** Endoscopic view of a suspected hypoplastic epiglottis that is "buckling" with an increase in negative pressure in the pharynx. The arytenoepiglottic folds have become more prominent.

horse has been coughing (Fig. 20–4). In a horse that has choked severely, a ring of submucosal hemorrhage may be visible around the pharynx, where it has collapsed, in the region of the nasopharyngeal sphincter.

During the endoscopic examination, the degree of lymphoid follicle proliferation and pharyngeal inflammation should be noted, as these are factors that may contribute to DDSP. An inflamed pharynx appears hyperemic and edematous and small mucosal hemorrhages may be observed where the endoscope has touched the pharyngeal wall. The epiglottis should be evaluated carefully for evidence of hypoplasia. A hypoplastic epiglottis will appear to fold or "buckle" with increased negative pressure in the pharynx allowing the palate to displace (Fig. 20–5). A DDSP associated with hypoplasia of the epiglottis usually becomes apparent in 2-year-old horses during race training or early in their racing career. Interpretation of the endoscopic findings, with regard to palate function, should be made prior to making endoscopic contact with the epiglottis or passing the endoscope into the trachea. These maneuvers can stimulate coughing and gagging and induce a DDSP, particularly in a horse that has an inflamed pharynx. The horse may not, however, have a palate problem when performing or racing and DDSP would be a misdiagnosis. Tracheal blood or exudate should also be noted.

If a horse is examined at rest, the endoscope is positioned in the pharynx and held in position at the nostril and the nostrils are manually occluded. As the horse becomes air hungry and the inspiratory efforts increase, the increased negative pressure in the pharynx may lead to DDSP. Horses with an abnormality of the palate or a hypoplastic epiglottis will displace the palate with relative ease. In some horses the rostral portion of the soft palate will billow and the horse will make an inspiratory noise prior to the dorsal displacement.

If the epiglottis appears hypoplastic, a lateral radiograph of the skull can be used to obtain epiglottic measurements for confirmation.[5] Although epiglottic measurements are useful, I rely more heavily on the endoscopic appearance of the epiglottis, particularly with increased negative pressure in the pharynx to make a diagnosis of hypoplastic epiglottis.

The heart and lungs should be examined in all horses suspected of intermittent DDSP. Frequently there is auscultatory evidence of bronchitis in conjunction with an increase in tracheal mucus or mucopurulent exudate. It is my opinion that most of the horses that develop DDSP and have no structural deformities, have some degree of upper and lower airway inflammation. A lung evaluation includes careful auscultation while making the horse breathe deeply with a rebreathing bag, and thoracic radiographs to evaluate the lung parenchyma. Many horses with intermittent DDSP have increased interstitial density and peribronchial infiltrates in the lung. A tracheal wash should be done in horses with mucopurulent material in the trachea. Occasionally, a significant heart murmur (i.e. tricuspid insufficiency) or arrhythmia (atrial fibrillation) is found as the likely cause of the exercise intolerance in a horse with a history of an upper respiratory tract obstruction.

If the DDSP is persistent, the diagnosis is obvious on an endoscopic examination. The epiglottis is not visible and despite repeated swallowing efforts, the palate remains dorsally displaced. Affected horses frequently show signs of dysphagia, particularly if there is neurologic damage, such as that encountered with guttural pouch mycosis, neoplasia of the pharynx, or following the infusion of irritating solutions into the guttural pouches. A horse with pharyngeal paralysis and DDSP cannot swallow properly, and food and water pass into the nasopharynx and reflux from the nose. The horse frequently coughs while eating. In addition, there may be laryngeal paralysis on the affected side and there is likely to be food material present in the trachea. The guttural pouches should be examined endoscopically for evidence of disease and a neurologic examination should be performed. Persistent DDSP may develop acutely in some horses with no other evidence of neurologic disease and produce signs of dysphagia.

Dorsal displacement of the soft palate and epiglottic entrapment may occur concomitantly. If the palate displacement is intermittent, then both conditions can be easily diagnosed. However, if the DDSP is persistent, the caudal margin of the soft palate obscures the view of the epiglottis. Careful inspection of the arytenoepiglottic area will reveal the arytenoepiglottic fold lying medial and ventral to the lateral and rostral borders of the ostium intrapharyngeum (Fig. 20–6). A lateral radiograph of the skull is useful to confirm the presence of an epiglottic entrapment hidden beneath the displaced soft palate.

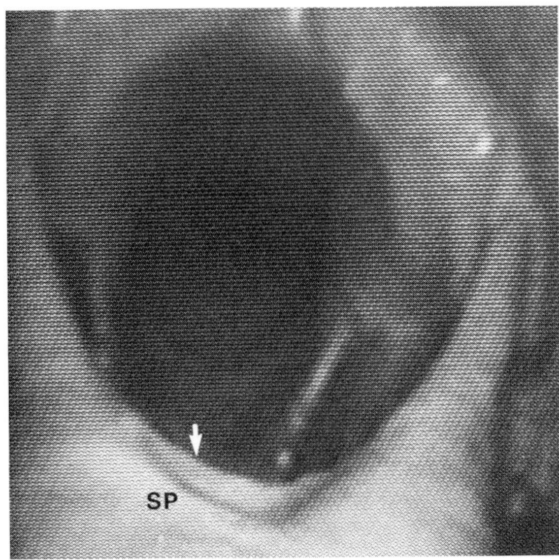


**FIG. 20–6.** This horse has both an entrapped epiglottis and a dorsal displacement of the soft palate. Endoscopic inspection of the arytenoepiglottic area reveals the arytenoepiglottic fold (arrow) lying ventral to the free border of the soft palate (SP).

## *Conservative Management of Intermittent DDSP*

### Tongue Tie

The tongue and the larynx are indirectly joined via their muscular attachments to the hyoid apparatus.[1] Retraction of the tongue during a race can cause upward pressure on the soft palate and caudal movement of the larynx resulting in laryngopalatal dislocation. Using a leather strap or a fabric strip, the tongue can be tied to the interdental space of the lower jaw to prevent this retraction. Many trainers routinely tie a horse's tongue when it trains or races. If a tongue tie has been used, and the horse still suffers from DDSP, advise the trainer to slip the tongue tie further back on the tongue in order to pull it more rostrally before tying it to the lower jaw. I have encountered two Standardbred trotters that had intermittent DDSP with one tongue tie in place that responded dramatically to the use of two tongue ties. Using the first tie to pull the tongue rostrally, the second was placed further back towards the frenulum and both were tied to the lower jaw.

### Equipment Changes

It is difficult to change the degree of poll flexion in horses that are ridden. In some show breeds, such as the Saddlebred, marked head flexion is desirable. In racehorses, a nose band can be used in combination with a tongue tie to keep the mouth closed. In Standardbred race horses with DDSP, the head can be checked up higher to extend the head and various types of leverage bits can be used to effect head extension rather than flexion when pressure is applied by the driver. A trainer of Standardbreds who is knowledgeable of the mechanics of "rigging" a horse with a breathing problem can significantly decrease the chances of a DDSP during the race in some horses. Some trainers attach a can under the throat latch to prevent excessive head flexion.

### Nebulization

If there is a significant degree of lymphoid follicular proliferation and pharyngeal inflammation, nebulization with an anti-inflammatory solution can be beneficial in certain cases. I recommend 20 to 30 minutes of nebulization daily with a solution of liquid furacin (350 ml), DMSO (125 ml) and prednisolone acetate (500 mg) for at least 7 to 10 days. The horse can be kept in light training while being treated. Once the upper respiratory tract inflammation has subsided the horse can resume full training. The nebulization can be continued daily for the entire racing season if necessary, being discontinued 72 hours prior to race time.

### Antibiotics and Bronchodilators

If there is mucopurulent material present in the trachea and increased lung sounds on inspiration, a tracheal wash should be performed. If there is significant bacterial growth on culture, the horse should be treated with an effective antibiotic at the appropriate dose for at least 7 days. Oral antibiotics are preferable to those that are injected IM or IV. It is preferable to rest the horse during the treatment period and limit exercise to walking. An expectorant or a bronchodilator can be used concurrently. If the culture is negative for bacterial growth, a bronchodilator given orally for 10 days is often effective. Horses that have obstructive lung disease are likely to have recurring problems during the racing season and may require repeated treatments with a bronchodilator. Every effort should be made to reduce the exposure to allergens and the horse should be turned out as much as possible.

## *Surgical Treatment of Intermittent DDSP*

### Sternothyrohyoid Myectomy

In horses that suffer DDSP, despite conservative management, a myectomy of the ventral "strap" muscles may be effective in preventing excessive caudal retraction of the larynx and laryngopalatal dislocation. The muscles that are responsible for caudal retraction of the larynx are the sternohyoideus, sternothyroideus and the omohyoideus muscles. The myectomy is usually confined to the sternothyrohyoideus group, although it may include the axial portions of the omohyoideus muscles.[6] I prefer to limit the resection to the sternothyrohyoideus muscles because they are easily isolated with minimal dissection and resected with little resultant hemorrhage in the standing patient. A myectomy that includes the omohyoideus muscles should be performed under general anesthesia because there is more dissection involved and a greater need for hemostasis. Major advantages of the sternothyrohyoid myectomy procedure (vs. staphylectomy) for treatment of DDSP are that the procedure can be done with the horse standing and training can be resumed at a week to 10 days after surgery. The results of the surgery can usually be judged after the first three to four races. Despite the fact that the action of these muscles may be desirable under normal circumstances, it has been my experience that a sternothyrohyoid myectomy has no detrimental effects on nasopharyngeal or laryngopalatal function.

In preparation for surgery, the ventral portion of the neck is clipped from the sternum to the throat latch. The horse is treated preoperatively with broad spectrum antibiotics particularly if the procedure is done standing. Following a surgical scrub, the horse is sedated with xylazine (0.44 mg/kg or .2 mg/lb IV) and butorphanol (.011 mg/kg or .005 mg/lb IV). Ten ml of 2% mepivacaine is infiltrated subcutaneously and intramuscularly into the sternothyrohyoideus muscles for a length of 10 cm, centered at the juncture of the upper one-third and lower two-thirds of the neck. A nose twitch is applied and the head is elevated and extended to tense the sternothyrohyoid muscles and expose the ventral aspect of the neck to the operator. It is important that the head and neck are extended straight out in front of the horse and not twisted to either side. A 10-cm skin incision is made on the ventral midline and extended through the cutaneous colli muscle to expose the sternothyrohyoideus muscles. Providing the head and neck are straight, the lateral margins of these paired muscle bellies are easily palpable and can be bluntly separated with scissors from the omohyoideus and the fascia on the ventral surface of the trachea. A 6- to 7-cm segment of the sternothyrohyoid muscles is freed from its fascial attachments and clamped with Pean forceps. Using the forceps to apply tension, the muscles are pulled down and sharply excised at the rostral margin of the incision, then the muscles are pulled up and the myectomy is completed by sharply excising the muscles at the caudal end of the incision. The cut muscle ends retract leaving considerable dead space. A drain is not necessary, providing hemorrhage is minimal and there was no intraoperative contamination. If a drain is desired, a 1.25 cm or ½ inch Penrose drain is placed through a stab incision, below the skin incision, at the level of the distal stump of the sternothyrohyoideus muscle. The drain is sutured to the skin. The cutaneous colli muscle layer is closed with 2-0 vicryl in a simple interrupted pattern, the subcutaneous tissue is closed similarly and the skin is closed with 0 vetafil in a simple interrupted pattern.

Following surgery, the wound should be covered with a sterile dressing and the neck wrapped with an elastic bandage. The bandage should be changed the following day and can be removed 3 days after surgery. Antibiotic treatment should continue for at least 3 days. If a drain was used, it can usually be removed within 3 days when drainage becomes negligible. Stall rest is recommended for 7 days and exercise is limited to hand walking. Light training is resumed after 7 days and full training after 14 days.

A low complication rate makes a sternothyrohyoid myectomy an appealing procedure.[6] The horse should be observed during the postoperative period for neck swelling or dyspnea. Hematomas and seromas may occur but are usually of little consequence and can be controlled by neck bandaging. However, I am aware of a horse that died within 24 hours after surgery as a result of development of a large hematoma that compressed the trachea at the thoracic inlet (Beech J, personal communication, 1990). Wound infection is rare, even if the procedure is done standing, providing careful attention is paid to asepsis. Damage to the recurrent laryngeal nerves is avoided by confining the dissection to the immediate vicinity of the sternothyrohyoid muscle group.

I feel that it is reasonable to expect that 50% of the race horses with performance induced DDSP will show improvement following a sternothyrohyoid myectomy.[7] The operation will be most successful in the horse with a normal larynx and epiglottis that has had some racing success but occasionally suffers DDSP near the end of a race. The procedure is least likely to improve a 2-year-old horse that has developed the problem during training or early in its racing career and has shown a progressive increase in the frequency and severity of "choking" episodes. A sternothyrohyoid myectomy may be of little value for correcting DDSP related to a hypoplastic epiglottis.

## Staphylectomy

If a sternothyrohyoid myectomy is not successful in correcting intermittent DDSP in a horse with a normal epiglottis and larynx, resection of a portion of the caudal margin of the soft palate is indicated. This procedure will improve some horses although there is no rational explanation for the fact that enlarging the ostium intrapharyngeum has a beneficial effect. In horses that have shown intermittent DDSP with a progressive increase in frequency and severity of signs, particularly 2-year-old race horses, I will perform both a sternothyrohyoid myectomy and a staphylectomy during one operation.

A horse affected with pharyngeal paralysis and a persistent dorsal displacement is not a candidate for and will not benefit from either a myectomy or a staphylectomy. Staphylectomy, however, may correct a persistent dorsal displacement that is secondary to trauma or inflammation of the soft palate when medical treatment has failed. DDSP that occurs as a complication following resection of the arytenoepiglottic folds can often be corrected by resecting the caudal free border of the soft palate, providing the epiglottis is not hypoplastic.

A staphylectomy is a short procedure and can be performed under intravenous anesthesia, if necessary. Prior to surgery, the horse can be given IV phenylbutazone, (4.4 mg/kg 2 mg/lb) to minimize postoperative swelling of the palate and larynx. A suitable drug combination for inducing anesthesia is IM xylazine, followed by glycerol guaicolate and ketamine, IV. The horse should be intubated after induction. If a deeper plane of anesthesia is desired, anesthesia can be maintained with halothane in oxygen. The horse is placed in dorsal recumbency with the head and neck extended and prepared for a laryngotomy. A routine laryngotomy is performed and the endotracheal tube is removed in order to view the soft palate. It is likely that the caudal portion of the palate will be in a displaced position and visible following removal of the endotracheal tube unless the horse has swallowed and returned it to a subepiglottic position. If it is not visible, the tube can be pushed back into the pharynx in order to displace the palate or if a tube is not used, a finger or a curved sponge forceps can be curled around the base of the epiglottis to elevate it and allow the palate to displace.

The appearance of the caudal portion of the soft palate varies greatly among horses. In some it may appear taut, while in others it appears flaccid with a great deal of mucosal redundancy. Raker has classified three types of palate conformation based on the appearance of the free border of the palate.[8] The free border of a Type A palate has a slight concavity, Type B has a marked concavity and is U shaped and Type C has a deep V shaped rostral concavity. The perceived "length" of the palate is also evaluated. The decision of how much tissue to remove from the free border is based on these subjective assessments of conformation and length of palate. Sponge forceps are passed through the laryngotomy and placed at the center of the free border, grasping no more than a 2.0-cm width of tissue in the jaws of the forceps. Much less tissue is grasped if there is a Type C concavity. Rather than tensing the palate by pulling the sponge forceps caudally, I prefer to move the sponge forceps laterally, tense half of the width of the palate and using long curved Metzenbaum scissors, cut from the caudal pillar towards the midline, trimming a crescent shaped segment of palate, widest at its midline and tapering laterally. The rostral limit of the resection is marked by the leading edge of the sponge forceps. When the incision reaches midline, the other half of the palate is tensed by shifting the sponge forceps to the opposite side and the resection is completed. Swallowing, when the palate is grasped, can be a problem when using intravenous anesthesia but this can be stopped by giving an IV bolus of a thiobarbiturate or swabbing the area with a sponge soaked in 2% mepivacaine. Hemorrhage is usually minimal and hemostasis is rarely necessary. Rather than scissors, an electrocautery knife can be used to cut the tissue to reduce bleeding although there is a greater risk of inadvertently damaging other structures. The cut margin of the palate is not sutured and heals by second intention. Some surgeons prefer to notch the palate by removing a wedge of tissue on each side of the midline in order to increase the aperture of the ostium intrapharyngeum.[9] In my opinion, this notching technique offers no advantages and is less beneficial than removing a crescent shaped segment.

In my experience, histopathologic examination of the resected portion of soft palate frequently shows some degree of submucosal inflammation which is characterized by edema and neutrophilic infiltration, and fibroplasia, particularly if there is focal ulceration. In one report, horses with DDSP had evidence of palatal myositis. The significance of this finding was unclear since a lesser degree of inflammatory myopathy was also found in a control group of horses with no respiratory problems.[10] It is also unclear whether these pathologic changes precede the development of DDSP or are secondary to palate displacement.

The laryngotomy incision is left to heal by second intention. In the recovery stall, narrow pads are placed under the horse's neck so that blood from the surgical site drains toward the nose and is not aspirated while the horse is in lateral recumbency. Once the horse is fully recovered from anesthesia, it can be returned to its stall and allowed to drink and eat hay. During the first few postoperative days, the horse may cough while eating or drinking. Hay and grain should be fed off the ground to help prevent aspiration. Usually by the third or fourth postoperative day the coughing and swallowing difficulties spontaneously resolve. The laryngotomy wound is cleaned daily with moist gauze sponges and is usually closed with granulation tissue by 14 days. Postoperative antibiotics are not routinely administered.

Periodic endoscopic examination should be performed, starting at 1 to 2 days following surgery, to evaluate healing and soft palate function. Intermittent DDSP may be observed during the healing period but the palate usually returns to its normal position with swallowing. If the palate does displace during the examination, the incision area along its free border is visible. A cause for concern is a persistent dorsal displacement during the entire endoscopic examination. If this is observed, the horse should be treated with phenylbutazone or flunixin meglumine and a topical anti-inflammatory throat spray. If the dorsal displacement persists despite 7 to 10 days of treatment, there is little hope of spontaneous improvement and the prognosis for successful athletic performance is poor. Those horses frequently cough when eating and are at risk for developing aspiration pneumonia. A second staphylectomy can be performed in an effort to correct the problem; however, the prognosis is poor and there is the risk of producing severe dysphagia and aspiration as a result of excessive shortening.

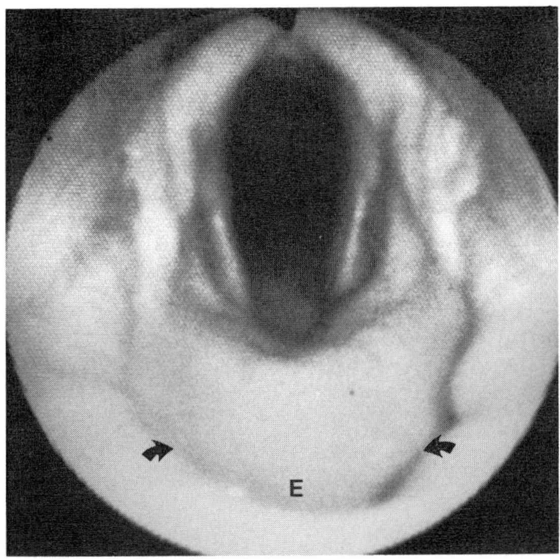


**FIG. 20–7.** Excessive shortening of the caudal margin of the soft palate (arrows). The resection has been so extensive that the epiglottis (E) no longer articulates with the soft palate.

The horse is stall rested for 3 weeks and can resume training 4 to 6 weeks following surgery. Prior to the resumption of training, an endoscopic examination should be performed to ensure that the palate is in its proper position and that healing is complete and uncomplicated. In horses suffering intermittent DDSP associated with the stress of performance, the effects of surgery cannot be evaluated until they resume racing. About 50% of these horses will be improved following a staphylectomy alone or in combination with a myectomy. A successful outcome is the ability to race or perform without developing signs of palate displacement. The prognosis for correcting a persistent dorsal displacement of the soft palate is guarded to poor.

Excessive shortening of the soft palate allows material to pass from the oropharynx into the nasopharynx during swallowing (Fig. 20–7). This produces coughing and discharge of food and water from the nose (Fig. 20–8).

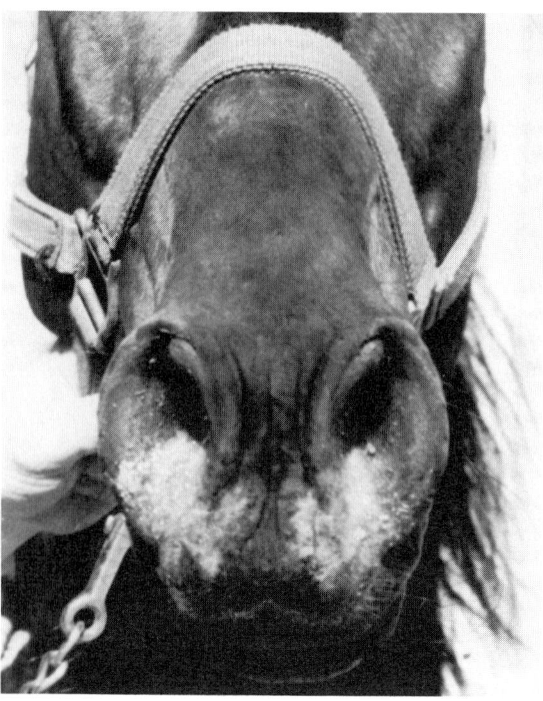

**FIG. 20–8.** Chronic nasal discharge of food material as a result of excessive resection of the caudal margin of the soft palate.

Aspiration pneumonia is usually a sequela. Raker cautions that removal of more than a 2.5-cm width of tissue from the free border can produce these disastrous complications.[8] I feel that in most cases, whether the problem is an intermittent DDSP or a persistent DDSP that is not neurologically related, it is possible to resect a much smaller segment of palate and still achieve the desired results. I came to this conclusion based on experience dealing with DDSP as a complication following resection of the arytenoepiglottic folds to correct epiglottic entrapment. In several horses that required further surgery, when it was apparent that the DDSP was persistent and likely permanent, I removed a crescent shaped section of the free border of the soft palate, measuring no more than 1 cm at midline, and the improvement was dramatic and immediate. Now, when performing a staphylectomy, I remove no more than a 1-cm width of palate and achieve the same results as when I removed a wider piece of tissue, with less risk of serious complications.

## Cleft Palate

Cleft palate, or palatoschisis, is a congenital condition that produces postprandial nasal discharge and dysphagia that usually results in aspiration pneumonia.[11,12] A cleft palate results from an interruption of the normal embryologic fusion of the palatal folds, a process which takes place on midline in a rostral to caudal direction and should be complete by the 47th day of gestation.[12–14] The extent and length of the cleft is dependent on the point of interruption of this process. Small clefts involve only a few centimeters of the caudal portion of the soft palate while the most extensive involve the soft and hard palates and may extend as far rostral as the incisive foramen. Almost all clefts occur on midline but occasionally a defect of the caudal margin of the soft palate will be asymmetrical with the tissue defect being primarily unilateral, or a bilateral hypoplasia of the soft palate may exist.[15] Clefts of the lip and maxilla have not been associated with cleft palate in horses.[12] The prevalence of cleft palate in horses is low.[12] Although the heritability of this anomaly is not known, genetics must be considered as an etiology along with nutritional, hormonal, mechanical and toxic factors that could affect palate development in the fetus.[11]

A cleft palate is usually suspected when milk is seen to reflux from a foal's nostrils after nursing (Fig. 20–9). The foal may also cough as a result of aspiration. Occasionally, particularly if the mare is a heavy milker, milk will reflux from the nostrils of a newborn foal with an apparently normal palate. This is usually a temporary problem and resolves within a few weeks. In foals with a cleft palate, the nasal reflux persists and eventually, within a few weeks, most of these foals develop aspiration pneumonia. An extensive cleft involving the entire length of the soft palate or the soft and hard palate can be seen on an oral examination. A less extensive cleft of the soft palate is usually not visible on an oral examination and must be viewed through a pediatric sized endoscope which is required for nasal passage in a newborn foal. The margins of the soft palate defect are visible, as are the epiglottis and the subepiglottic folds of

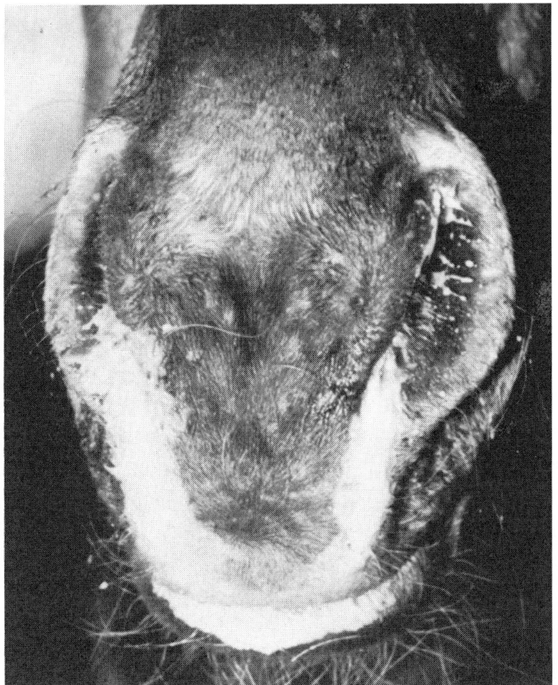

**FIG. 20–9.** Milk refluxing from the nostrils of a foal with a cleft palate.

mucosa and the floor of the oropharynx. Frequently, there is a concurrent arytenoepiglottic fold entrapment (Fig. 20–10). Auscultation and radiographic evaluation of the lungs usually reveals some degree of bronchopneumonia. In addition to the cleft palate, there may be a concomitant deviation of the premaxilla and the nasal septum (wry nose).

If left to grow, most foals with a cleft palate develop a chronic pneumonia that causes them to be unthrifty and unproductive. Some will die acutely but most can survive to adulthood. It is the remarkable horse that develops normally despite a cleft palate.[13,16]

When discussing surgical correction of a cleft palate with an owner, a number of points should be raised. The surgery should be considered a salvage procedure aimed at improving the horse's quality of life by eliminating the nasal reflux of ingested material and reducing the chances of developing recurrences of aspiration pneumonia. There is little chance that the surgical correction will restore athletic function since the laryngopalatal junction is likely to be unstable. The presence of a concurrent congenital abnormality such as a wry nose or an epiglottic entrapment may also limit athletic potential. If the horse is being salvaged for its breeding value, the owner should be cautioned about the potential heritability of the condition.[11] Since there are other nongenetic causes of a cleft palate, it is difficult to use ethics as a reason for refusing to operate on these individuals, particularly if an expensive stud fee must be paid. If an owner declines the option of surgical correction, euthanasia should be offered as an option.

Although there have been a few reports of successful repair of soft palate defects, it is generally conceded by most surgeons that palatoplasty almost always results in a degree of failure, from fistula formation to partial or complete dehiscence.[12] In my experience the prognosis for a successful correction of a soft palate cleft or a combination soft and hard palate cleft is poor although a successful repair can occasionally be achieved, providing certain selective criteria are met. The foal should be operated on as early as possible, preferably at 1 day of age. Delaying the repair for weeks or months only invites the inevitable aspiration pneumonia. It is also my impression that the surgical access offered by

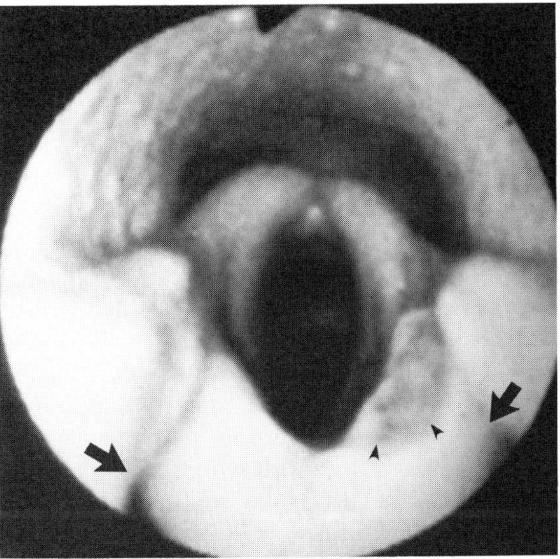

**FIG. 20–10.** Endoscopic view of a cleft soft palate and a concurrent entrapment of the epiglottis in a foal. The lateral margins of the cleft are denoted by large arrows, while the ulceration on the arytenoepiglottic fold is indicated by small arrowheads.

the mandibular symphysiotomy is greater in the newborn and it is easier to mobilize and appose the tissues of the palate. The type of cleft and the size of the tissue defect obviously affect the prognosis. Attempts to repair an asymmetrical soft palate defect will fail. Repair of a symmetrical, midline soft palate cleft with a minimal tissue defect has no greater than a 50% chance of success. Repairs of a cleft of both the soft and hard palate have no more than 20% chance of healing without dehiscence, providing there is not excessive tissue loss. A large tissue defect of either the hard or soft palate, approximately 20 to 25% of the total width or greater, requires that the palate edges be sutured under a degree of tension which inevitably leads to failure. An excessively wide defect will preclude a repair.[12]

Initial success is a resolution of the signs of dysphagia; nasal reflux of food and aspiration of food into the trachea. Long-term success is achieved if the palatoplasty remains intact and the horse grows normally and develops into a healthy individual. Endoscopically, at 1 year of age, I would hope to see the caudal margin of the soft palate in a subepiglottic position when the horse is breathing.

## *Palatoplasty*

Preoperatively, the foal is started on broad spectrum antibiotics which are maintained for 5 to 7 days following surgery. If aspiration pneumonia is present and the foal is ill, the foal should be fed through a nasogastric tube and treated for the pneumonia before the surgery is performed. In newborns, a test should be conducted to determine whether there was adequate colostral antibody absorption. If the IgG level is low, a plasma transfusion should be given prior to surgery.[17]

There are a number of surgical approaches to the hard and soft palate, but in my opinion, a mandibular symphysiotomy provides the best exposure.[11–13,18] Attempts to perform a palatoplasty through the mouth or buccal, pharyngeal or laryngeal incisions are needlessly frustrating. With the foal anesthetized in dorsal recumbency, in preparation for a mandibular symphysiotomy, a mid cervical tracheostomy is performed and a clean endotracheal tube is placed into the trachea. This allows removal of the endotracheal tube that was passed through the mouth. The lower lip is incised on midline through its full thickness and the skin incision is continued caudally on midline to the body of the hyoid. The mandibular symphysis can be separated with a scalpel, but carefully, to avoid accidental laceration of the roof of the mouth if the scalpel suddenly cuts through the symphysis. The dissection is continued along the ramus of one of the mandibles as the attachments of the geniohyoid, genioglossus and mylohyoid muscles are severed and the buccal mucosa is incised, leaving a rim of mucosa attached to the mandible to facilitate closure.[11] The mandibles are separated and the tongue is retracted to expose the palate defect. A curved narrow retractor, passed through a laryngotomy incision into the pharynx and under the base of the tongue, can be used to elevate the tongue and further increase exposure. Having an assistant retract the tongue in this fashion allows better access to the caudal portion of the soft palate, an area that is difficult to reach. Moist towels can be placed around the symphysis of each mandible and can be used to retract the mandibles. Antibiotic and saline solution can be intermittently sprayed on the exposed tissues to prevent drying.

A stay suture is passed through the soft palate on each side of the cleft at its most caudal limit. These two sutures are drawn through the laryngotomy incision and retracted slightly in order to tense the free edges of the soft palate. This facilitates preparation of the edges of the defect. A thin strip of mucosa is excised from each edge of the cleft and a narrow tangential incision is extended into the palatal musculature on each side with a hooked blade scalpel. This facilitates a more accurate apposition of tissue layers. Starting at the caudal margin of the cleft, the nasal mucosa is closed with a simple continuous layer using size 2-0 absorbable suture material. Rather than attempting to suture the muscle layer separately, I prefer to place a line of interrupted, vertical mattress sutures that incorporate the oral mucosa and the muscular layer but do not penetrate the nasal mucosal layer. These sutures provide good apposition of the muscle tissue and also act as tension sutures. Size 0 synthetic absorbable or silk sutures can be used in this layer. I prefer silk sutures because of the good handling characteristics of the suture and its knot security. Knot security in this area is important because the foal will constantly move its tongue against the suture line. The oral mucosa is closed with a continuous horizontal suture line using 3-0 synthetic absorbable suture material.

If there is a large soft palate defect or it becomes apparent during the repair that there is a good deal of tension on the suture lines, longitudinal, lateral mucosal relief incisions can be made. One group of surgeons recommends osteotomy and medial reflection of the hamulus of the pterygoid bone on each side in order to lessen the pull of the tensor muscle and relax the palate. They also suggest that if the soft palate defect involves greater than two-thirds of its length, that the levator veli palatini muscle may need to be dissected free of its attachment to the caudal edge of the hard palate in order to achieve a satisfactory closure.[12] If the foal has a concomitant epiglottic entrapment, I do not incise or resect the arytenoepiglottic folds.

If a hard palate cleft is also present, I prefer to first prepare the edges of the soft palate and then proceed with the dissection of the hard palate. Hemorrhage can be minimized by injecting small volumes of 2% xylocaine with epinephrine with a 25-gauge needle along the proposed lines of incision in the hard palate and nasal septum. On each side, a mucoperiosteal incision is made adjacent and parallel to the cheek teeth, extending from the caudal limit of the hard palate to a few centimeters beyond the rostral limit of the defect. Using a narrow bladed, periosteal elevator, the entire width of mucoperiosteum is elevated to the edge of the defect in a rostral to caudal direction. This dissection must be done carefully in order to preserve the palatine artery which is visible on the undersurface of the flap. As the dissection proceeds caudally, the artery is elevated from the palatine groove. At the caudal limit of the hard palate the artery can be seen to emerge from the major palatine foramen. Carefully, the dissection is continued around the foramen and with gentle pressure, the flap is elevated and the artery is stretched and actually drawn out of the foramen. Mobilizing the artery and mucoperiosteum in this area is necessary for tension free apposition of the flaps. The axial attachment of the mucoperiosteal flap, along the defect, is cut with a scalpel or scissors, thus completely freeing the flap from all but its rostral and caudal attachments. Two well-vascularized bipedicle mucoperiosteal flaps have been created. If the defect is quite wide, it may be necessary to separate the soft palate from its attachment to the caudal margin of the hard palate to accomplish closure of the defect.

Once the mucoperiosteal flaps are created, I then make a longitudinal ventral midline incision through the mucosa of the incomplete nasal septum. Using a periosteal elevator, two mucosal flaps are created on each side of this incision. The adjacent nasal mucosa along the cleft is similarly dissected free and the septal and palatal flaps of mucosa are apposed with size 3-0 synthetic absorbable suture material in a simple continuous pattern. Theoretically, a suture pattern that inverts these mucosal flaps into the nasal cavity is preferable but it is too difficult to accomplish. Once the nasal mucosal closure is completed, the oral mucoperiosteal flaps are sutured with interrupted horizontal mattress sutures using size 2-0 synthetic absorbable or non-absorbable suture material (Fig. 20–11). I prefer to use silk for the same reasons as in the soft palate repair. The large, lateral mucoperiosteal defects created by mobilizing the flaps towards midline are simply left to heal by second intention. The soft palate is repaired as previously described. In a few foals, following repair of a hard palate defect, I have moulded a dental wax retainer to fit between the cheek teeth and cover the roof of the mouth in order to protect the repair. The retainer is held in place by wires that cross between the cheek teeth. Although such a retainer protects the hard palate repair, it is difficult to secure these wires between the teeth of a newborn foal. The wires usually loosen within a few days.

When the palatoplasty is complete, a soft flexible nasogastric tube is placed and sutured to the nose. The mandibles are brought into

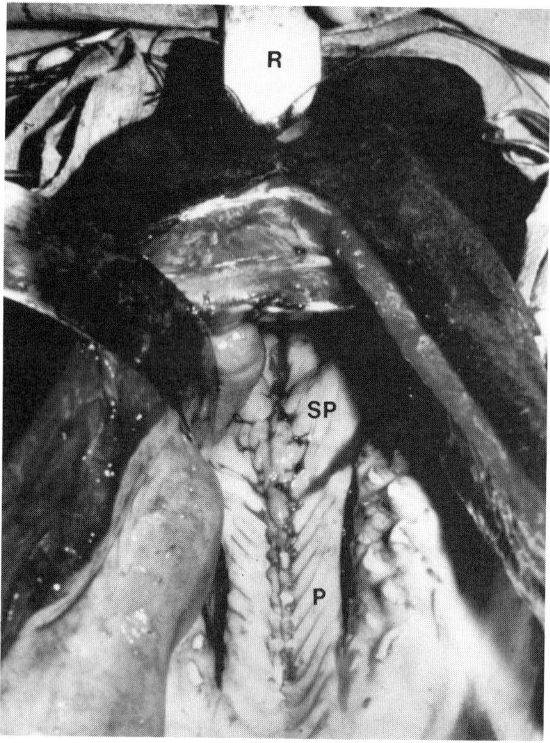


**FIG. 20–11.** Cleft hard palate (P) and soft palate (SP) repair as viewed through a mandibular symphysiotomy. The mucoperiosteal flaps of the hard palate have been sutured. The lateral defects created by mobilizing these flaps are visible adjacent to the cheek teeth. A curved narrow retractor (R) has been passed through a laryngotomy incision and under the base of the tongue in order to elevate the tongue and increase exposure to the caudal portion of the soft palate.

close approximation and the buccal mucosa and the incised muscles are sutured separately, with simple continuous suture lines using 2-0 synthetic absorbable suture material. The mandibular symphysis is stabilized with an ASIF cancellous lag screw, wire sutures placed through the ventral portion of the symphysis and a wire placed around the two central, lower incisors.

The mucosal, muscular and skin layers of the lower lip must be sutured carefully with three layers of interrupted sutures in order to avoid dehiscence. I prefer vertical mattress sutures using a size 0, monofilament nonabsorbable suture material, for closing the skin of the lower lip. The remainder of the skin incision is closed from the symphysis to the hyoid bone with simple interrupted sutures, leaving two or three 2 cm gaps in the suture line to allow for drainage. Placement of a subcutaneous drain is optional. The laryngotomy incision is not sutured. The endotracheal tube is removed and replaced by a self retaining tracheostomy tube which is removed in 12 to 24 hours providing the foal can breathe normally.

If the hard palate is repaired or a palatoplasty is performed on a horse that has already been weaned, I feel it is important that extraoral feeding be attempted for 7 to 10 days following surgery. It is easiest to do this through an indwelling nasogastric tube. This avoids the stresses placed on the repaired palate during nursing, chewing, and swallowing. The nasogastric tube should be fixed securely to the nostril to prevent it from being dislodged. If the tube has to be replaced, there is a significant risk of traumatizing the repaired palate and contributing to dehiscence. Allowing the foal to nurse the mare following surgery is an acceptable alternative only if the defect was limited to the soft palate.

Soft palate healing is evaluated endoscopically while the hard palate repair is best viewed through the mouth. Repeated endoscopic examinations are discouraged. Areas of dehiscence will be readily apparent by the fourteenth postoperative day and there will be recurrence of nasal reflux of milk or feed when the animal resumes nursing or eating. In most foals with a successful palatoplasty, there is no longer reflux of milk or feed. A small amount of nasal reflux of milk may persist if a small defect remains at the caudal limit of the soft palate. It is not necessary to remove the palatoplasty sutures, regardless of what type of suture material was used.

The most significant of the reported complications of palate repair are palate dehiscence and oronasal fistula formation.[12] These are more likely to develop as the length and breadth of the defect increase, particularly in the hard palate. Some of the factors that contribute to dehiscence are tension on the repair, avascularity as a result of improper suturing techniques or inappropriate dissection, inadequate tissue strength and the repetitive trauma produced by nursing, chewing, and swallowing. Even after eliminating most of these factors, dehiscence appears inevitable

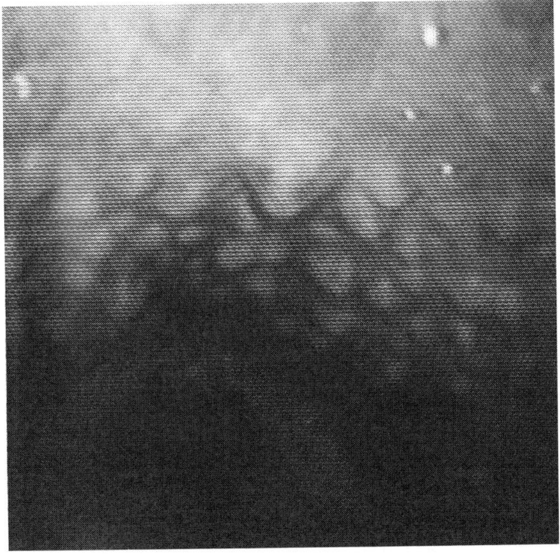

**FIG. 20–12.** Endoscopic view of dorsal pharyngeal lymphoid follicles in a young horse.

in the majority of these repairs.[12] Other reported complications include dehiscence of the lower lip, instability of the mandibular symphysis, osteomyelitis of the mandibular symphysis, submandibular abscessation and hypoglossal nerve damage.[12] These problems can usually be traced to technical errors and are avoidable. Recurrence of aspiration pneumonia can be expected following breakdown of a soft palate repair. Attempts at a second or even a third repair of the palate defect or an oronasal fistula invariably fail. When the mandibular symphysis is split for a second time, an osteotome is usually required.

## Pharyngeal Lymphoid Hyperplasia (PLH)

Pharyngeal lymphoid hyperplasia, also known as pharyngitis and lymphoid follicular hyperplasia, is a condition that is frequently observed during endoscopic examination of young horses. In most of these horses it is considered to be a normal physiologic finding. The mucous membrane of the dorsal and lateral walls of the nasopharynx and the dorsal surface of the soft palate contain numerous lymphoid follicles, a rather diffuse type of tonsillar tissue (Fig. 20–12). In the area of the pharyngeal recess, this lymphoid tissue forms a dorsal collection known as the pharyngeal tonsil.[2] Small lymphoid follicles may also be observed on the mucous membrane lining of the guttural pouches or on the surface of the epiglottis. Occasionally large accumulations of lymphoid tissue form a polyp-like mass, particularly in the area of the pharyngeal recess (Fig. 20–13). Horses less than 3 years of age possess the greatest population of pharyngeal lymphoid follicles. These follicles usually regress as the horse matures and by the time horses are 4 to 5 years of age they usually have few lymphoid follicles on the pharyngeal wall.[19] A grading system has been devised to describe the severity of the lymphoid hyperplasia and allow for some consistency in the interpretation of endoscopic fundings. The assigned grade is based on an endoscopic observation of the number of follicles present, their size and appearance (active vs. inactive) and the area of distribution within the pharynx[8,20] (Table 20–1).

The etiology of the PLH is not clear, although it appears to be multifactorial. It is generally thought that the lymphoid hyperplasia represents an immunologic response in the mucosa of the pharynx.[21] Histopathologic examination of biopsies of the wall of the pharynx in early cases of PLH show lymphoid

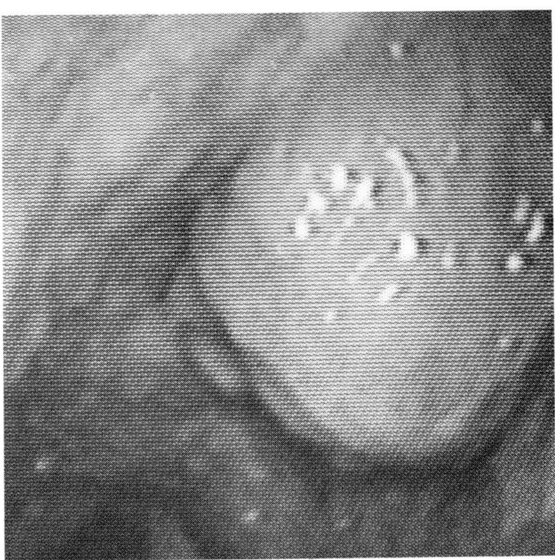

**FIG. 20–13.** Endoscopic view of a large lymphoid polyp in the area of the dorsal pharyngeal recess.

**TABLE 20–1.** ***Grading System for Pharyngeal Lymphoid Hyperplasia***

Grade I: A small number of inactive, white follicles are scattered over the dorsal pharyngeal wall.

Grade II: Many small, white and inactive follicles are distributed over the dorsal and lateral walls of the pharynx, to the level of the openings to the guttural pouch. Interspersed throughout these follicles are numerous follicles that are larger and are pink and edematous, indicating that they are active.

Grade III: Many large, pink follicles as well as some white follicles are distributed over the dorsal and lateral walls of the pharynx. The pharyngeal tonsillar tissue is frequently hyperplastic and the lymphoid follicles may extend on to the dorsal surface of the soft palate.

Grade IV: A more severe form of Grade III with more active, pink and edematous follicles packed closer together covering all of the surface of the pharynx and including the dorsal surface of the soft palate and occasionally the surface of the epiglottis and the lining of the guttural pouches. Large accumulations of lymphoid tissue that appear as polyps may be observed in the area of the pharyngeal recess or in the dorsal or lateral walls of the pharynx.

(Adapted from Raker and Boles[20] and Raker.[8])

proliferation and necrosis, while in chronic cases there is infiltration of fibrous connective tissue with lymphoid proliferation.[19] Clinically, pharyngeal lymphoid hyperplasia is observed following viral or bacterial respiratory tract infections.[19] Streptococcus zooepidemicus and Bordetella bronchiseptica have been isolated from bacterial cultures of the nasopharynx of affected horses although their significance is questionable.[21,22] Equine herpes virus 2 has been isolated from the nasopharynx of affected horses and it has been associated with development of chronic PLH. However, in a group of Thoroughbred race horses that were examined over a 14-month period, there was no association between the severity of PLH and the antibody titres to EHV-1 or the isolation of EHV-2.[23] In fact, EHV-2 was isolated in 5 of 13 clinically normal horses in this group. Clinically, some veterinarians including myself, believe that horses that are immunized every 30 to 60 days using vaccines against equine influenza and EHV-1 have a lower incidence of severe manifestations of PLH. A correlation between complement fixation antibody titres to EHV-1 and the severity of PLH has not been documented and it is only clinical impression that frequent immunization reduces the grade of PLH.[23]

It is likely that equine influenza viruses, herpes viruses, and such environmental factors as inhalation of irritants, pollutants and allergens can all contribute to the development of PLH.[19–21] Some horses appear to be far more reactive to these antigens and develop more severe PLH. Exercise, particularly speed training, also contributes to the development of PLH by repeatedly causing pharyngeal irritation as a result of the mechanical effect of airflow and air turbulence.

Endoscopic surveys of racing Thoroughbreds have shown that there is an inverse statistical relationship between the age of the horse and the prevalence of PLH.[21–24] Approximately 60 to 90% of all 2-year-old racing Thoroughbreds might be expected to have grade II or more PLH, while 35 to 65% of the 3 and 4 year olds and only 10 to 20% of the 5 years olds are similarly affected.

At one time, PLH was thought to be the most common cause of upper airway obstruction in the young race horse.[25] It was reasoned that pharyngeal edema and the mechanical obstruction produced by the pharyngeal lymphoid tissue limited airflow and increased the work of breathing. Frequently a diagnosis of PLH was made in a racehorse with decreased exercise tolerance and it was assumed that it was a cause of airway obstruction. Over time, we have come to realize that PLH, even Grades III and IV, may be present and have no obvious effect on racing performance.[21,23] In a study where arterial blood gas and acid base values were measured before and after experimental induction of PLH, it was shown that PLH did not inhibit gas exchange unless the lesions were severe.[26] If a horse has a history of exercise intolerance or respiratory noise, and PLH is observed, it is unlikely that it is the primary lesion. The horse should be examined carefully for other causes of upper airway obstruction and for evidence of lower airway disease. In my experience many of these horses with PLH and a history of poor racing performance or choking at the end of the race have small airway disease. This is not surprising considering that many of the factors implicated in the etiology of PLH could also contribute to producing bronchial inflammation. A complete respiratory examination of these horses should include lung auscultation using a rebreathing bag, thoracic radiographs, ultrasound scanning of the thorax, and tracheobronchial aspiration. Other causes of exercise intolerance should also be ruled out.

A diagnosis of PLH is made on endoscopic examination and the severity is graded (Table 20–1). There may be an increased amount of mucus present in the nasopharynx in association with the PLH. In horses with active PLH where the pharynx appears hyperemic and edematous, it is easy to produce small mucosal hemorrhages where the endoscope comes in contact with the wall of the pharynx. Also, horses with an inflamed pharynx are more likely to cough and suffer intermittent DDSP. External digital pressure placed over the caudal pharynx and larynx region may elicit a cough or a painful response, particularly if the pharyngitis is acute. The diagnosis of PLH as the cause of airway dysfunction is made by ruling out other causes of airway obstruction and exercise intolerance. The results of topical treatment of the pharynx with an anti-inflammatory solution can be used as a diagnostic aid. If the treatment reduces the inflammation in the pharynx and the severity of the PLH and the horse's racing performance improves, it is probable that the PLH was contributory to producing exercise intolerance. Lymphoid polyps, particularly those in the region of the pharyngeal recess, usually do not cause obstruction unless they become extremely large.

As previously mentioned, the pharyngeal lymphoid hyperplasia that is found in most racehorses rarely causes poor racing performance. In a few horses, however, a chronic Grade III–IV, PLH can cause a chronic cough and be related to decreased racing performances. Frequently, these horses have received medical treatment and periods of rest from training with only temporary improvement of the condition. In these horses, the condition usually persists throughout the 2-year-old year and into the 3-year-old racing season. Providing other causes of poor racing performance are ruled out, particularly a concurrent bronchitis, surgical treatment is indicated. Methods for surgical treatment of PLH include cryosurgery, chemical cautery, and electrocautery. Although some critics have likened these treatments to the firing of the roof of a horse's mouth for lampas, a widespread practice of centuries past, they can be effective in producing a permanent cure with minimal discomfort to the horse.[27]

Currently, cryosurgical treatment of PLH is popular with many racetrack veterinarians because it can be performed in the standing, sedated horse and little training time is lost. The cryogen, either liquid nitrogen or component coolant, is delivered through a catheter and sprayed onto the pharyngeal lymphoid tissue, while the pharynx is viewed through the endoscope. The main limitations of this technique are an inability to determine or control the depth of the freeze and the possibility of inadvertent damage to the normal tissues of the pharynx and larynx. Chemical cauterization of the pharynx can be accomplished with 50% trichloroacetic acid solution.[19] This treatment can be performed in the standing, sedated horse but requires daily treatment for 3 to 5 days. If the horse swallows during the procedure, the larynx, epiglottis, soft palate, or guttural pouch openings may be inadvertently cauterized. Chemical cautery produces an intense inflammatory response followed by sloughing of the nasopharyngeal mucosa. Postoperatively, 30 to 45 days of stall rest should be allowed for complete healing.

In my opinion, electrocautery of the pharynx, performed through a laryngotomy incision under general anesthesia, is a safe and effective form of surgical treatment for PLH. The endotracheal tube is withdrawn into the mouth and the pharynx is swabbed with a topical anesthetic such as 2% mepivicaine or butyn sulfate to inhibit swallowing. An endoscope is passed through the nose into the nasopharynx to provide illumination of the pharynx and to allow an assistant to view the procedure. The soft palate is elevated with curved sponge forceps, placed through the laryngotomy incision, and held by the surgeon.

A ball tipped electrocautery probe is held in the other hand and is introduced through the laryngotomy to make contact with the affected pharynx. With the electrosurgical unit setting on coagulate, the cautery is initiated and the hyperplastic lymphoid tissue is electrofulgurated by lightly sweeping the cautery tip across the roof and lateral walls of the pharynx. Cauterized mucosa turns a light tan color. Care should be taken to avoid cauterizing near the openings to the guttural pouches and the arytenoid cartilages should be retracted as necessary to prevent accidental cauterization.[25] An assistant viewing the procedure through the endoscope or guiding a video endoscope can direct the operator to ensure a complete coverage of the affected pharynx and to avoid cautery around the openings to the guttural pouches. The laryngotomy incision is left to heal by second intention.

Occasionally, severe pharyngeal lymphoid hyperplasia is seen in conjunction with other obstructive diseases of the upper respiratory tract. If the horse is 3 years of age, or older, and a laryngotomy is required for surgical correction of the primary problem, I feel there is some benefit to cauterizing the pharynx as well. Following the laryngotomy, the cautery should be completed first to avoid the bleeding associated with the other procedure (i.e. a sacculectomy).

Following cautery, a coagulum of necrotic tissue forms on the surface of the pharynx and forms a diphtheritic membrane (Fig. 20–14). Within 10 days, this tissue sloughs, leaving an inflamed, hyperemic mucosal surface. Healing is complete by 6 weeks and an endoscopic examination should reveal a smooth, slightly pale, pharyngeal mucosa that is permanently void of lymphoid follicles. If the pharyngeal cautery was incomplete or inadequate, lymphoid tissue may remain but the degree of PLH is generally reduced. Excessive cauterization or freezing of the pharynx results in cicatrix formation that can produce nasopharyngeal stenosis with distortion of the roof or walls of the pharynx. Full thickness necrosis of the pharyngeal wall can result in formation of a permanent fistula between the nasopharynx and guttural pouch. Cauterization around the pharyngeal openings to the guttural pouches can lead to scarring and deformity of the slit-like openings.

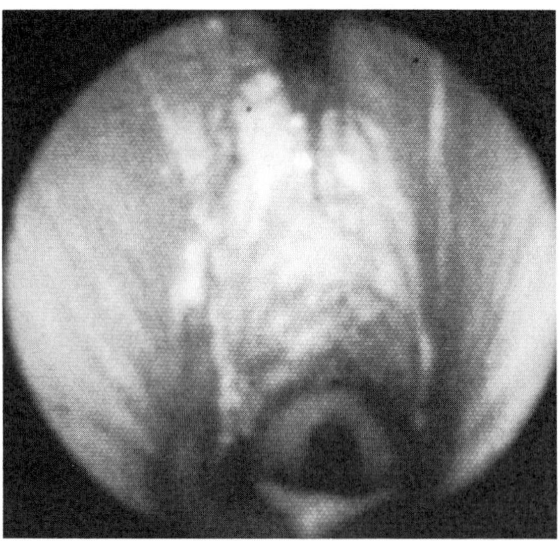

**FIG. 20–14.** Following a pharyngeal cautery, a diphtheritic membrane has formed over the cauterized mucosa. The pharyngeal cautery was performed the day before the endoscopy in conjunction with a left laryngoplasty and sacculectomy.

# Retropharyngeal Abscess

A retropharyngeal abscess can develop either as a sequel to a septic lymphadenopathy, often caused by Streptococcus equi, or following trauma to the pharynx.[28,29] The condition is usually unilateral and the enlarging abscess causes a lateral and dorsal swelling in the nasopharynx and ventral impingement on the medial compartment of the guttural pouch. Luminal compromise of the nasopharynx and larynx can be severe enough to cause inspiratory stertor at rest and necessitate an emergency tracheostomy. This condition may also produce dysphagia which is attributed to mechanical pressure around the pharynx and proximal esophagus, pain or damage to the glossopharyngeal and pharyngeal branch of the vagus nerves.[28]

In addition to dyspnea and/or dysphagia, other clinical findings can include anorexia, persistent fever, increased salivation, nasal discharge, coughing and aspiration pneumonia, as a sequel to the dysphagia. The throat latch area may appear normal or may be swollen on the affected side. External palpation of the caudal pharyngeal region may elicit a painful response.[29] A complete blood count (CBC) often reveals a leukocytosis and

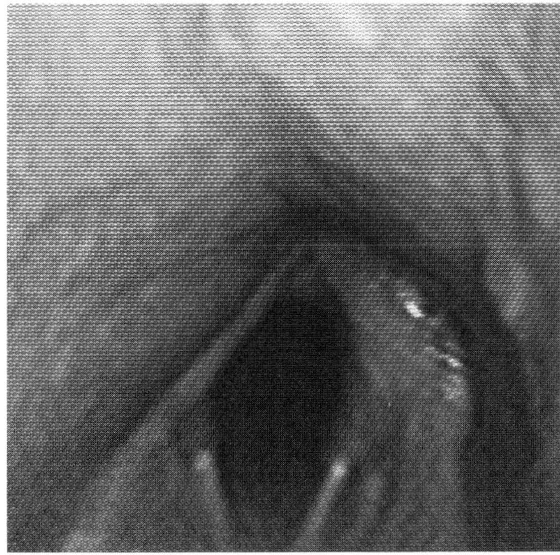

**FIG. 20–15.** Right-sided swelling of the nasopharynx as a result of a retropharyngeal abscess. This swelling impinges on the right corniculate process and makes it difficult to evaluate right arytenoid abductor function.

fibrinogen concentration is increased. On endoscopic examination, there is asymmetrical distortion of the nasopharynx with obvious swelling and compromise of the airway on the affected side. The swelling may also compress and distort the larynx causing medial displacement of the corniculate process on the affected side making it difficult to evaluate abductor function (Fig. 20–15). Endoscopic examination of the guttural pouch on the affected side usually reveals compression of the medial compartment, most frequently from a caudoventral direction (Fig. 20–16). In some cases, there may be purulent material in the guttural pouch as a result of leakage from the abscess. It is my opinion that the guttural pouch empyema and subsequent chondroid formation that follows some cases of strangles is a result of rupture of a retropharyngeal abscess into the guttural pouch on the affected side. Rarely, the abscess ruptures into the pharynx, in which case, the purulent material will be seen draining through the opening. It is also possible for a retropharyngeal abscess to rupture in the proximal cervical area and cause a dissecting infection in the neck. Penetrating pharyngeal wounds can also produce a retropharyngeal and proximal cervical cellulitis.[30,31]

On a lateral radiograph of the head, the abscess is seen as a retropharyngeal soft tissue density that impinges on the caudoventral aspect of the guttural pouch and causes a ventral depression of the roof of the pharynx and larynx[28] (Figs. 20–17 and 20–18). There may be a gas fluid interface if the abscess contains gas forming bacteria.[28] The roof of the pharynx frequently appears thickened. The abscess may extend from the level of the guttural pouch opening cranially to the area above the larynx and proximal esophagus caudally.[28,29] The cranial to caudal limits are variable among horses. A retropharyngeal cellulitis, usually the result of a pharyngeal laceration or trauma to the pharynx, would produce gas densities in the soft tissues surrounding the esophagus and trachea.[30,31] I feel that there is little benefit and a great deal of risk in attempting percutaneously to drain or aspirate pus from a retropharyngeal abscess, even with ultrasound guidance.

The treatment options can include one of, combinations of, or all of the following: (a) medical treatment with broad spectrum antibiotics which would be effective against both

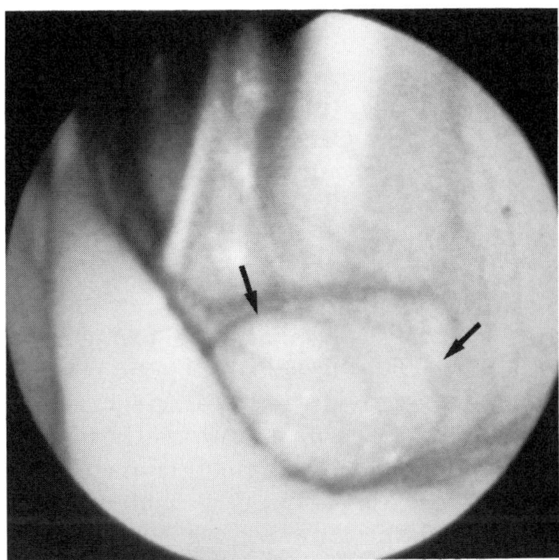

**FIG. 20–16.** Endoscopic examination of the right guttural pouch in this horse shows the abscess (arrows) projecting up into the floor of the medial compartment. This picture was taken 19 days after initial examination and treatment with antibiotics, as the abscess was resolving.

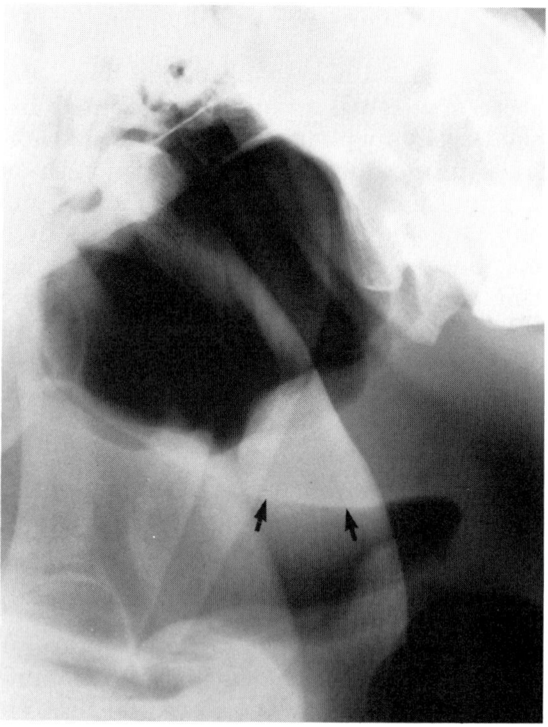

**FIG. 20–17.** On this lateral radiograph of the skull, the abscess is seen as a retropharyngeal soft tissue density that causes a ventral depression of the roof of the pharynx (arrows).

aerobes and anaerobes, a non-steroidal anti-inflammatory drug and an analgesic if the horse is in pain; (b) a tracheostomy in the horse that has a marked dyspnea and respiratory stertor; (c) surgical drainage of the abscess; (d) extraoral feeding of the severely dysphagic horse.

In my experience, there is no clear cut tactic for successful treatment. Those horses that are not obviously dysphagic or showing signs of dyspnea at rest usually respond to medical therapy. The response can be dramatic; within 3 days the horse's temperature may be normal and on endoscopic and radiographic examination the mass is smaller. Antibiotic treatment should be continued for 7 to 10 days. In horses in which the mass is large and causes more severe airway obstruction or where medical therapy alone has failed to resolve the abscess, I recommend surgical drainage under general anesthesia through an approach similar to the Modified Whitehouse approach. In the severely obstructed horse, a tracheostomy should precede any anesthetic premedication.

With the horse placed in dorsal recumbency and the head and neck extended, a skin incision is made along the medial border of the linguofacial vein. The incision extends cranially approximately 15 cm from the point where the linguofacial vein joins the jugular vein. The vein is separated from the omohyoideus muscle by blunt dissection using scissors and fingers and the incision is continued in a craniodorsal direction, lateral to the larynx and medial to the guttural pouch. During the deeper portion of this dissection, fibrous tissue may be encountered as a result of inflammation surrounding the abscess. At the craniodorsal aspect of the larynx, the dissection is continued cranially, to the retropharyngeal area. A 14-gauge needle on an extension set can be passed into the area where the abscess is located to confirm the presence of purulent material. Metzenbaum scissors are thrust into the abscess cavity, the scissors are opened, then withdrawn, creating a drainage opening. Usually a good quantity of pus fills the incision area. This material is removed with suction, the wound is lavaged with saline solution and the incision is left open to

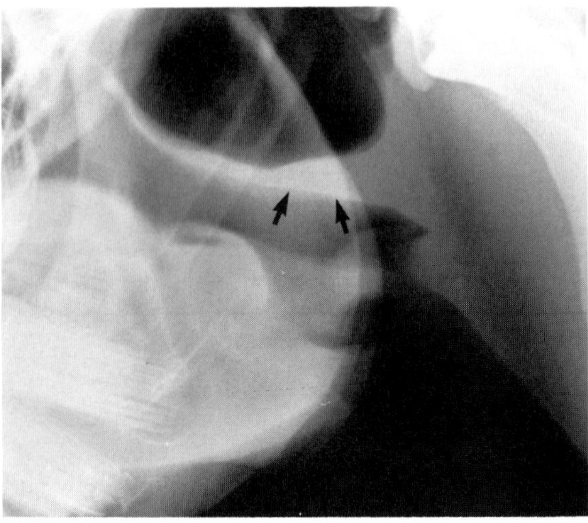

**FIG. 20–18.** This radiograph of the same horse as that shown in Figure 20–17 was taken 19 days after antibiotic treatment was initiated. The abscess (arrows) is resolving.

drain and heal by second intention. No drains or packing are necessary.

With medical treatment alone, it may take weeks or months for a retropharyngeal abscess to resolve completely. Following a combination of medical treatment and successful surgical drainage the abscess resolves quickly. Once the area has healed the horse should be examined endoscopically for any evidence of residual cranial nerve damage. In my experience, surgical intervention has not been a cause of cranial nerve dysfunction. Horses with severe dysphagia or an open wound in the pharynx should receive extraoral alimentation though an esophagostomy tube which can be placed under local anesthesia[28] with the horse standing. The tube can be removed when the clinical signs of dysphagia improve.

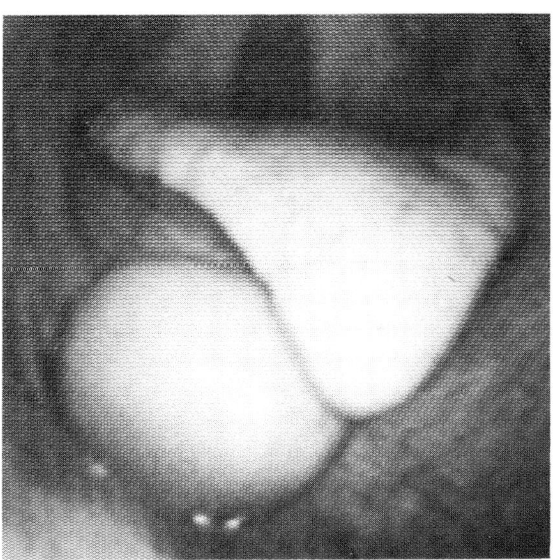

**FIG. 20–19.** Endoscopic view of a subepiglottic cyst.

## Pharyngeal Cyst

Pharyngeal cysts are an infrequent cause of airway obstruction and dysphagia in the horse.[32,33] They have been reported predominantly in Thoroughbreds and Standardbreds although they do occur in other breeds as well. The most common location for a pharyngeal cyst is the subepiglottic area. Rarely, they occur in the dorsal pharynx, larynx, and soft palate. Cysts that occur in the subepiglottic and dorsal pharyngeal regions are generally thought to originate from embryologic remnants of the thyroglossal and craniopharyngeal ducts, respectively. Subepiglottic cysts are usually smooth walled and fluctuant and contain a thick yellow mucus that may stain eosinophilic or contain foamy material and inflammatory cells.[32] The cysts are usually lined by stratified squamous, pseudostratified columnar or cuboidal epithelium or a combination of these epithelial types.[32] It has also been proposed that inflammation of the subepiglottic region can produce blockage of the mucus secreting glands and lead to development of a subepiglottic cyst.[33]

Subepiglottic cysts that develop in foals produce airway obstruction and dysphagia that causes aspiration of ingesta.[33] In addition to an abnormal respiratory noise, these foals have a chronic cough, a bilateral mucopurulent nasal discharge, and pneumonia. An endoscopic examination reveals a cystic mass that is often large enough to obscure the view of the epiglottis and larynx. In older horses (>1 year of age) the pharyngeal cyst produces an abnormal respiratory noise which is heard on inspiration and expiration and usually only during exercise. As the cyst slowly enlarges with time, the airway obstruction becomes more apparent. Subepiglottic cysts can also produce signs of dysphagia and nasal discharge in older horses but unlike foals, older horses do not develop aspiration pneumonia. In a review of 17 horses with pharyngeal cysts, the average age on admission to a referral hospital was 3½ years.[32]

The diagnosis of a pharyngeal cyst is based on an endoscopic visualization of the cyst. Subepiglottic cysts vary in size from 1 to 5 cm in diameter and are seen as smooth walled cystic masses situated under or slightly lateral to the epiglottis and above the caudal margin of the soft palate (Fig. 20–19). In some horses, however, the diagnosis is not so straight forward. It is possible for a subepiglottic cyst, even a large one, to be positioned under the caudal margin of the soft palate and hidden from endoscopic view. Fortunately, if the epiglottic area is viewed over a period of a minute or more and the horse is made to swallow, the cystic mass will come into view, often in

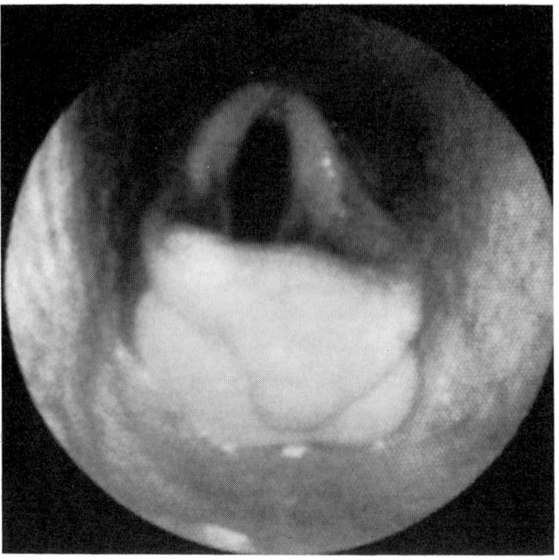

**FIG. 20–20.** A large, subepiglottic cyst is visible in this horse.

association with a temporary entrapment of the epiglottis (Figs. 20–20 and 20–21). I have encountered 3 such horses that on first glance through the endoscope appeared normal. The youngest was a yearling involved in a sale dispute. A subepiglottic cyst will also be hidden from view if the caudal margin of the soft palate is displaced above the epiglottis.

Occasionally, horses are referred to our

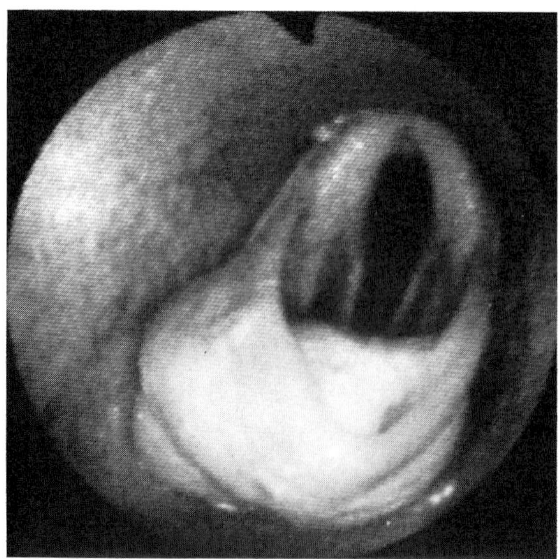

**FIG. 20–21.** Following a swallowing effort in the same horse as in Figure 20–20, the epiglottis has become temporarily entrapped.

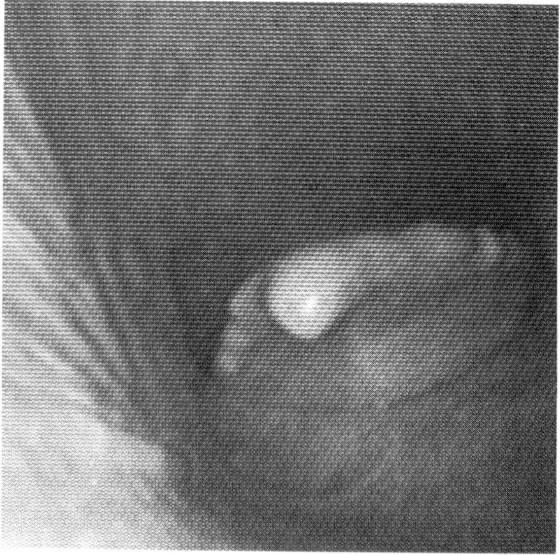

**FIG. 20–22.** Endoscopic view of an "upright" epiglottis.

hospital with an "upright" epiglottis which the referring veterinarians suspect is mechanically produced by a subepiglottic cyst that is situated under the soft palate and is not visible endoscopically (Fig. 20–22). In addition to an endoscopic examination, we take a lateral radiograph to evaluate the pharynx and larynx and under xylazine and ketamine anesthesia palpate the subepiglottic tissue. Invariably we conclude that a subepiglottic cyst is not present and the epiglottic conformation is a variation of normal.

Surgical resection of pharyngeal cysts can be achieved using a ventral midline laryngotomy to gain access to the pharynx.[32] A pharyngotomy approach has been described as an approach to subepiglottic cysts but in my opinion it offers no advantages over a laryngotomy.[6] The pharyngotomy approach to the subepiglottic region requires a deep incision that offers limited exposure and visibility. Recently, contact Nd:YAG laser assisted excision of subepiglottic cysts via an oral approach was reported.[34] Subepiglottic cysts may also be removed through the mouth using a wire snare. The method of removal of a subepiglottic cyst is the surgeon's preference.

If possible, I prefer to remove subepiglottic cysts using a snare. The procedure can be completed in only a few minutes under intravenous anesthesia with relatively little trauma to the subepiglottic area and if healing is uncomplicated, the horse can be returned to work within 1 to 2 weeks, as compared to 4 to 6 weeks, if the cyst is resected via a laryngotomy. A snare can be constructed using a long metal tube preferably with two chambers and obstetric or stainless steel surgical wire. The horse is anesthetized with xylazine, glycerol guiacolate, and ketamine and placed in lateral recumbency with the head and neck extended. A mouth speculum is secured in place and the operator's hand and the snare are passed into the pharynx. The cyst is placed through the loop of the snare with one hand, while the other manipulates the opposite end of the snare. Only the cyst and its mucosal covering should be incorporated into the snare. Once the cyst is ensnared, the operator has an assistant pull on the ends of the wire with a needle holder or pliers to effect an amputation of the cyst. Excessive traction on the snare during the amputation should be avoided as it can result in tearing of the subepiglottic tissue.

If the horse has a small head and it is difficult to manipulate the cyst or if it cannot be ensnared or amputated successfully and relatively atraumatically, the horse should be intubated, placed in dorsal recumbency, and a laryngotomy performed. The epiglottis is everted into the larynx and the cyst is brought into view by applying traction to the arytenoepiglottic folds and the subepiglottic tissue using Allis tissue forceps. This may be accomplished with the endotracheal tube in place although it may be necessary to temporarily remove the endotracheal tube in order to evert the epiglottis. The endotracheal tube can be replaced when the cyst is exposed. Direct manipulation of the epiglottis with sponge forceps or tissue forceps is not necessary and should be avoided. If additional exposure is required, the body of the thyroid cartilage can be split. The mucosa over the cyst is incised with a scalpel and the cyst is carefully dissected free of the surrounding loose connective tissue using scissors. If the cyst is punctured or ruptures during this dissection, a small hemostat can be used to close the defect to prevent evacuation of the entire contents of the cyst. The cyst is freed circumferentially and excised through its stalk at the base of the epiglottis. The cyst should be examined to insure that all cystic tissue has been removed. If the cyst is removed intact, the mucosa can be apposed with a few buried, simple interrupted sutures that are absorbable. Alternatively, the mucosa can be left unsutured. If the cyst ruptures during removal and a complete excision of all secretory tissue is not possible, the area where the tissue remains can be carefully swabbed with 2% aqueous iodine solution to prevent cyst recurrence.[32] Resection of the arytenoepiglottic folds is indicated if an epiglottic entrapment is associated with the cyst. In foals, where the cyst may have an inflammatory etiology, the arytenoepiglottic folds and redundant mucosa around the cyst are removed to prevent cyst recurrence.[33]

Following resection of a pharyngeal cyst through a laryngotomy approach, the horse should be rested for 4 to 6 weeks before work is resumed.[32] The prognosis for a successful, uncomplicated return to work is good providing the cyst is removed completely. Scarring of the subepiglottic region has been observed to result in lateral deviation of the epiglottis, but there is no apparent interference with swallowing or soft palate function. If the cyst is removed with a snare passed through the mouth, the horse can return to work when the swelling and inflammation in the subepiglottic area has subsided. This is determined endoscopically and in many horses can be as early as 1 week following the surgical procedure. Raker states that there is a greater risk of developing adhesions that interfere with epiglottic function if the cyst is removed with a snare.[8] This has not been my experience, although I think that it is important to minimize subepiglottic trauma and excise only the cyst and the mucosa surrounding it and not remove an excessive amount of subepiglottic mucosa.

## Hypoplasia of the Epiglottis

Normal epiglottic length has been determined to be in the 8- to 9-cm range based on measurements obtained from pharyngeal radiographs of adult Thoroughbreds. The term hypoplastic has been applied if the epiglottic cartilage measures less than 7.0 cm in length from base to apex.[5,35] I feel that the term should also be applied if the epiglottic cartilage appears flaccid and seems to lack the rigidity necessary to hold the palate in a subepiglottic position, regardless of its length. A shortened epiglottis or one that lacks rigidity is likely to allow laryngopalatal dislocation during maximal exercise.[35] A hypoplastic epiglottis is also more apt to become entrapped by the arytenoepiglottic tissue than one that is normal.[5]

It is likely that hypoplasia of the epiglottis is a developmental abnormality rather than an acquired one.[35] The condition usually becomes apparent in young horses during training, when they start to make a respiratory noise associated with dorsal displacement of the soft palate. This can be early or late in the training period depending on the degree of hypoplasia. Some horses can tolerate a degree of epiglottic hypoplasia and race or perform successfully without developing dorsal displacement of the soft palate, while others occasionally have intermittent DDSP when racing, particularly near the end of the race.

On endoscopic examination, a hypoplastic epiglottis will appear flaccid and may be obviously shortened. If the hypoplasia is severe, the soft palate may be dorsally displaced at rest. Usually, however, the epiglottis is in a normal position at rest. Following training, the soft palate can be seen to displace easily and the epiglottis appears to buckle or fold from the upward pressure exerted by the soft palate. The same effect can be achieved in the resting horse by occluding the nostrils and forcing the horse to breathe against an obstruction thereby increasing the negative pressure in the pharynx. One gets the impression that the epiglottis provides little resistance to the upward movement of the soft palate (Fig. 20–23). The horse may also experience difficulty in replacing the palate to the normal breathing position, despite repeated swallowing efforts. As mentioned previously, a lateral radiograph of the larynx can be taken to determine the length of the epiglottis.[5] Although the epiglottic length is useful in helping to document hypoplasia, I feel that the subjective endoscopic evaluation of the epiglottis is the basis for arriving at the diagnosis.

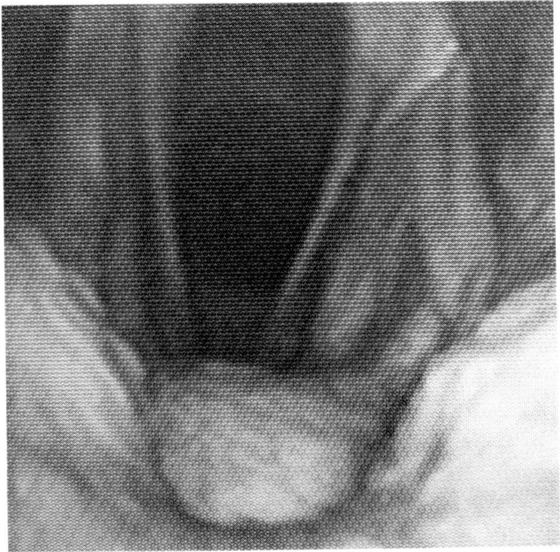

**FIG. 20–23.** In this 2-year-old Thoroughbred that has intermittent, dorsal displacement of the soft palate, the epiglottis appears hypoplastic. With slight increases in negative pressure, the soft palate "swells" around the small epiglottis.

Conservative management will help some horses that have a hypoplastic epiglottis and occasional DDSP. Efforts should be made to minimize the amount of pharyngeal inflammation and a tongue tie should be used when training or racing. If possible, the head should be kept in an extended position to maximize the nasopharyngeal diameter and streamline airflow. A sternothyrohyoid myectomy is useful in some horses with a marginally small epiglottis. Resection of the caudal margin of the soft palate is contraindicated and may even make the condition worse.

A procedure developed by Dr. Chris Koch has been used to successfully augment the bulk of the epiglottis and prevent dorsal displacement of the soft palate (Koch C. Personal Communication, 1988). With the horse under general anesthesia, a laryngotomy is performed and the epiglottis is everted into the larynx by grasping the arytenoepiglottic tissue. Teflon paste is deposited along the epiglottic cartilage in the subepiglottic tissue and along the lateral margins of the epiglottis in the arytenoepiglottic tissue in order to strengthen the epiglottis and increase its size. Many of the horses treated have improved and it would appear that providing the hypoplasia is not severe, the prognosis for the horse racing is good.

The owner or trainer of a horse that has a hypoplastic epiglottis that develops a dorsal displacement of the soft palate during training frequently asks if the condition could have been detected at the time of purchase at a yearling sale. It is my opinion that unless the epiglottis is severely hypoplastic, resulting in a dorsal displacement of the soft palate at rest, it is difficult to assess epiglottic size in young horses, endoscopically. A yearling may have what appears to be a hypoplastic epiglottis yet go on and race without ever having a problem. The heritability of the condition is unknown.

## Nasopharyngeal Cicatrices

In this condition, the lumen of the nasopharynx is narrowed by transverse or longitudinal bands of scar tissue that may involve the dorsal and lateral walls of the pharynx and the soft palate.[36] The condition is usually seen in conjunction with other upper airway abnormalities such as chondritis of the arytenoid cartilages, epiglottic deformity, and deformity of the guttural pouch openings. The nasopharyngeal stenosis is usually not severe enough to produce respiratory obstruction and the presenting signs of exercise intolerance and abnormal respiratory noise production are usually caused by the coexisting laryngeal and nasopharyngeal lesions. Abnormal vocalization and dysphagia have also been reported in association with a nasopharyngeal cicatrix. The etiology and pathogenesis are as yet undefined although ulcerative nasopharyngitis has been proposed as a cause of cicatrix formation. The condition is seen more frequently in aged horses (>10 year of age) and females. Surgical correction of nasopharyngeal cicatrix has not been performed. Horses with a concurrent arytenoid chondritis that are severely compromised will benefit from an arytenoidectomy or a permanent tracheostomy.[36]

## Nasopharyngeal Neoplasia

Neoplasms of the nasopharynx are rarely encountered. Squamous cell carcinoma may arise from the nasal mucosa and invade the nasopharynx or it may metastasize to the retropharyngeal lymph nodes from a primary site in the oral cavity or oropharynx.[37] Lymphosarcoma may also be found to involve the nasopharynx or larynx.[38,39] Fibrosarcoma and melanoma have also been reported in the pharyngeal area.[40]

Signs associated with nasopharyngeal or laryngeal neoplasia are dependent on the size and location of the tumor masses and the degree of tissue destruction. Large masses in the nasopharyngeal area or tumorous infiltration of the larynx will produce airway obstruction. Neoplasms of the oropharynx and those involving the retropharyngeal region produce signs of dysphagia and metastatic spread of the neoplasm will produce regional lymph node enlargement. Nasopharyngeal tumors that cause tissue necrosis will produce nasal discharge. Neoplastic destruction of the palate can lead to the formation of an oral-nasal fistula that results in a persistent, ingesta-stained nasal discharge.[38] In a case of multicentric lymphosarcoma, the subcutaneous lymph nodes may be swollen.

Endoscopically, tumor masses that protrude from the mucosal surface of the nasopharynx may appear smooth or irregular and their surface may be covered with mucosa or ulcerated, depending on the tumor type. Tumors occupying the retropharyngeal space produce a dorsolateral swelling in the pharynx which compresses the lumen of the nasopharynx and impinges on the caudoventral aspect of the guttural pouch of the affected side(s) (Figs. 20–24 and 20–25). Neoplasms of the larynx produce thickening of its cartilaginous and soft tissue structures and must be differentiated from arytenoid chondritis. Lymphosarcoma of the nasopharynx may appear similar to the nasopharyngeal polyps associated with severe lymphoid hyperplasia. Soft tissue masses of the nasopharyngeal, retropharyngeal, and laryngeal regions are usually visible on standing lateral radiographs of this area and the radiographs can be useful

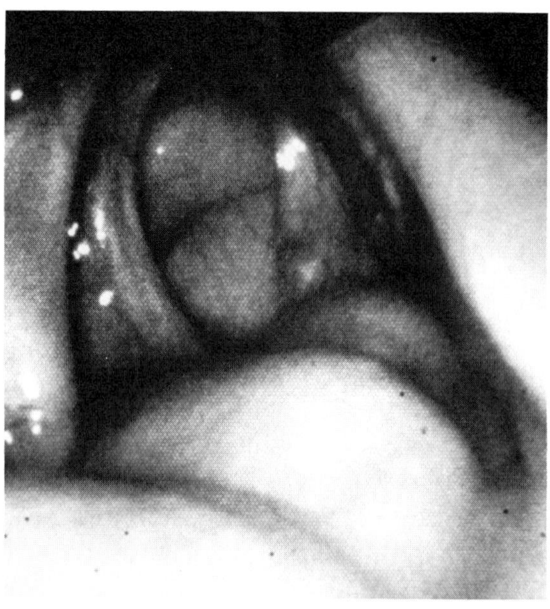

**FIG. 20–24.** Retropharyngeal tumor masses (squamous cell carcinoma) can be seen impinging on the floor of the left guttural pouch.

for determining the size of the neoplasm and the degree of involvement of surrounding structures. A definitive diagnosis of neoplasm is made following a histopathologic examination of a core specimen from the intrapharyngeal mass or an excisional biopsy of a regional lymph node.[39] Small surface biopsies obtained through a fiberoptic endoscope may show evidence only of chronic inflammation.

Unfortunately, due to the aggressive nature of most of these tumors and the likelihood of metastasis, treatment is rarely attempted and if it is, it is invariably unsuccessful. Complete surgical excision is usually impossible due to the extent of the lesion and its inaccessibility. At best, radiation or chemotherapy is palliative only for a short period of time. However, more discrete and non-metastatic tumors of the nasopharynx or larynx may be successfully removed with an Nd:YAG laser (Tate LP, personal communication, 1988). The laser fibers are passed through a flexible fiberoptic endoscope and the patient can be treated standing. In horses in which salvage is attempted, a tracheostomy tube may be necessary if the nasopharynx or larynx becomes obstructed.

## Epiglottic Entrapment

Entrapment of the epiglottis is a condition that can produce exercise intolerance, respiratory noise, and occasional coughing.[41] An entrapment is produced when the arytenoepiglottic and subepiglottic tissues envelop the epiglottis. The arytenoepiglottic folds are thick bands of mucous membrane that attach to the ventral surface of the epiglottis along its lateral free borders and then extend caudodorsally along the lateral aspects of the arytenoid cartilages to blend dorsally with the mucous membrane that covers the corniculate processes.[41] The arytenoepiglottic folds are supported by the cuneiform cartilages, and laterally form the boundaries of the laryngeal opening.[41] They are continuous with the redundant mucosa of the glossoepiglottic fold on the lingual side of the epiglottis and with the mucous membrane on its laryngeal sur-

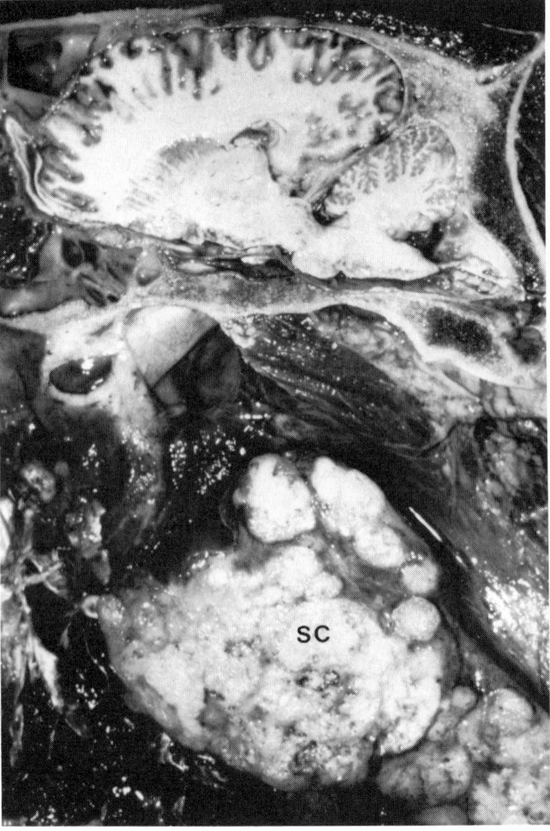


**FIG. 20–25.** An extremely large retropharyngeal squamous cell carcinoma (SC) as seen on a sagittal section of the head at post mortem.

face. The subepiglottic epithelium is quite loose and redundant which allows for epiglottic elevation during deglutition.[9] Entrapment develops when the subepiglottic tissue and the arytenoepiglottic folds roll up and around the apex and lateral margins of the epiglottis.

Horses with a congenitally hypoplastic epiglottis appear to be predisposed to developing epiglottic entrapment since it is easier for the arytenoepiglottic tissue to envelop a small epiglottis.[41] In these horses, signs of airway obstruction usually become apparent during early race training. Other abnormalities of the epiglottis that have been found in association with arytenoepiglottic entrapment include epiglottic cysts, cartilage thickening or deformity, lateral deviation along the long axis of the epiglottis, and necrosis of the tip of the epiglottis.[41] It is questionable whether these deformities predispose to an epiglottic entrapment or whether they develop secondary to a long-standing entrapment. Epiglottic entrapment may also be acquired in horses of any age that have a normal epiglottis. Inflammation and swelling of the arytenoepiglottic and subepiglottic tissue may be a predisposing factor. In some horses with entrapment of the epiglottis, particularly those with a hypoplastic or deformed epiglottis, there may be a concurrent dorsal displacement of the soft palate (DDSP). The DDSP may be intermittent or persistent, obscuring the entrapment from view (see DDSP). Epiglottic entrapment is also seen in foals with cleft soft palate, as early as 1 day of age.

The entrapping membrane usually acts as an impediment to airflow and creates air turbulence which may produce noise both on inspiration and expiration. The degree of reduction of the cross-sectional area of the airway, just rostral to the laryngeal opening, is dependent on the severity of the entrapment, the amount of inflammation in the entrapping membrane, and whether there is a concurrent dorsal displacement of the soft palate. Epiglottic entrapment can cause obstruction and exercise intolerance without a respiratory noise. It can also affect swallowing and cause a chronic cough, particularly when the horse is eating.

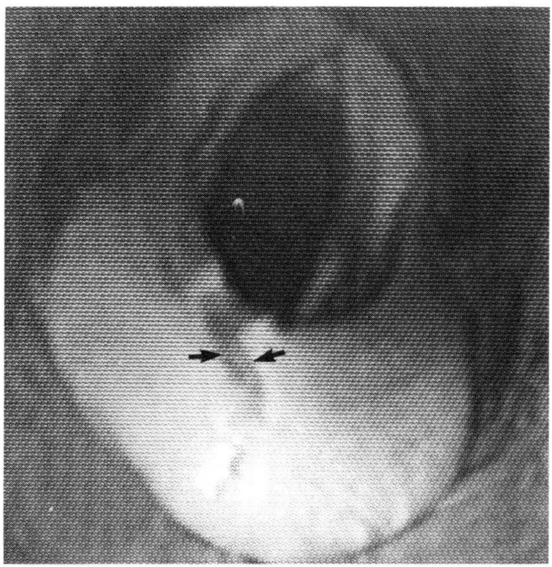

**FIG. 20–26.** Endoscopic view of an entrapped epiglottis. The outline of the epiglottis is visible; however, the serrated edges of the epiglottis and its surface vasculature are covered. There is a mucosal ulceration on the surface of the entrapping membrane (arrows).

In some horses, epiglottic entrapment is asymptomatic and causes no respiratory impairment. In an endoscopic survey of 479 horses, mostly racing Thoroughbreds, 10 horses were discovered to have epiglottic entrapment.[24] None of the affected horses had decreased exercise tolerance or made a respiratory noise. There was no apparent congenital predisposition to the epiglottic entrapment, since there was no association between the age of the horse and the prevalence of the entrapment and none of the horses appeared to have a hypoplastic epiglottis or an epiglottic deformity.

Epiglottic entrapment is diagnosed on endoscopic examination. The gross outline of the epiglottis is visible, however, the serrated edges of the epiglottic cartilage and the vasculature on the laryngeal surface of the epiglottis are covered by the entrapping membrane (Fig. 20–26). The entrapment may form a small rim of tissue that covers only the apex and the lateral borders or it may be more complete, covering most of the laryngeal surface of the epiglottis. It may also be incomplete, covering only the apex and one lateral border of the epiglottis (Fig. 20–27). The caudal mar-

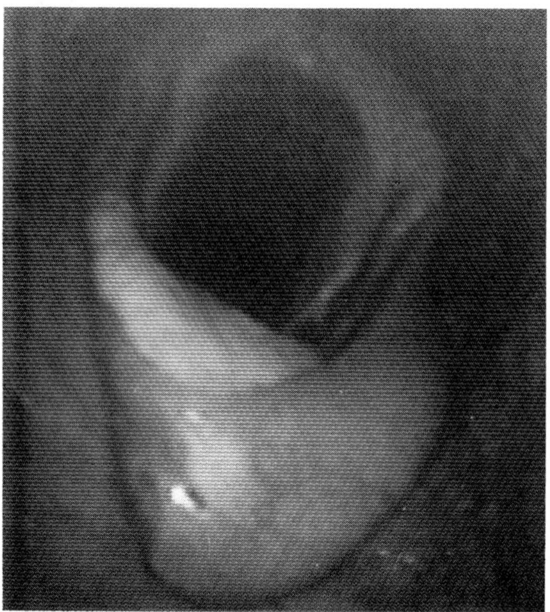

**FIG. 20–27.** Incomplete entrapment of the epiglottis. The arytenoepiglottic tissue covers the apex and the left lateral border of the epiglottis. The right lateral border of the epiglottis is visible.

gin of the entrapping membrane is always visible. Granulating ulcerations are frequently seen on the surface of the aryteno-epiglottic tissue in horses with a long-standing entrapment. Occasionally an ulcer over the apex of the epiglottis will erode completely through the membrane and the tip of the epiglottis will protrude through the defect. The entrapment may be intermittent and in some cases the epiglottis may become entrapped and unentrapped as the horse swallows during the examination. If an intermittent entrapment of the epiglottis is suspected, the horse should be examined after racing or training or during exercise on a high speed treadmill when there is a greater likelihood of observing the condition.

Surgical correction of an epiglottic entrapment is usually indicated if the diagnosis coincides with a decrease in racing performance and an apparent compromise in respiratory function. Other causes of exercise intolerance should be ruled out. An entrapment of short duration may correct spontaneously if the horse is removed from training and given stall rest for 1 week, but it is likely to recur once training is resumed. There are a number of different techniques for surgical relief of epiglottic entrapment and a method is selected after considering the age of the horse, the stage of training or racing, the economic factors involved, and the experience and preferences of the surgeon.

In general, there are two basic methods for surgical correction.[4] The entrapped epiglottis can be approached through a ventral midline laryngotomy and the arytenoepiglottic tissue resected. Following this resection, the horse requires at least 30 days of stall rest before training is resumed. An alternative approach is to simply divide the entrapping membrane along its midline, allowing the arytenoepiglottic folds to fall to each side of the epiglottis thereby correcting the entrapment. Utilizing this principle, various tools including hooked cutting instruments, electrosurgical cutting electrodes and Nd:YAG lasers have been employed in various ways to effect a correction without the need for a laryngotomy.[4,42,43] Successful application of one of these techniques allows the horse to resume training within 10 to 14 days, which means that the horse misses only a few races.

If a concurrent dorsal displacement of the soft palate is observed prior to surgery or the epiglottis appears hypoplastic or deformed, there is an increased likelihood of postoperative displacement of the soft palate. In addition to a subjective evaluation of the size and shape of the epiglottis during the endoscopic examination, a preoperative measurement of epiglottic cartilage length can be made from a lateral pharyngeal radiograph to determine if the epiglottis is shorter than normal.[5] It has been hypothesized that a small or deformed epiglottis is unable to hold the caudal margin of the soft palate in a subepiglottic position, particularly once the additional bulk of the entrapping membrane is removed. An owner or trainer must be made thoroughly aware of the risks associated with surgery and the possible postoperative complications prior to the operation.

## *Methods of Dividing the Entrapping Membrane*

The most recently described method for correction of arytenoepiglottic fold entrapment involves the use of an Nd:YAG laser and the surgery is performed in the standing horse[42] (Tate LP, personal communication, 1988). The horse is placed in stocks, sedated with xylazine, and a topical anesthetic is sprayed over the entrapping membrane. A flexible, contact or free cutting Nd:YAG laser fiber is passed through the biopsy port of a fiberoptic endoscope and the entrapping membrane is divided on its midline, starting at the apex of the epiglottis and working caudally. This ensures that the entire length of the midline incision, from the apex of the epiglottis to the caudal margin of the entrapping membrane, is incised before the entrapment is reduced. Surgery time is reported to be in the 30- to 50-minute range and hemorrhage is negligible. The results of the transendoscopic contact Nd:YAG laser correction of epiglottic entrapment are encouraging. In a report of 24 horses, 1 horse reentrapped within 1 week but was successfully corrected with a second laser procedure and only 2 horses developed persistent dorsal displacement of the soft palate following surgery. Most horses returned to training within 1 to 2 weeks and raced within 1 month after surgery.[42] The advantages of transendoscopic correction of an epiglottic entrapment with the Nd:YAG laser are numerous. The procedure can be performed in the standing horse on an outpatient basis; there is minimal hemorrhage associated with the surgery and minimal postoperative swelling; healing is rapid (2 weeks), ensuring an early return to work; there are few complications associated with the procedure and the equipment is relatively safe for both the patient and surgeon providing an experienced operator is performing the surgery. The primary disadvantage is the major expenditure required to purchase the laser equipment.

Monopolar electrosurgical cutting has also been used to correct epiglottic entrapment.[4] The active electrode is passed through the biopsy chamber of a flexible fiberoptic endoscope and the surgery is conducted in a fashion similar to that just described for the Nd:YAG laser surgery. Five horses with epiglottic entrapment were treated with transendoscopic electrosurgery with relatively good long-term results. Two of the horses developed a minor degree of reentrapment but none of the horses had dorsal displacement of the soft palate. Despite the favorable outcome of these cases there is a major disadvantage to using transendoscopic electrosurgery in the standing horse; the potential for serious electrical accidents and burns to both the operator and patient. In my opinion, the meticulous preoperative attention which must be paid to insulating the stocks, floor, twitch and the assistants, inspecting the equipment for safety and the worry that faulty equipment or inappropriate application of the patient plate could cause an electrical accident and serious burns to the operator or patient make this technique impractical.

The most common, and simplest, method for dividing the entrapping membrane involves using a long, gently curved wire with a hook and cutting edge at one end to engage the membrane and slit it by pulling the instrument in a rostral direction. This can be performed in the standing, sedated horse by passing the instrument up the nasal passage and into the nasopharynx, using the endoscope in the opposite nasal passage to guide the operation or it can be performed through the oral cavity in the horse anesthetized with xylazine, glycerol guiacolate, and ketamine. If the operation is performed in the standing horse, there is potential for lacerating the soft palate with the bistoury if the horse rears unexpectedly, or inadvertently hooking other structures if the horse swallows. The chances of this occurring are low with an experienced operator.[43] Performing the procedure through the mouth under anesthesia reduces the chances of inadvertently damaging other structures, allows more accurate placement of the hook through the entrapping membrane and allows a more controlled cutting of the entrapping membrane.

I prefer the oral approach for these stated advantages. With a large dental speculum securely fastened in the mouth, the operator's hand and the hooked end of the instrument are passed into the oral pharynx. After palpating the entrapment, the hook of the instrument is passed between the caudal margin of the entrapment and the epiglottis and advanced rostrally until it engages the membrane covering the tip of the epiglottis (Fig.

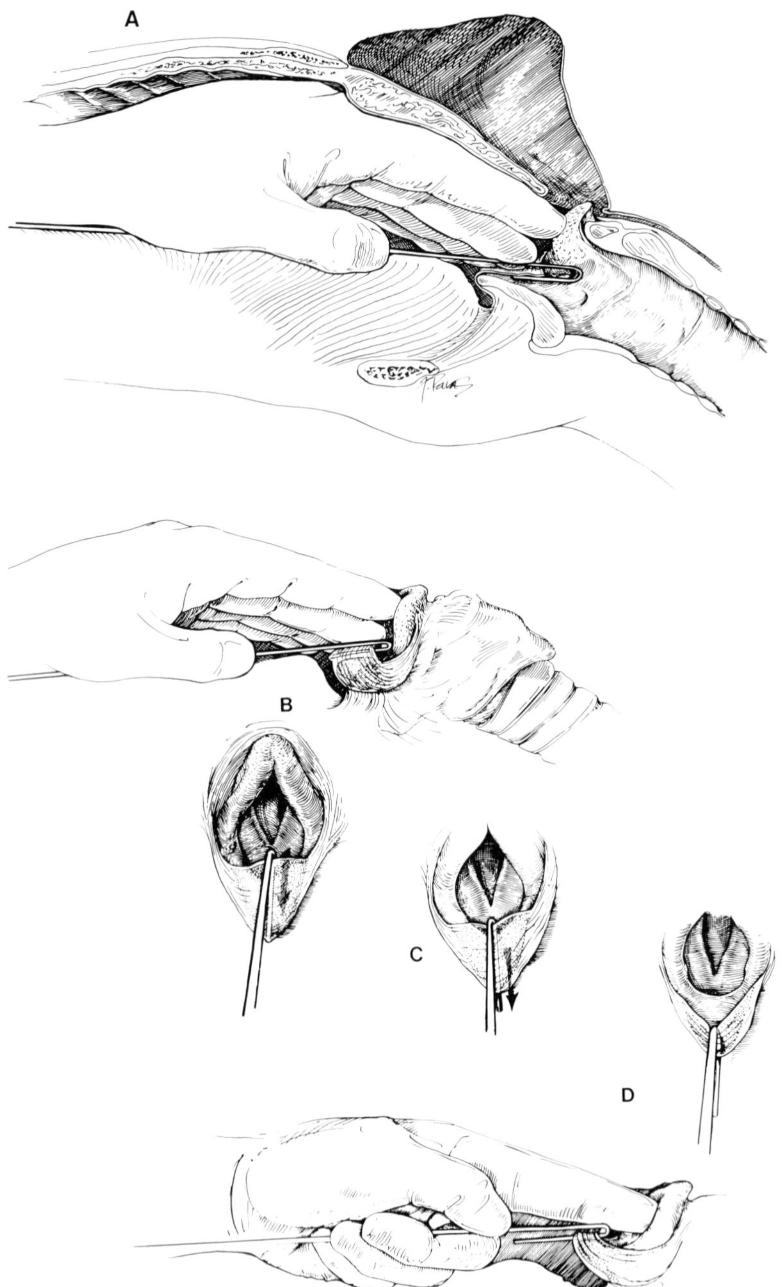


**FIG. 20–28.** Division of the arytenoepiglottic tissue—oral approach. A. The hook of the cutting instrument is passed between the caudal margin of the entrapment and the epiglottis. B. The tip of the hook is advanced rostrally until it engages the membrane covering the tip of the epiglottis. C. The tip of the hook is pulled through the entrapping membrane. D. The instrument is pulled in a rostral direction and the membrane is divided by the cutting edge on the inside bend of the hook.

20–28A–D). The position of the hook is determined by palpation. The tip of the hook is pulled through the entrapping membrane and the membrane is divided as the instrument is pulled in a rostral direction. If the epiglottis becomes unentrapped during digital manipulation, prior to placement of the hook, it can usually be reentrapped by manually "rolling" the aryepiglottic tissue over its dorsal surface.

The design of the hooked bistoury is important to ensure complete division of the entrapping membrane. The cutting surface is situated on the inside bend of the hook. This sharp edge can be created by filing the inside edge with a small circular file. The length of the hook should be slightly longer than the length of the entrapping membrane, from the apex of the epiglottis to the caudal margin. The hook should securely engage the membrane over the midline of the epiglottis before cutting begins, thus ensuring a complete cut

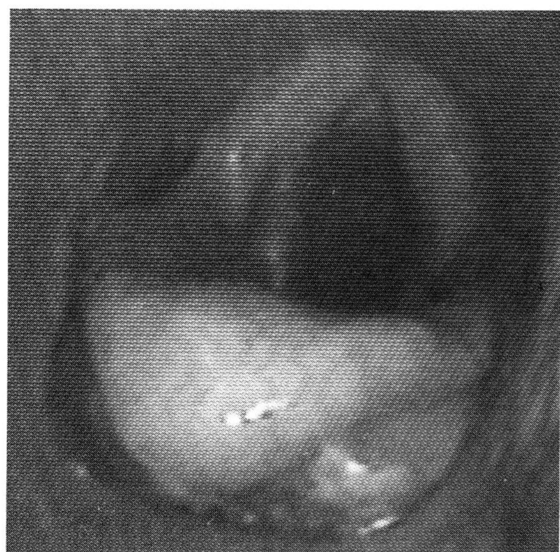

**FIG. 20–29.** Endoscopic examination of a horse, 5 days following division of an entrapped membrane with a hooked bistoury. The subepiglottic tissues remain considerably swollen.

and minimizing the chances of postoperative recurrence. If the hook at the end of the instrument is short and engages only the caudal margin of the entrapping membrane most of the entrapment is disengaged before the membrane is cut.[4] This produces only a small notch on the caudal margin of the entrapping membrane and the entrapment will likely recur.

In my experience there is a great deal of variability in the postoperative appearance of the epiglottic area following transection using a hooked bistoury. In the first few days after surgery, the epiglottis has a "bordered" appearance, the lateral folds of the arytenoepiglottic membrane appear to be rolled up and over the lateral margins of the epiglottis, however the apex of the epiglottis is clearly visible. This should not be misinterpreted as a recurrence of the entrapment. As the swelling and inflammation subside, these lateral folds retract to the ventral surface of the epiglottis. The amount of postoperative swelling ranges from mild to severe and subepiglottic swelling can persist for as long as 2 weeks (Fig. 20–29). Pre- and postoperative administration of phenylbutazone and postoperative nebulization with an anti-inflammatory solution help reduce the degree of swelling. Training can be resumed when the swelling has subsided, usually at 7 to 10 days following surgery. If the entrapment recurs, the procedure can be repeated or another surgical technique can be applied.

## *Resection of Arytenoepiglottic Folds*

The entrapped epiglottis is approached through a ventral laryngotomy incision with the horse in dorsal recumbency, under inhalation anesthesia. If the procedure is performed using only intravenous anesthetics, swallowing can seriously interfere with the surgery. The exposure offered through a routine laryngotomy incision is adequate and it is rarely necessary to split the thyroid cartilage. Withdrawal of the endotracheal tube allows direct visualization of the caudal margin of the entrapping membrane, just dorsal to the caudal edge of the soft palate. The edge of this membrane is grasped on its midline with a sponge forceps or an Allis tissue forceps and retracted into the larynx. This also everts the apex of the epiglottis into the lumen of the larynx as the membrane is attached to the ventral margins of the epiglottis. It is possible for the epiglottis to become unentrapped during intubation, in which case, the entrapping membrane will not be visible when the endotracheal tube is removed. If this occurs, the end of a curved sponge forceps can be hooked under the base of the epiglottis and used to turn the epiglottis back toward the larynx. The arytenoepiglottic tissue is then grasped with Allis tissue forceps and retracted into the larynx. It is possible to evert the epiglottis without having to directly grasp the epiglottic cartilage. Trauma to the epiglottic cartilage can lead to chondroma formation or a cartilage deformity (Fig. 20–30).

Allis tissue forceps are attached to the free edge of the retracted membrane on each side of midline in order to symmetrically spread out the tissue before resection. The apex and the lateral margins of the epiglottis are identified by digital palpation. Using Metzenbaum scissors, the membrane is divided on its midline down to the tip of the epiglottis and the incision is continued along both

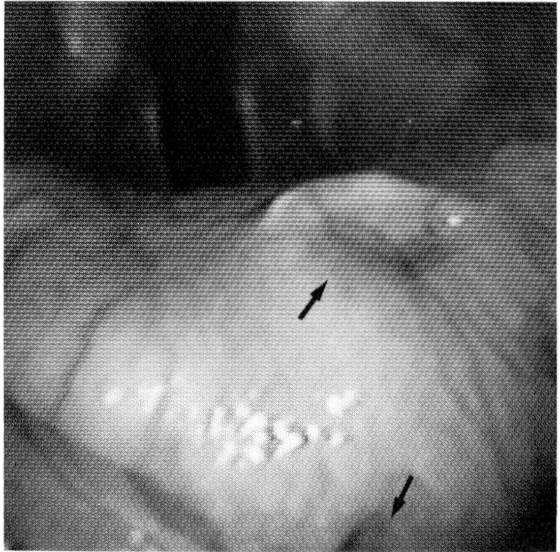

**FIG. 20–30.** Epiglottic deformities (arrows) secondary to trauma associated with resection of the arytenoepiglottic folds.

edges of the epiglottis for approximately one-third the length of the epiglottis, at which point the folds are amputated. The incisions along the epiglottis are made at least 5 mm from its lateral margins to avoid damage to the cartilage. Some surgeons remove only the central portion of the fold and do not excise along the lateral margins of the epiglottis.[6] It is difficult to give dimensions for the precise amount to resect because there is such a wide variation between horses. Knowing that some horses will develop DDSP regardless of the amount resected, some surgeons also perform a staphylectomy in conjunction with the arytenoepiglottic fold resection. In my opinion, if the epiglottis appears to be hypoplastic, a staphylectomy should not be performed. The laryngotomy incision is left to heal by second intention (Fig. 20–31).

It is generally accepted that the postoperative occurrence of dorsal displacement of the soft palate is much greater following resection of the arytenoepiglottic folds than after simple division of the entrapping membrane.[4] The frequency of DDSP following resection of the arytenoepiglottic tissue may be as high as 20%.[44] DDSP may be observed immediately following surgery or it may develop as late as 1 week postoperatively perhaps suggesting different etiologies. The DDSP observed may be intermittent or persistent, despite swallowing efforts.

The DDSP may occur for two reasons. When the added bulk and support provided by the entrapping membrane is suddenly removed, a hypoplastic or deformed epiglottis may no longer be able to resist the upward pressure exerted by the soft palate and a DDSP develops. This is likely to be observed immediately after surgery. It has also been postulated that creation of a subepiglottic mucosal defect produces inflammation and scarring that limits the mobility of the epiglottis and leads to DDSP. The area of the subepiglottal mucosal defect created and the chance of a postoperative DDSP are directly proportional to the amount of tissue resected.[4] This hypothesis would explain why a DDSP can develop despite the presence of a normal epiglottis and why soft palate function may appear normal for 4 to 5 days before the development of a dorsal displacement. It would seem, therefore, that the surgeon who wishes to minimize the chances of a postoperative DDSP should select one of the techniques that divides the entrapping membrane. If resection through a laryngotomy is necessary because of recurrence following one of the sim-

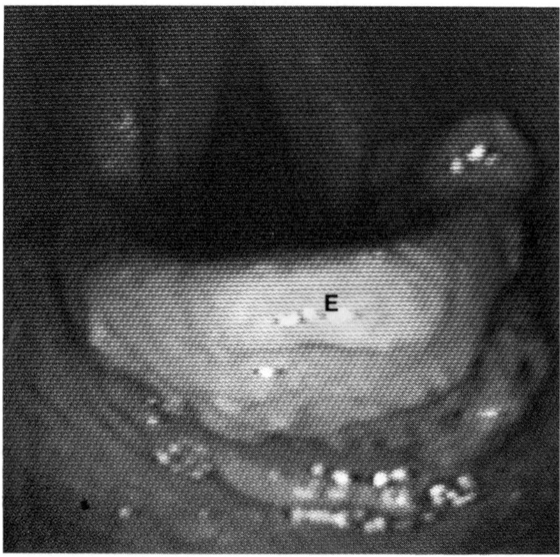


**FIG. 20–31.** Endoscopic view of the epiglottis 1 week following liberal resection of the aryepiglottic tissue via laryngotomy. The tip of the epiglottis (E) is visible; however, swelling and granulation tissue are visible lateral and ventral to the epiglottis.

pler procedures, the central portion of the entrapping membrane and only a minimal amount of tissue along the lateral margins of the epiglottis should be removed. Enough of the membrane must be removed, however, to prevent recurrence of the entrapment.

The dorsal displacement of the soft palate that develops following epiglottic entrapment surgery can be intermittent or persistent. Intermittent DDSP frequently resolves without treatment and is not a cause for great concern unless the epiglottis is hypoplastic. What is worrisome is a persistent DDSP. If this is observed, the horse should be nebulized or have its throat sprayed with an anti-inflammatory spray for at least 1 week in an attempt to relieve the inflammation around the epiglottis. I have found that the horse that develops a DDSP later in the postoperative period, at 5 to 7 days, is more likely to respond to medical treatment than the one that develops a DDSP earlier or immediately after surgery.

If the DDSP persists beyond 2 weeks following surgery, there is a good chance that it will be permanent unless an attempt is made to correct it surgically. If there is a marked hypoplasia of the epiglottis, there is little hope of correcting the problem with surgery. I have found, providing there has not already been a staphylectomy performed, that resection of a narrow strip off the caudal margin of the soft palate will correct the DDSP about 50% of the time. A sternothyrohyoid myectomy is of little use in attempting to correct a persistent DDSP.

Although I usually make the decision to trim the soft palate for a persistent DDSP at about 2 weeks after resection of the epiglottal entrapment, it would not be unreasonable to recommend that a definitive evaluation of the condition and a decision for further surgery be deferred until the healing around the epiglottis is complete. I have had a few horses that developed a persistent DDSP after resection of an epiglottal entrapment that recovered palate function without the benefit of further surgery. I would be more inclined to take a "wait and see" approach in horses that (a) had a concurrent DDSP associated with the epiglottic entrapment, (b) had a staphylectomy performed already or (c) had a hypoplastic epiglottis.

## Rostral Displacement of the Palatopharyngeal Arch

In this condition, the caudal margin of the ostium intrapharyngeum, also referred to as the palatopharyngeal arch, is displaced rostral to the corniculate processes of the arytenoid cartilages producing dorsal laryngopalatal dislocation.[45–47] It has been proposed that a developmental abnormality of the fourth branchial arch causes anatomic changes in the thyroid cartilage that lead to the displacement. The thyroid cartilage is shaped abnormally, with shortened lateral and posterior laminae that are tilted dorsally and do not articulate with the cricoid cartilage. The abnormally conformed laminae of the thyroid cartilage, in effect, limit the normal excursion of the arytenoid cartilages. In addition, the cricopharyngeus muscles are absent.

The effect of this condition seems to vary among horses, perhaps because there are varying degrees of deformity. In those that are severely affected there is both respiratory compromise and dysphagia. Some horses only show signs of airway obstruction during exercise. The airway obstruction is caused by the palatopharyngeal tissue causing physical blockage to airflow and the limited ability of the arytenoid cartilages to abduct as a result of the thyroid cartilage deformity. An absence of the cricopharyngeus muscles and a loss of the normal co-ordination between the pharynx, larynx and the upper esophageal sphincter during swallowing contribute to producing dysphagia.[45]

Clinical signs in those horses that are severely affected include dysphagia, nasal discharge of food material, chronic coughing, and an abnormal inspiratory noise during exercise.[46] The condition may become apparent shortly after birth. In less severely affected horses, the only abnormality noted is a respiratory noise that is associated with exercise intolerance. Endoscopically, the palatopharyngeal arch is seen covering the apical area of the corniculate cartilages (Fig. 20–32). It appears as though there is a hood of tissue over the top of the larynx. The displacement can be accentuated by making the horse breathe deeply or by tranquilization. In most

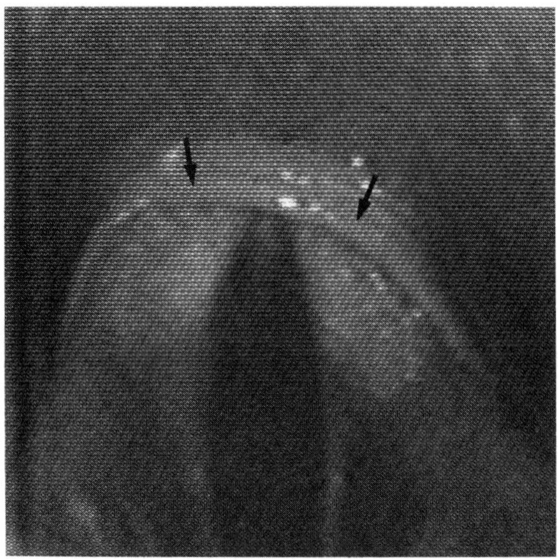

**FIG. 20–32.** Rostral displacement of the palatopharyngeal arch over the apical area of the corniculate cartilages (arrows).

of these horses, the arytenoid cartilages appear incapable of abducting maximally. This has been attributed to a mechanical limitation of movement caused by the anomaly. In some horses, however, left laryngeal hemiplegia may be found in conjunction with a rostral displacement of the palatopharyngeal arch. In one yearling Thoroughbred, I found a rostral displacement of the palatopharyngeal arch, left laryngeal hemiplegia, and a ventricular septal defect in the heart. Digital palpation and radiographic evaluation of the larynx might be of some value in assessing whether the thyroid cartilage is deformed. On a lateral radiograph, the rostrally displaced palatopharyngeal arch is visible cranial to the larynx and the cranial esophagus is usually filled with air.

Surgical treatment is of no use in those horses that are severely affected, showing signs of dysphagia and airway obstruction. Those horses generally are euthanized. Affected horses that are not dysphagic but have airway obstruction may benefit from surgical resection of the palatopharyngeal arch. This is accomplished through a ventral laryngotomy incision with the horse in dorsal recumbency under general anesthesia. The endotracheal tube is removed and the palatopharyngeal arch, which is visible immediately anterior to the dorsum of the larynx is grasped with Allis tissue forceps and excised flush with the roof of the pharynx using long curved scissors. The palatopharyngeal tissue is not sutured. Postoperatively, the horse is rested for 6 weeks before resuming training.

A guarded prognosis must be given. Even following removal of the obstructing tissue of the palatopharyngeal arch, the deformity of the larynx remains and arytenoid function is limited. If left laryngeal hemiplegia is diagnosed in conjunction with the condition, a grave prognosis should be given for successful performance because it is unlikely that a laryngoplasty will successfully abduct the affected arytenoid.

## Laryngeal Hemiplegia

There are few diseases of the horse that inspire as many differences of opinion, as much spirited debate, or evoke the citation of more historical references and quotes from antiquity as laryngeal hemiplegia.[48–52] Although this important disease has been widely recognized for over two centuries and volumes of clinical information have been recorded, it remains one of the most frequently diagnosed but least understood diseases of the upper airway. We do know that with this condition, the horse cannot fully dilate the larynx on the affected side and this produces an obstruction to airflow. Most horses with laryngeal hemiplegia are presented with a complaint of decreased exercise tolerance and abnormal inspiratory noise production at exercise. The noise is usually characterized as a whistle or a roar, hence the term "roarer" has become synonymous with laryngeal hemiplegia. The paralysis is usually left sided and may be partial or complete. Right sided and bilateral paralyses are occasionally encountered.[53–55] In the majority of horses with left laryngeal hemiplegia, no precise cause is evident hence the term idiopathic is applied. An iatrogenic cause, such as a perivascular injection, can frequently be found for a right sided laryngeal hemiplegia, while CNS disease is the usual cause of a bilateral laryngeal paralysis.[53]

The primary lesion associated with idiopathic laryngeal hemiplegia (ILH) is damage to the left recurrent laryngeal nerve.[54] This results in neurogenic atrophy of the intrinsic laryngeal musculature supplied by that nerve, the most important of which is the cricoarytenoideus dorsalis muscle which abducts the arytenoid cartilage. The adductor muscles are similarly affected, with the cricoarytenoideus lateralis being more severely affected than the abductor.[56] The lesion in the recurrent laryngeal nerve is characterized by a distal, progressive loss of large myelinated nerve fibers. These pathologic changes are not limited to the left recurrent laryngeal nerve and are also found in the right recurrent laryngeal nerve as well as in some long peripheral nerves of the distal hindlimb.[56] However, the changes are most severe in the left recurrent laryngeal nerve and the degree of neurogenic myopathy correlates strongly with the severity of the nerve damage.[57] It is interesting to note that this neuropathy and the neurogenic atrophy of the laryngeal muscles supplied by the left recurrent laryngeal nerve have been found in horses that are clinically normal with no endoscopic evidence of laryngeal hemiplegia.[57,58] These horses have been classified as being subclinical, however, there is no evidence that they have a progressive condition.[49] In these subclinical horses, the left cricoarytenoideus lateralis, an adductor, was more severely affected than the abductor. It has been concluded from the study of nerves from normal as well as subclinically and clinically affected horses that left laryngeal hemiplegia can be attributed to a distal axonopathy that is the result of repeated episodes of segmental demyelination.[56]

The condition of ILH can be encountered in horses of all ages, from a few months to 10 years of age or older but the incidence is highest in young horses, particularly 2- and 3-year-old racehorses. In one study, nearly half of a group of affected Thoroughbreds showed clinical signs of the disease before they were 3 years old.[59] ILH has become quite a frequent observation in yearlings and this has led to problems at sales, where these horses often become the subjects of dispute between buyers and sellers. At present, the documented incidence of ILH in Thoroughbred sales yearlings is no less than 2.75%, but the incidence in the entire yearling population is likely to be higher.[51] Endoscopic surveys of racehorses, 2 years of age and older, showed a prevalence of ILH that ranged from 2.6 to 4.7%.[51] Another study of 169 Thoroughbreds of all ages on one farm showed ILH to be present in 8.3% of the population.[61] It would appear, therefore, in light of recent publications which estimate that over 90% of Thoroughbreds have some degree of recurrent laryngeal neuropathy (based on external laryngeal palpation and diagnosis of muscle atrophy), that the prevalence of ILH in any population of horses is dependent primarily on the bias of the diagnostic criteria established by the individual making the diagnosis.[50,52,60]

In some cases of acquired laryngeal hemiplegia, a specific etiology can be identified. Damage to the recurrent laryngeal nerve can occur as a sequel to perivascular inflammation, guttural pouch mycosis, strangles abscessation, neoplasms of the neck or chest and injuries to the neck, and as complications of surgical procedures of the neck, such as esophagostomy or tracheal reconstruction. Other conditions that have been documented as direct causes of laryngeal paralysis include plant poisoning, lead intoxication, and organophosphate intoxication.[53,55] Bacterial and viral toxins and thiamine deficiency are also proposed causes.[55,61] As mentioned previously, horses with right sided laryngeal hemiplegia often have an iatrogenic cause such as a perivascular injection or there may be an intrathoracic lesion such as a lung abscess causing the disease. Horner's syndrome may be seen in conjunction with the laryngeal paralysis produced by perivascular inflammation if the cervical sympathetic nerve trunk has also been damaged.

The cause of ILH is speculative and appears to be related to a number of factors. Large breed horses such as Thoroughbreds and draft horses, heavy horses, and horses greater than 16 hands tall are all more likely to be affected. There may be a higher incidence of ILH in males, although this has not been proven conclusively.[50,59] Long necked horses are purported to be predisposed to developing ILH by virtue of the tensile forces placed on the left recurrent laryngeal nerve when the horse moves its head and neck up or bends it to the right.[55] Repeated stretching of the nerve may lead to ischemic nerve damage.[63] Other proposed causes of left recurrent laryngeal nerve degeneration include trauma from pulsation of the aortic arch or compression from enlarged thoracic lymph nodes. As a result of the more recent findings that the left recurrent nerve damage is only part of a more generalized peripheral neuronal axonopathy that affects the right recurrent laryngeal nerve as well, one is tempted to dismiss the hypothesis of repeated stretching of trauma of the left recurrent laryngeal nerve due to its differing anatomic pathway. Certain management practices such as severe and premature training have also been implicated in predisposing horses to ILH.[55]

It is possible that ILH is a congenital condition that is heritable.[52,64–66] Although there is evidence to support this theory, and a dominant gene has been suggested, the mode of inheritance has not yet been elucidated. A recent study showed that out of 47 offspring from an affected stallion 47% were judged to be suspect or affected compared to 10% of a control group.[66] In this study endoscopic and clinical examinations were used, and pathologic findings also confirmed the sire's status; other studies have not shown such a high percentage of affected offspring by a stallion with laryngeal hemiplegia. Even if it is genetic, non-genetic factors may be a cause in some cases.

The dysfunction caused by ILH has been eloquently explained and illustrated by Cook.[52,60,67] In response to sustained exercise, the larynx of a normal horse dilates maximally to accommodate the increased inspiratory and expiratory airflows. Prolonged and constant dilatation is necessary to prevent dynamic collapse of the larynx in the face of increased negative inspiratory pressure. In a horse affected with laryngeal hemiplegia, there is a collapse of the affected arytenoid into the airway producing an obstruction. As the inspiratory pressure increases, there is a passive adduction of the affected arytenoid, further narrowing the laryngeal lumen. The arytenoid cartilage and the vocal fold on the affected side provide an impedance to inspiratory airflow which limits flow rates and increases the work of breathing. The exercise intolerance that is associated with laryngeal hemiplegia may be attributable to a more rapid development of hypoxemia, hypercarbia, and metabolic acidosis than in a normal horse doing the same work. It may also be related to an increased oxygen cost of breathing.[26] The abnormal inspiratory noise produced with exercise is the result of air turbulence created by the asymmetric larynx. The characteristic "whistle" sound is produced by air passing over the patent left lateral ventricle and saccule which act as resonators.

Clinically, horses with laryngeal hemiplegia are presented because of making an abnormal inspiratory noise at exercise and/or showing some degree of exercise intolerance. The horse generally makes a roaring or whistling sound that gets louder the longer and harder the horse works. The degree of noise production and the capacity for exercise can vary greatly between horses with the same apparent degree of paralysis. The history may indicate that the condition was apparent from the time the horse was first broken as a yearling and became more apparent as training progressed or it may reveal that the condition was recently acquired. In a horse with an acquired ILH, the onset of signs may be relatively acute or slowly progressive over months of time. Horses with bilateral laryngeal paralysis have severe respiratory compromise and frequently require an emergency tracheostomy.

If possible, a horse suspected of having ILH should receive a physical and endoscopic examination at rest and following exercise, and be observed at exercise for evidence of a respiratory noise. Endoscopic examination of the horse while it is exercising on a treadmill may be indicated in some cases. The horse should not be tranquilized or sedated and should be minimally restrained with a nose twitch for the endoscopic examinations. In the case of a yearling being examined for sale, particularly in North America, it may not be possible to perform an exercise test and the diagnosis

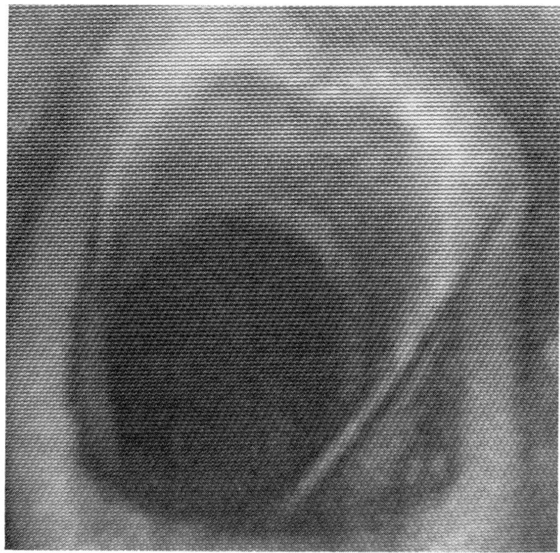

**FIG. 20–33.** Maximal abduction of the arytenoid cartilages.

must be made solely on the basis of physical and endoscopic examinations at rest. It is definitely preferable to exert the yearling until it is breathing deeply and rapidly so any abnormal respiratory noises might be heard.[51,69]

In addition to an endoscopic examination of a horse being evaluated for laryngeal hemiplegia, the evaluation can also include palpation of the larynx, the arytenoid depression test, the "grunt" test and the "slap" test, and a measurement of intermandibular width.[52,60]

1. Endoscopic Evaluation. During an endoscopic evaluation, the range of motion of the arytenoid cartilages is evaluated (Fig. 20–33). In the resting horse, arytenoid abduction is evaluated during deep inspiration produced by occlusion of the nostrils or injection of a respiratory stimulant and following induced swallowing. Full adduction of the arytenoids may be observed if the horse vocalizes or closes the glottis to strain. Slapping the saddle area of the horse's thorax produces what has been described as an adductory flicker on the contralateral side (thoraco-laryngeal reflex).[60] This is known as the "slap test" and in normal horses the response of both arytenoids should be symmetric.[70] The test should be performed while the horse is breathing quietly and during the expiratory phase of respiration.[60]

It has been estimated that 40% of all horses show some degree of asynchronous abduction at rest.[71] This asynchronous movement, however, can cause some interpretive problems. On initial viewing through the endoscope, the left arytenoid may be resting in a more medial position than the right or may adduct more quickly than the right following abduction. Occasionally the right arytenoid is in question. Some veterinarians view asynchronous movement of an arytenoid cartilage as an abnormality and refer to the condition as laryngeal hemiparesis. However, unless contradictory evidence can be produced and both arytenoid cartilages can abduct maximally, asynchronous movement of the arytenoids should be considered to be a variation of normal and of no current clinical significance.[49,71] The controversy surrounding the endoscopic interpretation of laryngeal asynchrony (hemiparesis) and its significance will not be settled until prospective studies conclusively correlate its effect on laryngeal function during performance.

In a horse with laryngeal hemiplegia, the endoscopic appearance of the larynx at rest and following exercise is dependent on the degree of paralysis. If paralysis is complete, the affected arytenoid cartilage exhibits little or no movement and is displaced towards midline (Figs. 20–34 and 20–35). Its position lies in the median or fully adducted to the

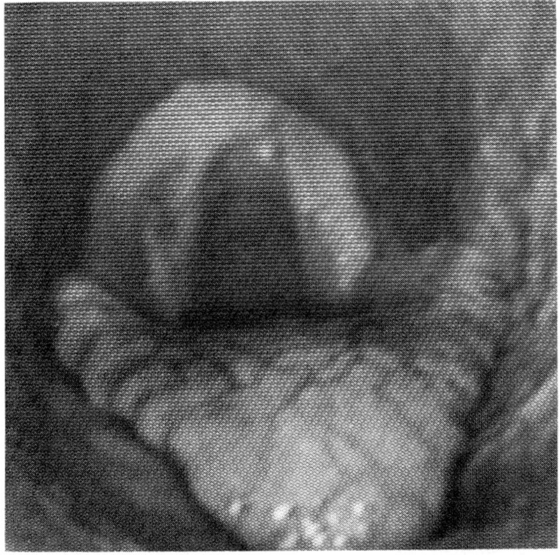

**FIG. 20–34.** Left laryngeal hemiplegia. The left arytenoid is displaced toward midline.

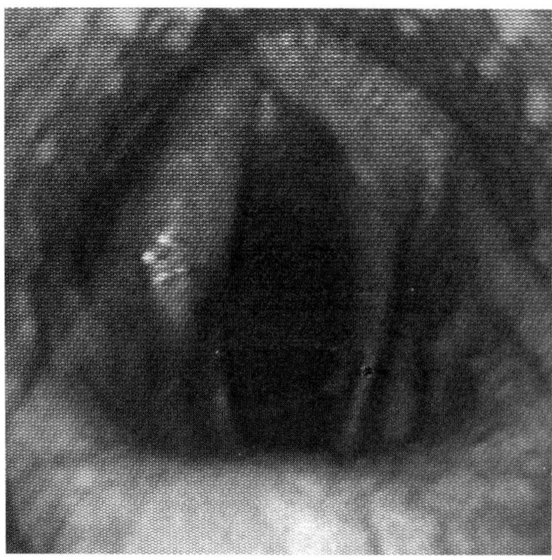

**FIG. 20–35.** Right laryngeal hemiplegia caused by a perivascular reaction following a right jugular injection.

intermediate range. The vocal fold on the affected side is more obvious as is the opening into the lateral ventricle. The piriform recess, lateral to the corniculate process of the paralyzed arytenoid, is also visible. In horses that have incomplete laryngeal paralysis, there is a loss of abductor function, however, the degree of collapse of the affected cartilage will vary depending on the severity of the neurogenic muscle atrophy. All horses with laryngeal hemiplegia should be carefully examined for evidence of arytenoid chondritis.

In horses that are subtly affected, a loss of abductor function may be difficult to detect with endoscopy at rest. However, in most horses with ILH there is some degree of reduced abductor function even at rest. If it is questionable whether there is normal abductor function, the horse should be exercised and examined immediately after exercise or even during exercise if a high speed treadmill is available. As the horse exercises and fatigues, so will the affected cricoarytenoideus dorsalis muscle. During or immediately following hard exercise, a horse should have a symmetrically dilated larynx with both arytenoids fixed in maximal abduction. In a horse with ILH there will be some loss of abductor function of the affected arytenoid and any asymmetry observed in the resting state will be exaggerated.[49]

2. Palpation of the Larynx. Using the index finger of each hand, both sides of the larynx are palpated in the region of the muscular process. In more advanced cases of neurogenic atrophy of the cricoarytenoideus dorsalis, the muscular process on the affected side will be more prominent and there will be a slight depression over the dorsal aspect of the cricoid cartilage. Cook believes that laryngeal palpation is a reliable and sensitive method for evaluating the degree of muscle atrophy associated with recurrent laryngeal neuropathy.[52,60] He grades the disease from I to IV with Grades I to III representing increasing degrees of muscle atrophy associated with hemiparesis (incomplete paralysis) and Grade IV representing hemiplegia (complete paralysis) with no response to the slap test.[60]

The horse should also be examined for scars suggestive of a previous laryngotomy or laryngoplasty. If a laryngotomy was performed, there is likely to be some thickening in the skin beneath the larynx as well as adhesion of the skin to the subcutaneous tissue along the scarline. Clipping of the hair usually enables positive identification of incisional scars.

3. Arytenoid Depression Test. The examiner is positioned in front of the horse with the horse's chin resting on his shoulder and his ear next to the horse's nostril. Using one or two fingers, the muscular process of each arytenoid is depressed. In a horse with laryngeal hemiplegia, pressure on either arytenoid may produce an inspiratory stertor, although less force is required on the affected side to produce a noise, and depression of both arytenoids will produce a much louder inspiratory noise.[49,55]

4. Grunt Test. Atrophy of the adductor muscles in the laryngeal hemiplegic leads to an inability of the horse to close its glottis and maintain an airtight seal.[64] This may result in a prolonged grunt when the horse is threatened with a stick.

5. Slap Test. As previously mentioned, the slap test is performed to evaluate adductor function during the endoscopic examination.[70] The test can also be performed without the benefit of an endoscope by palpating for

movement of the muscular process while an assistant slaps the horse's thorax.[60] In a horse with laryngeal hemiplegia, a slap on the contralateral thorax during expiration will elicit either no response if the paralysis is complete or a diminished, asymmetrical response if the paralysis is incomplete.

6. Intermandibular Width. With the back of the right hand in contact with the ventral surface of the neck, the flexed fingers of that hand are inserted to the level of the first knuckle into the intermandibular space at the angle of the jaw. The intermandibular width is commonly expressed as a finger width, with each finger representing approximately 1.8 cm.[52,60] Horsemen have long believed that a young horse with an intermandibular width of less than 4 fingers is an undesirable prospect as a racehorse. They reason that a narrow jaw indicates an equally narrow pharynx and feel that a horse with a narrow jaw will have a limited ability to move air, a situation which would compromise racing performance. Cook has taken this idea even further and has postulated that not only is there a direct correlation between intermandibular width and racing performance, but there is also an inverse relationship between the intermandibular width and the degree or grade of recurrent laryngeal neuropathy.[52,60] On the basis of his examination of a large number of horses of all ages, primarily Thoroughbreds, he suggests that the wide jawed horse has a lower degree of recurrent laryngeal neuropathy. This hypothesis, however, has not gained universal acceptance.

Another indication of abnormal adductor function is an inability to vocalize normally. Although this is not a consistent finding in all roarers, many will sound hoarse when they phonate. Horses that have had laryngeal "tie-back" surgery also vocalize abnormally.

The type of surgical treatment chosen for left laryngeal hemiplegia is dependent on the intended use of the horse and the surgeon's preference. Surgical options include a laryngeal "tie-back," utilizing an abductor muscle prosthesis; ventriculectomy—unilateral or bilateral, alone or in combination with a laryngoplasty; arytenoidectomy; and nerve implantation. In my opinion, arytenoidectomy should be reserved for treatment of arytenoid chondritis and failure of laryngoplasty. Implantation of the second cervical nerve or a pedicle formed from a portion of the omohyoideus muscle and second cervical nerve into the cricoarytenoideus muscle and anastomosis of the first cervical nerve to the severed abductor branch of the recurrent laryngeal nerve are experimental techniques that have failed to restore functional abductor ability.[72] None of these surgical procedures will ever restore complete and normal function to the larynx; however, some do provide obvious salvage value.

Despite the pessimism of a noted veterinary researcher,[73] "In my opinion, these surgical prostheses have about as much value for an equine athlete in respiratory terms as a wooden leg has for a human athlete in orthopedic terms," most veterinary surgeons, at least in North America, feel that a prosthetic laryngoplasty, usually in combination with a ventriculectomy, can be quite effective for restoring performance and reducing airway noise.[74] In racehorses, in which airflow rates are high and movement of a large volume of air is critical for a sustained performance, stabilization of the affected arytenoid cartilage in an abducted position minimizes inspiratory resistance and reduces the work of breathing. The flow limitations associated with left laryngeal hemiplegia can be significantly improved with a prosthetic laryngoplasty but not with a ventriculectomy alone.[75] Although the degree of abduction achieved with an abductor muscle prosthesis may vary greatly between horses, it is my opinion that moderate to full abduction is considered optimal (Fig. 20–36), particularly in high speed horses if they are to compete successfully with horses of equal ability. In other types of performance horses, where the effort is less strenuous or long, sustained maximal effort is not necessary, a lesser degree of abduction may be acceptable. Generally, a successful laryngoplasty also reduces noise production, frequently to a level that is acceptable in the show ring. However, the results with regard to decreasing noise are somewhat unpredictable.

Although ventriculectomy alone is of questionable value as the sole treatment for laryngeal hemiplegia in a racehorse, it can be quite

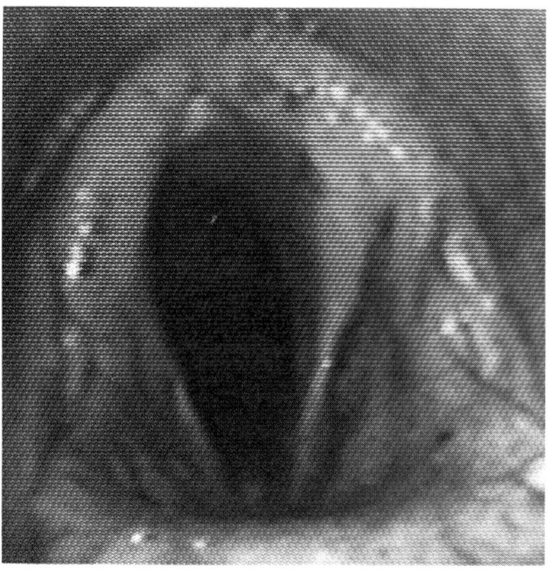

**FIG. 20–36.** Endoscopic examination of a horse 1 day following a left laryngoplasty shows good abduction of the left arytenoid cartilage.

effective in restoring exercise tolerance and reducing noise production in work horses, particularly pulling horses of the draft breeds. Although there is a scar formed over the opening to the lateral ventricle following a ventriculectomy, the procedure does not create a permanent adhesion between the arytenoid and thyroid cartilages nor does it produce abduction of the affected arytenoid.[67] Rather, the benefits of a ventriculectomy can be attributed to a smoothing of the contour of the lumen of the larynx, thereby reducing air turbulence, and to increasing the resistance of the paralyzed arytenoid to passive adduction during maximal inspiration.[67,77]

Generally, there is no reason to delay surgical treatment of laryngeal hemiplegia once the diagnosis is made. Horses with ILH have a progressive deterioration over time and those with an iatrogenic laryngeal hemiplegia rarely show improvement. I have had experience with only one horse that showed nerve regeneration. This was a young foal with left laryngeal hemiplegia induced by irritating guttural pouch flushes. Over a period of 12 months, the foal regained over 80% abductor function of the left arytenoid as evaluated endoscopically. I do have reservations, however, about performing a laryngoplasty on a horse that is clinically affected but has greater than 75% range of arytenoid motion and would advise the client to wait at least 1 to 2 months with the hope that the paralysis progresses considerably. I think there is a greater chance of suture pull out if a great deal of adductor and abductor muscle function remains. Although some surgeons feel that the failure rate of laryngoplasty is greater in 2-year-old horses, because of decreased cartilage holding power, I do not delay surgery until they are 3 years of age, primarily for economic reasons.

A laryngoplasty is usually performed in combination with a ventriculectomy in an attempt to optimize the potential for streamlined airflow. If the laryngoplasty successfully fixes the arytenoid in near maximal abduction, the vocal fold is tight and the opening to the saccule is effectively closed. In this situation, providing that abduction is maintained, a ventriculectomy is not necessary and would offer little improvement to airflow. However, if the laryngoplasty effects only moderate abduction, a ventriculectomy could augment the effectiveness of the surgery. Therefore, since a laryngoplasty does not always produce the desired degree of abduction, I perform both procedures, with some exceptions. In situations when resting the horse 45 to 60 days following surgery is economically unacceptable to the owner, I have performed a laryngoplasty alone and allowed the horse to resume training in 10 to 14 days when the incisional swelling had subsided. The owner should be warned of the increased chances of failure in this situation.

## *Laryngeal Abductor Muscle Prosthesis—Laryngoplasty*

The original laryngoplasty technique described by Marks et al. was well conceived and featured the placement of an extraluminal, elastic suture from the caudal border of the cricoid to the muscular process of the arytenoid that served to simulate the pull of the cricoarytenoideus dorsalis muscle.[74] Since the introduction of this laryngoplasty technique in 1970, various modifications have been reported including the use of nonelastic prosthetic suture material. It has since been shown that there is less acute and chronic tissue reaction to an inelastic, braided nonabsorbable suture material than to an elastic fiber suture.[76]

Prior to surgery, I treat the horse prophylactically with broad spectrum antibiotics. Phenylbutazone may also be administered to minimize postoperative swelling. The horse is anesthetized and placed in lateral recumbency with the affected side up and the head and neck fully extended. A 15-cm skin incision, extending from the cranial aspect of the larynx to the level of the first tracheal ring, is made parallel and slightly ventral to the linguofacial vein. The linguofacial vein and the omohyoideus muscle are separated bluntly with Metzenbaum scissors, leaving enough connective tissue attached to the vein to hold sutures for closure. This plane of dissection is continued lateral to the larynx by blunt digital separation of the surrounding fascial attachments. In some cases it is necessary to ligate the vascular pedicle from the linguofacial vein that supplies the omohyoideus muscle in order to increase exposure. A wide, malleable retractor is placed into the incision to retract the tissues dorsally and the dorsal ridge and the caudal notch of the cricoid are identified by palpation. The thyropharyngeus and cricopharyngeus muscles are bluntly separated with scissors to allow access to the muscular process of the arytenoid cartilage. Careful dissection minimizes the trauma to the blood vessels and cranial laryngeal nerve which supply these muscles. The next step is to place the prosthesis.

I prefer No. 2 Mersilene for the prosthesis although other nonabsorbable suture materials such as No. 5 Dacron, Polydek and Ethibond are currently used by other surgeons.[6,9] A double strand of No. 2 Mersilene is threaded through a ½ circle, trochar point Torrington needle and the ends are tagged with a small forceps. The needle is then grasped in needle holders and placed into the incision with its point positioned in the notch on the caudal aspect of the cricoid cartilage. This notch is situated slightly lateral to the dorsal midline. The index finger of the operator's hand should be placed over the notch and the point of the needle to maintain tactile appreciation of the position of the needle and to ensure that no other structures are inadvertently incorporated in the suture bite. The point of the needle is then "walked" off the back of the cricoid, until the inner surface is reached. With a turn of the wrist, the needle is advanced rostrally through the lamina of the cricoid to emerge just lateral to the dorsal ridge, located on midline, approximately 1 to 1.5 cm rostral to the caudal border. It is critical that the needle point penetrate no deeper than the submucosa of the inner surface of the cricoid cartilage in order to avoid penetration of the lumen of the larynx.[6] If the lamina of the cricoid feels particularly thin, I try to increase the width of the suture bite. Axial placement of the suture is important to simulate accurately the forces applied by the cricoarytenoideus dorsalis muscle. If the suture is placed too far laterally, greater than 1.0 cm from midline, tension in the suture is liable to produce inadequate abduction or even adduction of the arytenoid and the suture may slip laterally and loosen.

As the needle emerges from the cricoid, the surgeon can locate the point of emergence with an index finger and guard the needle point. The suture is drawn through the cricoid, the needle is cut off, and the suture ends are tagged with a small forceps. A curved Kelley hemostat is passed under the cricopharyngeus muscle and the soft tissue covering the larynx from rostral to caudal, to the point where the leading end of the prosthesis has perforated the soft tissue overlying the cricoid. The hemostat is then pushed through this tissue, immediately adjacent to the prosthesis, and the leading end of the prosthesis is grasped and drawn under the cricopharyngeus muscle. The prosthesis is threaded on a smaller trochar point needle and this needle is passed through the muscular process of the arytenoid in a medial to lateral and slightly caudal to rostral direction; the surgeon must be careful to have the point of the needle penetrate the lateral aspect of the muscular process above the level of the thyroid cartilage. Another method for placement of the prosthesis through the muscular process involves drilling a hole with a 16-gauge needle and inserting a crochet hook which is used to draw the suture through the hole.[74] The trailing end of the prosthesis is drawn under the cricopharyngeus muscle and both strands of the suture are tightened maximally and tied together. The suture is digitally examined to ensure that it is tight and it is palpated as it curves around the caudal border of the cricoid lamina to ensure that it has not cut through the cartilage. At this time, if the surgeon is not confident that the suture will hold, the suture should be removed and replaced or a second suture should be placed adjacent to the first to provide reinforcement.

Simple interrupted sutures of 3-0 synthetic absorbable material are used to oppose the cricopharyngeus and thyropharyngeus muscles. The connective tissue and fascia adjacent to the linguofacial vein are sutured to the omohyoideus muscle with simple interrupted sutures of 2-0 synthetic absorbable suture material and the skin is closed with a size 0, monofilament nonabsorbable suture material. Drains are not necessary.

Intraoperative problems associated with a laryngoplasty include:

1. Hemorrhage. This usually results from perforation of a laryngeal vessel during placement of the suture in the cricoid cartilage. Bleeding can be slowed by applying digital pressure or packing the area with sponges. Hemorrhage usually ceases when the prosthesis is tied.

2. Broken Needle. If a fine cutting needle is used or excessive bending forces are applied to the needle during passage through the cricoid or muscular process of the arytenoid, the needle may break. Broken needles should be retrieved, although it is not always possible. Use of a trochar point Torrington needle minimizes the chances of needle breakage.

3. Penetration of the Lumen of the Larynx. This will occur if too deep a bite is taken through the cricoid cartilage. Penetration of the lumen will result in contamination of the suture and granuloma formation at the point of penetration and usually necessitates future removal of the prosthesis. This complication can be avoided by careful placement of the needle through the cricoid cartilage.

4. Suture Pulling through the Cartilage. While the suture is being tied, the operator may feel a sudden release of tension if the suture pulls through either of the cartilages. I have experienced this when a prosthesis was tightened; it pulled through the cricoid cartilage and I attributed it to the horse having an inherently weak cartilage. If it happens, the suture should be replaced in a slightly different location and less tension should be applied to the suture prior to tying it. This suture may also be reinforced with a second, adjacent prosthetic suture or a suture can be placed from the muscular process to the adjacent wing of the thyroid cartilage in order to further stabilize the abducted arytenoid.

5. Incorporation of the Esophagus in the Prosthesis. Although rare, this complication produces immediate postoperative signs of choke. A stomach tube or endoscope cannot be passed beyond the obstruction. If this occurs, a second operation is required and the suture replaced. This can be avoided by guarding the needle point with the left index finger as it passes through the cricoid cartilage.

6. Inadequate Abduction of the Arytenoid Cartilage. Often this can be attributed to inaccurate placement of the prosthesis. In some horses, however, even with an accurately placed prosthesis, satisfactory abduction is not achieved. Long standing hemiplegics may develop some degree of ankylosis of the cricoarytenoid joint that limits abductor motion, or structural abnormalities of the arytenoid cartilage may preclude abduction.[67]

7. Excessive Abduction. It is possible to exert too much tension on the prosthetic suture and over abduct the arytenoid cartilage. This happens infrequently, but can result in postoperative aspiration that can lead to a chronic cough and aspiration pneumonia. It is difficult to advise on how to avoid this problem because even the most experienced surgeons may create an over abduction of the arytenoid. Intraoperative endoscopic viewing of the larynx, while the suture is being tied, is thought by some to be useful to evaluate the degree of abduction but it has been my experience that there is not a good correlation between the perceived degree of intraoperative abduction and the actual position of the arytenoid following surgery.

## *Ventriculectomy*

The modern day ventriculectomy procedure was described by Williams in 1907 and popularized by Hobday, for whom the operation was named.[77] The operation is best performed under anesthesia with the horse in dorsal recumbency and the head and neck extended straight from the body. Usually the procedure is being done following a laryngoplasty while the horse is under general anesthesia. Ventriculectomy alone, however, can be performed under intravenous anesthesia or if anesthesia is considered to be too great a risk, it can be performed with the horse standing.

A 10-cm skin incision, centered over the larynx, is made on the ventral midline. The sternothyrohyoideus muscles are bluntly separated to expose the ventral surface of the larynx. At this point, the position of the head and neck should be checked to ensure they are straight and not tilted because it is important to make a perpendicular incision into the larynx to avoid lacerating the vocal folds. A self-retaining Weitlaner retractor is then used to retract the muscles and the cricothyroid membrane is sharply incised with a scalpel, from the cricoid cartilage to the body of the thyroid cartilage. The retractor is then placed into the larynx to provide exposure of the lumen. It is not necessary to split the body of the thyroid cartilage and incision of the cricoid cartilage should be avoided. The endotracheal tube is removed in most horses and a roaring burr is introduced into the depths of the ventricle of the affected side and turned to engage its mucosal lining. With traction on the burr, the mucosa is completely everted and excised, flush with the opening to the ventricle, being careful not to cut the vocal fold. The opening to the ventricle is not sutured. Some surgeons perform a bilateral ventriculectomy although there appears to be little justification for removing the saccule on the normal side. The caudodorsal mucosal surface of the larynx should also be inspected for evidence of prosthetic suture penetration into the lumen.

If the sacculectomy is performed in the standing horse, the horse should be sedated with a light dose of acepromazine, xylazine, or a combination of xylazine and butorphanol and restrained in stocks. The area over the larynx is surgically prepared and approximately 20 ml of 2% carbocaine is infiltrated subcutaneously and intramuscularly into the sternothyrohyoideus muscles along the proposed incision line. With the head elevated slightly and extended straight out in front of the horse by an assistant, the right-handed operator positions himself on the right side of the horse and makes a 7-cm skin incision on the ventral midline that is centered over the larynx. The center of the larynx is generally located near a line dropped from the vertical ramus of the mandible. The sternothyrohyoideus muscles are bluntly separated on midline with Mayo scissors and can be further separated digitally by exerting lateral retractive force. Once the muscles are separated, the cricoid and thyroid cartilages and the cricothyroid membrane are palpable.

Using the left hand to separate the muscles over the cricothyroid membrane, the operator takes a scalpel in the right hand and introduces it into the incision until its point rests on the cricothyroid membrane. The scalpel should be grasped at a point near the blade and positioned so the back of the blade rests against the cricoid cartilage. At this point the operator should ensure that the horse's head and neck are straight and that the knife is not angled laterally. During inspiration, the blade is thrust into the lumen of the larynx and the membrane is incised from the cricoid to the body of the thyroid cartilage. The feeling as the blade penetrates the mucosa of the larynx is unmistakable and if it is not experienced, it is likely that the knife was angled laterally and the incision has not extended into the lumen. If the operator suspects this is the case, the blade should be withdrawn and another attempt made slightly rostral to the first. Having the incision into the larynx stray off midline can make the sacculectomy more difficult and also contributes to more postoperative swelling in the larynx. The scalpel should not be thrust deeply into the larynx in order to avoid lacerating the vocal folds or the arytenoid cartilages.

A gauze sponge is cut into small pieces that are grasped securely in the jaws of Allis tissue forceps to create a small swab. This gauze is soaked in local anesthetic and then introduced into the lumen of the larynx and the affected saccule. The mucosa is swabbed repeatedly with these anesthetic soaked sponges until swallowing ceases. Although a roaring burr can be utilized, I prefer a finger technique to evert the saccule. The surgical glove is removed from the left hand and the index finger is introduced into the laryngeal saccule until the dorsal rim of the opening to the saccule rests on the back of the first knuckle. The finger is then slowly withdrawn until the end of the fingernail comes to rest in a narrow furrow that is situated between the opening to the saccule and the ventral border of the arytenoid cartilage. Using a sawing motion, the fingernail is used to make a mucosal incision at this point. The fingertip is introduced through the incision and is used to bluntly separate the saccule from its loose connective tissue attachments. When the saccule is freed of its attachments, it is everted through the mouth of the saccule by flexing and rotating the index finger. Traction is applied with the finger as the saccule is completely everted. Metzenbaum scissors are then grasped in the operator's right hand, the tips are introduced into the larynx, and the tensed, everted saccule is resected along its attached margin.

Regardless of whether the sacculectomy is performed with the horse standing or under anesthesia, the laryngotomy incision is left to heal by second intention. Suturing a laryngotomy incision only promotes the development of incisional infection, cellutitis, and subcutaneous emphysema.

Recently, Tate and Shires have reported on the use of the Nd:YAG laser for ablation of the laryngeal ventricle[78] (Tate LP, personal communication, 1988). The laser fiber is passed through the biopsy port of a flexible fiberoptic endoscope which is inserted into the larynx via the nasal passage. The opening to the ventricle and part of its mucosal lining are ablated. There are minimal intraoperative hemorrhage and postoperative swelling. The benefits of this technique are obvious: a laryngotomy incision is not required and if the procedure is being done in conjunction with a laryngoplasty, the horse does not need to be repositioned. It is possible to perform ventricular ablation in the standing, sedated horse with the use of laser contact points.[78] One of the limitations of the procedure is an inability to ablate completely the ventricular mucosa although preliminary reports would indicate that mucosal remnants do not complicate healing.[78]

## Aftercare

Following a laryngoplasty and/or a ventriculectomy, the horse can be allowed to eat and drink as soon as it is fully recovered from anesthesia. During the first few days following surgery the horse is likely to cough while eating and water, saliva, and feed material may drain from the laryngotomy incision (Fig. 20–37). The laryngotomy incision should be wiped daily with a moist gauze sponge but it is not necessary to scrub the incision with antiseptic solutions. By 3 weeks, the laryngotomy incision is sealed and requires no further care. The laryngoplasty incision should be observed for swelling and signs of infection. Many horses develop a postoperative seroma that causes a swelling lateral to the larynx, above the incision and caudal to the ramus of the mandible but this usually is resolving by 1 week. The horse should receive 6 weeks stall rest with handwalking for exercise and training can be resumed following this rest period. Apparent mild slackening or decreased abduction of the arytenoid is commonly seen if the horse is examined endoscopically following a laryngoplasty, but it is not considered abnormal.

Problems encountered following laryngoplasty and ventriculectomy:

1. Infection. If the laryngotomy incision becomes swollen, has a foul odor, and there is obvious evidence of muscle necrosis, the area between the muscles is packed with nitrofurazone soaked gauze and the horse is started on broad spectrum antibiotics. There is some cause for concern if there is an extensive cellutitis associated with the laryngotomy incision because of its proximity to the laryngoplasty incision. Rarely, a clostridial infection of the laryngotomy incision will cause extensive tissue necrosis.

If progressive swelling develops around the laryngoplasty incision and the horse develops a fever, infection should be suspected. The infected seroma must be drained. This can be accomplished by removing the skin sutures,

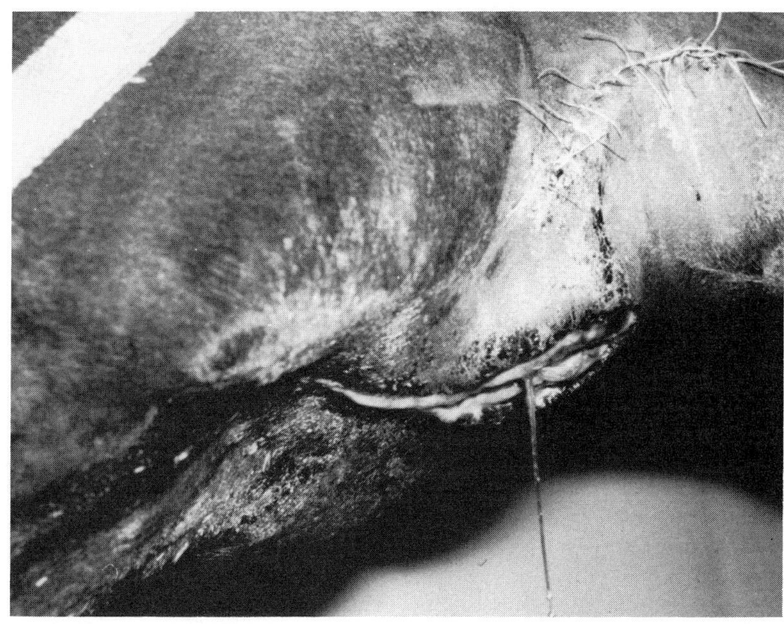

**FIG. 20–37.** Appearance of a laryngotomy incision 1 week after a left laryngoplasty and bilateral sacculectomy. Some saliva can be seen draining from the incision.

surgically preparing the area, and creating a drainage opening by bluntly separating the skin edges and perforating the suture line between the linguofacial vein and the omohyoideus muscle with a mosquito forceps. The fluid that is evacuated should be cultured and antibiotic sensitivities determined. If the prosthesis has become infected, drainage will continue and a chronic draining fistula will develop. Infection of the prosthesis may or may not lead to a failure of laryngoplasty. If the arytenoid remains abducted, despite the infection, the suture should be left in place as long as possible in the hope that fibrous tissue infiltration around the muscular process will fix it in a permanent position, even if the suture must be removed.

2. Chronic Coughing. Some horses develop a chronic cough, particularly during eating. This is likely due to a low grade aspiration of food material into the trachea. In most horses this is not a significant problem, however, the client should be forewarned. Some of the horses that cough also will intermittently have food and water return from the nose, likely as a result of pharyngeal dysfunction related to the surgery.[79]

3. Aspiration Pneumonia. Rarely, a horse will develop a severe aspiration problem following laryngoplasty. These horses develop a persistent cough and a nasal discharge, are febrile, and have an aspiration pneumonia. On endoscopic examination, food material is seen in the trachea. Although this is more likely to occur in a horse where the arytenoid cartilage has been overabducted, it may also develop in horses that have less than a maximally abducted arytenoid. The prognosis in these horses is poor even if the prosthesis is removed.

4. Failed Laryngoplasty. The suture may pull through either the cricoid cartilage or the muscular process of the arytenoid following surgery. If this occurs within the first few days following surgery, the horse can be operated on again immediately. If the prosthesis fails during training or once the horse resumes racing, there are two surgical options: repeat the laryngoplasty or perform a unilateral arytenoidectomy. If the cartilage appears normal endoscopically and has normal structure and minimal calcification radiographically, I prefer to attempt a second laryngoplasty. Even a year later, the laryngoplasty approach is difficult because of the scar tissue surrounding the larynx and there is likely to be a great deal of hemorrhage produced by the dissection. If the first prosthesis can be found, it is removed and the scar tissue around the muscular process is cut with scissors. Using scissors, I also sever adhesions between the lateral aspect of the arytenoid and the lamina of the thyroid in an attempt to mobilize the arytenoid cartilage.

A video endoscope placed in the nasal passage prior to the start of surgery with a view of the larynx can be used to evaluate whether the arytenoid cartilage can be abducted. This is the only time that I use an endoscope during laryngoplasty and I feel that if the arytenoid can be elevated away from the endotracheal tube when tension is placed in the suture, then a successful abduction is likely to be achieved. If the prosthesis does not appear to abduct the arytenoid cartilage, I will place the horse in dorsal recumbency, perform a laryngotomy and proceed with an arytenoidectomy. Although I have had some success with arytenoidectomy following failure of a laryngoplasty, I feel that a successful laryngoplasty is more desirable than an arytenoidectomy. The prognosis for racing success is greater and there are fewer potential complications.

The success rates reported for laryngoplasty and ventriculectomy range from 5 to 90%.[49,80,81] Variables that could account for such a wide range of success include the criteria used to measure success, case selection, and the surgeon's experience and ability. I think that an experienced surgeon can expect that 50 to 75% of the horses with left laryngeal hemiplegia that have a laryngoplasty and ventriculectomy will show marked improvement following surgery. The best prognosis can be given to those horses that have demonstrated ability and performed successfully prior to acquiring ILH. The prognosis is lower in young horses that develop signs of laryngeal hemiplegia early in the training process. I have found in this group that the results of a laryngoplasty are less predictable. Unless the surgeon is left-handed the prognosis is also lower in horses with right laryngeal hemiplegia because of the technical difficulty in placing the prosthetic suture in a "backhanded" fashion. Horses with a concomitant Horner's syndrome have a poor prognosis for racing success because of the obstruction produced by the unilateral nasal obstruction. Those with bilateral laryngeal paralysis can be salvaged with a unilateral laryngoplasty or a permanent tracheostomy.

## Arytenoid Chondritis

The term chondritis has been used to describe a variety of pathologic changes of arytenoid cartilage that produce progressive cartilage enlargement and laryngeal obstruction. Arytenoid chondritis is seen most frequently, although by no means exclusively, in young Thoroughbred race horses and can involve one or both of the arytenoid cartilages. The abnormality occurs most often unilaterally with an equal distribution between the right and left sides. The pathogenesis of arytenoid chondritis is not clearly understood although infection and trauma have been proposed as two etiologic factors in some horses.[9,82–84] Pathologic examination of the diseased cartilages consistently reveals decreases in the craniocaudal and dorsoventral dimensions with increases in the width of the body of the arytenoid cartilage.[84,85] This thickening frequently extends into the corniculate process. The central portion of the arytenoid may be cavitated and communicate with the lumen of the larynx via sinus tracts (Fig. 20–38). Granulomas frequently form around the openings of these tracts and project into the airway. Mucopurulent material may drain from these tracts. A severe infection involving the arytenoid cartilage can also extend into the musculature adjacent to the arytenoid car-

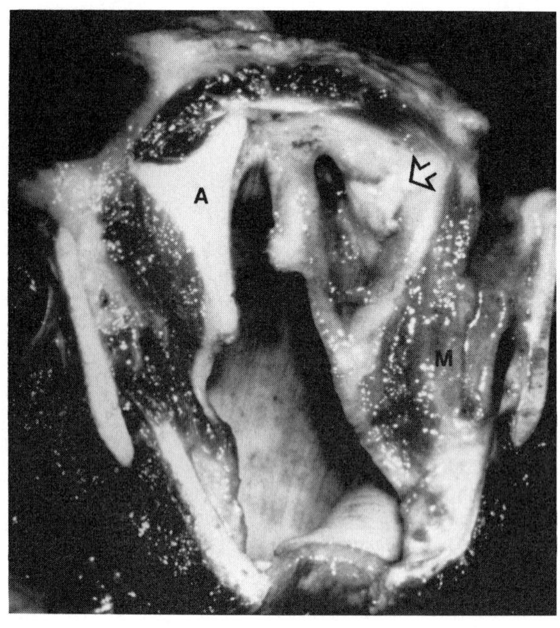


**FIG. 20–38.** Rostral view of a cross section through the larynx of a horse with left arytenoid chondritis. The chondritic cartilage (arrow), which can be compared to the normal arytenoid (A), is enlarged and cavitated. The abaxial musculature (M) is also inflamed.

tilage as well as the cricoid cartilage.[83,84] Paralaryngeal abscessation has also been observed[83] (Fig. 20–39).

The histopathologic descriptions of diseased cartilage vary among cases and even between areas of the same arytenoid cartilage. Chondritic changes in the body of the arytenoid feature a loss of normal hyaline cartilage and replacement with granulation tissue infiltrated with neutrophils, lymphocytes, and macrophages.[82] Chondrosis with hypertrophied chondrocytes and areas of excessive matrix, matrix fibrillation or matrix loss and replacement with vascular connective tissue is also commonly found. Frequently, the affected cartilages and surrounding soft tissues become mineralized as a result of osseous metaplasia.[84]

The overall effect of an arytenoid chondropathy is a reduction in the cross-sectional area of the aditus laryngis as a result of the space occupying effect of the enlarged cartilage and decreased abduction. This loss in the range of abduction is attributed to three factors: thickening of the arytenoid cartilage, inflammation of the musculature surrounding the arytenoid, and involvement of the cricoarytenoid articulation.[9] The severity of clinical signs produced by arytenoid chondritis is dependent on the degree of laryngeal obstruction. The onset of signs may be sudden and severe, particularly with an acute suppurative form of chondritis, or gradual with progressive deterioration over many months. The disease is likely to be discovered in its earliest stages in race horses because they are required to perform at high speed, at which a relatively minor laryngeal airway obstruction will cause the production of an inspiratory noise and exercise intolerance. The initial signs of arytenoid chondritis are similar to those produced by left laryngeal hemiplegia. With progressive enlargement of either one or both arytenoid cartilages, the obstruction becomes more severe. In the most advanced cases of chondritis or chondroma, dyspnea is apparent at rest or with minimal exercise and the obstruction can be life-threatening, necessitating a tracheostomy. In the sedentary or less closely scrutinized horse, a broodmare for example, the condition may be well advanced before signs of an airway obstruction are observed.

A diagnosis of arytenoid chondritis is confirmed, based on the findings of an endoscopic examination. With subtle, unilateral changes, the condition may appear similar to laryngeal hemiplegia, with axial displacement of the affected arytenoid cartilage and reduced abductor function. Closer examination usually reveals ulcerative erosions in the mucous membrane over the medial aspect of the corniculate process, one or more small projections of granulation tissue from the luminal surface, thickening or distortion of the corniculate process and a prominent palato-

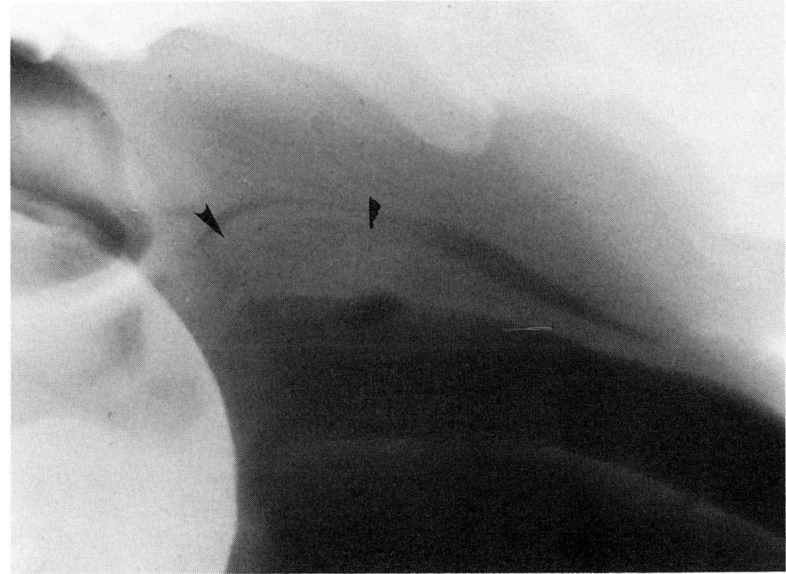

**FIG. 20–39.** Lateral radiograph of the head of a horse with an acute suppurative form of chondritis. A perilaryngeal abscess (arrowheads) is seen as a soft tissue density situated dorsal to the larynx. A small gas pocket can be seen over the caudodorsal aspect of the larynx. A fistulous tract communicated between the lumen of the larynx and the abscess.

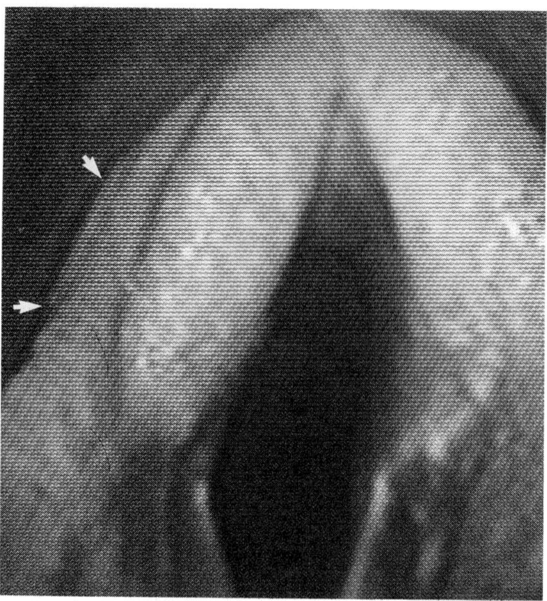

**FIG. 20–40.** On initial inspection, this yearling may appear to have right laryngeal hemiplegia; however, the increased prominence of the right arytenoepiglottic fold and palatopharyngeal arch (arrows) and the presence of a small ulcerative erosion in the mucous membrane on the luminal surface of the arytenoid (not visible on this view) signaled an arytenoid chondritis.

pharyngeal arch on the affected side.[9,82,84] A horse suspected of having right laryngeal hemiplegia should be examined carefully for evidence of chondritis because right arytenoid chondritis occurs far more frequently than right laryngeal hemiplegia[9] (Fig. 20–40). In advanced cases of chondritis, the thickened arytenoid obviously projects into the airway and reduces the size of the laryngeal lumen. Intraluminal projections of granulation tissue frequently produce a contact ulcer on the opposing arytenoid (Fig. 20–41). If both arytenoids are affected, the rima glottis may be reduced to a mere slit. Other endoscopic abnormalities such as entrapment of the epiglottis, dorsal displacement of the soft palate and hypoplasia of the epiglottis may be observed concurrently in a small percentage of cases.[82]

External, digital palpation of the larynx may reveal an enlargement of the affected cartilage with a loss of the normal resiliency.[82] Pressure over the affected arytenoid frequently produces a pronounced dyspnea and a respiratory noise.[82] A lateral radiograph of the larynx of affected horses usually reveals mineralization of the affected cartilages. This must be differentiated from the normal process of laryngeal calcification and ossification that takes place with aging.[86,87] Other radiographic abnormalities include obliteration of the lateral ventricle by the expanded cartilage and soft tissue mass, an enlarged corniculate process, and increased and irregular tissue densities associated with the affected arytenoid cartilage.[84]

In addition to laryngeal hemiplegia, other differential diagnoses for arytenoid chondritis include laryngeal neoplasms, polyps, granulomas, and hypertrophic ossification of the laryngeal cartilages.[87,88] Arytenoid chondroma is occasionally encountered and is usually benign and can be successfully treated with arytenoidectomy.[88] Other tumors of the larynx are rare but include squamous cell carcinoma and lymphosarcoma. These tumors are invasive and have a grave prognosis because they usually metastasize and recur following surgical resection.

When arytenoid chondritis renders a performance horse useless for competition or becomes life threatening to a horse, an arytenoidectomy is indicated. Some horses with

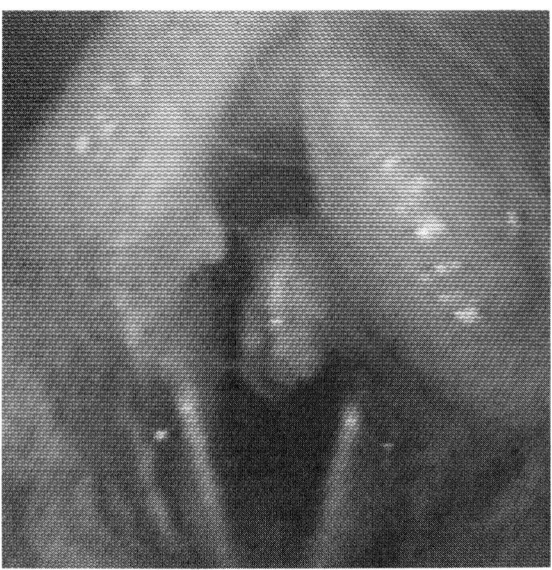

**FIG. 20–41.** An advanced left arytenoid chondritis with an intraluminal projection of granulation tissue. There is a contact ulcer on the opposing arytenoid.

the acute suppurative form of arytenoid chondritis will improve with antibiotic and systemic anti-inflammatory therapy, in combination with a temporary tracheostomy. Although the response is sometimes dramatic, medical treatment palliates the condition but never completely resolves it. Some of these horses even return to work after conservative treatment but the problem usually recurs, often necessitating an arytenoidectomy.

## *Arytenoidectomy*

Beginning in 1843, for a period of approximately 60 years, arytenoidectomy procedures were used for treatment of left laryngeal hemiplegia.[77,82,85,89] Although some horses were returned to work, most suffered from severe postoperative dysphagia and aspiration pneumonia.[89] In the early 1900's arytenoidectomy fell into disuse as a result of the combination of unsatisfactory results and frequent complications and was replaced by the ventriculectomy procedure.[77,89] Within the last 10 years there has been a renewed interest in arytenoidectomy to treat horses with arytenoid chondropathy and a failed laryngoplasty.[77,82,84,85,89–91]

Terms applied to describe the types of arytenoidectomy are total, partial, and subtotal and are based on the extent of the cartilage resection. Removing the entire arytenoid cartilage, including the corniculate and muscular process comprises a total arytenoidectomy. A partial arytenoidectomy involves removing all but the muscular process. With a subtotal arytenoidectomy, there is retention of the corniculate and muscular processes and occasionally the articular facet. Total arytenoidectomy produces a high incidence of serious dysphagia, therefore it is not used except in cases of arytenoid neoplasia when a total resection is desired. Partial and subtotal arytenoidectomy procedures are safer than the total arytenoidectomy and are currently used to treat horses with unilateral or bilateral chondritis, chondroma, ossification of the larynx, neoplasia of the larynx, and those with left laryngeal hemiplegia where a prosthetic laryngoplasty has failed. It would appear from published reports that exercise tolerance can be restored postoperatively with either a partial or a subtotal arytenoidectomy, but that partial arytenoidectomy has a greater potential for producing coughing and dysphagia.[82,85,89,91] If both arytenoids are diseased, a bilateral arytenoidectomy can be performed, however, the prognosis for successful restoration of exercise tolerance is poor and there are increased risks of postoperative complications.[82,92]

Prior to surgery, the ventral neck area is clipped and shaved in preparation for a midventral cervical tracheostomy. A standing tracheostomy should be performed in the severely obstructed horse that is dyspneic and making a respiratory noise. The horse should be oxygenated through the tracheostomy tube prior to induction of anesthesia. Otherwise, the tracheostomy is performed after induction of anesthesia. If an endotracheal tube cannot be passed through the larynx as a result of a luminal obstruction, a tracheostomy should be performed immediately to ensure adequate ventilation during induction of anesthesia. The tracheal incision is made transversely, between adjacent cartilage rings. The cuffed endotracheal tube is introduced through this space and gas anesthetic is administered through this tube (Fig. 20–42). Ordinarily, the tracheostomy is performed once the horse is positioned on the table. A routine laryngotomy is performed and if additional exposure is needed, the thyroid and cricoid cartilages can be incised. The body of the thyroid should be incised on ventral midline with sharp bone-cutting forceps because in many horses this region is ossified.[9] An index finger is inserted into the lumen of the larynx to determine the rostral limit of the body of the thyroid to avoid damage to the base of the epiglottis. The cricoid cartilage can be incised on ventral midline with a scalpel, even if it is mineralized or ossified. Self retaining Weitlaner retractors are used to expose the lumen (Fig. 20–43). The arytenoid cartilages and the luminal surface of the larynx should be visually and manually inspected for mucosal ulcerations and projections, sinus tracts, exudate and cartilage thickening. The width of the affected arytenoid is estimated as the distance between the index finger inserted into

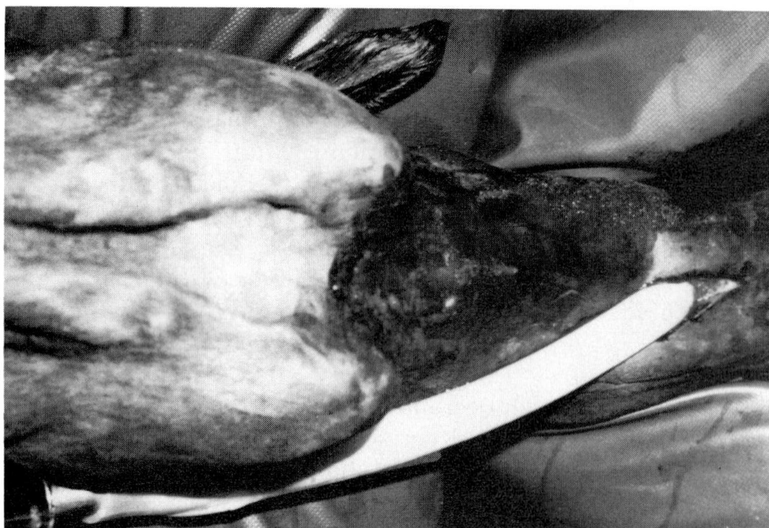

FIG. 20–42. An endotracheal tube is introduced into the tracheostomy incision in preparation for an arytenoidectomy.

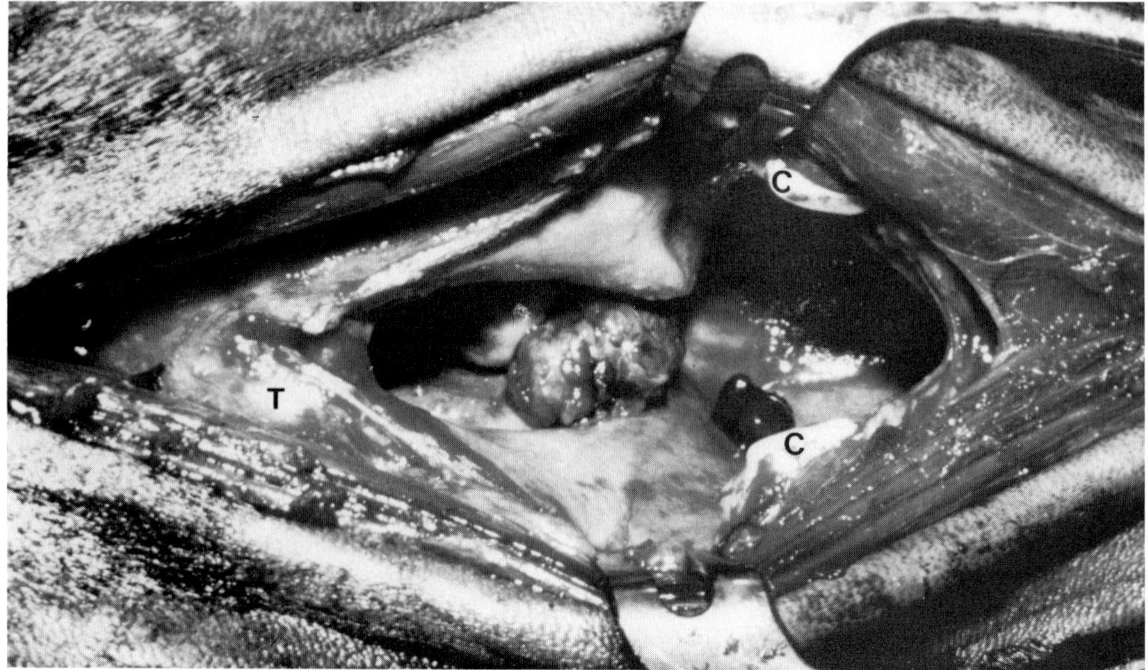


FIG. 20–43. Intraoperative view of the lumen of the larynx just prior to an arytenoidectomy. The body of the thyroid (T) and the cricord cartilage (C) have been incised to increase exposure. A large granulation mass can be seen originating from the chondritic right arytenoid cartilage.

the laryngeal saccule and the opposing thumb in the lumen.

Saline solution (0.9% NaCl) or an epinephrine in saline solution (1:10,000) can be injected submucosally on the luminal side of the arytenoid to elevate the mucosa and reduce hemorrhage.[91] The mucosa overlying the luminal surface of the arytenoid is then incised with a scalpel to allow submucosal dissection over the portion of the arytenoid to be removed.

## Subtotal Arytenoidectomy

A mucosal incision is made vertically along the caudal border of the arytenoid cartilage, from the articular facet, dorsally, to the vocal process, ventrally. This incision is extended rostrally, along the ventral border of the arytenoid to the level of the corniculate process.[9] The mucosa is separated from the underlying cartilage with a periosteal elevator. Efforts are usually made to preserve the mucosa, although this is not possible in areas where it is scarred or ulcerated and adhered to the cartilage or where there are large granulomatous projections. In these areas, the abnormal mucosa is excised. The submucosal dissection is extended to the dorsal midline of the larynx. Using the periosteal elevators or scissors, the abaxial surface of the arytenoid cartilage is then separated from its attachments to the vocalis, vestibularis and cricoarytenoideus lateralis muscles, and the lateral ventricle.[9] If a previous ventriculectomy was performed, the adhesions between the arytenoid and the thyroid cartilages are severed. The cartilage is then incised vertically along the junction of the corniculate process and the body of the arytenoid using scissors or a scalpel. The body of the arytenoid is grasped with Allis tissue forceps and elevated axially and rostrally and using long curved scissors, the muscular process is severed. If the muscular process is ossified, it may be necessary to use a large blade scalpel or rongeurs to complete the amputation. The cricoarytenoid joint can be disarticulated or transected and left in place along with the muscular process.[9] Remaining attachments to the dorsal, abaxial portion of the body of the arytenoid are carefully cut as close to the cartilage as possible using the long curved scissors. Bleeding from the depths of the resection can be controlled with digital pressure. Ragged edges of cartilage or fragments from the muscular or corniculate process should be removed with rongeurs. The lateral ventricle is removed using a laryngeal burr or is dissected free following excision around the opening to the ventricle. If possible, the mucosa is closed over the defect, using size 2-0 synthetic absorbable suture material in a simple interrupted pattern. A mucosal gap should be left to allow for ventral drainage from the considerable dead space and to prevent against development of a hematoma or seroma.

## Partial Arytenoidectomy

In most descriptions of partial arytenoidectomy, the mucosa overlying the axial surface of the arytenoid cartilage is incised vertically, from the level of the laryngeal ventricle to the dorsal midline, and the mucosa is circumferentially freed from the axial surface of the corniculate process and body of the arytenoid.[77,82,85] Alternatively, I prefer to make a vertical mucosal incision, more rostrally, over the corniculate cartilage and extend it along the ventral and caudal margins of the arytenoid, creating a large three-sided mucosal flap. This increases the submucosal exposure of the arytenoid and allows a more careful submucosal dissection around the rostral border of the corniculate process (Fig. 20–44). It is critical that the mucosa overlying the corniculate process be preserved and not be accidentally lacerated or excised during the resection of the corniculate process. This mucosa is thicker than that overlying the axial surface of the body of the arytenoid and is easily separated from the corniculate process with a periosteal elevator. The arytenoid is dissected free of its mucosal and abaxial soft tissue attachments and the muscular process is amputated. The rostral portion of mucosa which folded around the corniculate process should be maintained as a cuff of tissue at the rima glottis rather than being pulled caudally and sutured in an effort to close the mucosal

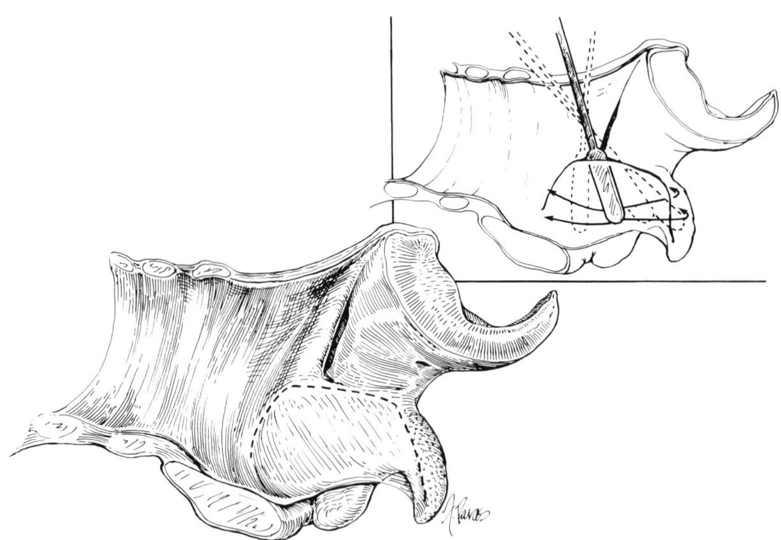

**FIG. 20–44.** Schematic view of a sagittal section of the larynx, showing placement of the mucosal incision (dotted line) and elevation of the mucosa (inset) during a partial arytenoidectomy.

defect and streamline the airway. I feel it is critical that this cuff of mucosa is preserved in order to maintain the contour of the piriform recess and to prevent spillage of material into the larynx. The incised margin of the mucosal cuff can be tacked to the soft tissues laterally with a few simple interrupted sutures of 3-0 absorbable synthetic suture material to eliminate dead space and reduce postoperative swelling. The remaining mucosa is then apposed with a consideration for allowing ventral drainage of the dead space.

Large mucosal gaps can be left to heal by second intention with no untoward effects. In fact, it has been demonstrated experimentally that the healing following unilateral, partial arytenoidectomy without preservation of the mucosa is uncomplicated and completed by 16 weeks. The complications associated with suturing the preserved mucosa such as suture granulomas, hematoma and seroma formation in the submucosal dead space, wound dehiscence, and postoperative airway obstruction are avoided.[93] With a bilateral arytenoidectomy, every effort should be made to preserve the mucosa in the dorsal laryngeal region. If a bilateral mucosal defect is left in the interarytenoid area, the opposing wound surfaces heal together, producing a web of scar tissue in the dorsal larynx. The resultant dorsal glottal stenosis may seriously reduce the cross-sectional area of the rima glottis.[92]

An alternative to a subtotal or a partial arytenoidectomy is simple excision of the protruding, obstructive masses of tissue. In those cases with a central core of necrosis or cavitation of the arytenoid cartilage, the cavity can be opened with a small curette and the lining can be curetted carefully. The only indications for this form of treatment are in a bilaterally affected larynx where the most severely affected arytenoid is removed and the remaining arytenoid is treated in this fashion and in a larynx where a discrete laryngeal polyp is easily excised, leaving a relatively normal arytenoid cartilage.

If the cricoid cartilage was incised, the cut ends should be apposed with simple interrupted sutures (size 2-0, synthetic absorbable material) placed in the soft tissues immediately adjacent to the cartilage. Suture material that passes through the cricoid cartilage may promote chondroma formation. The remainder of the laryngotomy incision is not sutured. The cuffed endotracheal tube is left in place in the trachea while the horse recovers from anesthesia and is replaced with a self retaining tube once the horse is standing. Following a unilateral arytenoidectomy, the tracheostomy tube can usually be removed within 24 hours. After a bilateral arytenoidectomy, where swelling is severe, a tracheostomy tube may be required for as long as a week in order to ensure a patent airway. An

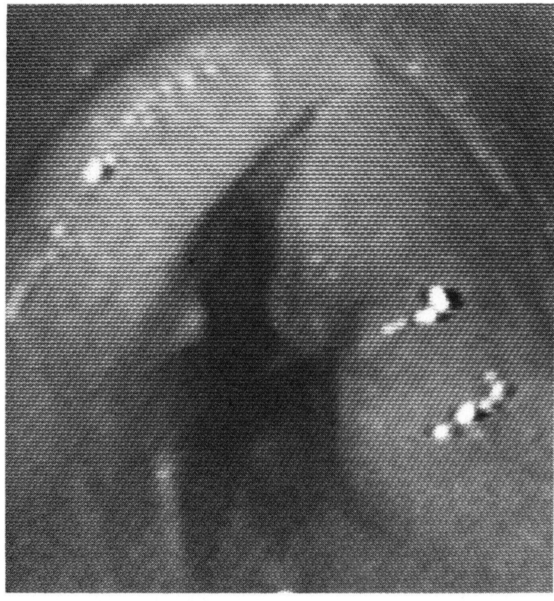

**FIG. 20–45.** Endoscopic view of a larynx (see Fig. 20–41, for preoperative view), 4 days following a partial left arytenoidectomy. There is a great deal of mucosal and soft tissue swelling at the operative site.

endoscopic examination of the surgery site should be performed prior to removal of the tube. Postoperative phenylbutazone, 4.4 mg/kg, IV, s.i.d., will help minimize the degree of laryngeal swelling.

Stall rest is recommended for 60 days following surgery, during which time intermittent endoscopic examinations can be performed to evaluate healing. The mucosa at the arytenoidectomy site remains quite swollen for at least 14 to 21 days (Fig. 20–45). Granulomas may develop around the mucosal sutures or in areas of mucosal dehiscence (Fig. 20–46). As healing progresses, these projections usually disappear, the swelling subsides and at 60 days, healing is usually complete. Rarely, a granuloma that develops around a suture does not resolve and must be resected via laryngotomy. A frequent observation following a partial arytenoidectomy is slight rostral displacement of the palatopharyngeal arch on the affected side. The lumen of the larynx and trachea should be examined for evidence of aspiration of saliva or food material. If this is observed, the prognosis for a successful racing career must be guarded.

The most recent innovation with regard to arytenoidectomy is the use of the Nd:YAG laser to perform partial arytenoidectomy in the standing horse. Early results would indicate that this treatment modality is useful for removing luminal masses as well as portions of the arytenoid cartilage.[94]

Following either a unilateral or bilateral arytenoidectomy, it is common to observe signs that are related to problems with swallowing: coughing, nasal discharge of food and water, and aspiration of food, water, and saliva.[82,85,89] These problems develop because of a loss of the protective function of the larynx during swallowing, after removal of the arytenoid cartilage(s).[77] From some reports, it would appear that these complications occur more frequently following partial arytenoidectomy than subtotal arytenoidectomy.[77,89] It is my opinion, however, that if the thick mucosa that covers the rostral portion of the corniculate process is left intact and in situ, rather than being retracted caudally into the larynx, that the reported incidence of dysphagia associated with partial arytenoidectomy, 36%, can be greatly reduced. Many horses can tol-

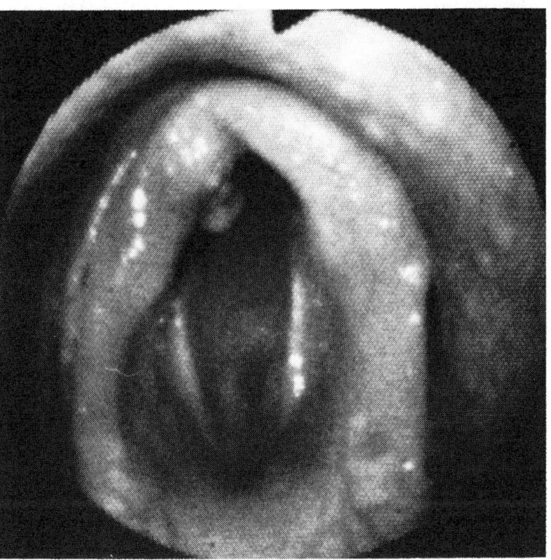

**FIG. 20–46.** View of a larynx 2 weeks following a right partial arytenoidectomy for chondritis. There is a minimal amount of residual mucosal swelling and a granuloma has formed around one of the mucosal sutures.

erate some degree of dysphagia and aspiration and perform successfully. In others, the chronic cough and recurrent bouts of low grade aspiration pneumonia render them useless as performance horses.

Other reported long-term complications include rostral displacement of the palatopharyngeal arch and advanced laryngeal cartilage mineralization.[82]

From the published reports of arytenoidectomy, it is difficult to extract precise figures with regard to the prognosis for a successful return to racing or other performance activities.[82,85,89] The methods of case selection, the criteria established to judge success, the statistical analysis of data, and the surgical techniques employed vary greatly with each study. Some generalizations, however, can be made with regard to arytenoidectomy.

1. It would appear that a unilateral arytenoidectomy procedure meets the goals of increasing the cross-sectional area of the rima glottis, increasing the resistance of the affected side to dynamic collapse and improving the geometry of the airway.[82]

2. The prognosis for return to racing or other performance activity following a unilateral arytenoidectomy would appear to be in the 50 to 60% range.[82,85,89] In my opinion, and as a recent report would suggest, the success rate following unilateral partial arytenoidectomy for treatment of arytenoid chondritis is greater than that for failure of laryngoplasty.[82] This might be because the residual intrinsic muscle activity, which is usually absent in the hemiplegic, provides some support and retraction on the affected side during the healing process and also helps prevent against dynamic collapse during maximal exercise.

3. A significant number of these horses (as high as 50% in one study) develop postoperative complications related to swallowing.[82,85,89]

4. A bilateral arytenoidectomy should be considered as a salvage procedure since the prognosis for a successful return to racing is poor.[82]

It is not clear which arytenoidectomy technique, partial or subtotal, is superior for successfully returning horses to the racetrack. Empirically, the efficacy of each treatment needs to be evaluated in an exercise physiology laboratory by measuring airflows, airway resistance, and metabolic and blood gas changes in exercising horses. In one study, it was demonstrated that subtotal arytenoidectomy had no beneficial effect in the treatment of experimentally induced left laryngeal hemiplegia.[95]

## References


1. Cook WR. Some observations on form and function of the equine upper airway in health and disease: 1. The pharynx. In: Proceedings of 27th Annual Convention of American Association of Equine Practitioners, 1981, p 355.
2. Sisson S. Equine digestive system. In: Sisson and Grossman's The Anatomy of the Domestic Animals. 5th Ed. R Getty (ed). Philadelphia, WB Saunders Co, 1975.
3. Heffron CJ, Baker GJ. Observations on the mechanism of functional obstruction of the nasopharyngeal airway in the horse. Equine Vet J, *11*:142, 1979.
4. Jann HW, Cook WR. Transendoscopic electrosurgery for epiglottal entrapment in the horse. J Am Vet Med Assoc, *187*:484, 1985.
5. Linford RL, O'Brien TA, Wheat JD, et al. Radiographic assessment of epiglottic length and pharyngeal and laryngeal diameters in the Thoroughbred. Am J Vet Res, *44*:1660, 1983.
6. McIlwraith CW, Turner AS. Surgery of the upper respiratory tract. In: Equine Surgery: Advanced Techniques. Philadelphia, Lea & Febiger, 1987, pp 202–259.
7. Harrison IW, Raker CW. Sternothyroidhyoideus myectomy in horses: 17 cases (1984–1985). J Am Vet Med Assoc, *193*:1299, 1988.
8. Raker CW. The nasopharynx. In: Equine Medicine and Surgery, Vol. 3. RA Mansmann and ES McAllister (eds). Santa Barbara, American Veterinary Publications, 1982, p 747.
9. Haynes PF. Surgery of the equine respiratory tract. In: The Practice of Large Animal Surgery. PB Jennings (ed). Philadelphia, WB Saunders, 1984.
10. Blythe LL, Cardinet GH, Meagher DM, et al. Palatal myositis in horses with dorsal displacement of the soft palate. J Am Vet Med Assoc, *183*:781, 1983.
11. Scott EA. Surgery of the oral cavity. In: Veterinary Clinics of North America Large Animal Practice Symposium on Equine Gastrointestinal Surgery. CW McIlwraith (ed). Philadelphia, WB Saunders Co, 1982, pp 3–31.
12. Bowman KF, Tate LP Jr, Evans LH, et al. Complications of cleft palate repair in large animals. J Am Vet Med Assoc, *180*:652, 1982.
13. Mason TA, Speirs VC, Maclean AA, et al. Surgical repair of cleft soft palate in the horse. Vet Rec, *100*:6, 1977.
14. Jones RS, Maisels DO, DeGeus JJ, et al. Surgical re-

pair of cleft palate in the horse. Equine Vet J, *7*:86, 1975.

15. Bertone JJ, Traub-Dargatz JL, Trotter GW. Bilateral hypoplasia of the soft palate and arytenoepiglottic entrapment in a horse. J Am Vet Med Assoc, *188*:727, 1986.
16. Haynes PF, Qualls CW. Cleft soft palate, nasal septal deviation, and epiglottic entrapment in a Thoroughbred filly. J Am Vet Med Assoc, *179*:910, 1981.
17. Becht JL, Semrad SD. Hematology, blood typing, and immunology of the neonatal foal. In: Veterinary Clinics of North America. Equine Practice Symposium on Neonatal Equine Disease. J Beech (ed). Philadelphia, WB Saunders Co, *1*:91, 1985.
18. Nelson AW, Curley BM, Kainer RA. Mandibular symphysiotomy to provide adequate exposure for intraoral surgery in the horse. J Am Vet Med Assoc, *159*:1025, 1971.
19. McAllister S, Blakeslee JR. Clinical observations of pharyngitis in the horse. J Am Vet Med Assoc, *170*:739, 1977.
20. Raker CW, Boles CL. Pharyngeal lymphoid hyperplasia in the horse. J Equine Med Surg, *2*:202, 1978.
21. Auer DE, Wilson RG, Groenendyk S. Pharyngeal lymphoid hyperplasia in Thoroughbred race horses in training. Aust Vet J, *62*:124, 1985.
22. Baker GJ. Diseases of the pharynx and the larynx. In: Current Therapy in Equine Medicine 2. NE Robinson (ed). Philadelphia, WB Saunders Co, 1987, pp 607–612.
23. Burrell MH. Endoscopic and virological observations on respiratory disease in a group of young Thoroughbred horses in training. Equine Vet J, *17*:99, 1985.
24. Raphel CF. Endoscopic findings in the upper respiratory tract of 479 horses. J Am Vet Med Assoc, *181*:470, 1982.
25. Raker CW. Diseases of the pharynx. Mod Vet Pract, *57*:396, 1976.
26. Bayly WM, Grant BD, Breeze RG. Arterial blood gas tension and acid base balance during exercise in horses with pharyngeal lymphoid hyperplasia. Equine Vet J, *16*:435, 1984.
27. Clarke AF, Madelin TM, Allpress RG. The relationship of air hygiene in stables to lower airway disease and pharyngeal lymphoid hyperplasia in two groups of Thoroughbred horses. Equine Vet J, *19*:524, 1987.
28. Todhunter RJ, Brown CM, Stickle R. Retropharyngeal infections in five horses. J Am Vet Med Assoc, *187*:600, 1985.
29. Sweeney CR, Sweeney RW, Raker CW, et al. Upper respiratory tract obstruction caused by a pharyngeal abscess in a filly. J Am Vet Med Assoc, *187*:268, 1985.
30. Koch DB. The oral cavity, oropharynx and salivary glands. In: Mansmann RA, McAllister ES (eds). Equine Medicine and Surgery. 3rd ed. Vol. 2. Wheaton, American Veterinary Publications Inc, 1982, pp 458–476.
31. Brock KA. Pharyngeal trauma from endotracheal intubation in a colt. J Am Vet Med Assoc, *187*:944, 1985.
32. Koch DB, Tate LP. Pharyngeal cysts in horses. J Am Vet Med Assoc, *173*:860, 1973.
33. Stick JA, Boles CL. Subepiglottic cyst in three foals. J Am Vet Med Assoc, *77*:62, 1980.
34. Tulleners EP. Contact Neodynium: YAG laser-assisted excision of upper airway obstructions in the horse. Scientific Meeting Abstracts. ACVS 24th Annual Meeting. Vet Surg, *18*:68, 1989.
35. Haynes PF. Persistent dorsal displacement of the soft palate associated with epiglottic shortening in two horses. J Am Vet Med Assoc, *179*:677, 1981.
36. Schumacher J, Hanselka DV. Nasopharyngeal cicatrices in horses: 47 cases (1972–1985). J Am Vet Med Assoc, *191*:239, 1987.
37. Schuh JCL. Squamous cell carcinoma of the oral, pharyngeal and nasal mucosa in the horse. Vet Pathol, *23*:205, 1986.
38. Lane JG. Palatine lymphosarcoma in two horses. Equine Vet J, *17*:465, 1985.
39. Adams R, Calderwood-Mays MB, Peyton LC. Malignant lymphoma in three horses with ulcerative pharyngitis. J Am Vet Med Assoc, *193*:674, 1988.
40. Boulton CH. Alimentary Tract Neoplasia. In: Current Therapy in Equine Medicine 2. NE Robinson (ed). Philadelphia, WB Saunders Co, 1987, pp 107–109.
41. Boles CL, Raker CW, Wheat JD. Epiglottic entrapment by arytenoepiglottic folds in the horse. J Am Vet Med Assoc, *172*:338, 1978.
42. Tulleners EP. Transendoscopic contact YAG laser correction of arytenoepiglottic fold entrapment in the standing horse: 24 cases. In: Scientific presentation abstracts. ACVS 23rd Annual Meeting. Vet Surg, *17*:44, 1988.
43. Honnas CM, Wheat JD. Epiglottic entrapment. A transnasal surgical approach to divide the aryepiglottic fold axially in the standing horse. Vet Surg, *17*:246, 1988.
44. Haynes PF. Surgical failures in upper respiratory surgery. In: Proceedings of 24th Annual Convention of American Association of Equine Practitioners, 1978, p 233.
45. Wilson RG, Sutton RH, Groenendyk S. Rostral displacement of the palato pharyngeal arch in a Thoroughbred yearling. Aust Vet J, *63*:99, 1986.
46. Goulden BE, Anderson LJ, Davies AS, et al. Rostral displacement of the palatopharyngeal arch: a case report. Equine Vet J, *8*:95, 1976.
47. Cook WR. Some observations on diseases of the ear, nose and throat in the horse, and endoscopy using a flexible fiberoptic endoscope. Vet Rec, *94*:533, 1974.
48. Baker GJ. Roaring, Whistling, Cornage, Siffleurs; Kehlkopfpfeifen, Pfeiferdampf. Equine Vet J, *19*:373, 1987.
49. Baker GJ. Laryngeal hemiplegia in the horse. Comp Cont Ed, *5*:S6, 1983.
50. Cook WR, Williams RM, Kirker-Head, CA, et al. Upper airway obstruction (Partial asphyxia) as the possible cause of exercise-induced pulmonary hemorrhage in the horse: an hypothesis. Eq Vet Sci, *8*:11, 1988.
51. Lane JG, Ellis DR, Greet TRC. Observations on the examination of Thoroughbred yearlings for idiopathic laryngeal hemiplegia. Equine Vet J, *19*:531, 1987.

52. Cook WR. Recent observations on recurrent laryngeal neuropathy in the horse: applications to practice. In: Proceedings of 34th Annual Convention of American Association of Equine Practitioners, 1988, p 427.
53. Duncan ID, Brook D. Bilateral laryngeal paralysis in the horse. Equine Vet J, *17*:228, 1985.
54. Duncan ID, Griffiths IR, McQueen A, et al. The pathology of equine laryngeal hemiplegia. Acta Neuropath, *27*:337, 1974.
55. Marks D, MacKay-Smith MP, Cushing LS, et al. Etiology and diagnosis of laryngeal hemiplegia in horses. J Am Vet Med Assoc, *157*:429, 1970.
56. Cahill JI, Goulden BE. Equine laryngeal hemiplegia Part I. A light microscopic study of peripheral nerves. NZ Vet J, *34*:161, 1986.
57. Cahill JI, Goulden BE. Equine laryngeal hemiplegia Part IV. Muscle pathology. NZ Vet J, *34*:186, 1986.
58. Gunn HM. Histochemical observations on laryngeal skeletal muscle fibers in "normal" horses. Equine Vet J, *4*:144, 1972.
59. Goulden BE, Anderson LJ. Equine laryngeal hemiplegia. Part I: Physical characteristics of affected animals. NZ Vet J, *29*:150, 1981.
60. Cook WR. Diagnosis and grading of hereditary recurrent laryngeal neuropathy in the horse. J Equine Vet Sci, *8*:432, 1988.
61. Hillidge CJ. Prevalence of laryngeal hemiplegia on a Thoroughbred horse farm. J Equine Vet Sci, *5*:252, 1985.
62. Cymbaluk NF, Fretz PB, Loew FM. Thiamine measurements in horses with laryngeal hemiplegia. Vet Rec, *101*:97, 1977.
63. Rooney JR, Delaney FM. An hypothesis on the causation of laryngeal hemiplegia in horses. Equine Vet J, *2*:35, 1970.
64. Cook WR. The diagnosis of respiratory unsoundness in the horse. Vet Rec, *77*:516, 1965.
65. Gunn HM. Further observations on laryngeal skeletal muscle in the horse. Equine Vet J, *5*:77, 1973.
66. Poncet PA, Montavon S, Gaillard C, et al. A preliminary report on the possible genetic basis of laryngeal hemiplegia. Equine Vet J, *21*:137, 1989.
67. Cook WR. Some observations on form and function of the equine upper airway in health and disease: II Larynx. Proceedings of the 27th AAEP, 1981, pp 393–451.
68. Attenburrow DP. Resonant frequency of the lateral ventricle and saccule and "whistling." In Equine Exercise Physiology. Snow DH, Persson SG, Rose RJ (eds). Cambridge, Granta Editions, 1983, pp 27–32.
69. Frank C. Wind examinations. Vet Rec, *121*:156, 1987.
70. Greet TRC, Jeffcott LB, Whitwell KE, et al. The slap test for laryngeal adductory function in horses with suspected cervical spinal cord damage. Equine Vet J, *12*:127, 1980.
71. Baker GJ. Laryngeal asynchrony in the horse: definition and significance. In: Equine Exercise Physiology. Snow DH, Persson SG, Rose RJ (eds). Cambridge, Granta Editions, 1983, pp 46–50.
72. Ducharme NG, Horney FD, Partlow GD, et al: Attempts to restore abduction of the paralyzed equine arytenoid cartilage. I. Nerve muscle pedicle transplants. Can J Vet Res, *53*:202, 1989.
73. Cook WR. Tufts researcher works to develop way to predict racehorse performance. From Tufts University Office of Communications. July 15, 1988.
74. Marks D, Mackay-Smith MP, Cushing LS, et al. Use of a prosthetic device for surgical correction of laryngeal hemiplegia in horses. J Am Vet Med Assoc, *157*:157, 1970.
75. Shappell KK, Derksen FJ, Stick JA, et al. Effects of ventriculectomy, prosthetic laryngoplasty, and exercise on upper airway function in horses with induced laryngeal hemiplegia. Am J Vet Res, *49*:1760, 1988.
76. Merriam JG. Laryngoplasty—an evaluation of three abductor muscle prosthetics. In: Proceedings of 17th Annual Convention of American Association of Equine Practitioners, 1973, p 123.
77. Speirs VC. Laryngeal surgery—150 years on. Equine Vet J, *19*:377, 1987.
78. Shires GM, Adair HS, Patton CS. The use of the Nd:YAG Laser for removal of the laryngeal ventricles in the equine. A pilot study. Unpublished material, 1988.
79. Greet TRC, Baker GJ, Lee R. The effect of laryngoplasty on pharyngeal function in the horse. Equine Vet J, *11*:153, 1979.
80. Goulden BE, Anderson LG. Equine laryngeal hemiplegia. Part III. Treatment by laryngoplasty. NZ Vet J, *30*:1, 1982.
81. Speirs VC, Bourke JM, Anderson GA. Assessment of the efficacy of an abductor muscle prosthesis for treatment of laryngeal hemiplegia in horses. Aust Vet J, *60*:294, 1983.
82. Tulleners EP, Harrison IW, Raker CW. Management of arytenoid chondropathy and failed laryngoplasty in horses: 75 cases (1979–1985). J Am Vet Med Assoc, *192*:670, 1988.
83. Barber SM. Paralaryngeal abscess with laryngeal hemiplegia and fistulation in a horse. Can Vet J, *22*:389, 1981.
84. Haynes PF, Snider TG, McClure JR, et al. Chronic chondritis of the equine arytenoid cartilage. J Am Vet Med Assoc, *177*:1135, 1980.
85. Speirs VC. Partial arytenoidectomy in horses. Vet Surg, *15*:316, 1986.
86. Orsini PG. Radiographic examination of the head and neck. ACVS Surgical Forum, 1987.
87. Shapiro J, White NA, Schlafer DH, et al. Hypertrophic ossification of the laryngeal cartilages of a horse. J Eq Med Surg, *3*:370, 1979.
88. Trotter GW, Aanes WA, Snyder SP. Laryngeal chondroma in a horse. J Am Vet Med Assoc, *178*:829, 1981.
89. Haynes PF, McClure JR, Watters JW. Subtotal arytenoidectomy in the horse: an update. In: Proceedings of the 30th Annual Convention of American Association of Equine Practitioners, 1984, p 21.
90. Wheat JD. Pathology and related surgery of the larynx. ACVS Surgical Forum, Chicago, 1978.
91. White NA, Blackwell RB. Partial arytenoidectomy in the horse. Vet Surg, *9*:5, 1980.
92. Harrison IW, Raker CW. Dorsal glottic stenosis after

bilateral arytenoidectomy in two horses. J Am Vet Med Assoc, *192*:202, 1988.
93. Tulleners EP, Harrison IW, Mann P, et al. Partial arytenoidectomy in the horse with and without mucosal closure. Vet Surg, *17*:252, 1988.
94. Tate LP. Neodynium (Nd):YAG laser surgery in the equine larynx: A pilot study. Lasers in Surgery and Medicine, *6*:473, 1986.
95. Belknap J, Derksen FJ, Nickels FA. Evaluation of subtotal arytenoidectomy as a surgical treatment for left laryngeal hemiplegia in the horse. Scientific Meeting Abstract, ACVS 24th Annual Meeting. Vet Surg, *18*:57, 1989.

CHAPTER 21

# TRACHEA

DAVID E. FREEMAN

Diseases of the trachea are not common in horses. Although tracheal diseases are tolerated well in sedentary horses, most cause severe airway obstruction during work and can limit athletic ability.

## Anatomy

The trachea is a flexible tube composed of 48 to 60 hyaline cartilaginous plates that are circular to elliptical in cross section.[1] It bifurcates into right and left principal bronchi at the level of the 5th and 6th intercostal space, dorsal to the base of the heart.[1] The cervical portion of the trachea is enclosed in deep cervical fascia that is continuous with endothoracic fascia in the mediastinum.[1] The cervical part is related dorsolaterally to the carotid artery, the recurrent laryngeal nerve, and the vagosympathetic trunk.[1] The sternothyroideus and sternohyoideus muscles lie on the ventral aspect of the cervical trachea and the esophagus lies dorsal to it at its origin.[1] In the lower part of the neck, the esophagus lies to its left side. The trachea receives its blood supply from the common carotid artery and bronchoesophageal artery and is drained by the jugular vein and bronchoesophageal veins.[1] Smooth muscle of the trachea is innervated by the autonomic nervous system and sensory impulses involved with pain and cough reflex are carried by the vagus nerve.[2]

Cartilaginous plates of the trachea are incomplete dorsally and each plate is connected to the next by fibroelastic tissue, the annular tracheal ligament. The tracheal smooth muscle is attached dorsally to the inner surface of the cartilaginous plates[1] and combines with the mucosa and adventitia to form the dorsal tracheal membrane.[2] The tracheal mucosa is composed of pseudostratified columnar ciliated epithelium and numerous goblet cells, and it forms longitudinal folds that allow expansion.[1] Hyaline cartilage of the trachea is partly calcified and ossified in older animals.[1]

Dust particles and other foreign material that enter the trachea are entrapped by mucus and removed rapidly by cilia that propel the gel layer of mucus cranially.[3] Whereas the action of cilia is independent of mucosal innervation, denervation interrupts activity of mucus-forming cells.[3,4] The mucociliary clearance mechanism is also impaired by epithelial loss, toxic agents, and infections, and can be overwhelmed by excess secretions from the lungs.[3]

## Examination

Many diseases of the trachea produce nonspecific clinical signs. The trachea should be palpated throughout its course in the neck and the skin overlying its ventral aspect should be palpated to detect adhesions or subcutaneous fibrosis, indicative of a previous wound or surgery. On auscultation, it may be possible to detect abnormal sounds at the site of tracheal stenosis;[5] however, care must be taken to avoid misinterpretation of abnormal sounds referred from other parts of the respiratory tract. Stenotic diseases of the cervical trachea cause greater dyspnea and abnormal sounds on inspiration and a greater than normal ratio of inspiratory to expiratory times.[6] This is in contrast to obstruction of the thoracic segment which causes changes in expiration.[6] Abnormal sounds can be episodic in some horses[7] and in unusual cases they are not induced by work.[8]

Tracheobronchoscopy can be performed on the conscious horse. The most commonly used endoscope is 100 to 110 cm long but a 2-meter endoscope is necessary to reach the thoracic trachea and bifurcation in an adult horse.[9] Radiographs are useful for detecting tracheal stenosis and other obstructive lesions; however, endoscopic examination generally allows more complete evaluation of the lesion and the extent to which tracheal circumference is involved. Xeroradiographs are superior to black and white films because of improved soft tissue detail.

## Diseases of the Trachea

### *Acquired Tracheal Stenosis*

The most common causes of acquired tracheal stenosis in the horse are technical errors in performance of a tracheotomy (Fig. 21–1). The most common error is a longitudinal incision through the ventral part of the trachea rather than a transverse incision through the annular tracheal ligament. Because each tracheal ring is incomplete dorsally, the dorsal tips override when ventral support is interrupted. The trachea then collapses from side to side and the cut mucosal edges heal to form a web across the lumen (Fig. 21–1).

Another cause of acquired tracheal stenosis is transection through the tracheal annular ligament for a greater part of its circumference than 180°. An incision of this size will allow adjacent tracheal rings to retract from each other and create a large defect. Without cartilaginous support, mucosa that fills this defect can collapse into the lumen during deep inspiration (Fig. 21–2).

***Clinical Signs and Diagnosis.*** Mild tracheal stenosis may be tolerated well and may be clinically nondetectable in a sedentary horse, but can cause inspiratory dyspnea during exercise or excitement. The level of stenosis can be detected by palpation and by auscultation along the trachea. If available, history of recent surgery or wounding of the trachea facilitates diagnosis. On endoscopic examination, it may be possible to see the severed ends of tracheal rings protruding into the lumen (Fig. 21–3) and there may also be associated mucosal defects. On radiographs, it may be possible to see fractured, severed and overriding tracheal rings, soft tissue and cartilaginous thickening, tracheal ring separation, and stenosis (Fig. 21–4).

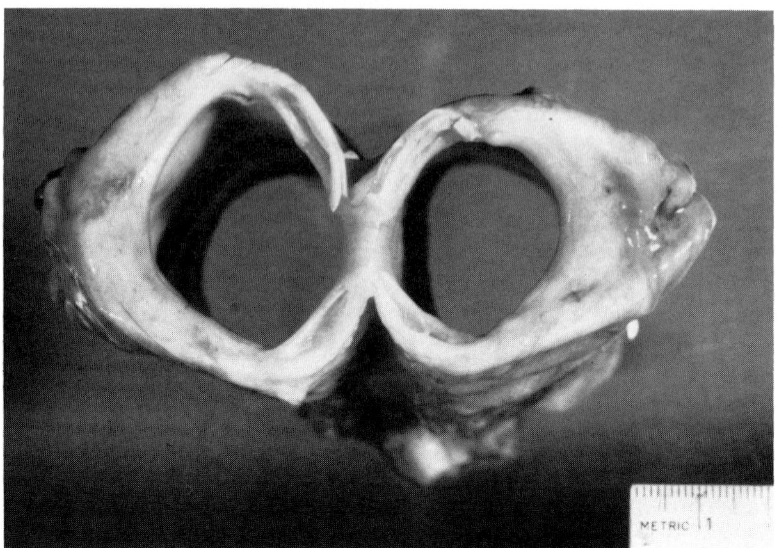


**FIG. 21–1.** Tracheal rings of a yearling that had three tracheotomies through the same site as a foal. Tracheal ring on the right was severed ventrally during one procedure, so that its dorsal ends overlapped and the ring collapsed from side to side. Mucosa that healed across the severed segment formed a web that further reduced airway diameter. Tracheal ring on the left is of more normal configuration and diameter.

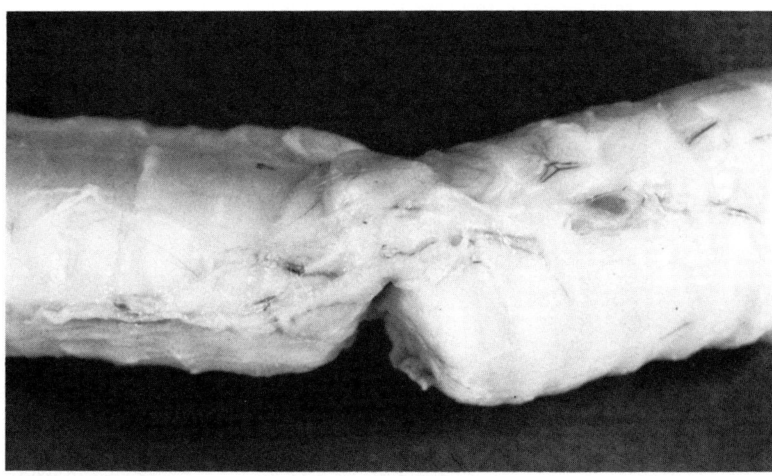

**FIG. 21–2.** Stenosis caused by almost complete transection of the trachea by tracheotomy through the annular ligament. Note that tracheal rings on each side are distracted and the healed mucosa between them projects into the lumen. This horse had stertorous breathing during mild activity or excitement.

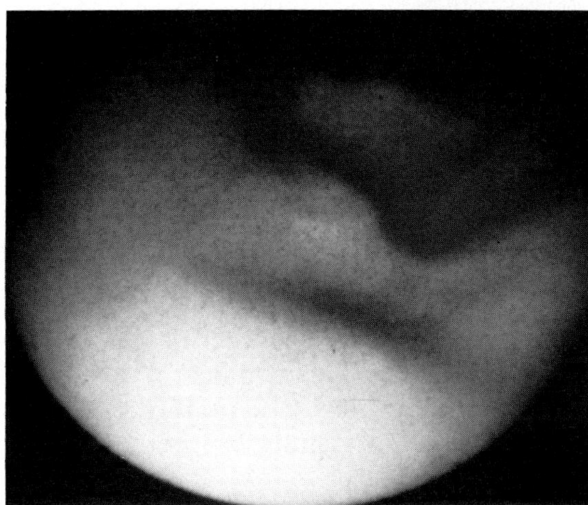

**FIG. 21–3.** Endoscopic view of floor of trachea in which severed ends of tracheal rings project into the tracheal lumen following tracheotomy. The overall effect of these intraluminal projections on performance could not be assessed because the horse had severe laryngeal problems.

***Treatment.*** Treatment of tracheal stenosis is difficult, especially in those horses in which athletic potential must be restored. Treatment is not required in sedentary horses that can tolerate the stenosis well. Methods of correction include resection and anastomosis, extraluminal support, and imbrication procedures (see below).

***Prognosis.*** Prognosis is largely determined by the severity of stenosis, which in turn determines the complexity of surgical repair. Satisfactory outcomes, including return to racing, have been recorded after surgical repair,[5,10] but a poor to guarded prognosis for competition must be issued in many cases.

## *Open Wounds*

Open wounds involve all layers from the tracheal mucosa to the skin and can be caused by tracheotomy and, less frequently, by blunt, penetrating trauma.

***Clinical Signs and Diagnosis.*** Diagnosis of open wounds is often straightforward because of location and obvious tracheal involvement. Depression, respiratory distress, fever, subcutaneous emphysema, and cellulitis can develop depending on the severity of trauma and adequacy of ventral drainage.

***Treatment.*** Treatment of traumatic open wounds of the trachea involves debridement, daily wound cleaning, and creation of ventral drainage. In one report, an open wound was repaired by apposing adjacent tracheal rings with fine monofilament wire that encircled each ring without penetrating the mucosa.[11] In that horse, primary repair eliminated a large separation between two adjacent tracheal rings that could have caused stenosis.[11] Horses with cellulitis and extensive subcutaneous emphysema should be treated with broad spectrum antibiotics, nonsteroidal anti-inflammatory drugs, and stall rest.

***Prognosis.*** The most serious complication of planned or accidental wounds of the trachea is stenosis. Subcutaneous emphysema and cellulitis can resolve over a period of 1 to 2 weeks, provided that adequate drainage is

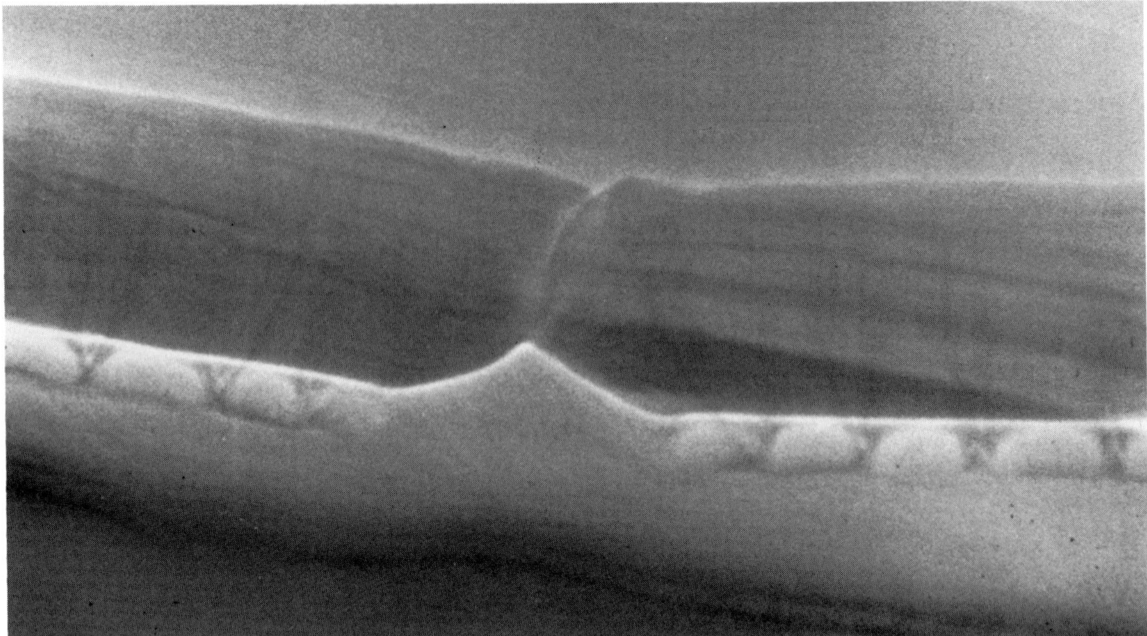

**FIG. 21–4.** Xeroradiograph of tracheal stenosis caused by almost complete transection of the tracheal annular ligament with subsequent distraction of tracheal rings above and below the incision. The intervening segment of mucosa healed, but in doing so formed a constriction at the tracheotomy site.

established. Pneumomediastinum can develop following any wound in the trachea but usually resolves in less than a week and rarely causes pneumothorax.[12] Open wounds of the trachea should seal within approximately 2 weeks and should be completely healed by 1 month after injury.

## Closed Wounds

Closed wounds are usually caused by blunt trauma to the ventral part of the neck, such as from a kick or collision, that compresses the trachea against cervical vertebrae. Overlying skin, muscle, and fascia remain intact but linear and longitudinal defects are inflicted along the dorsal, ventral, or lateral aspects of the trachea.[13,14]

***Clinical Signs and Diagnosis.*** Closed tracheal wounds can be difficult to diagnose but should be suspected in a horse that develops acute, severe subcutaneous emphysema. Stridor may be evident on inspiration if edges of the tracheal wound project into the airway.[13] A seroma may be evident on the ventral aspect of the neck at the level of injury.[14] Radiographs and endoscopic examination should be used to detect mucosal defects.

***Treatment.*** Small wounds of the trachea can be managed successfully by pressure bandages at the level of injury, stall rest, and a course of systemic antibiotics and nonsteroidal anti-inflammatory drugs.[13,14] If edematous fat and fascia prolapse through a wound in the dorsal ligament of the trachea, prolapsed tissues should be trimmed and the wound edges apposed with simple interrupted absorbable sutures.[13]

***Prognosis.*** Subcutaneous emphysema, cellulitis and mild, transient pneumomediastinum usually resolve within 1 to 2 weeks after spontaneous or surgical closure of the wound. Prognosis for complete recovery after small closed tracheal wounds is good, but affected horses should be closely monitored for worsening subcutaneous emphysema and cellulitis. Pneumothorax is a potential complication of severe emphysema.

## Mucosal Wounds

Tracheitis and pressure necrosis can be caused by orotracheal and nasotracheal intubation for delivery of inhalant anesthetics.[15,16] Although most horses are intubated without any apparent adverse effects on tracheal mucosa, it was shown in one study that superficial mucosal damage may be detected on endoscopic examination shortly after intubation in a larger proportion of horses than might be expected.[16]

Stiff endotracheal tube cuffs require high inflation pressures and are likely to damage tracheal mucosa.[17] These cuffs become round in cross section as they assume their final shape in the trachea but, because the tracheal cross section is elliptical, undue pressure may develop at isolated points of contact between the tracheal wall and tube.[16,17] Cuffs that expand in an eccentric fashion can also inflict damage at isolated points in the tracheal mucosa.[17] Even low cuff pressures can cause venous and capillary stasis in the tracheal mucosa, and mild cellular damage, transient ciliary loss, and delayed mucociliary clearance.[18] High pressures can cause cartilage damage, necrosis and mucosal ulceration, and formation of a pseudomembrane of fibrin and necrotic epithelial debris.[16] Factors that can contribute to cuff-induced injuries include localized pressure against the tracheal wall from a deflected endotracheal tube tip, residual ethylene oxide, cold sterilization agents and antiseptics on the tracheal tube, and tubes from materials that are not of medical grade.[15,17]

Large residual volume, low pressure cuffs are recommended to prevent iatrogenic mucosal injury. They apply little pressure to the tracheal mucosa when fully inflated and they conform evenly to the tracheal wall.[17,18] Although tracheal wall pressure may be more important in production of mucosal damage than length of intubation,[16] both should be kept to a minimum.[15]

***Clinical Signs and Diagnosis.*** Possibly because this complication is rare in horses, clinical signs have not been well described. Mild, serous nasal discharge can develop but some affected horses may not have clinical signs. Diagnosis is made by endoscopic examination.

***Treatment.*** Mild cuff-induced tracheitis can resolve without treatment. Moderate to severe injuries should be treated with systemic antibiotics and anti-inflammatory agents.

***Prognosis.*** Prognosis for minor mucosal injuries appears to be good, but there is little information on long-term consequences of severe post-intubation injury in horses.[16]

## Collapsed Trachea

Collapsed trachea in horses is most likely a congenital defect and bears several similarities to the disease in dogs. Unlike acquired tracheal stenosis, which usually involves a short segment of cervical trachea, collapsed trachea usually involves the entire cervical and thoracic portions. The condition is also referred to as dorsoventral flattening of the trachea and "scabbard" trachea. The affected tracheal rings form half circles with widely separated ends and the dorsal membrane that spans this space is thin and flaccid. In the cervical segment, the esophagus lies in a groove on the dorsal membrane.

As in dogs,[19] miniaturization appears to be a factor in development of collapsed trachea in horses because ponies and miniature horses are predominantly affected.[20–24] Structural changes that have been identified in dogs, such as cartilage fibrodystrophy[19] and inflammation, desquamation and metaplasia in the mucosa,[25] have not been fully investigated in horses; however, chondrodysplasia has been described in affected tracheal rings in a miniature foal.[20]

***Clinical Signs.*** Most affected animals are 10 years old or older, but the condition has been reported in a 2-month-old miniature foal.[20] The disease is frequently diagnosed as an incidental finding at necropsy in horses or ponies that appeared clinically normal, in spite of their pronounced and extensive tracheal collapse. This can be attributed largely to the sedentary lifestyle of those horses that are most frequently affected. Clinical signs may develop or worsen in later life because aging changes in affected cartilages, such as calcification and inflammation, can exacerbate the obstruction.[20,21] A "honking" respiratory noise can become evident on inspiration and expiration[21] and is usually exacerbated by exercise, although not consistently.[7] Some horses cough[20] and have signs similar to those of "heaves."[22] Severe cases can become debilitated and have cyanotic mucous membranes.[22,23]

***Diagnosis.*** It may be possible to palpate the ends of flattened tracheal cartilages as sharp ridges along the course of the cervical trachea.[23,24] The severe dorsoventral flattening of the trachea and flaccid dorsal membrane can be seen through the endoscope[20,24] and on radiographs.

***Treatment.*** Treatment has been generally unsuccessful. The entire trachea is involved and most treatment efforts have been directed at correction of the problem in the cervical segment. Unsuccessful treatment methods in the cervical trachea include tracheal imbrication,[24] extraluminal support,[20] and replacement of a segment of the cervical trachea with a prosthesis.[23]

***Prognosis.*** If clinical signs develop only during exercise or excitement, the condition may be well tolerated if the horse or pony is retired to a more sedentary lifestyle. Enlargement of the right ventricle has been reported in one pony[22] and any secondary changes in heart and lungs might worsen the prognosis.[25]

## Tracheobronchial Foreign Body

Horses can readily cough out and expel foreign bodies in the trachea,[26] but aspirated thorn and conifer twigs up to 70 cm in length have become lodged in the right mainstem bronchus[27–29] and less often in the left mainstem bronchus.[9] If the thorns or branches of the aspirated twig are directed cranially, deep penetration and fixation are enhanced.[27] Pneumonia and pleuritis can develop.[28]

***Clinical Signs.*** The most common clinical sign of tracheobronchial foreign body is a chronic cough of several months' duration.[29] Coughing can be spontaneous or can be induced by tracheal manipulation.[29] The frequency and severity of coughing can vary and in 2 reported cases, was regarded as mild and only occasional.[28,30] Other signs that can develop are fetid breath, intermittent bilateral purulent nasal discharge, epistaxis, hemoptysis, and reduced exercise tolerance.[27,30,31] Signs of severe pneumonia may also be evident.[27,28] There may be a history of favorable but transient response to antibiotics.[27]

***Diagnosis.*** Abnormal lung sounds may be heard on auscultation and chest radiographs are indicated to determine if pneumonia and pleuritis have developed. Diagnosis can be made on endoscopic examination, but affected horses may have to be sedated heavily to control the severe coughing induced by introduction of the endoscope. In addition, an endoscope of at least 2 meters should be used to examine the mainstem bronchi. An accumulation of purulent material and, less frequently, blood can be seen draining from the affected bronchus.

***Treatment.*** The biopsy forceps of the flexible fiberoptic endoscope is usually inadequate for removal of tracheobronchial foreign bodies. Successful removal has been reported with long grasping forceps[27,29] and with a flexible retrieval basket.[30] A low cervical tracheotomy is needed to allow introduction of these long handled instruments because of the curvature that must be followed to enter the mainstem bronchus.[30]

***Prognosis.*** A complete recovery can be expected following successful removal of a tracheobronchial foreign body,[27,29,30] provided that severe pulmonary complications have not developed.[28]

## Extraluminal Causes of Stenosis

Tracheal compression by extraluminal masses, such as lymph node abscesses,[32] lipoma,[33] mediastinal masses and tumors,[9] is rare. Clinical signs and methods of diagnosis are similar to those described for acquired tracheal stenosis. Removal of the impinging mass or drainage of abscesses may not provide relief because the involved tracheal rings may remain collapsed after compression is removed.[32,33] Tracheal reconstruction may be required in such cases.[33]

## *Intratracheal Prolapse of the Cricotracheal Membrane*

This is a rare cause of abnormal respiratory noise and reduced exercise tolerance in horses.[34,35] In affected horses, the space between the cricoid cartilage and first tracheal ring may be 5 cm long and the intervening segment of tracheal mucosa appears to be redundant and flaccid.[34,35] It has been proposed that this mucosal segment is aspirated into the airway during strenuous activity.[35] Recommended treatment is imbrication of the cricotracheal membrane;[35] however, this condition is poorly defined and the response to treatment in a large number of cases is unknown.

## *Neoplasia*

Tumors of the trachea are rare in mammals.[36] A round cell sarcoma has been described in the trachea of a 6-year-old gelding[36] and tracheal mastocytosis has been described in a 21-year-old gelding.[8] In the latter case, the horse had a cutaneous mastocytoma removed previously and lesions were also evident in the nasal cavity and pharynx.[8] The tracheal lesion was removed through a laryngotomy and the horse recovered completely.[8]

# Surgery of the Trachea

## *Tracheotomy*

### Indications

Tracheotomy is frequently required in horses that develop a life-threatening obstruction of the upper respiratory tract. Severe nasal septal deformities, fractures of nasal and conchal bones, extensive tumors of the upper respiratory tract, complete bilateral laryngeal paralysis, severe arytenoid cartilage deformities, parotitis, acute laryngeal or pharyngeal edema, severe guttural pouch distention, abscessation of retropharyngeal lymph nodes, and complications of smoke inhalation and snakebite are examples of conditions that may require a tracheotomy.[37] The procedure is also used prophylactically in horses that undergo extensive upper respiratory tract surgeries in which postoperative swelling could occlude the upper airway or in which tamponade of the nasal passages is required to control postoperative hemorrhage.

In horses that require ventilatory support, a tracheotomy may be useful because it reduces anatomic dead space and allows easy delivery of oxygen in the conscious animal.[25,38] A tracheotomy can be used for delivery of gas anesthetics in horses undergoing complicated surgical procedures in the upper respiratory tract. Less common indications for tracheotomy are retrograde endoscopic examination of lesions in the pharynx and larynx, removal of tracheobronchial foreign bodies,[30] and oxygen delivery after recovery from general anesthesia.[39]

### Surgical Procedure

Tracheotomy can be performed on the standing horse using local infiltration of the surgical site or with the horse under general anesthesia. Exact location of the ventral midline of the neck and subsequent dissection to the trachea are easier in the standing horse than in the anesthetized horse in dorsal or lateral recumbency. In the recumbent horse, incisions through successive layers may be staggered when the horse stands.

In an adult horse, a tracheotomy is performed at the junction of the upper and middle thirds of the neck, and in the pony, in the middle of the neck. In these sites, the trachea is superficial and also subsequent tracheotomies can be made distal to any obstructions that develop in the original site. A 6- to 8-cm long incision is made through the skin, the underlying cutaneous colli muscle or fascia, and the septum of the paired sternothyroideus and sternohyoideus muscles. The ventral part of the trachea is then freed from the surrounding fascia and a transverse incision is made through the annular ligament attaching two adjacent tracheal rings. The site for this incision should correspond to the center of the skin opening in the standing horse and should be one ring proximal to this level if the horse is anesthetized with its head extended. The skin and underlying incisions should provide good exposure to the trachea and should correspond to each other in location and direction.

In the awake horse, the tracheal annular ligament should be incised with a one-piece scalpel, such as a cartilage knife, because the blade of a conventional scalpel can become detached or broken in the trachea.[40] The point of the scalpel is inserted perpendicularly to the ligament and it should be thrust into the lumen of the trachea for a depth of 1.5 to 2 cm in a single motion. In this way, the scalpel penetrates the membrane and underlying mucosa in one movement and thus avoids the risk of dissecting mucosa away from the ligament. The point of the scalpel is kept within the lumen of the trachea and the incision is enlarged. If the scalpel is removed before the incision is extended, it may not be possible to find the initial site of entry. The incision into the tracheal lumen should encompass approximately 120° (from 4 o'clock to 8 o'clock) of the tracheal diameter and should not exceed 180°. A small opening makes tube insertion and replacement too difficult. The tracheotomy tube is held in position with two tapes tied around the neck and secured to the mane to prevent the tube falling out when the horse lowers its head.

Preparation of the surgical site and incision placement may be difficult when a tracheotomy must be performed on a conscious horse that is struggling because of airway obstruction. It may be necessary to allow the horse to collapse, but there should be no subsequent delay because a horse can die shortly after this stage is reached. A tracheotomy should be done as soon as signs of impending airway obstruction become evident because warning signs precede death by a short interval, usually minutes. For this reason, a tracheotomy tube and the necessary surgical instruments always should be placed outside the stall of a horse at risk for airway obstruction. In general, a tracheotomy should always be performed as a prophylactic procedure if there is a significant risk of obstruction.

## Tracheotomy Tubes

The preferred tube for adults is metal and is curved from its flange at almost a right angle (Fig. 21–5). This tube is flattened dorsoventrally to facilitate insertion and reduce pressure on tracheal rings. The tube should be small because the loss in diameter is offset by reduction in anatomic dead space gained by a tracheotomy[25,38] and large tubes cause pressure damage and stricture. In addition, small tubes are usually adequate if the upper airway is partly patent. If necessary, a tube can be improvised from a segment of stomach tube or the handle of a plastic gallon container.

Human pediatric or small animal tracheotomy tubes of soft material are used for foals but any form of tracheotomy tube can rapidly damage a foal's trachea. Tubes with an inflated cuff carry risks of mucosal damage similar to that inflicted by cuffed endotracheal tubes (see above) and result in complete airway obstruction if they become blocked with secretions.

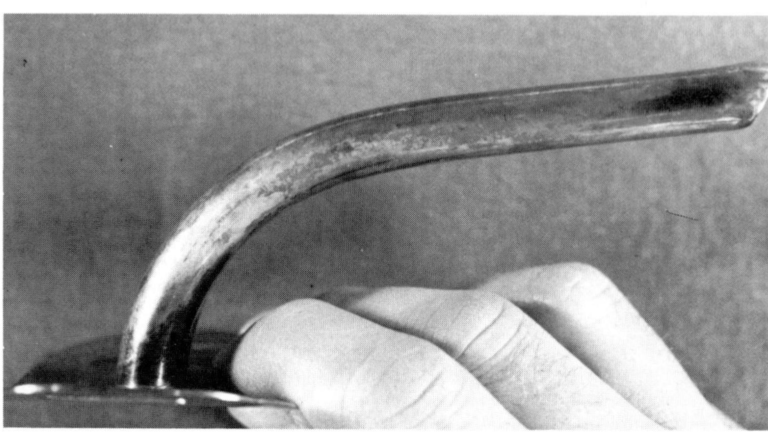

**FIG. 21–5.** Stainless steel tracheotomy tube recommended for use in horses. Note the flange for securing ties to the neck and the angle and beveled tip that facilitate insertion.

## Aftercare

The tracheotomy tube should be replaced with a sterile tube daily and the wound should be cleaned with warm water and a dilute antiseptic solution. The tube can become partially occluded with secretions over a short period of time so that frequent aspiration or replacement may be needed. If superficial wound infection and cellulitis develop, systemic antibiotic treatment may be indicated. To minimize risks of complications, a tube should be left in place for a maximum of 3 days and, unless absolutely necessary, not more than 10 days.

The tracheotomy tube is removed permanently when the clinician is completely satisfied that the upper airway is patent. Patency is assessed by obstructing the tube and stoma for approximately 2 to 3 minutes with one hand while feeling air movement through the nostrils with the free hand. The tracheotomy tube should be removed early in the day so that the horse can be checked frequently and kept under close observation for any signs of respiratory distress. The open wound is allowed to heal by second intention and exuberant granulation tissue can be controlled by application of 1% hydrocortisone in antibiotic ointment.

A tracheotomy can close completely 10 to 14 days after a 3-day cannulation and heal completely by 1 month. During healing, polypoid masses of granulation tissue can form in the tracheotomy wound but can resolve without treatment.[41]

## Complications

Complications are most likely if tracheotomy is done as an emergency on a struggling patient or if tracheal rings are incised. Superficial infection and some cellulitis are frequent complications that are usually mild and respond to topical treatment, cleaning, and hydrotherapy. Air can dissect through peritracheal fascial planes (Fig. 21–6), and, although the resulting subcutaneous emphysema is alarming in appearance, it usually resolves within a couple of weeks. Factors that increase the risk of cellulitis and emphysema are large airflows through the tracheotomy because of upper airway obstruction, and poor drainage because incisions through successive layers are staggered. Major complications following tracheotomy are pneumothorax and necrotizing or granulomatous tracheitis, usually terminating in stenosis of the trachea.

The role of any single factor in development of tracheal stenosis is controversial.[42,43] The risk of stenosis is greater in foals than in adult horses because they have soft and pliable cartilaginous rings that are easily traumatized. Tracheal stenosis can be expected if tracheal cartilages are incised or if they are damaged by large, tight-fitting tubes, intubation for too long, or repeated tracheotomies through the same site[41–43] (Fig. 21–1).

If a transverse incision through the tracheal annular ligament exceeds 180°, there is a risk of wide separation of tracheal rings on each side of the incision and the intervening mucosa can project into the tracheal lumen (Figs. 21–2 and 21–4). This complication is most likely when a large incision is made to accommodate an endotracheal tube.

Pulmonary complications are rare following tracheotomy but may arise because normal filtering mechanisms of the upper respiratory tract are bypassed and inspired air is not warmed and humidified before it reaches the lower respiratory tract.[44] An efficient cough reflex is also lost.[44]

# Permanent Tracheostomy

## Indications

A permanent tracheal opening may be indicated in horses with a severe, nontreatable upper airway obstruction, such as bilateral chondrosis of the arytenoid cartilages with poor response to arytenoidectomy.[45] However, a horse cannot race in the United States with a tracheostomy.[37] The life of a horse with an inoperable upper airway tumor can be briefly extended with a tracheostomy and the procedure can be used under such conditions to allow a mare to complete gestation. A self-retaining tracheostomy tube, composed of interlocking segments and a plug, can be used for permanent tracheostomy in the horse; however, the tube may need frequent clean-

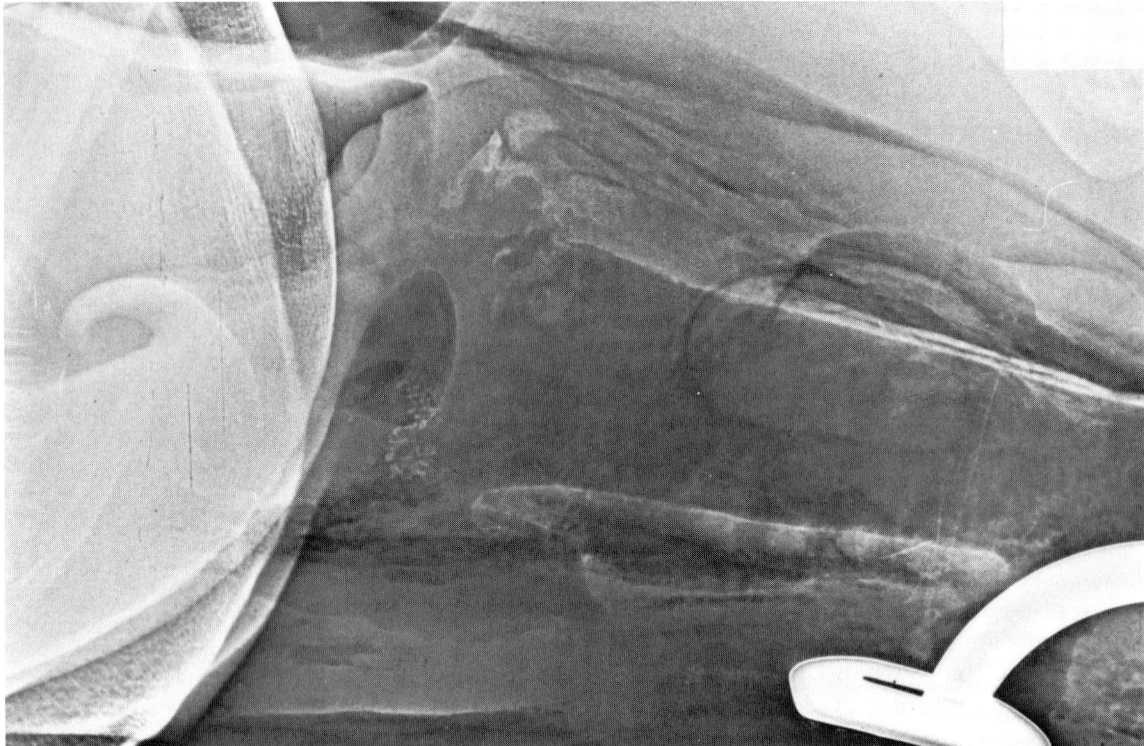

**FIG. 21–6.** Xeroradiograph showing extensive peritracheal dissection of air and subcutaneous emphysema following a tracheotomy.

ing and inspection. The procedure described below has been used successfully in a horse and ponies and required minimum aftercare for periods ranging from 2 to 59 months.[45]

## Surgical Procedure

The horse is placed under general anesthesia in dorsal recumbency and the ventral part of the neck prepared for an aseptic surgical procedure. In the cranial third of the neck (horse) or central third (pony), four tracheal rings are exposed through a 10-cm long ventral midline incision.[45] These rings are incised on the midline and 15 mm on both sides of it.[45] The eight rectangles of cartilage created in this way are dissected from the tracheal mucosa, which is left intact.[45] Segments of the paired sternothyroideus and sternohyoideus muscles are excised at the proposed stoma site to reduce tension on the mucocutaneous suture line.[45] The exposed mucosa is then incised on the midline except at the proximal and distal ends, where it is incised to form V-shaped flaps.[45] The mucosal edges are sutured to adjacent skin edges with 2-0 polypropylene to complete the stoma.[45] Careful mucosa-to-skin apposition without tension is necessary to reduce risks of wound infection, inflammation, dehiscence, and stenosis. Care must be taken to avoid rotating the trachea because a stoma created at the free ends of the rings, where they are weakest, will collapse.[45] If the stoma is made too wide, the trachea will collapse, and if it is too narrow, skin edges can heal together and seal the opening.[45]

### Aftercare

Polypropylene skin sutures are removed 10 to 14 days after surgery.[45] Before that time, the stoma may need to be cleaned with warm water or saline solution and dilute antiseptic solution twice daily and then once daily. Cleaning may need to be continued once daily over the following week or so, but then further aftercare is not required.[45] Although mucus may continue to collect around the stoma and mat hair at the stomal edges, this usually does not require attention.[45]

## Complications

The most serious complications of permanent tracheostomy is lumen obstruction. If the stoma seals, it can be opened by incising skin along the line of apposition.[45]

# *Resection and Anastomosis*

## Indications

Resection and anastomosis of the trachea are difficult in horses and should be reserved for those acquired tracheal stenoses in which other reconstructive techniques have failed. Severe damage such as mucosal fibrosis, induration, granulation, polyp formation, intraluminal webbing, thickening of cut cartilage rings, dystrophic changes in affected cartilages, and telescoping of cut edges of cartilages over each other, may warrant resection.

Three tracheal rings can be resected in a horse without much difficulty but the force required to appose the ends has been shown to double when five rings are removed compared with three.[5] Greater elasticity in the trachea allows for a longer resection in young animals, but young cartilage is soft and cannot withstand the same tension in an anastomosis that can be tolerated by adult cartilage.[19]

## Procedure

The goal of tracheal resection and anastomosis is to establish an airtight union between two ends of trachea and to preserve lumen diameter, tracheal rigidity, and mucosal lining.[25,46] These goals can be accomplished by minimizing tension on the suture line, precise anatomic reconstruction of the mucosa and cartilage, and use of a monofilament suture material that induces minimal tissue reaction.[2,25] Risks of infection, granuloma formation, and mucosal ulceration increase if braided material enters the tracheal lumen.[2,25] To minimize tension on the suture line, a martingale apparatus is used after surgery to maintain head and neck flexion.[5] This is applied in the week beforehand to allow the horse to become adjusted to it.[5]

With the horse in dorsal recumbency, the trachea from the cricoid cartilage to the thoracic inlet is exposed and mobilized through a 40-cm long ventral midline incision.[5] Damage to the vagosympathetic trunk or recurrent laryngeal nerve is carefully avoided during this step. Two large traction sutures are placed around the ventral portion of two tracheal rings (without entering the tracheal lumen) at least two cartilages proximal and distal to the damaged segment. The affected segment is resected but a cuff of normal mucosa of 360° circumference is left extending beyond the ends of trachea to be apposed.[5] A sterile endotracheal tube is placed in the distal end of the transected trachea. The mucosal cuffs are then turned back over the normal tracheal cartilages and sutured to the adventitia with fine, absorbable suture material in a simple continuous pattern.[5] The horse's head is then flexed and the endotracheal tube in the distal part of the trachea is removed. The original orotracheal tube is then passed through the two severed ends of the trachea and advanced towards the lungs. The severed ends of trachea are brought into apposition by means of traction sutures and are held together by four Backhaus towel clamps. The approximated tracheal rings are anastomosed with simple interrupted sutures of 25-g stainless steel wire or nylon swaged to a curved cutting needle. Sutures are placed 0.5 to 1 cm apart and through half the width of each tracheal ring, without entering the tracheal lumen.[5] The trachea is checked for air leaks by flooding the surgical site with antibiotic in saline solution and forcing air through the endotracheal tube with a ventilator. A continuous suction drain is then placed for 3 to 4 days adjacent to the trachea and the overlying muscles and skin are opposed in routine fashion.

## Aftercare

Antibiotics are given for up to 10 days and the horse is kept in the martingale apparatus for 3 weeks after surgery.

## Complications and Prognosis

In a small number of horses that underwent the above procedure, tracheal diameter was restored to approximately 90% of normal and the horses did not make an abnormal noise at work.[5] Small buds of granulation tissue developed in the mucosa at the site of anastomosis, but there was no evidence of reaction where stainless steel suture penetrated the tracheal cartilage.[5] Based on the outcome in these cases, it was also concluded that the trachea can tolerate extensive mobilization and that it has good collateral blood supply.[5]

The most common cause of failure is anastomosis under tension. This can cause dehiscence and, in young animals, may retard growth of tracheal rings.[19] Even minor dehiscence of the suture line allows separation of the tracheal ends followed by subcutaneous emphysema and eventually stenosis.[2,25,46] Wide separation reduces mucociliary clearance.[2]

Errors in suture placement also cause complications. Sutures placed directly through cartilaginous rings can fracture the cartilage, but sutures that encircle the cartilage tend to telescope apposed tracheal rings.[25] Long tension sutures tend to buckle intervening segments of trachea and thereby misalign the anastomosis.

# *Extraluminal Support of Collapsed Cartilages*

## Indications

Collapsed or deformed tracheal rings can be reshaped and maintained in a normal configuration by extraluminal supports that conform to the shape of normal trachea. This approach is preferable to resection and anastomosis whenever possible because complications are less severe. However, it is of limited value if there is mucosal damage and severe cartilage injury.

## Surgical Procedure

The most popular material for extraluminal support is a 60-ml polypropylene syringe case, cut in half longitudinally and with many small holes drilled in it.[10,19,25,33] If a long segment of trachea is involved, several individual plastic rings may be preferable to one solid piece because they would permit more normal tracheal flexibility and movement.[19] An alternative support is a wire spring covered with polyethylene tubing and spiraled onto the affected segment.[37,47]

The support is applied through a ventral midline incision with the horse under general anesthesia, in dorsal recumbency. Several partial or full-thickness incisions may be necessary across the width of each affected tracheal ring to allow reshaping.[10] Fine, monofilament, nonabsorbable sutures, such as polypropylene, are preplaced as needed around the affected segments of tracheal rings to elevate them to a normal position.[10,19] Intraoperative endoscopic examination should be used to help avoid mucosal penetration with sutures and to ensure satisfactory lumen expansion. The support is then applied, taking care to insert it under the recurrent laryngeal nerves, and preplaced sutures are tied through the holes. A continuous, closed suction drainage device can be buried close to the trachea and the incision is closed in routine fashion.[10,33]

## Aftercare

The horse should receive preoperative and postoperative antibiotics, the latter for 7 to 10 days, or as indicated by clinical progress. Nonsteroidal anti-inflammatory drugs can be given, if needed, to reduce postoperative inflammation. The closed suction drainage device should be removed at 3 days or earlier to eliminate the risk of bacterial migration to the implant.[10,33]

## Prognosis and Complications

Extraluminal supports in horses can eliminate noise and dyspnea[33] and allow return to a successful racing career.[10] Implants that encircle the trachea, such as coiled springs, may have to be removed from a young animal to allow tracheal growth.[47] Failures with external supports can be attributed to infection, soft tissue damage from movement against an unyielding implant, and damage to adjacent nerves.[19]

## *Miscellaneous Procedures*

A silicone rubber Montgomery T-tube has been used to provide a patent airway and to serve as an intraluminal stent in young animals with collapsed tracheas or chondromalacia of tracheal rings after tracheotomy. The tube is suitable only for short-term use because it can become obstructed with secretions or dislodged;[19] however, long-term use (12 months) is possible.[48] There are few options for treatment of acquired tracheal stenosis in very young animals because any reduction in tracheal diameter can cause complete obstruction. The purpose of a T-tube in these patients is to provide some support to damaged tracheal rings until the trachea grows and damaged rings stabilize at a larger diameter.

When tracheal stenosis develops because of partial transection through a transverse tracheotomy (Figs. 21–2 and 21–4), tracheal diameter can be restored by imbrication. Interrupted sutures of #2 nylon or polypropylene are preplaced around the distracted rings ventrally without penetrating the mucosa. Fine, absorbable, submucosal sutures are preplaced through redundant submucosa and, when tied around the strands of heavy material, they draw the mucosa out of the tracheal lumen. Mucosal resection may be necessary if there is concurrent mucosal stricture (Fig. 21–4).

Laser surgery offers a new and promising approach to many intraluminal diseases of the trachea in horses.[49,50] The advantages are easy application by a transendoscopic approach, excellent hemostasis, reduced convalescence time, improved accuracy, and suitability for use as a standing, outpatient procedure.[49,50]

## *Tracheal Healing*

Surface damage to tracheal mucosa heals rapidly and in a similar fashion to damage in the epidermis.[4] Cell migration from the wound margin followed by mitosis produces a transitional epithelium without normal mucosal architecture.[4] Ciliated columnar cells and goblet cells develop from this transitional epithelium to complete epithelial regeneration.[4] Deeper loss of mucosa and underlying supportive structures causes scarring and replacement with poorly differentiated epithelium.[4]

Mild subperichondrial formation of new cartilage and cartilage proliferation can occur in tracheal rings adjacent to a transverse tracheotomy.[41] Cartilage does not regenerate if a segment of tracheal ring is removed.[42] Replacement of damaged cartilage with a prosthesis is not recommended because mucosa that covers the prosthesis is composed of undifferentiated epithelium and mucociliary clearance is damaged sufficiently to cause severe pulmonary complications.[4]

## References


1. Hare WCD. Equine Respiratory System. In: Sisson and Grossman's The Anatomy of the Domestic Animal. 5th Ed. R. Getty (ed). Philadelphia, WB Saunders Co, 1975.
2. Tangner CH, Hedlund CS. Tracheal surgery in the dog—part I. Comp Cont Ed Pract Vet, *5*:599, 1983.
3. West JB. Respiratory Physiology—The Essentials. Baltimore, Williams & Wilkins, 1981.
4. Peacock EE. Wound Repair. 3rd Ed. Philadelphia, WB Saunders Co, 1984.
5. Tate LP, Koch DB, Sembrat RF, et al. Tracheal reconstruction by resection and end-to-end anastomosis in the horse. J Am Vet Med Assoc, *178*:253, 1981.
6. Robinson NE, Sorenson PR. Pathophysiology of airway obstruction in horses: A review. J Am Vet Med Assoc, *172*:299, 1978.
7. Hanselka DV. Tracheal collapse and laryngeal hemiplegia in the horse. VM/SAC, *68*:859, 1973.
8. Wenger IE, Caron JP. Tracheal mastocytosis in a horse. Can Vet J, *29*:563, 1988.
9. Lane G. Fibreoptic endoscopy. In Pract, *3*:24, 1981.
10. Robertson JT, Spurlock GH. Tracheal reconstruction in a foal. J Am Vet Med Assoc, *189*:313, 1986.
11. Scott EA. Ruptured trachea. VM/SAC, *73*:485, 1978.
12. Farrow CS. Pneumomediastinum in the horse: A complication of transtracheal aspiration. J Am Vet Radiol Soc, *19*:192, 1976.
13. Fubini SL, Todhunter RJ, Vivrette SL, et al. Tracheal rupture in two horses. J Am Vet Med Assoc, *187*:69, 1985.
14. Caron JP, Townsend HGG. Tracheal perforation and widespread subcutaneous emphysema in a horse. Can Vet J, *25*:339, 1984.
15. Heath RB. Complications associated with general anesthesia of the horse. Vet Clin North Am [Large Anim Pract], *3*:45, 1981.
16. Holland M, Snyder JR, Steffey EP, et al. Laryngotra-

cheal injury associated with nasotracheal intubation in the horse. J Am Vet Med Assoc, *189*:1447, 1986.
17. Grillo NC. Tracheostomy and its complications. In: Davis-Christopher Textbook of Surgery. 12th Ed. D.C. Sabiston (ed). Philadelphia, WB Saunders Co, 1981.
18. Sanada Y, Kojima Y, Fonkalsrud EW. Injury of cilia induced by tracheal tube cuffs. Surg Gynecol Obstet, *154*:648, 1982.
19. Nelson AW. Lower respiratory system. In: Textbook of Small Animal Surgery. D.H. Slatter (ed). Philadelphia, WB Saunders Co, 1985.
20. Simmons TR, Petersen M, Parker J, et al. Tracheal collapse due to chondrodysplasia in a miniature horse foal. Equine Pract, *10*:39, 1988.
21. Martin JE. Dorsoventral flattening of the trachea in a pony. Eq Pract, *3*:17, 1981.
22. Rothenbacher H. Interesting differential diagnosis in a case of "heaves" in a horse. VM/SAC, *60*:211, 1965.
23. Carrig CB, Groenendyk S, Seawright AA. Dorsoventral flattening of the trachea in a horse and its attempted surgical correction: a case report. J Am Vet Rad Soc, *14*:32, 1973.
24. Delahanty DD, Georgi JR. A tracheal deformity in a pony. J Am Vet Med Assoc, *125*:42, 1954.
25. Hedlund CS, Tangner CH. Tracheal surgery in the dog—part II. Comp Cont Ed Pract Vet, *5*:738, 1983.
26. Mansmann RA. Evaluation of transtracheal aspiration in the horse. J Am Vet Med Assoc, *169*:631, 1976.
27. Brown CM, Collier MA. Tracheobronchial foreign body in a horse. J Am Vet Med Assoc, *182*:280, 1983.
28. Hultgren BD, Pearson EG, Lassen ED, et al. Pleuritis and pneumonia attributed to a conifer twig in a bronchus of a horse. J Am Vet Med Assoc, *189*:797, 1986.
29. Urquhart KA, Gerring EL. Tracheobronchial foreign body in a pony. Equine Vet J, *13*:262, 1981.
30. Duckett WM, Baum JL, Cook WR. Bronchial foreign body in a horse. Equine Pract, *5*:8, 1983.
31. Lane JG. Fibreoptic endoscopy of the equine upper respiratory tract: a commentary on progress. Equine Vet J, *19*:495, 1987.
32. Randall RW, Myers VS. Partial tracheal stenosis in a horse. VM/SAC, *68*:264, 1973.
33. Yovich JV, Stashak TS. Surgical repair of a collapsed trachea caused by a lipoma in a horse. Vet Surg, *13*:217, 1984.
34. Goulden BE. Some unusual cases of abnormal respiratory noises in the horse. NZ Vet J, *25*:389, 1977.
35. Pouret E. Laryngeal ventriculectomy with stitching of the laryngeal saccules. In: Proceedings of 12th Annual Meeting of the American Association of Equine Practitioners, 1966, p 207.
36. Moulton JW. Tumors in Domestic Animals. 2nd Ed. Berkeley, University of California Press, 1978.
37. Raker CW. Trachea and tracheostomy. In: Equine Medicine and Surgery. R.A. Mansmann, and E.S. McAllister (eds). Santa Barbara, American Veterinary Publications, 1982.
38. Nunn JF. Applied respiratory physiology. 2nd Ed. Boston, Butterworths, 1977.
39. Moore JN, Johnson JH, Traver DS, et al. Tracheostomy. Arch ACVS, *6*:35, 1977.
40. Delahanty DD. A tracheotomy with complications in surgery. J Am Vet Med Assoc, *124*:265, 1954.
41. Harvey CE, Goldschmidt MH. Healing following short duration transverse incision tracheotomy in the dog. Vet Surg, *11*:77, 1982.
42. Natvig K, Olving JH. Tracheal changes in relation to different tracheostomy techniques. J Laryngol Otol, *95*:61, 1981.
43. Lulenski GC, Batsakis JG. Tracheal incision as a contributing factor to tracheal stenosis. An experimental study. Ann Otol, *84*:781, 1975.
44. Comroe JH, Forster RE, Dubois AB, et al. The Lung. 2nd Ed. Chicago, Year Book Medical Publishers Inc, 1962.
45. Shappell KK, Stick JA, Derksen FJ, et al. Permanent tracheostomy in Equidae: 47 cases (1981–1986). J Am Vet Med Assoc, *192*:939, 1988.
46. Hedlund CS. Tracheal anastomosis in the dog. Comparison of two end-to-end techniques. Vet Surg, *13*:135, 1984.
47. Horney FD. Tracheal prosthesis in a calf. J Am Vet Med Assoc, *167*:463, 1975.
48. Levine SA, Lindsay WA, Beck KA. The use of a silicone T-tube to treat tracheal stenosis in a llama. Vet Surg, *16*:241, 1987.
49. Tate LP. Laser application in large animals. Proceedings of ACVS 16th Veterinary Surgery Forum, 1988, p 24.
50. Tulleners EP. Contact neodymium: YAG laser-assisted excision of upper airway obstructions in the horse. Vet Surg, *18*:68, 1989.

CHAPTER 22

# DISORDERS OF THE NEONATAL FOAL

*ANNE M. KOTERBA*

Diseases associated with the respiratory system are particularly common during the neonatal period, as both primary conditions and conditions which occur secondary to other disease processes. In many instances, abnormalities result from failure of the lungs to make a complete transition from a collapsed, fluid-filled organ to an air-filled structure responsible for sufficient gas exchange for the entire body. Even if the lungs are reasonably normal at birth, pathologic conditions of the lungs often develop during the course of treatment for other neonatal diseases or dysfunction, most notably prematurity, birth asphyxia, neonatal maladjustment syndrome, and septicemia. The onset of the pulmonary component of the syndrome, however, may be extremely insidious and therefore difficult to diagnose on physical examination alone. Failure to identify pulmonary disease early often results in an unfavorable outcome, with chronic, severe pneumonia and/or respiratory failure resulting.

## Diagnostic Approach to Respiratory Dysfunction in the Neonatal Foal

### *History*

Important historic parameters include the gestational age and maturity of foal at birth, prenatal maternal problems, such as vaginal discharge, fever, etc., systemic illness in the mare prior to or following foaling, abnormal delivery, placental abnormalities, meconium staining, suboptimal passive transfer of immunity, and possible exposure to infectious diseases, such as equine herpesvirus-1 and equine influenza.

### *Physical Examination*

#### Limitations of the Physical Examination

Diagnosis of respiratory abnormalities in the equine neonate by physical examination can be straightforward or difficult. Signs of respiratory distress and hypoxemia may be rather vague. Some severely affected individuals show only restlessness and considerable resistance and struggling when handled. Fever, cough, and nasal discharge are inconsistently observed in neonatal respiratory disease. There are also nonrespiratory conditions that cause clinical signs, such as increased respiratory rate, which mimic respiratory disease and these must be distinguished as well (Table 22–1).

Physical examination is usually not particularly useful in identifying the cause of the respiratory disorder, even when clinical signs are present. Physical findings are best interpreted in conjunction with blood gas analysis, radiographic findings, and other laboratory

**TABLE 22–1.** ***Conditions Associated with Respiratory Distress in the Neonate***[58]

1. Airway obstruction
   - Malformations (e.g., choanal atresia)
   - Laryngeal edema
   - Tracheal malformation; stenosis, collapse
   - Trauma
2. Developmental disorders
   - Pulmonary hypoplasia
   - Diaphragmatic hernia
3. Lung parenchymal diseases
   - Pneumonia (bacterial or viral)
   - Atelectasis
   - Hyaline membrane disease
   - Pulmonary edema, congestion
   - Aspiration
   - Air leaks (e.g., pneumothorax)
   - Pulmonary hemorrhage
4. Non-pulmonary causes
   - Birth asphyxia
   - Congestive heart failure
   - Central nervous system lesions
   - Metabolic derangements (e.g., acidosis, hypoglycemia)
   - Severe anemia, hypovolemia
   - Persistent pulmonary hypertension
   - Pain
   - Abdominal crisis
   - Fever, high environmental temperatures
   - Excitement
   - Pleural effusion (e.g., pleuritis)
   - Transient tachypnea syndrome (cause unknown)

parameters. There should be a high index of suspicion of pulmonary complications in conditions such as prematurity, sepsis, and post-asphyxial injury. Careful assessment of the respiratory system should take place early in the disease course, and the animal should be monitored closely for worsening respiratory function.

## Breathing Pattern

Assessment of the pattern and effort of breathing is an important part of the examination of the respiratory system. Any obvious abnormal noises associated with respiration should be noted.

Inspiratory noises are most commonly associated with upper airway obstruction, but if obstruction is severe, noise may be present throughout the breathing cycle. Upper airway malformations which result in obstruction to air flow can cause respiratory distress. Deviation of the nasal septum, stenotic nares, choanal atresia, masses in the respiratory passages, or malformations of the pharynx, soft palate or larynx may all be associated with signs of upper airway obstruction. Tracheal collapse during breathing may also obstruct respiration and predispose to lower respiratory tract disease. Any problem which interferes with swallowing (botulism, cleft palate, guttural pouch tympany, neurologic disease) may result in aspiration pneumonia. If noises are associated with breathing or dysphagia is noted, radiography and/or endoscopy is usually indicated to make a more specific diagnosis.

Expiratory grunting has been associated with active laryngeal throttling in both human infants and neonatal foals. This laryngeal activity acts to retard expiratory air flow with a greater end-expiratory lung volume resulting. A larger end-expiratory lung volume aids gas exchange, decreases the work of breathing, and is thus particularly advantageous to the neonate with pulmonary diseases such as atelectasis and pneumonia.

The respiratory rate and amount of rib retraction, abdominal muscle activity, and paradoxical movement of the chest and abdomen (chest moving in and abdomen moving out on inspiration) should also be noted. Although the respiratory rate can be increased as a result of many factors unrelated to the respiratory system, a trend of increasing respiratory rate may indicate a worsening pulmonary condition and should not be ignored. The normal pattern of breathing in the healthy, awake neonate is regular, while during rapid eye movement (REM) sleep, extremely erratic breathing patterns may be noted. Irregular breathing patterns, often characterized by periods of tachypnea or normal breathing alternating with 10 to 30 second periods of apnea and resulting in hypercapnia and hypoxemia, have also been observed in the awake premature or asphyxiated foal, or in the foal suffering from neonatal maladjustment syndrome. In the standing position, a small abdominal component is normally observed at end-expiration. Any marked abdominal effort, however, is an abnormal finding.

Normal values for respiratory rate, tidal

volume, and other respiratory parameters in the neonatal foal are listed in Tables 22–2 and 22–3.

## Mucous Membrane Color

Mucous membrane color can be extremely misleading in the evaluation of the respiratory system. Cyanosis is not a reliable indicator of adequacy of oxygenation in the neonate, as the partial pressure of oxygen may reach low levels (<35 to 40 mmHg) before cyanosis is observed. In the cyanotic foal, pulmonary causes must be differentiated from cardiac causes.

## Lung Auscultation

Lung sounds are normally much easier to hear in the neonate than in the adult. They may sound abnormally loud and harsh, particularly if the respiratory rate is elevated. In many cases, the number and type of abnormal lung sounds auscultated do not seem to correlate well with the degree of pulmonary dysfunction. Individuals with no auscultable abnormalities may have severe pulmonary disease, while resolution of an interstitial disease process may actually be accompanied by worsening nasal discharge and adventitial sounds, with increased secretions into the alveoli. Marked differences between the sounds of the upper and lower lung in lateral recumbency have been appreciated in neonatal foals with no detectable respiratory disease. In addition, a change from lateral to sternal recumbency may be associated with crackles in the previously down lung. These findings may be secondary to the increased tendency of the immature lung to collapse. In summary, lung auscultation can be a misleading indicator of pulmonary function and must be interpreted together with other data.

# *Thoracic Radiology*

Thoracic radiographs are often helpful in establishing that respiratory disease is present and in determining the type and extent of pulmonary involvement. In human neonatology, thoracic radiographs have been useful in identification of certain diseases with characteristic radiographic appearances, including hyaline membrane disease and meconium aspiration. In equine neonatology, interpretation has not yet advanced to that point.

## Evaluation of Thoracic Radiographs

Shortly after birth, there should be good vascular clarity of the smaller vessels posterior to the heart and in the caudodorsal lung fields. The heart, posterior vena cava, and aorta should be clearly defined, and a thymic shadow is usually visible cranial to the heart. Other tissue structures (including the heart, vessels, and diaphragm) and bones (ribs, vertebrae, long bones) should also be evaluated. Evaluate the type (interstitial, nodular, alveolar, mixed), severity, and location (diffuse, cranioventral, caudodorsal) of the pulmonary infiltrate.

Diffuse infiltrates are commonly associated with atelectasis, interstitial bacterial, or viral pneumonia (Fig. 22–1) and hyaline membrane disease. A cranioventral and/or caudoventral distribution is suggestive of aspiration or inhalation bronchopneumonia, but patchy atelectasis can also result in ventral interstitial densities. A primarily caudodorsal distribution has been observed in several cases of suspected in utero acquired infections in premature foals, the significance of which is unknown (Fig. 22–2).

Unfortunately, there are large voids in our

**TABLE 22–2.** ***Ventilatory Parameters and Pressure Changes During Normal Tidal Breathing in the Standing Foal Less Than 1 Week of Age***[59]

| *Day of Age* | *n* | $V_T$ *(L)* | $V_T$*/kg (ml/kg)* | *f (bpm)* | $V_E$ *(L/min)* | $V_E$*/kg (ml/kg)* | $T_I$ *(sec)* | $T_E$ *(sec)* |
|---|---|---|---|---|---|---|---|---|
| 2 | 7 | 0.65±0.15 | 15.8±2.5 | 53.9±9.9 | 34.8±12.0 | 848±231 | 0.51±0.15 | 0.72±0.09 |
| 7 | 9 | 0.90±0.17 | 17.6±3.0 | 40.9±5.2 | 33.9±7.5 | 717±157 | 0.65±0.10 | 0.75±0.17 |

Values are means ± s.d.

$V_T$ = tidal volume; f = frequency of breathing, bpm = breaths per minute, $\dot{V}_E$ = minute ventilation, $T_I$ = inspiratory time, $T_E$ = expiratory time.

**TABLE 22–3.** ***Subdivisions of Lung Volumes in the Anesthetized Neonatal Foal*[59]**

| *Day* | *n* | *TLC (L)* | *FRC (L)* | *OCW (L)* | *FRC/TLC (%)* | *OCW/TLC (%)* | *TLC/kg (ml/kg)* | *FRC/kg (ml/kg)* |
|---|---|---|---|---|---|---|---|---|
| 2 | 4–5 | 3.23 ± 0.56 | 1.26 ± 0.24 | 1.88 ± 0.22 | 39.2 ± 2.8 | 58.8 ± 5.0 | 79.5 ± 4.5 | 32.0 ± 3.2 |
| 7 | 6 | 4.14 ± 0.43 | 1.65 ± 0.22 | 2.20 ± 0.30 | 39.8 ± 3.5 | 53.5 ± 6.6 | 83.2 ± 4.7 | 33.1 ± 3.2 |

Values are means ± s.d.

BW = body weight; TLC = total lung capacity; FRC = functional residual capacity; OCW = resting volume of chest wall.

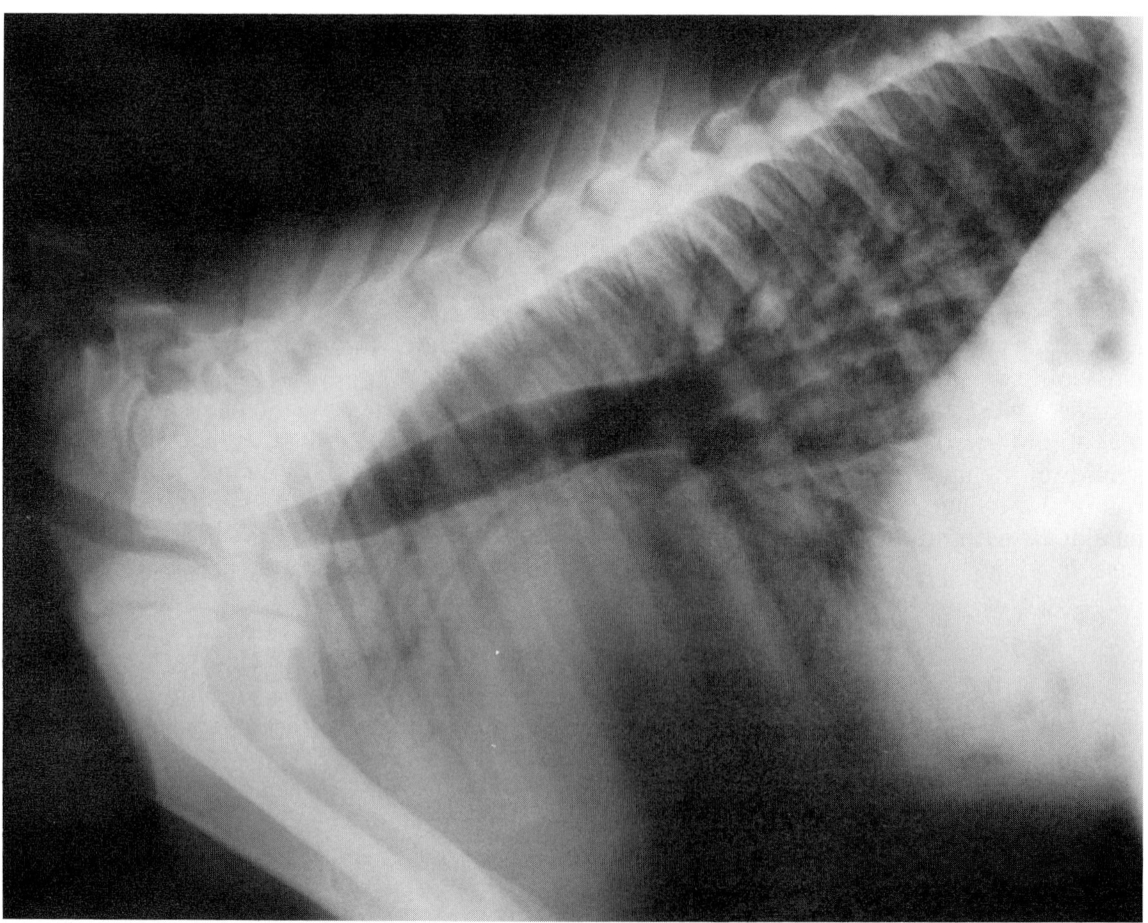

**FIG. 22–1.** Standing chest radiograph of a 3-day-old term Arabian foal with a history of acute onset of respiratory distress and cyanosis ($Pa_{O_2}$ = 22 mmHg). The foal was normal for the first 48 hours of life, and the CBC was normal on presentation. Diffuse pulmonary interstitial and alveolar infiltrates are present. On necropsy, severe interstitial pneumonia with syncytial cell formation was suggestive of viral infection. No bacterial or viral agents were cultured, and the etiology remains unknown.[58]

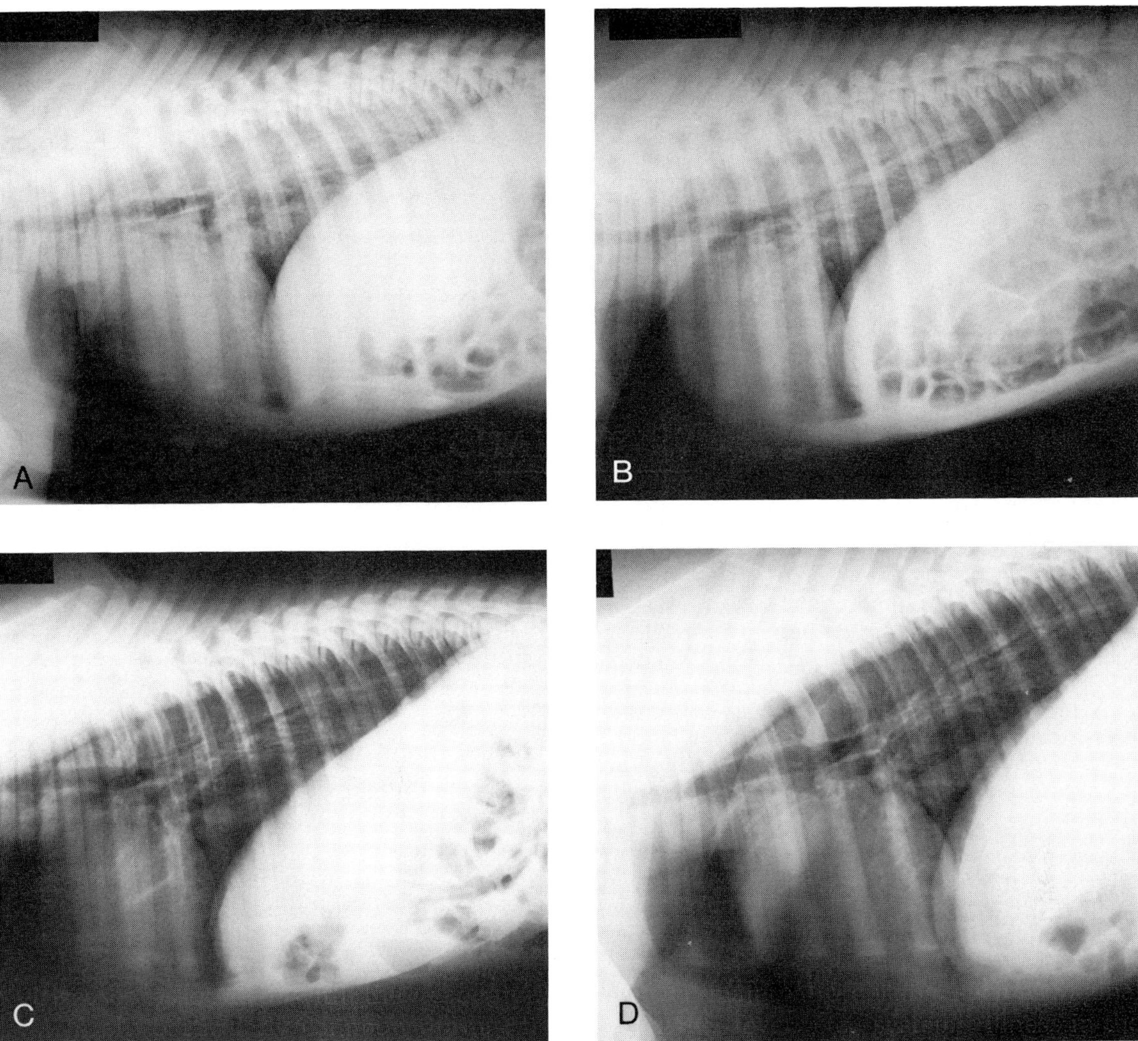


**FIG. 22–2.** A. Thoracic radiograph taken in lateral recumbency of a 305-day gestational age foal with suspected in utero acquired pneumonia (WBC count 48,000; blood cultures negative; $PaO_2$ = 48 mmHg). There is a diffuse increase in pulmonary interstitial infiltrates, particularly in the caudodorsal lung lobes. There is also poor mineralization of sternebral bodies and incomplete ossification of dorsal spinous processes. B. Thoracic radiograph of the same foal 3 days later. Little change has occurred in the diffuse pulmonary interstitial infiltrate. C. Thoracic radiograph of the same foal at 7 days of age. Appearance of the lungs has improved. The interstitial density appears to be resolving, but a small amount remains. D. Thoracic radiograph of the same foal at 3 weeks of age. The interstitial infiltrate continues to improve.[58]

knowledge of normal thoracic radiographic appearance at different gestational and postnatal ages. Therefore, the diagnosis of lung "immaturity" vs. "disease" is virtually impossible. It can be impossible to distinguish bacterial pneumonia accurately from atelectasis or pulmonary edema based on radiographic appearance alone. In these cases, other diagnostic aids (cultures, hematologic studies) must be used in conjunction with radiography to reach an accurate diagnosis. Similar problems in interpretation of lung radiographs have been reported in human neonatology, particularly in distinguishing neonatal pneumonia from hyaline membrane disease.[1] If the neonate has been in lateral recumbency for extended periods of time, atelectasis may result in diffuse or localized interstitial infiltrates which usually resolve once overall strength is regained and lung expansion recurs. Abnormal chest radiographs (increased interstitial density) are frequently ob-

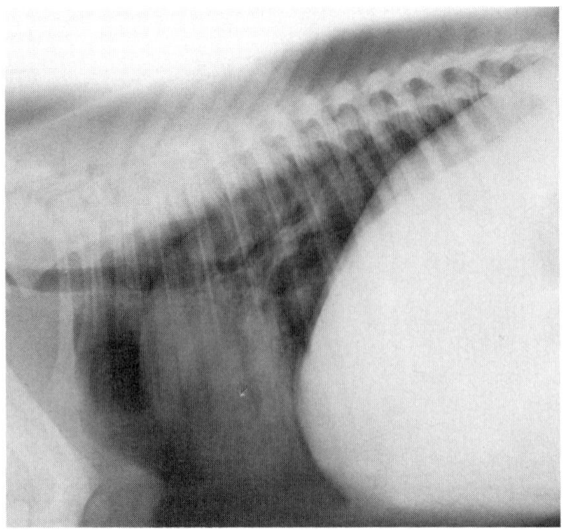

**FIG. 22–3.** Thoracic radiograph (lateral recumbency) of a 36-hour-old pony foal with atresia coli and a grossly distended abdomen (see Fig. 21–5). There is an increase in pulmonary interstitial density, especially in the caudal lung lobes. The interpretation of these radiographs was either atelectasis due to the inability to inspire fully and/or bacterial pneumonia. On histologic examination, atelectasis and an inflammatory cell infiltrate were present.[58]

served with abdominal distension, and it can be difficult to differentiate simple atelectasis as a result of pressure of the abdominal viscera through the diaphragm from an ongoing pneumonic process (Fig. 22–3).

Serial chest radiographs are useful in monitoring the progress of a respiratory condition. Radiographic changes may either follow or precede changes in clinical condition, and sometimes major changes can occur rapidly (Fig. 22–4). Clinical signs of pneumonia frequently resolve long before chest radiographs and hemogram show a return to normal (Fig. 22–2). Because premature cessation of antibiotic therapy has resulted in relapse in a number of cases, sequential radiographs and hematologic studies are highly recommended prior to stopping antibiotic therapy.

### Technique

For the safety of handlers and equipment, thoracic radiographs are routinely taken only in the standing or lateral position in foals, with dorsoventral positioning reserved for the anesthetized or depressed foal. Thus, interpretation can be limited because of positioning constraints. With the use of rare earth screens, thoracic radiology of the foal and calf is feasible using a portable x-ray machine in the field. The major disadvantage of the use of portable x-ray equipment is that motion is often present, particularly when the respiratory rate is high, and there is a tendency to overread such films. Alternatively, most small animal x-ray units are capable of taking good quality chest films, if the patient can be transported to such a facility.

## *Arterial Blood Gas Analysis*

Arterial blood gas analysis is useful in defining the severity of respiratory system dysfunction and the type of respiratory therapy required, as well as monitoring the response to therapy. It is difficult to administer respiratory support safely and effectively to neonates without means to monitor the partial pressures of oxygen ($PaO_2$) and carbon dioxide ($PaCO_2$). Even the simple technique of oxygen insufflation is potentially hazardous because if high oxygen partial pressures are inadvertently maintained, resorption atelectasis and pulmonary oxygen toxicity may result. Thus, although blood gas analysis can be associated with some problems, including difficulty of sampling and interpreting the results, and the inconvenience and expense of analyzing the sample, the advantages of obtaining this information often outweigh the disadvantages.

### Technique of Arterial Blood Gas Sampling in the Neonatal Foal

*Sites for Sampling.* If the pulse quality is reasonably strong, the great metatarsal artery is preferred for sampling. The likelihood of mistakenly acquiring venous blood from this area is fairly low, because in most foals the vein running with the artery is small. With proper care, this artery can be preserved for multiple samples. The brachial artery, as it crosses the medial aspect of the foreleg, is usually easy to palpate, even when the pulse quality is poor in the more peripheral arteries. However the brachial vein may be inadver-

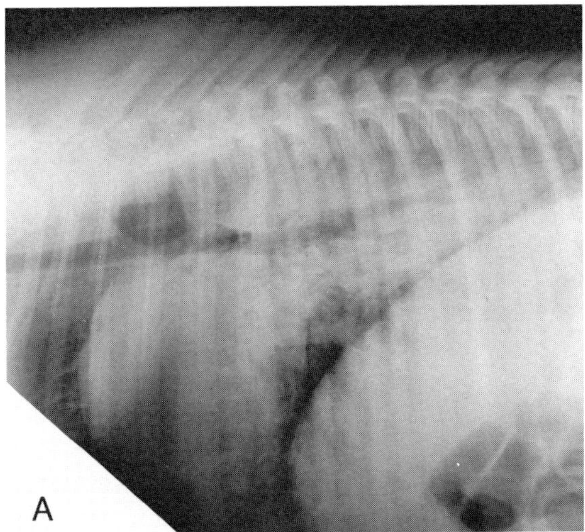


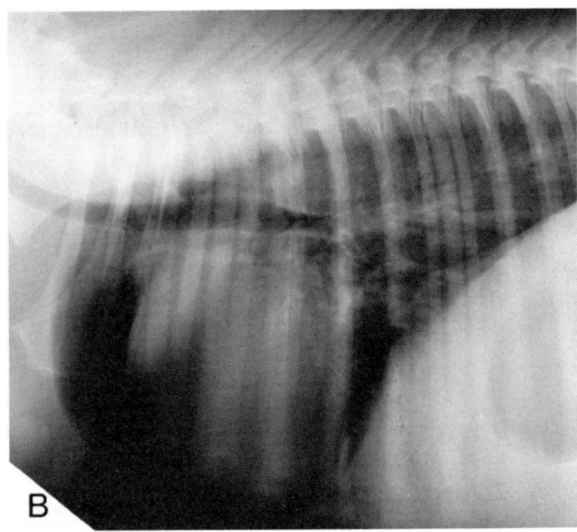


**FIG. 22–4.** A. Chest radiograph of a 6-day-old Thoroughbred foal in respiratory distress secondary to Staphylococcus aureus septicemia and pneumonia. B. Chest radiograph of same foal 5 days later, when the clinical condition was markedly improved. Note the almost complete resolution of the previously extensive pulmonary infiltrate. The hemogram remained abnormal, however, for the first month of age. (From Kosch PE, Koterba AM, Coons TJ, et al. Developments in the management of the newborn foal in respiratory distress. 1: Evaluation. Equine Vet J, *16*:312, 1984.)

tently sampled because it runs close to the artery. The carotid artery is easily palpated in the jugular furrow. However, hematomas readily form after a few samples are drawn and the artery becomes progressively more difficult to locate. Other sites that may be sampled include the facial and femoral arteries.

***Procedure.*** The sample is usually collected while the patient is restrained in sternal or lateral recumbency. The position is noted as $Pa_{O_2}$ may be lower in lateral vs. sternal recumbency (see interpretation of blood gases, below). The site of arterial puncture is clipped and thoroughly cleaned, and the pulse quality is assessed. A small bleb of local anesthetic (2% lidocaine, without epinephrine) placed subcutaneously over the artery can greatly facilitate proper collection technique and minimizes needless struggling and subsequent hyperventilation. A small gauge needle (25 gauge, ⅝ inch) attached to a 1 or 3 ml syringe previously flushed with heparin is used for arterial blood sampling. Ideally, the needle used for the heparin flush is replaced with a sterile needle before the artery is punctured. The needle is advanced through the skin, the artery is located and stabilized, and blood is withdrawn slowly, taking care to introduce as little air as possible into the syringe. Following removal of the needle, direct pressure is placed on the artery for 1 to 2 minutes to minimize hematoma formation and to preserve the artery for future sampling. Any air bubbles are removed promptly from the syringe, and the syringe is sealed with a cork and placed in ice slush until the analysis is carried out. A sealed blood gas sample may be stored on ice for 6 hours without major changes in $Pa_{O_2}$.

***Problems Associated with Direct Arterial Puncture and Alternate Methods.*** Problems caused by poor compliance by the patient and vessel trauma after multiple punctures can be serious limitations to adequate blood gas monitoring. In most cases, if good technique is used, arteries can be maintained for many days of frequent sampling. If pulse pressure is poor, however, it can be difficult to maintain an artery for frequent sampling.

Alternatively, percutaneous placement of an indwelling arterial catheter is not difficult, but maintenance of catheter position and patency can be extremely difficult. A slow constant infusion of saline* is often helpful in preventing clotting. An umbilical arterial

*Infusor, Baxter Healthcare Corp.

catheter may also be placed if the birth is attended. In each case, the advantages of continuous access to arterial blood must be weighed against the possible disadvantages, including infection and hemorrhage.

Various methods for noninvasively monitoring oxygen tension in the body have been developed. Unfortunately, although transcutaneous oxygen monitors are widely used in human neonatology, they were not valid when tested in the neonatal foal.[2] A transconjunctival oxygen monitor was found to yield more accurate results in the anesthetized foal,[3] but the development of a suitable probe for the awake foal posed serious technical difficulties, and the instrumentation is no longer available. A relatively recent development in oxygen monitoring has been the wide adoption of pulse oximetry. This technology can be easily used and gives a continuous measure of arterial oxygen saturation. The equipment is expensive, however, and the technique has not been rigorously tested in the foal. One general problem with all of these noninvasive oxygen monitoring systems is that since they estimate the oxygenation status of the peripheral tissues, when perfusion and hypotension develop, they tend to become much less accurate in reflecting arterial oxygen concentration.

Capnography allows analysis of expired carbon dioxide concentrations and provides an estimate of $Paco_2$. The end-tidal $CO_2$ corresponds to the partial pressure of $CO_2$ in alveolar gas, which is assumed equal to the partial pressure of $CO_2$ in mixed pulmonary venous blood, and approximately equal to $Paco_2$. Capnographs measure expired $CO_2$ concentration using infrared spectroscopy. End-tidal $CO_2$ measurements are made over several respiratory cycles or continuously. Clinical applications of capnography include monitoring of both patients receiving mechanical ventilation and those which are spontaneously breathing but have severe lung disease with precarious gas exchange. In cases of uneven ventilation, however, end-tidal $CO_2$ may not accurately reflect the $Paco_2$. Noninvasive monitors do not replace arterial blood gas analysis, but can markedly reduce the frequency of sampling.

## Interpretation of Arterial Blood Gas Results

Factors influencing the interpretation of arterial blood gas results include the sampling technique, measurement techniques, the position and amount of struggling of the foal when the sample is drawn, gestational and postnatal age of the foal, and the inspired oxygen concentration.

Introduction of room air into the blood sample is one of the most common sampling errors. The presence of room air artificially increases $Pao_2$ and decreases $Paco_2$, resulting in a more alkaline pH. Faulty measurement techniques include improper calibration of the blood gas machine and introduction of air when the machine aspirates the sample. The position of the neonate when the sample is taken (lateral vs. sternal) can exert an important effect on blood oxygen concentration. In many neonatal foals, particularly those with immature or diseased lungs,[4] but also in the normal, term foal,[5] a significant decrease in the $Pao_2$ can result from repositioning from sternal or standing to lateral recumbency (Table 22–4). Clearly, this observation also becomes important in treatment considerations. With supplemental oxygen, $Pao_2$ will be increased variably, depending on the age of the foal, inspired oxygen concentration and the amount of disease present, particularly the extent of right to left shunting, and possibly, the foal's position.[7] While a $Pao_2$ of 85 mmHg would be considered normal in a foal breathing room air, it would be abnormal if 100% oxygen is being inspired. A flow rate of 10 L/min increased the $Pao_2$ to 298 $\pm$ 68.7 mmHg (mean $\pm$ SEM) in the normal term, 4 to 11 hour old foal, but to only 110.6 $\pm$ 34.8 mmHg in the prematurely induced, 0.5 to 10 hour old foal.[8] In another study,[7] a greater response was noted in older neonatal foals breathing 100% oxygen. Although values obtained at 12 hours of age were similar to the above values, at 48 hours, the mean oxygen tension was 363.8 $\pm$ 36.0 mmHg, 368.9 $\pm$ 52.6 mmHg at 4 days of age, and 484.0 $\pm$ 43.2 mmHg at 7 days of age. All foals were restrained in lateral recumbency for the studies.[7]

If the $Pao_2$ of a hypoxemic patient remains low ($<$200 mmHg) while the patient is breath-

**TABLE 22–4.** ***Normal Arterial Blood Gas Values. X ± SEM[58]***

| *Gestational Age/Status* | *Postnatal Age* | *Position* | *pH* | *$Paco_2$ mmHg* | *$Pao_2$ mmHg* | *$HCO_3$* | *n* | *Ref* |
|---|---|---|---|---|---|---|---|---|
| Normal | 3–168 hr | Lateral | 7.354 ± 0.011 | 47.5 ± 2.6 | 80.0 ± 3.8 | | 10 | 60 |
| Normal | 1–12 hr | Lateral | 7.378 ± .015 | 42.2 ± 1.8 | 77.3 ± 3.1 | | 6 | 61 |
| | 12–48 hr | | 3.374 ± .004 | 44.5 ± 1.2 | 83.2 ± 3.1 | | 6 | |
| | 48–168 hr | | 7.384 ± .014 | 42.4 ± 1.0 | 88.2 ± 5.9 | | 5 | |
| Normal | 4–11 hr | Lateral | 7.367 ± .010 | 39.5 ± 1.8 | 83.8 ± 6.3 | | 5 | 6 |
| Normal | 24 hr | Standing | 7.41 ± .03 | 45.2 ± 2.5 | 84.6 ± 6.9 | | 3 | 5 |
| | 24 hr | Lateral | 7.38 ± .05 | 48.1 ± 3.8 | 72.69 ± 14.2 | | 3 | |
| | 48 hr | Standing | 7.40 ± .03 | 47.5 ± 3.7 | 106.6 ± 3.9 | | 3 | |
| | 48 hr | Lateral | 7.37 ± .00 | 49.5 ± 2.8 | 89.6 ± 12.7 | | 3 | |
| | 72 hr | Standing | 7.39 ± .07 | 49.6 ± 1.5 | 104.5 ± 4.8 | | 5 | |
| | 72 hr | Lateral | 7.44 ± .14 | 51.6 ± 7.2 | 94.1 ± 4.3 | | 5 | |
| | 144 hr | Standing | 7.42 ± .03 | 47.3 ± 2.3 | 98.8 ± 4.8 | | 5 | |
| | 144 hr | Lateral | 7.41 ± .03 | 46.9 ± 2.1 | 84.2 ± 6.9 | | 5 | |
| Premature | .5–11 hr | Lateral | 7.208 ± .048 | 55.3 ± 3.6 | 53.7 ± 1.5 | | 7 | 61 |
| Term | Birth | Lateral | 7.413 ± 0.019 | 45.7 ± 1.1 | 39.7 ± 2.1 | 26.3 ± 1.1 | 8 | 62 |
| | 2 min | Lateral | 7.312 ± 0.016 | 54.1 ± 2.0 | 56.4 ± 2.3 | 24.0 ± 1.2 | 10 | |
| | 15 min | Lateral | 7.322 ± 0.025 | 50.4 ± 2.7 | 57.5 ± 3.6 | 24.4 ± 1.6 | 9 | |
| | 30 min | Lateral | 7.354 ± 0.010 | 51.5 ± 1.5 | 57.0 ± 1.8 | 25.3 ± 0.7 | 10 | |
| | 60 min | Lateral | 7.362 ± 0.013 | 47.3 ± 2.2 | 60.9 ± 2.7 | 25.3 ± 1.0 | 9 | |
| | 2 hr | Lateral | 7.362 ± 0.012 | 47.7 ± 1.7 | 66.5 ± 2.3 | 25.0 ± 0.9 | 8 | |
| | 4 hr | Lateral | 7.355 ± 0.017 | 45.0 ± 1.9 | 75.7 ± 4.9 | 23.6 ± 1.1 | 10 | |
| | 12 hr | Lateral | 7.357 ± 0.024 | 44.3 ± 1.2 | 73.5 ± 3.0 | 23.2 ± 1.3 | 10 | |
| | 24 hr | Lateral | 7.393 ± 0.012 | 45.5 ± 1.5 | 67.6 ± 4.4 | 26.2 ± 1.1 | 9 | |
| | 48 hr | Lateral | 7.398 ± 0.008 | 46.1 ± 1.1 | 74.9 ± 3.3 | 25.7 ± 0.6 | 8 | |
| | 96 hr | Lateral | 7.396 ± 0.012 | 45.8 ± 1.1 | 81.2 ± 3.1 | 23.2 ± 2.1 | 8 | |

ing 100% oxygen, some degree of right to left shunting must be present. The other causes of hypoxemia (ventilation/perfusion mismatch, hypoventilation, diffusion impairment) are considerably more responsive to 100% oxygen (Table 22–5). Intracardiac causes of shunt must be distinguished from intrapulmonary causes.

Both the gestational and postnatal age of the animal influence the expected blood gas results. Table 22–4 lists previously reported normal values from days 1 to 7 of life in term, awake foals in lateral and standing position. The values listed for premature foals should not be considered "normal" because many of these individuals were compromised following induction of parturition.

## Patterns of Arterial Blood Gas Derangement

If an abnormality is detected on blood gas analysis, one of two patterns of derangement is usually encountered:

***Hypoxemia.*** ($Pao_2$ <70 mmHg) with low or normal $Paco_2$. Hypoxemia may result from:

1. Right to left vascular shunting (intrapulmonary or cardiac shunt); common.
2. Ventilation-perfusion mismatch; common.
3. Inadequate alveolar ventilation (hypoventilation; $Paco_2$ is also increased); common.
4. Diffusion impairment (uncommon).
5. Low inspired oxygen (rare).

**TABLE 22–5.** ***Interpretation of Arterial Blood Gases in Newborn Foals***[58]

| *Functional Problem* | $Pao_2$ | $Paco_2$ | *pH* | $P(A\text{–}a)O_2$ | *Response to 100% $O_2$* | *Typical Clinical Conditions* |
|---|---|---|---|---|---|---|
| $\dot{V}$–$\dot{Q}$ mismatch | ↓ | Normal or ↓ from hypoxic drive | Normal or ↓ from tissue hypoxia | ↑ | Good | Pneumonia<br>Aspiration<br>HMD |
| Right to left shunt | ↓ | Normal or ↓ from hypoxic drive | Normal or ↓ from tissue hypoxia | ↑ | Poor | Atelectasis<br>PFC<br>Congenital heart disease |
| Alveolar hypoventilation | ↓ | Increased | Decreased unless full metabolic compensation | Normal | Very good | CNS depression, upper airway obstruction, fatigue |
| Diffusion impairment | ↓ | Normal or ↓ from hypoxic drive | Normal or ↓ from tissue hypoxia | ↑ | Good | Common with most parenchymal conditions |
| Low inspired oxygen | ↓ | Normal or ↓ from hypoxic drive | Normal or ↓ from tissue hypoxia | Normal | Very good | Iatrogenic |

$P(A\text{–}a)O_2$ = alveolar-arterial $O_2$ difference; HMD = hyaline membrane disease; CNS = central nervous system; PFC = persistent fetal circulation. Note: Normal values have not been determined from different ages of neonatal foals. Values will depend on the "normal" degree of venous admixture (right to left shunt, $\dot{V}/\dot{Q}$ mismatch). Normal values for adults would be less than 20 mmHg.

*Hypoxemia with Hypercapnia.* If hypercapnia is present, hypoventilation is diagnosed. Respiratory acidosis may or may not be compensated, depending on the duration of the disease process. In the neonate, hypoventilation may occur for several different reasons.

1. One of the most common reasons is the inability of the neonate's respiratory muscles to work hard enough to ventilate abnormal lungs adequately.
2. In animals with neurologic dysfunction, chemosensitivity also may be altered, resulting in an inappropriate ventilatory response to changes in blood gas values.
3. In foals with botulism and other neuromuscular diseases, hypoventilation occurs primarily because the respiratory muscles become too weak to ventilate normal lungs adequately.

Clinical signs must be evaluated in addition to blood gas analysis in order to choose the appropriate therapy. Certain hypoxic and/or hypercapnic neonates do not display signs of respiratory distress, while others with similar or worse blood gas parameters will be markedly distressed. The reasons for these discrepancies may include the rapidity of the development of the problem, developmental or pathologic variation in chemoreceptor function, and the type of lung disorder present.

## *Venous Blood Gas Analysis*

Interpretation of blood gas values of venous blood can be notoriously deceptive and is properly restricted to evaluation of peripheral conditions and not pulmonary gas exchange. Venous blood gas analysis may be useful in the following circumstances:

***Tissue Hypoxia Due to Insufficient $O_2$ Delivery.*** This would most commonly reflect poor tissue perfusion due to cardiac failure. To avoid problems associated with regional blood sampling, peripheral venous blood should be taken from a free flowing jugular vein since the metabolic status of the head is usually stable. In order to obtain a sample representative of the whole body, mixed venous blood is drawn from the right atrium. Determination of mixed venous blood oxygen saturation is a good test for assessing the overall adequacy of oxygen delivery to tissues because it reflects the balance between oxygen delivery and oxygen utilization.

***Tissue Hypoxia Due to Arterial Hypoxemia.*** When an arterial puncture is not possible without a cut-down, a jugular venous sample combined with clinical impressions may be used to estimate the extent of the clinical problem. If jugular venous $P_{CO_2}$ is >60 mmHg, arterial hypercapnia is probably present, and if venous $PO_2$ is <20 mmHg, arterial hypoxemia or cardiac failure (poor tissue perfusion, therefore inadequate oxygen delivery to tissues) is suspected. A normal venous $PO_2$ does not rule out severe gas exchange abnormalities with arterial hypoxemia. If venous blood is obtained from a poorly perfused and/or cold site, such as a leg vein, the results probably do not reflect the overall status of the individual.

# *Bacterial Cultures*

## Blood Cultures

When respiratory infection is acquired via the hematogenous route, failure of passive transfer is present, or if infection is well established, blood cultures are often useful in identifying the responsible bacteria.[8] If pneumonia is acquired through the respiratory tract via aspiration (infected amniotic fluid or meconium) or inhalation, and localized to that area, blood cultures may not identify the pathogen. In these situations, bacterial cultures should be acquired from additional locations (see below). Details of blood culture technique are provided in other references.[8,9] If neonatal infection is suspected, blood cultures are taken regardless of body temperature and previous antibiotic therapy. Fever is inconsistently associated with neonatal sepsis, and cultures may still be positive even with previous use of antibiotics.[8] Although taking several blood cultures over a period of time may improve the sensitivity of the technique, the necessity of instituting antibiotic therapy promptly often precludes the acquisition of a series of blood cultures.

## Transtracheal Aspiration

***Procedure.*** The ventral cervical skin overlying the trachea is clipped and a sterile scrub is performed. Local anesthetic (lidocaine) is injected subcutaneously over the trachea and a stab incision is made in the skin. With the foal adequately restrained (lateral or standing), a 14-gauge 2-inch intravenous catheter (Abbocath, Abbott Hospital Inc., St. Louis, Mo.) or a 16- to 19-gauge, 6-inch intravenous catheter is inserted between the tracheal rings into the tracheal lumen. After removal of the stylet (if the 2-inch catheter is used, a 5-French polypropylene canine catheter [Monoject, St. Louis, Mo.] is passed through the catheter down to the area of the carina), a syringe is attached to the catheter and 10 to 15 ml of nonbacteriostatic sterile saline is injected into the tracheal lumen and rapidly aspirated. If no fluid is recovered, additional fluid is injected and then aspirated.

***Sample Analysis.*** The sample should be divided into two portions; one for cytology, one for microbiology. Direct smears are also examined with a Gram stain, for an early indication of the type of bacteria present. Cytology and bacteriology of tracheal washes of normal foals have not been well delineated. Although the lower airways of the adult horse are expected to have little or no resident bacterial flora, it is not known if this is true for the foal. Based on preliminary evidence,[10] although the airways of normal neonatal foals are presumably sterile at birth, early bacterial colonization of the trachea and lower airways probably does occur. Therefore, mixed microbiologic cultures from tracheal aspirates of ill foals must be cautiously interpreted. Pure bacterial cultures accompanied by cytologic evidence of infection (intracellular bacteria, degenerative neutrophils, etc.) are considered indicative of infection. Unfortunately, nosocomial pneumonias in intubated human patients, intubated baboons, and baboons with diffuse lung injury tend to be polymicrobial.[11] The same probably is true for the hospitalized foal. Quantitative bacteriology has been useful in human medicine to distinguish likely pathogens from upper respiratory tract contaminants and from tracheal colonizers. A "bacterial index," which takes into account the bacterial concentration of the separate bacterial isolated species, may become useful in diagnosis of lower respiratory disease in the foal and horse.

Possible complications of tracheal washes include local reactions, such as cellulitis and abscess formation, subcutaneous emphysema, and pneumomediastinum. The sample obtained may not accurately reflect what is occurring in the lung parenchyma. The procedure may also be excessively stressful to the foal in respiratory distress. Complications are rare.

### Guarded Brush Catheter Cultures

An important advance in human medicine was the development of the protected specimen brush. The brush is generally passed through an endoscope to collect secretions from a selected airway, but it may be passed through an endotracheal tube as well. The configuration of the brush protects it from upper airway contamination. It has been reasonably accurate in diagnosing both community acquired and nosocomial pneumonias in humans and animal models.[11] Most studies have employed quantitative methods to identify bacterial pathogens (usually using a finding of $\geq 10^3$ colony-forming units [cfu]/ml to distinguish pathogens from contaminants).

***Procedure.*** The foal is restrained in either standing or lateral position. A flexible fiberoptic bronchoscope or endotracheal tube is passed via the nares into the trachea. In most neonatal foals, this is met with little resistance. If a bronchoscope is used, it is passed into a second order bronchus of the right caudal lung lobe. Cultures are obtained by passing a double sheathed brush catheter* through the inner channel of the bronchoscope and advanced beyond the end of the bronchoscope. The inner telescoping cannula containing the specimen sampling brush is advanced about 2 cm, the protective polyethylene glycol plug is ejected, and the specimen is obtained by advancing the brush into the airway secretions. The brush is retracted, the device is removed, and the secretions on the brush are cultured. If an endotracheal tube is used, the brush catheter is blindly passed through it into the trachea, and the wall of the trachea gently brushed with a swirling motion. One advantage to this technique is that if an endotracheal tube is used, an airway is already established if a foal becomes distressed by the procedure. Most neonatal foals tolerate nasotracheal intubation well. However, as in the transtracheal aspiration technique, interpretation may be difficult unless a pure culture is obtained or quantitative cultures are performed.

*Micro Vasive, Milford, MA

### Endotracheal Tube Cultures

In intubated foals receiving some type of positive pressure ventilation, the normal upper airway defense mechanisms are bypassed, and the endotracheal tube serves as a potential portal of entry of bacteria into the lungs. In human infants, endotracheal tubes are rapidly colonized, and cultures obtained after the tube has been in place for more than 12 hours are likely to be misleading. The ratio of colonization of mucosal surfaces to disease is approximately 300 or 400 to 1.[12] Although we have routinely cultured secretions from endotracheal tubes after removal from the animal, the correlation between these culture results and those obtained at necropsy has not been particularly good. In several foals, however, the same organism was recovered from other culture sites as well, leading us to believe that the result was significant.

### Other Cultures

In the foal with evidence of in utero acquired aspiration pneumonia, it can be difficult to identify the pathogen from blood cultures and tracheal aspirates alone, particularly if cultures are delayed until after antibiotic therapy is instituted. In these cases, additional sites should be cultured, including the urine, gastric contents (pre-suckle), placenta, and uterus of the mare (shortly after foaling). Such cultures should be taken as early in the foal's life as possible.[13]

## *Bronchoalveolar Lavage*

***Procedure.*** The foal is well restrained in standing or lateral position. Sedation usually facilitates the procedure, depending on the awareness and temperament of the foal. The bronchoscope (7 to 8 mm O.D.) is passed through the nasal passages and directed into the trachea. It is directed into the right or left caudal lobe and advanced into a smaller airway to obtain lobar washings for cell counts. The airway is occluded and 200 ml of sterile, pyrogen-free, phosphate-buffered saline solution maintained at body temperature is introduced through the catheter port in 30 ml aliquots. Aspiration by syringe is then immediately performed, and the lung washings are immediately chilled on crushed ice. For details on processing and analysis of this fluid, see Chapter 4.

***Normal Values.*** Complete and definitive descriptions of normal bronchoalveolar lavage fluid analysis in the growing foal are not yet available. In one study, the concentration of alveolar macrophages (cells/ml) in the lavage fluid was considered to be low ($\bar{x} = 3.9 \times 10^3$) in 2-day-old foals, but by 14 days of age, the macrophage numbers approached values considered normal for adult horses ($\bar{x} = 57.6 \times 10^3$). The average distribution of cell types in the fluid retrieved from 2-day-old foals was 84.2% macrophages, 10.44% neutrophils and 5.56% lymphocytes, vs. 69.67% macrophages, 1.86% neutrophils and 28% lymphocytes in the adult horse.[14] The alveolar macrophage was also the predominant cell type (89 ± 7.5% macrophages, 3.7% ± 2% lymphocytes, 7.6% ± 7% neutrophils) in foals <4 days old.[15] The chemotactic function of alveolar macrophages from young foals (<2 weeks of age) was significantly impaired compared to older foals,[14] and alveolar macrophages showed little if any evidence of intracellular killing.[15] It was speculated that these deficiencies could predispose the neonatal foal to respiratory disease.

## *Endoscopy*

Endoscopy of the respiratory tract is performed in the foal in much the same manner as in adult. Most young foals tolerate endoscopy without sedation. Indications for endoscopy include an abnormal pattern of breathing or noises during breathing suggestive of obstruction, milk observed at one or both nostrils, and unexplained external swellings (such as near the guttural pouch) or nasal discharges. A 7 mm outer diameter endoscope is usually small enough to pass through the ventral meatus of most horse and large pony foals.

# Specific Respiratory Conditions

## *Lung Maturity and the Surfactant System in the Neonate*

Surfactant, a mixture of phospholipids (primarily dipalmitoyl phosphatidylcholine [DPPC] and phosphatidylglycerol [PG]) and proteins, is produced and stored in the type II alveolar pneumocytes of the mammalian lung. It is an extremely active surfactant mixture, and under dynamic compression is capable of lowering surface tension dramatically.[16]

The biophysical properties of lung surfactant allow it to reduce the work of breathing by increasing lung compliance, stabilize alveoli, enhance alveolar fluid clearance, decrease the driving force for pulmonary edema, and protect epithelial cell surfaces. In 1959 Avery and Mead[17] reported that saline extracts of lungs removed from premature babies dying of respiratory distress syndrome (RDS) lacked the capacity to reduce surface tension effectively. They suggested that RDS was caused by either the absence or delayed appearance of pulmonary surfactant, due to an immaturity of the type II alveolar epithelial cell. Since that time, the biochemical and physiologic aspects of the fetal and newborn surfactant system have been studied extensively, and many review articles are available.[16,18,19]

Briefly, the time period for maturation of the type II alveolar cells and surfactant system is during the last quarter of gestation. Both DPPC and PG are secreted into the fluid-filled alveoli in the fetal lung and are then carried into the amniotic fluid. Prenatal determination of the likelihood of RDS in premature human infants is largely based on assays of selected phospholipids in the amniotic fluid. There is considerable evidence which suggests that cortisol, thyroxine, β-adrenergic agonists, and other agents stimulate maturation of the surfactant system.[20] The corticosteroids accelerate epithelial maturation of the lung, with increased phospholipid synthesis, and may affect other aspects of lung maturation as well, such as the permeability characteristics of the lung.[21] Their effects are probably mediated at least in part by a local hormone, fibroblast pneumocyte factor, which is produced by local fibroblasts following stimulation by corticosteroids.[16] Other compounds, including insulin and phenobarbital, appear to delay maturation of the fetal lung.

Maturation of the lung involves not only maturation of the surfactant system, but also thinning of the alveolar capillary barrier, a decrease in alveolar epithelial permeability, and maturation of the chest wall.[21] Although lack of surfactant is an important factor in the initiation of RDS, a highly compliant chest wall, altered permeability characteristics of the lung, and the type of perinatal treatment also play important roles in its expression (Fig. 22–5).

The highly compliant chest wall of the premature human neonate predisposes to a low end-expiratory lung volume (EEV), even in the presence of surfactant. This results in an increased tendency for airway collapse and atelectasis and necessitates high pressures to reopen closed airways, increasing the work of breathing. When the neonatal lung is deficient in surfactant, FRC may be further decreased and the work of breathing is increased accordingly. The respiratory muscles must generate more pressure for inflation to any given lung volume, and respiratory muscle failure may result.

The permeability characteristics of the lung may be directly influenced by many factors in addition to surfactant, including the fluid balance of the patient, cardiovascular function, the presence of a patent ductus arteriosus, the degree of pulmonary hypertension, and the extent of ischemic injury (Table 22–6; Figure 22–5). Hyaline membrane formation, the typical pathologic lesion associated with respiratory distress syndrome, is caused by aggregations of protein and cellular debris which accumulate in the alveoli as a result of increased alveolar permeability. This protein not only disrupts alveolar architecture, but also interacts directly with surfactant and inactivates it.[21] Therefore, while a deficiency of surfactant predisposes to increased capillary permeability and a "wet" lung, many other factors can worsen the permeability characteristics, which results in further deterioration in surfactant and pulmonary function (Fig. 22–5). Small airway edema causes narrowing of bronchioles, increasing airway resistance, and interstitial edema decreases lung compliance and FRC. These abnormalities contribute to further impairment in gas exchange. Improvement in lung function in infants with RDS has long been associated with a spontaneous diuresis of extracellular water.[22]

## Primary vs. Secondary Surfactant Deficiency

Surfactant system dysfunction may occur as a result of primary deficiency (as in respiratory distress syndrome of premature infants) or secondary deficiency. A number of other conditions are known to interfere with the activity of surfactant. These include asphyxia, acidosis, hypercarbia, pulmonary edema with protein leak into the alveoli, sepsis, shock, hypoperfusion, prolonged atelectasis, and overinflation.[23]

Determining the relative importance of immaturity (primary deficiency) vs. insults causing surfactant dysfunction (secondary deficiency) in the pathogenesis of neonatal respiratory distress has been the topic of much debate over the years. Various animal models of diffuse lung injury secondary to septic shock, toxins, and asphyxia have been used to study the response of surfactant to alveolar damage. It appears that the response is variable, depending on the severity of injury to the type II alveolar cells.[20]

Reynolds et al[24] investigated the relative influences of gestational age and asphyxia on the development of RDS in neonatal lambs and concluded that immaturity was the most important factor. Although lesions compatible with hyaline membrane disease could be produced by subjecting neonatal lambs to severe asphyxia, the term lambs appeared to be considerably more resistant to asphyxial damage than the younger lambs. Since asphyxia enhances the risk of development of RDS,

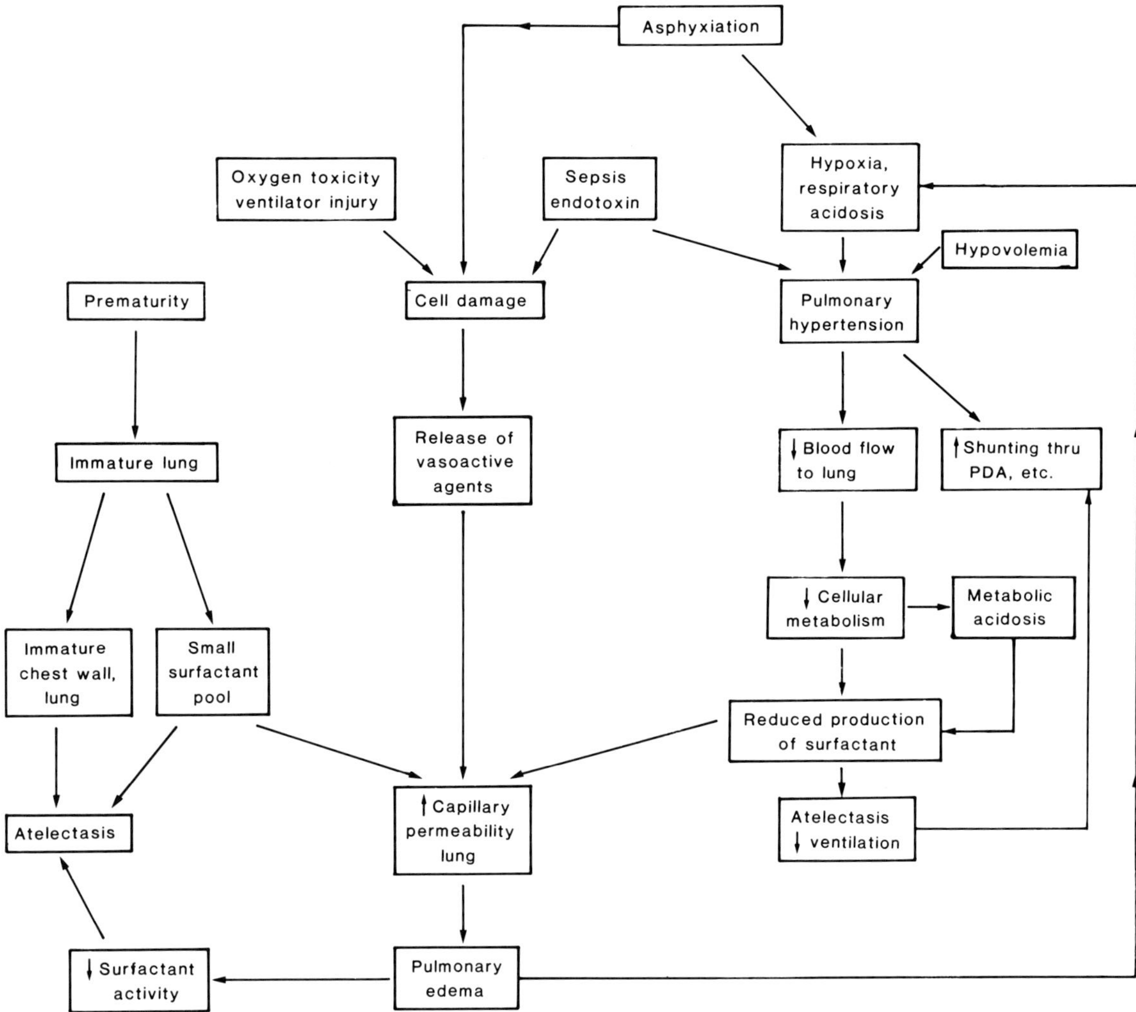


**FIG. 22–5.** Pathophysiology of respiratory distress syndrome in the premature neonate, showing the interactions of an immature chest wall, incomplete surfactant lining, and asphyxial damage.[58]

prevention of birth asphyxia remains of great importance in reducing the incidence of RDS.

Hyaline membrane formation and atelectasis are not pathognomonic for primary surfactant deficiency; they can be observed in human neonates in whom the presence of surfactant is documented.[25] In term human infants, pulmonary infection with group B Streptococcus can cause a syndrome clinically, radiographically, and pathologically similar to hyaline membrane disease.[1] It was theorized that hyaline membrane formation resulted from damage to alveolar pneumocytes and capillary endothelial cells as a result of bacterial growth, with subsequent exudation of plasma protein into the alveoli and formation of hyaline membranes. Injury to the type II alveolar cells could have resulted in the diffuse atelectasis observed.

Although the adult respiratory distress syndrome (ARDS) is not a disease of primary surfactant deficiency, there is evidence to suggest that there are alterations in the lipid to protein ratio with aggregation and impaired function of surfactant.[26] This dysfunction is probably a reflection of generalized lung injury mediated by many factors, including complement activation, neutrophil aggregation, lung prostaglandin production, etc. Surfactant dysfunction may result from direct damage to type II alveolar cells or by the release of substances into the alveoli which in-

**TABLE 22–6.** ***Factors Contributing to Pulmonary Edema in Infants***[58]

1. Pulmonary endothelial injury, leading to capillary leak:
   a. Endotoxin
   b. Asphyxia
   c. Oxygen toxicity
   d. Atelectasis and overinflation
   e. Barotrauma
2. ↑ hydrostatic pressure
   a. Hypoxia-induced increase in pulmonary resistance
   b. ↑ Pulmonary blood flow secondary to expansion of circulating volume
   c. Left to right shunt (through ductus)
   d. Myocardial dysfunction
3. ↓ oncotic pressure
   a. Prematurity
   b. Excessive fluid administration
   c. Protein loss (secondary to diarrhea)
   d. Poor nutritional status
4. Impaired lymphatic drainage
   a. Pulmonary air leak
   b. Interstitial emphysema

terfere with the surface tension reducing properties of surfactant.[20]

## Lung Development and Clinical Syndromes of Hyaline Membrane Disease

Hyaline membrane disease (HMD) or respiratory distress syndrome (RDS) has been reported in the premature infant, premature lamb, pig, calf, and foal. Respiratory distress syndrome has been defined as progressive respiratory failure in a premature infant caused by inadequate surfactant function superimposed on a structurally immature lung.[21] It should not be confused with the generic term "respiratory distress," which simply describes the clinical signs of increased respiratory effort and/or rate.

Following birth, the human infant with RDS may have little or mild evidence of respiratory distress. Over the next 24 to 48 hours, increasingly severe respiratory distress is noted, followed by a plateauing of clinical signs. This period is then followed by a period of rapid improvement over the next few days. Diagnosis is based on the following criteria in human infants:

1. The characteristic clinical course, as outlined above.
2. Negative blood cultures.
3. A typical diffuse, ground-glass radiographic appearance, with air bronchograms.
4. Lecithin-sphingomyelin ratio of <2:1 and absence of phosphatidylglycerol in the amniotic fluid is suggestive of lung and surfactant immaturity.

The relatively mild clinical signs often seen in the human infant with RDS shortly after birth can be explained by a rapid release of all available tissue-associated surfactant pools. Progressive respiratory failure (decreased $PaO_2$, increased $PCO_2$) may result from compromise of function of a pool of surfactant which is only slowly increasing.[21]

All piglets affected by the "barker" syndrome or HMD were sired by the same boar and analysis of breeding data suggested that the condition was inherited. The three major features of these "barker" piglets were abnormally immature lungs with hyaline membranes, a deficiency of surfactant in lung washings, and abnormally small thyroid glands accompanied by clinical signs of hypothyroidism. The relationship between the abnormalities in the thyroid glands and pulmonary immaturity in these piglets remains unknown.[27,28]

There have been several reports of respiratory distress syndrome in the calf. In one study,[29] 35 calves were delivered by cesarian section near term (range of 247 to 284 days), lecithin/sphingomyelin (L/S) ratios were measured in calves with and without evidence of respiratory distress, and the lungs of calves that died were examined histologically. Twenty of the 35 calves developed signs of respiratory dysfunction within the first hours following birth. In the normal calves, there were no deaths and the average L/S ratio was 2.6, while in the calves showing signs of respiratory disease, 11 died and the average L/S ratio was 1.5, statistically lower than in the normal individuals. Only two calves with an L/S ratio greater than 2.0 developed respiratory distress, while 18 of 19 calves with a ratio less than 2.0 developed respiratory disorders during the first hour of life. There was a fairly poor correlation between gestational age and L/S ratio. The most striking findings on postmortem examination were pulmonary lesions (hyaline membranes, interstitial and alveolar edema) and intracranial hemorrhages. Thus, the syndrome of RDS in the calf seems to be similar to that in the human infant. Similar studies in the foal have not yet been conducted.

The results of one study of surfactant in the foal[30] suggest, based on limited numbers, that maturation of surfactant occurs late in gestation, at or after 300 days (88%) of gestation. Traces of surfactant and occasional lamellar bodies, representing intracellular surfactant stores, were present at 150 days' gestation, 40 to 50 days before the transition from the glandular to the canalicular stage of lung development. Reserves of surfactant were present at day 250 but formation of a lining film was incomplete at 300 days and sometimes incomplete at full term. However, only one fetus was studied at 300 days. This compares with full development of the surface lining in the sheep at around 90% of gestation and 75 to 80% in human infants. This information in the foal should be considered preliminary pending further investigations.

Primary surfactant deficiency as a cause of respiratory distress has not been well documented in the foal. The only report of respiratory disease accompanied by low surfactant levels concerned a full-term foal which was normal at birth but showed signs of central nervous system derangement at 32 hours of age.[31] Pathologic findings included atelectasis and edema, no true hyaline membrane formation, but a decrease in lung lining film. Respiratory distress in foals has been associated with neonatal asphyxia, hypovolemia, prematurity, dysmaturity, and bronchial obstructions,[32] but there has been little effort to correlate these conditions with surfactant quantity or function. Analysis of L/S ratios and phosphatidylglycerol (PG) levels in equine amniotic fluid yielded conflicting results.[33] In amniotic fluid of 12 normal term foals, the mean L/S ratio was 2.2 (range 1.5 to 3.0) and PG was present in 9 of 11 samples tested. However, five premature foals which were delivered via premature induction of labor or cesarian section and showed signs of severe respiratory dysfunction shortly after birth had a mean L/S ratio of 3.0 (range 1.8 to 3.6). PG levels were variable. All foals died within 72 hours of age, and severe pulmonary consolidation was present on postmortem examination. In contrast, two spontaneously born premature foals (300 and 310 days gestation) which did not show signs of severe respiratory compromise had L/S ratios of 1.4, and PG was weakly positive. The significance of these findings are not well understood, and additional studies are indicated.

Observations of RDS in one equine neonatal intensive care unit suggest that the classic presentation of RDS as described in the human premature infant is fairly uncommon in foals presented for critical care. Only one foal showed a characteristic radiographic appearance (diffuse alveolar pattern) coupled with the typical clinical course and histopathologic appearance (Fig. 22–6). A number of spontaneously born premature foals (gestational ages 290 to 320 days), however, have displayed signs of respiratory distress which were more attributable to in utero acquired infections than to RDS, on the basis of placental examination, hematologic parameters, radiographic appearance, and culture results. Most of these individuals survived. It has been speculated that fetal maturation (including lung maturation) is accelerated by adverse in utero conditions, enhancing the viability of the newborn. In other premature and term foals which were usually victims of complicated deliveries (cesarian section, early induction of labor), certain signs, such as progression of respiratory distress over the first 24 to 48 hours, diffuse interstitial infiltrates on radiographs, and diffuse atelectasis on postmortem examination were suggestive of RDS. However, air bronchograms were rarely observed radiographically, hyaline membrane formation was rarely observed on postmortem examination, and the outcome was usually poor, with progressive neurologic and cardiovascular deterioration, in spite of mechanical ventilation and intensive care.

Atelectasis, with or without inflammatory cell infiltrate, has been a prominent postmortem finding in foals with a variety of clinical syndromes, including septicemia, pneumonia, and neonatal maladjustment syndrome.[34] Dubielzig[35] also noted an association between lung atelectasis and central nervous system dysfunction associated with asphyxial injury

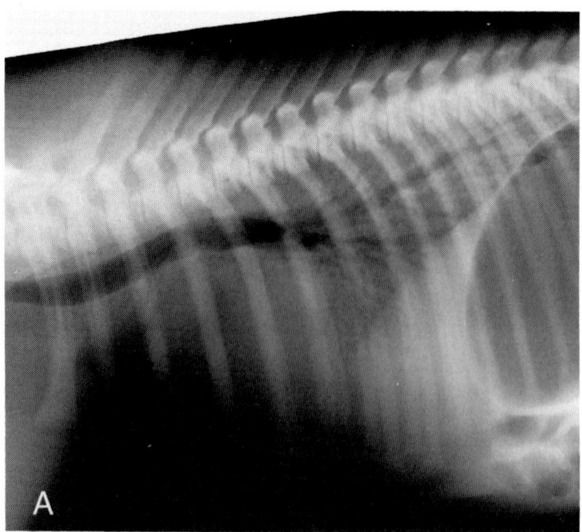


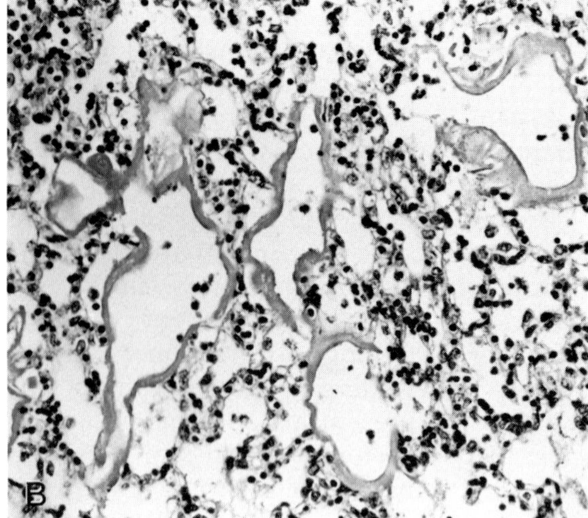


**FIG. 22–6.** A. Lateral thoracic radiograph of a 305-day gestational age, 3-hour-old foal in respiratory distress. A severe diffuse alveolar pattern is present throughout the lung fields and is suggestive of hyaline membrane disease. B. Lung from the same foal, approximately 24 hours after the radiographs were taken. Many alveoli are lined by hyaline membranes. Interstitial areas are widened by inflammatory cells, primarily neutrophils (hematoxylin and eosin, ×85). (From Koterba AM, Drummond WH, Kosch PC. Intensive care of the neonatal foal. Vet Clin North Am, *1*:3, 1985.)

in neonatal foals undergoing postmortem examination. Unfortunately, surfactant measurements have not been made in any of these cases, and the role of primary or secondary surfactant deficiency in the pathophysiology of respiratory distress in the neonatal foal remains to be determined.

## Prevention of Respiratory Distress Syndrome

Prevention of RDS in the premature human infant includes prevention of premature delivery, prevention of birth asphyxia, and maternal corticosteroid therapy. While investigating corticosteroid induction of parturition in the sheep, Liggins found that lambs that had been infused with steroids or ACTH in utero were viable and showed alveolar stability at 118 to 123 days gestation, while previous studies had indicated that RDS normally developed in lambs less than 125 days gestation at delivery.[36] Because of these studies and further work in the sheep, which showed that the appearance of surfactant was accelerated in lungs of cortisol-treated fetal lambs,[37] maternally administered steroids were given in human pregnancies to enhance fetal lung maturation.

In the years since these discoveries, the use of steroids for this purpose is widespread in human medicine but still somewhat controversial. Some groups feel that the prevention of birth asphyxia is of greater importance in preventing RDS than steroid administration to the mother. There was a much better effect observed in female infants than male infants whose mothers received steroids. The use of steroids is usually avoided if amnionitis is present and if birth is likely to take place in less than 24 hours. Although there is no one dose that is universally agreed upon, dexamethasone at 5 mg IM q 12 hours for four doses is one regimen used in human mothers.[38]

## Artificial Surfactant Therapy

Large, multicenter studies are currently under way to study the effectiveness of surfactant replacement therapy in reduction of the severity of clinical signs of RDS and the incidence of adverse long-term complications of RDS, such as bronchopulmonary dysplasia, in the premature human infant.[39] To date, a number of published studies have reported statistically significant improvements in respiratory function (improved oxygenation, easier ventilation, and fewer complications) noted after natural surfactant administration to premature infants. Sources of surfactant have included the calf, cow, pig, and human amniotic fluid. Positive effects have also been observed following the use of certain artificial surfactants, but the results of these studies generally have not been as encouraging as with the natural products.

### Treatment of RDS in Human Infants

Therapy has been aimed at preventing atelectasis and maintaining adequate end-expiratory lung volume and gas exchange. This usually involves some combination of oxygen therapy, continuous positive airway pressure, and mechanical ventilation. Fluid therapy is managed carefully to avoid volume overloading the patient and causing a worsening of respiratory function. In humans, complications such as infection and air leaks are fairly common, but the prognosis for RDS is generally good with modern ventilator management. Surfactant replacement therapy has been shown to be an effective treatment for RDS in animal models and human infants; some neonatologists predict that it will revolutionize the management of RDS in premature infants.[39] It may also be of use in treating conditions associated with secondary surfactant deficiencies.

## *Bacterial Respiratory Infections*

Equine neonatal respiratory infection most commonly takes the form of bacterial pneumonia, and in many cases, is only part of a generalized infection affecting many different organ systems. Pleuritis has also been observed in association with septicemia and peritonitis, but the incidence appears to be much lower than pneumonia. Infection in other parts of the respiratory tract, such as bronchiolitis or laryngotracheitis, appears to be relatively rare in the neonate.

### Factors Predisposing to Neonatal Pneumonia

Lung immaturity, an immature immune system and inadequate passive transfer of immunity are all factors predisposing the neonate to respiratory infections. Little has been reported about the developmental anatomy of the foal lung. In human infants, an immature ciliary apparatus leads to inefficient removal of bacteria and inflammatory debris. Many neonatal mammalian species, including the foal, have lower numbers of alveolar macrophages than the adult during the first few days of life,[14] and bacterial clearance is probably considerably reduced.

Several studies have shown that complement values in newborn calves are less than 50% of the values in adult cows, with levels decreasing to even lower values the day after birth, possibly as a result of an increase in plasma volume.[40] Information regarding the complement system in the foal is not yet available. The complement system plays an important role in host defense, being the first humoral barrier against invading organisms.

If colostrum intake is insufficient and serum IgG values are low, the individual is at even higher risk of acquiring a severe bacterial infection. When IgG levels are low, not only is the neonate deprived of specific antibody protection, but neutrophil function, as measured by the chemiluminescence assay, is also seriously impaired.[41] The environment also provides predisposing factors that may lead to neonatal pneumonia. Exposure to pathogenic bacteria, use of invasive procedures such as intravenous catheters and endotracheal tubes which interrupt the normal physical barriers to infection, and exposure to contaminated equipment, such as humidifiers and other respiratory equipment, may all lead to an increased risk of respiratory infections.

### Etiology

Pneumonia may be acquired in utero, during the birth process, or at some time following the delivery.

***In utero acquired bacterial infections*** are not uncommon in the foal. Pneumonia is probably the most common manifestation of the disease process but may be accompanied by uveitis and/or diarrhea. Chronic placental dysfunction may cause fetal growth retardation, but the stresses associated with an abnormal uteroplacental environment may also help to speed maturation of the fetus and exert a beneficial effect on survival.[42] Early in life, localizing signs of respiratory infection may be absent, even in the presence of extensive disease, with weakness and depression the only abnormal physical examination findings. A complete blood count during the first 24 hours of life usually reveals an elevated plasma fibrinogen concentration with a variable total white blood cell count. Although the fetus may be infected by hematogenous transmission of bacteria across the placenta, it appears that ascending infection of the placenta occurs more frequently, with aspiration of infected amniotic fluid being the most common route of infection.

***Infection Acquired During or After Birth.*** During the delivery process, the fetus becomes colonized by bacteria living in the vagina. Initial colonization probably occurs on the skin and mucosal surfaces, including the nasopharynx. Although bacteria may proliferate at these sites, they rarely cause disease unless other predisposing factors are present. In human infants, pneumonia may result from aspiration of pharyngeal secretions and seems to occur more commonly in infants born after difficult deliveries.[12] In the equine neonate, the respiratory system may serve as the primary portal of entry of bacteria into the body or be infected secondarily as a result of septicemia and hematogenous spread of bacteria. Foals which acquire pneumonia postnatally are usually presented for treatment on or after day 2 to 3 of life.

## Organisms Involved

Bacteria causing pneumonia are essentially the same as those causing neonatal septicemia.[43] More specifically, any gram-negative enteric organism (E. coli, Klebsiella, Salmonella, etc.), Actinobacillus or Pasteurella, Streptococcal spp. etc. may cause pneumonia.

## Clinical and Laboratory Assessment

As in most neonatal infections, the clinical presentation of pneumonia can be nonspecific. Signs of respiratory distress may or may not be present. If respiratory distress is present, bacterial pneumonia should be differentiated from the other causes of respiratory distress, but in some cases this can be difficult. Arterial blood gases and thoracic radiographs are extremely helpful in establishing that there is a respiratory problem, but usually cannot pinpoint infection as the cause. Radiographic interpretation is difficult because of the similarities between the abnormalities associated with pneumonia and other respiratory conditions, such as atelectasis. A complete blood count and computation of a sepsis score may be of more use in distinguishing infection.[44] However, even with the use of the sepsis score, it can be difficult to distinguish pneumonia from atelectasis in the compromised, "nonviable" premature foal, in which the WBC count is low regardless of whether infection can be confirmed.[45]

## Microbial Cultures

Bacterial cultures are important in confirming the diagnosis of pneumonia. In in utero acquired infections in foals, blood cultures are frequently negative, while signs of pneumonia are prominent. In these individuals, cultures and cytology (including Gram stain) of tracheal secretions (obtained via placement of a nasotracheal tube and use of a protected brush catheter or via transtracheal aspiration), gastric aspirate and pharynx (if newborn), and urine should be performed, in addition to blood cultures. See preceding section for additional information on the interpretation of respiratory system cultures. If pneumonia is postnatally acquired, blood cultures have been helpful in identifying the pathogen. In the distressed neonate, transtracheal aspiration can be a difficult, hazardous procedure.

## Treatment of Bacterial Pneumonia

***Antibiotic Therapy.*** Antibiotic therapy is an essential part of the medical treatment of pneumonia. Pending culture results, broad-spectrum antibiotic therapy should be instituted. The combination of ampicillin (or penicillin) and gentamicin is a reasonable initial empiric treatment. In a hospital setting, with the documentation of a resident population of resistant bacteria, a combination of ampicillin and amikacin or cefotaxime may be a better choice. The third generation cephalosporins present certain advantages over aminoglycosides in the treatment of neonatal pneumonia. They have been found to have good penetration into lung tissue, with the concentrations achieved greatly exceeding the concentrations needed to kill susceptible bacteria.[46] Aminoglycosides penetrate lung tissue in amounts equal to 10 to 45% of serum levels,[47] but in the acidic environment of infected airways, the activity of the drugs is markedly reduced and levels attained may not be sufficient to kill the offending bacteria.[48] One major disadvantage of the routine use of the third generation cephalosporins seem to be the rapid induction of resistance in a hospital setting.[49]

As stated earlier, antibiotic therapy should not be discontinued prematurely. In many instances, pulmonary infection is well established prior to its diagnosis, and white blood cell count, plasma fibrinogen level, and chest radiographs may not return to normal for several weeks. We generally do not discontinue antibiotic therapy until all parameters (WBC count and differential, fibrinogen, and chest radiographs) are normal. If blood cultures are positive, a minimum of 2 weeks of antibiotic therapy is recommended. The duration of antibiotic therapy for established pneumonia has ranged from 2 to 5 weeks. The premature or debilitated foal should be monitored carefully for the development of infection due to multiple resistant bacteria and chronic pneumonia. The most critical period is the first 3 months of life. If there is suspicion that a pneumonic process is not responding appropriately to treatment (fever spikes, increasing plasma fibrinogen, worsening clinical signs, etc.) additional bacterial cultures are strongly recommended.

If failure of passive transfer of immunoglobulins is present, the patient is routinely treated with plasma. Depending on the IgG levels of the patient and the donor plasma, 20 to 50 ml/kg of plasma is administered intravenously. In the foal with severe respiratory and/or renal compromise, the infusion rate of the plasma should be conservative to avoid volume overload and pulmonary edema.

***Respiratory Supportive Care.*** Respiratory physiotherapy is an extremely important part of the treatment of pneumonia. Commonly used techniques include: (1) Maintenance of the foal in a sternal position, or at least frequent turning from side to side to avoid progressive atelectasis and hypoxemia, (2) routine coupage and (3) good airway hygiene, including suction, if an endotracheal tube is present. Physical examination findings combined with blood gas results determine the need for oxygen or other more aggressive mechanical or pharmacologic support of respiratory function.

## *Viral Respiratory Disease in the Neonatal Foal*

Viral pneumonia may also be acquired in utero or postnatally. In the horse, equine herpesvirus (EHV-1) may cause interstitial pneumonia or bronchopneumonia and lymphoid depletion and result in an aborted fetus or in a live, healthy, or weak neonate.[50] The influenza virus has been incriminated as a cause of severe interstitial pneumonia in neonatal foals.[51] Neonatal foals (2 to 7 days of age) with suspected viral interstitial pneumonia had a normal CBC count and only mildly elevated fibrinogen, marked respiratory distress, and chest radiographs with a diffuse, severe interstitial pattern. Treatment, including mechanical ventilation, was not successful in reversing the condition. Virus could not be isolated from the lungs, but in two cases, rising maternal serum titers together with typical clinical signs in the mares provided circumstantial evidence of influenza infection. Fatal adenovirus pneumonia has been primarily associated with combined immunodeficiency syndrome in Arabian foals. Experimental infection of normal and colostrum deprived neonatal foals 24 to 48 hours of age resulted in signs of pneumonia (fever, cough, nasal discharge) within 7 days postinoculation, but no foals died of the infection, and marked lymphoid depletion was not observed.[52]

Unfortunately, definitive diagnosis of viral interstitial pneumonia can be difficult. Although virus isolation is probably the quickest and most efficient way to diagnose viral infection, many laboratories do not have the capacity to perform viral isolation. In addition, compared to human medicine, we know little about which viruses infect the equine fetus and newborn foal. Virus isolation is often attempted late in the clinical course, when secondary bacterial infection is usually present, and the primary viral agent may be gone or extremely difficult to isolate.

Although intranuclear inclusion bodies in the lung and liver are considered diagnostic of equine herpesvirus infection in aborted fetuses, infected foals which were born alive did not consistently demonstrate inclusion bodies.[50] The postmortem findings of interstitial pneumonia are not specific and can be caused by a number of conditions, including bacterial infection, shock, and toxic injury (for example, oxygen toxicity).

Currently, serology is also not dependable in diagnosing fetal or neonatal virus infection, as passively derived antibody titers may be acquired from the dam's colostrum. The presence in the newborn of serum IgM antibody specific for a particular agent may be useful in the future in diagnosing selected congenital viral infections. It is clear that much improvement is needed in methods to diagnose viral respiratory and/or systemic disease in neonatal foals.

## *Meconium Aspiration Syndrome*

Hypoxia of the fetus in utero or during the birth process may result in passage of meconium into the amniotic fluid. Gasping secondary to hypoxia can cause aspiration of the meconium-contaminated amniotic fluid. The fluid may obstruct airways, interfere with gas exchange, cause severe respiratory distress, and promote the growth of bacteria. It may be difficult to differentiate this condition from bacterial pneumonia, especially if the birth was unattended. Occasionally, if chronic placentitis is present, both bacterial pneumonia and meconium aspiration may be present.[53]

A diagnosis of meconium aspiration is based on a history of meconium-contaminated amniotic fluid and a meconium-stained newborn. Radiographs typically show a cranioventral distribution of pulmonary infiltrate characteristic of aspiration. Clear, brownish fluid may drip from the nose.

The best treatment of meconium aspiration, intubation and suction, is accomplished while the animal is still in the birth canal, before it has taken its first breath. Once meconium has been aspirated, broad spectrum antibiotic therapy is indicated and an appropriate level of ventilatory support is provided, based on clinical signs and blood gas results. Good airway hygiene and coupage are crucial. Multiorgan dysfunction may result from the hypoxic episode.

## *Pneumothorax*

Pneumothorax may occur as an iatrogenic sequela of positive pressure ventilation of diseased lungs, may occur spontaneously, or may be a result of birth trauma.[54] During mechanical ventilation, uneven alveolar ventilation leads to alveolar rupture and dissection of air into the interstitium. The air moves along bronchioles and other lung structures to pleural surfaces, forming blebs. This air may rupture into the pleural space.

Pneumothorax should be suspected if the respiratory condition suddenly worsens while an animal is being ventilated (decreased $PaO_2$, increased peak inspiratory airway pressure). Clinical signs may include respiratory distress, shift of cardiac point of maximum impulse, cyanosis, and hypotension. Auscultation may reveal decreased breath sounds on one or both sides of the thorax. Auscultation may be misleading because of wide referral of breath sounds. Percussion may be fairly unremarkable if the condition is mild, but hyperresonance may be detected in severe cases. Radiographs are indicated to confirm the diagnosis, but if radiography is unavailable or the animal is distressed, a direct needle aspirate is both diagnostic and therapeutic.

Pneumothorax may be treated conservatively if no distress is associated with the air leak and the condition appears stable. Stress should be minimized. Chest tube insertion is indicated in human infants with continuing air leak if underlying pulmonary disease is causing respiratory distress, and in patients receiving mechanical ventilation. A trocar catheter is sterilely introduced into the chest cavity. The catheter is secured with an "argyle sock" pattern, with the suture material wrapped tightly around the catheter. Suction is applied at $-15$ cm $H_2O$ after confirmation of chest tube position by chest radiograph. Suction is discontinued when the tube has drained no air for 24 to 48 hours and when extrapulmonary air has been resolved radiographically for 24 to 48 hours. The tube may then be placed under water seal for an additional 24 hours and if no air accumulates, the tube may be removed.

# *Disorders of Breathing Pattern*

## Idiopathic Tachypnea in the Neonatal Foal

One syndrome observed in a small number of Clydesdale, Thoroughbred and Arabian neonatal foals has been the combination of fever and tachypnea. The condition appears to be more frequent during hot, humid weather conditions. The pathogenesis of the condition is unknown, but it is speculated that it results from a transient problem in central or peripheral control of thermoregulation and/or respiratory rate and pattern. Unfortunately, we know little about these control mechanisms in the normal foal.

Affected foals are usually of normal gestational age and experience a normal birth. Most display normal activity for a variable period after birth, with a sudden onset of clinical signs. Occasionally, a foal may show mild signs of maladjustment. Body temperature is variable among foals, ranging from 38.9° to 42.2°C (102°–108°F). A generally poor response to antipyretics has been noted, while the best control of fever has been body clipping, alcohol baths, and provision of cooler environmental temperatures. The respiratory rate and breathing pattern often resembles panting (respiratory rate >80 BPM). In human infants, transient tachypnea syndromes have been attributed to a delay in resorption of lung liquid, but in foals there is usually no sign of pulmonary abnormalities on chest radiographs and blood gas analysis. The condition usually resolves spontaneously within a few days to weeks.

Before idiopathic tachypnea is diagnosed, it is extremely important to rule out a pneumonic process or other pulmonary abnormality, other forms of infection, metabolic acidosis, and other causes of an increased respiratory rate (Table 22–1). Hematology, thoracic radiographs, and arterial blood gases should be normal, and bacterial cultures should be negative.

Treatment is directed toward controlling the body temperature by body clipping, alcohol baths and maintenance in a cool environment if possible. If infection cannot be ruled out entirely, antibiotic therapy should be strongly considered.

## Neonatal Apnea and Irregular Breathing Patterns

Periods of apnea in the neonate are commonly associated with nonrespiratory factors, including infection, central nervous system disorders, hypothermia, and metabolic causes, such as hypoglycemia. Seizure activity may be expressed by changes in breathing rate and pattern. Neonatal asphyxia may induce respiratory depression whether or not cerebral lesions are present.[55] Neonatal respiratory distress may also cause apnea resulting from respiratory center depression or diaphragmatic fatigue.

There are two mechanisms of apnea, both of which have been observed in the neonatal foal: (1) Central apnea, resulting from cessation of diaphragmatic activity, and (2) Obstructive apnea, resulting from obstruction of the airway, usually at the pharyngeal level.

Foals with irregular breathing patterns characterized by frequent pauses in breathing activity often show evidence of hypoventilation and hypoxemia on blood gas analysis. Oxygen therapy usually corrects the mild hypoxemia, but has no effect on hypercapnia. Treatment of the condition in human infants includes increasing the amount of external stimulation, continuous positive airway pressure, pharmacologic treatment with doxapram, and the methylxanthines, such as theophylline, and intermittent positive pressure ventilation if prolonged apnea persists in spite of other treatments. In human infants, a serum theophylline concentration of about 70 μmol/L (12.7 mg/L) was effective in reducing the frequency of apnea in 75 to 80% of treated infants.[56] In most foals with the condition, resolution of the neurologic problem has resulted in resolution of the abnormalities in breathing pattern.

## Treatment of Respiratory Distress in the Neonatal Foal

It is beyond the scope of this book to provide detailed information on the respiratory support of the equine neonate, and the reader is referred to other articles and text for additional information.[4,57,58]

### *Oxygen Therapy*

Oxygen therapy is extremely useful in the treatment of the equine neonate with respiratory disease. The decision as to when to institute oxygen therapy is somewhat subjective, and is based on clinical signs as well as blood gas analysis. Increased respiratory rate, labored respiration, increased intercostal and abdominal muscle activity, and restlessness are considered indications for a trial of oxygen therapy. A $PaO_2$ of less than 55 to 60 mmHg in lateral recumbency is considered an objective indication for oxygen therapy, although many foals recovering from pneumonia apparently do well on room air with a $PaO_2$ of 50 to 55 mmHg. If blood gas analysis is not available, clinical signs indicating a favorable response to oxygen therapy include a decrease in effort of breathing, decrease in respiratory rate and a foal that appears more comfortable. Lack of response may indicate a nonrespiratory origin of the clinical signs, severe lung disorder, or a cardiac malformation, resulting in right-to-left shunting of blood.

The inspired oxygen concentration is most easily increased by insufflation using a bias flow of humidified oxygen. Depending on the severity of disease and size of the individual, oxygen is initially delivered at a flow rate of about 5 L/minute and the response is noted. The actual oxygen concentration delivered to the alveoli is dependent on several factors, including the position of the tube and the depth and rate of breathing. Oxygen therapy should be directed at maintaining a $PaO_2$ of 80 to 100 mmHg and the flow rate should be adjusted according to blood gas results. Oxygen therapy should be on a continuous basis and weaning from it should be gradual.

### *Treatment of Hypoventilation*

Unfortunately, oxygen therapy is not effective in correcting hypoventilation, and if hypercapnea is progressive and accompanied by signs of increasing respiratory distress, some type of mechanical ventilatory support is usually indicated. This decision to provide mechanical ventilation must take into account several considerations including the economic value of the individual, the commitment of the owners, the facility and manpower availability, and the type of disease process present. Methods of ventilatory support include continuous positive airway pressure, intermittent mandatory ventilation, and high frequency ventilation. If hypoventilation is secondary to neurologic dysfunction, it can often be managed conservatively with respiratory supportive techniques and/or provision of intermittent signs using an ambu bag and endotracheal tube to reverse any atelectasis.

### *Respiratory Supportive Techniques*

Regardless of the level of respiratory support provided, the importance of meticulous respiratory supportive technique cannot be overemphasized. Maintenance in sternal position, frequent turning from side to side, regular coupage, and use of proper suction technique are all important components of respiratory support.

## Persistent Pulmonary Hypertension

Persistent pulmonary hypertension (PPH) or persistent fetal circulation (PFC) is a perinatal syndrome, caused by pulmonary vascular abnormalities, that affects both human neonates and foals.[63–65] In human infants it has been associated with prenatal treatment with anti-prostaglandin drugs, placental insufficiency that causes intrauterine hypoxemia, postmaturity, pulmonary infection, meconium aspiration, and sometimes hyaline membrane disease (particularly in later gestation neonates).

PPH is characterized by marked elevation of the pulmonary artery pressure and cyanosis caused by right to left shunting through the ductus arteriosus and foramen ovale. An audible murmur is inconsistent but the second heart sound is characteristically loud and "single" without a clear differentiation between the aortic and pulmonic components. Thoracic radiographs may show clear lung fields or evidence of pneumonia, hyaline membrane disease, or pneumothorax in cases in which the pulmonary vasospasm is secondary to stressful factors such as hypoxemia, acidosis, or bacterial toxins.

Other causes of cyanosis from which it must be differentiated include cardiac anomalies, hyaline membrane disease, and meconium aspiration. The latter two conditions may be complicated by pulmonary hypertension. Thoracic radiographs and cardiac ultrasonography aid differentiation. Diagnosis of right to left ductal shunting is made by blood gas analysis of samples simultaneously obtained from the right brachial artery and from a hind limb vessel and finding a higher oxygen saturation in the right brachial arterial blood sample.

As hypoxemia stimulates pulmonary vasoconstriction, and acidosis accentuates it, treatment for PPH includes the administration of high oxygen concentrations and correction of acid-base abnormalities. If administration of 100% oxygen and correction of the pH to 7.4 does not improve systemic oxygenation, metabolic and respiratory alkalosis may relieve pulmonary vasospasm. This can sometimes be achieved by mechanical hyperventilation combined with $NaHCO_3$ administration, but neither technique is necessarily safe. PPH can be rapidly fatal and a favorable outcome requires a fully equipped and staffed intensive care unit. If PPH resolves by 2 to 4 days of age, complete recovery without recurrence of pulmonary hypertension is possible. Sequelae of treatment include lung and brain damage.

## References


1. Katzenstein A, Davis C, Braude A. Pulmonary changes in neonatal sepsis due to group B beta-hemolytic streptococcus: Relation to hyaline membrane disease. J Infect Dis, *133*:430, 1976.
2. Warren RG, Webb AI, Kosch PC, et al. Evaluation of transcutaneous oxygen monitoring in anesthetized pony foals. Equine Vet J, *16*:358, 1984.
3. Webb AI, Daniel RT, Miller HS, et al. Preliminary studies on the measurement of conjunctival oxygen tension in the foal. Am J Vet Res, *46*:2566, 1985.
4. Kosch PC, Koterba AM, Coons TJ, et al. Developments in the management of the newborn foal in respiratory distress. 1: Evaluation. Equine Vet J, *16*:312, 1984.
5. Madigan J, Thomas WP. Cardiopulmonary function in normal newborn foals from 1–14 days of age. Proc Am Coll Vet Int Med, *10*:101, 1986.
6. Rose RJ, Hodgson DH, Leadon DP, et al. Effect of intranasal oxygen administration on arterial blood gas—acid-base parameters in spontaneously delivered, term-induced, and induced premature foals. Res Vet Sci, *34*:159, 1983.
7. Stewart JH, Rose RJ, Barko AM. Response to oxygen administration in foals: Effect of age, duration and method of administration on arterial blood gas values. Equine Vet J, *16*:329, 1984.
8. Brewer BD. Neonatal infection. In: Equine Clinical Neonatology, Koterba AM, Drummond WH, Kosch PC (eds). Philadelphia, Lea & Febiger, 1990.
9. Koterba AM, Brewer BD. The diagnosis and treatment of equine neonatal septicemia. Proceedings of American Association of Equine Practitioners, 1985, p 127.
10. King R. Unpublished data. University of Florida, 1988.
11. Failing LJ. New advances in diagnosing nosocomial pneumonia in intubated patients Part I. (editorial). Am Rev Reşpir Dis, *137*:253, 1988.
12. Dennehy PH. Respiratory infections in the newborn. Clin Perinatol, *14*:667, 1987.
13. Sherman MP, Goetzman BW, Ahlfors CE, et al. Tracheal aspiration and its clinical correlates in the diagnosis of congenital pneumonia. Pediatrics, *65*:258, 1980.
14. Liu IKM, Walsh EM, Bernoco M, et al. Bronchoalveolar lavage in the newborn foal. J Reprod Fert, Suppl *35*:587, 1987.
15. Fogarty U, Leadon DP. Comparison of systemic and local respiratory tract cellular immunity in the neonatal foal. J Reprod Fert, Suppl *35*:593, 1987.
16. Notter RH, Shapiro DL. Lung surfactants for replace-

ment therapy: Biochemical, biophysical and clinical aspects. Clin Perinatol (Respir Syst), *14*:433, 1987.
17. Avery ME, Mead J. Surface properties in relation to atelectasis and hyaline membrane disease. J Dis Child, *97*:517, 1959.
18. Notter RH, Finkelstein JN. Pulmonary surfactant: An interdisciplinary approach. J Appl Physiol, *57*:1613, 1984.
19. Perelman RH, Engle MJ, Farrell PM. Perspectives of fetal lung development. Lung, *159*:53, 1981.
20. Kikkawa Y, Smith F. Cellular and biochemical aspects of pulmonary surfactant in health and disease. Lab Invest, *49*:122, 1983.
21. Jobe A. Respiratory distress syndrome—New therapeutic approaches to a complex pathophysiology. Adv Pediatr, *30*:93, 1983.
22. Costarino AT, Baimgart S. Controversies in fluid and electrolyte therapy for the premature infant. Clin Perinatol, *15*:863, 1988.
23. Kotas RV. Surface tension forces and liquid balance in the lung. In: Neonatal Pulmonary Care, 2nd Ed. Thibeault DW, Gregory GA (eds). Menlo Park, CA, Addison-Wesley Publishing, 1986, p 125.
24. Reynolds EO, Jacobson HN, Motoyama EK, et al. The effect of immaturity and prenatal asphyxia on the lungs and pulmonary function of newborn lambs: The experimental production of respiratory distress. Pediatrics, *35*:382, 1965.
25. Reynolds EO, Roberton NR, Wigglesworth JS. Hyaline membrane disease, respiratory distress and surfactant deficiency. Pediatrics, *42*:758, 1968.
26. Petty TL, Reiss OK, Paul GW, et al. Characteristics of pulmonary surfactant in adult respiratory distress syndrome associated with trauma and shock. Am Rev Respir Dis, *115*:531, 1977.
27. Slauson DO. Naturally occurring hyaline membrane disease syndromes in foals and piglets. J Pediatr, *95*:889, 1979.
28. Gibson EA, Blackmore RJJ, Wijeratne WVS, et al. The "barker" (neonatal respiratory distress) syndrome in the pig: Its occurrence in the field. Vet Rec, *98*:476, 1976.
29. Eigenmann UJE, Schoon HA, Jahn D, et al. Neonatal respiratory distress syndrome in the calf. Vet Rec, *114*:141, 1984.
30. Pattle RE, Rossdale PD, Schock C, et al. The development of the lung and its surfactant in the foal and in other species. J Reprod Fert, Suppl *23*:651, 1975.
31. Rossdale PD, Pattle RE, Mahaffey LW. Respiratory distress in newborn foals with failure to form lung lining film. Nature (Lond), *215*:1498, 1967.
32. Sonea I. Respiratory distress syndrome in neonatal foals. Comp Cont Ed Pract Vet, *7*:462, 1985.
33. Paradis MK. Lecithin/sphingomyelin ratios and phosphatidylglycerol in term and premature equine amniotic fluid. Proc Am Coll Vet Int Med, 1987, p 789.
34. Koterba AM. Equine neonatal intensive care at the University of Florida 1982–1987. An update. Proceedings of American Association of Equine Practitioners, 1988, p 807.
35. Dubielzig RR. Pulmonary lesions of neonatal foals. J Equine Med Surg, *1*:419, 1977.
36. Liggins GC. Premature delivery of foetal lambs infused with glucocorticoids. J Endocrinol, *45*:515, 1969.
37. DeLemos R, Shermeta DW, Knelson JH, et al. Acceleration of appearance of pulmonary surfactant in the fetal lamb by administration of glucocorticoids. Am Rev Respir Dis, *102*:459, 1970.
38. Coustan DR. Clinical aspects of antenatal enhancement of pulmonary maturation. Clin Perinatol, *14*:697, 1987.
39. Shapiro DL, Notter RH. Controversies regarding surfactant replacement therapy. Clin Perinatol, *15*:891, 1988.
40. Mueller R, Boothby JT, Carroll EJ, et al. Changes in complement values in calves during the first month of life. Am J Vet Res, *44*:747, 1983.
41. LeBlanc MM. Responses to plasma transfusion in clinically healthy and clinically ill foals. Proceedings of American Association of Equine Practitioners, 1988, p 755.
42. Hack M, Fanaroff AA. How small is too small? Considerations in evaluating the outcome of the tiny infant. Clin Perinatol, *15*:773, 1988.
43. Koterba AM, Brewer BD, Tarplee FA. Clinical and clinicopathological characteristics of the septicemic neonatal foal: Review of 38 cases. Equine Vet J, *16*:376, 1984.
44. Brewer BD, Koterba AM. The development of a scoring system for the early diagnosis of equine neonatal sepsis. Equine Vet J, *20*:18, 1988.
45. Koterba AM, Chase JP, Bain FT. Development and evaluation of a scoring system predicting mortality in premature and immature equine neonates undergoing intensive care. Equine Vet J Suppl, *5*:56, 1988.
46. Cohen SH, Hoeprich PD, Demling R, et al. Entry of four cephalosporins into the bovine lung. J Infect Dis, *149*:264, 1984.
47. Pennington JE. Penetration of antibiotics into respiratory secretions. Rev Infect Dis, *3*:67, 1981.
48. Bodem CR, Lampton LM, Miller DP, et al. Endobronchial pH: Relevance to aminoglycoside activity in gram-negative bacillary pneumonia. Am Rev Respir Dis, *127*:39, 1983.
49. Bryan CS, John JF Jr, Pai MS, et al. Gentamicin vs. cefotaxime for therapy of neonatal sepsis. Relationship to drug resistance. Am J Dis Child, *139*:1086, 1985.
50. Bryans JT, Swerczek TW, Darlington RW, et al. Neonatal foal disease associated with perinatal infection by equine herpes virus I. J Eq Med Surg, *1*:20, 1977.
51. Buergelt CD, Hines SA, Cantor G, et al. A retrospective study of proliferative interstitial lung disease of horses in Florida. Vet Pathol, *23*:750, 1986.
52. McChesney AE, England JJ, Whiteman CE, et al. Experimental transmission of equine adenovirus in Arabian and non-Arabian foals. Am J Vet Res, *35*:1015, 1974.
53. Koterba AM, Haibel GK, Grimmett J. Respiratory distress in a premature foal secondary to hydrops

allantois and placentitis. Comp Cont Ed Pract Vet, *16*:312, 1983.

54. Stiles AD. Airleak: Pneumothorax, pneumomediastinum, pulmonary interstitial emphysema, pneumopericardium. In: Manual of Neonatal Care. Cloherty JP, Stark AR (eds). Boston, Little, Brown & Co. 1985, p 185.
55. Marchal F, Baltram A, Vert P. Neonatal apnea and apneic syndrome. Clin Perinatol, *14*:509, 1987.
56. Muttitt SC, Tierney AJ. The dose response of theophylline in the treatment of apnea of prematurity. J Pediatr, *112*:115, 1988.
57. Webb AI, Coons TJ, Koterba AM, et al. Developments in management of the newborn foal in respiratory distress: Treatment. Equine Vet J, *16*:319, 1984.
58. Koterba AM, Drummond WH, Kosch PC. Equine Clinical Neonatology, Philadelphia, Lea & Febiger, 1990.
59. Koterba AM, Kosch PC. Respiratory mechanics and breathing pattern in the neonatal foal. J Reprod Fert, Suppl *35*:575, 1987.
60. Rossdale PD. Some parameters of respiratory function in normal and abnormal foals with special reference to levels of $PaO_2$ during air and oxygen inhalation. Res Vet Sci, *11*:270, 1970.
61. Rose RJ, Rossdale PD, Leadon DP. Blood gas and acid-base status in spontaneously delivered, term-induced, and induced premature foals. J Reprod Fert, Suppl *32*:521, 1982.
62. Stewart JH, Rose RJ, Barko AM. Respiratory studies in foals from birth to seven days old. Equine Vet J, *16*:323, 1984.
63. Drummond WH. Neonatal pulmonary hypertension. Equine Vet J, *19*:169, 1987.
64. Cottrill CM, O'Connor WN, Cudd T, Rantanen NW. Persistence of foetal circulatory pathways in a newborn foal. Equine Vet J, *19*:252, 1987.
65. Drummond WH. Persistent pulmonary hypertension of the neonate (persistent fetal circulation syndrome). Adv Pediatr, *30*:61, 1984.

# *Appendix A*

# Stains

## Wright's Stain[1]

Solutions required:
- Wright's stain
- 6.4 pH buffer

*Procedure:*

1. Fix slide in 95% methyl alcohol for 1 hour or longer.
2. Air dry and stain immediately.
   - A. Cover with Wright's stain.
   - B. Dilute stain with buffer of 6.4 pH, approximately equal volume, and allow to stand until a metallic scum appears—2 to 5 minutes.
     Buffer: $KH_2PO_4$-6.63 Gm; $Na_2HPO_4$-2.56 g. Then add distilled water to 1000 ml total volume.
   - C. Gently rinse slide with a stream of buffer from wash.
   - D. Rinse the slide under a thin stream of running tap water until thinner parts of smear turn pale purple or pinkish red.
3. Allow slide to dry. Dip dry slide in xylene and mount in gum damar in xylene or other suitable mounting media.

   NOTE: The addition of 1% of 2,6-di-tert.-butyl-p-cresol to gum damar or Permount prevents fading of basophilic elements and loss of stain intensity.

## Wright's-Giemsa Stain

Solutions required: Wright's-Giemsa stain

*Procedure:*

1. Fix slides in clean, fresh methanol for 3 minutes.
2. Air dry.
3. Filter stain.
4. Flood slide with 20 drops of Wright's Giemsa for 4 minutes.
5. Flood slide for 20 drops phosphate buffer for 10 minutes. Mix by blowing on slide a few seconds. A green sheen should appear.
6. Rinse with water several seconds.
7. Clean back of slide.
8. Air and blot dry.
9. Check for stain precipitate before coverslipping.

## Gram's Staining[2]

Solutions required:
- Crystal Violet solution
  - (2 g certified crystal violet + 20 ml 95% ethyl alcohol)
  - $NH_4$ oxalate 0.8 g + 80 ml $H_2O$ (distilled) mixed with crystal violet solution and filtered.
- Iodine solution
  - (1 g Iodine [I] + 2 g KI + 300 ml $H_2O$ (distilled):
  - grind iodine and KI adding $H_2O$ slowly to dissolve and then store in dark bottle.)
- 10 ml Counterstain of Safranine (2.5% solution in 95% ethyl alcohol).
- Distilled $H_2O$, 100 ml.

*Procedure:*
1. Dry and heat fix slide.
2. Stain 1 minute with crystal violet solution.
3. Wash briefly in tap $H_2O$.
4. Add iodine solution and let stand for 1 minute.
5. Wash with tap $H_2O$.
6. Decolorize until solvent runs clear from slide. Wash briefly with equal parts acetone and alcohol or acetone.
7. Counterstain for 10 seconds with Safranine.
8. Wash in tap $H_2O$.
9. Examine for blue staining gram-positive microorganisms and red gram-negative microorganisms.

Modifications of Gram's stain are Burke's and Hucker's modification.

## *Burke's Modification*[2]

This modification of Gram's stain has the advantage that all solutions are aqueous and the decolorization is more vigorous, resulting in easier differentiation of the organisms in thick preparation.

*Solutions*
1. Alkaline crystal violet
   SOLUTION A
   Crystal violet 1 g
   Distilled water 100 ml
   SOLUTION B
   $NaHCO_3$ 5 g
   Distilled water 100 ml
   Add merthiolate (1:20,000)
2. Iodine solution
   Iodine 1 g
   KI (potassium iodide) 2 g
   Distilled water 200 ml
3. Decolorizing solution
   Ether 1 volume
   Acetone 3 volumes
4. Counterstain
   Safranine O (85% dye content) 0.5 g
   Distilled water 100 ml

*Procedure:*
1. Flood slide with Solution A. Then add 3 to 5 drops of Solution B, depending on the size of the flooded area, and allow to stand 1 minute. Wash well with water.
2. Cover with iodine solution and let stand 1 minute or longer.
3. Rinse with water.
4. Decolorize at once with the ether-acetone mixture, adding it to the slide drop by drop until no more color comes off in the drippings. Care must be taken to avoid excessive decolorization.
5. Wash with water.
6. Counterstain 10 to 15 seconds with the safranine O.
7. Wash in tap water.

## *Hucker's Modification of Gram's Stain*[2]

*Solutions:*
1. Ammonium oxalate crystal violet
   SOLUTION A
   Crystal violet (certified) 2 g
   Ethyl alcohol (95%) 20 ml
   SOLUTION B
   Ammonium oxalate 0.8 g
   Distilled water 80 ml
   Mix solution A and B, store for 24 hours and filter through paper.
2. Iodine solution (mordant)
   Iodine 1 g
   Potassium iodide 2 g
   Distilled water 300 ml
   Grind iodine and potassium iodide in mortar, adding a few milliliters water at a time until dissolved. Store in dark bottle.
3. Counterstain
   Safranine O (2.5% solution in 95% ethyl alcohol) 10 ml
   Distilled water 100 ml

*Procedure:*
After the smear has been dried and heat-fixed, proceed as follows:
1. Stain smears 1 minute with the crystal violet solution.
2. Wash briefly in tap water.
3. Add iodine solution and let stand for 1 minute.
4. Wash in tap water.
5. Decolorize until the solvent flows colorlessly from the slide. Wash briefly

with acetone, or a mixture of equal parts of acetone and alcohol.
6. Counterstain 10 seconds with safranine.
7. Wash in tap water.

*Results:*
Gram-positive organisms stain blue; gram-negative, red.

## Acid-Fast Stain
(Ziehl-Nielsen for mycobacteria)

*Solutions*

CARBOL FUCHSIN STAIN

| | |
|---|---|
| Basic fuchsin | 0.3 g |
| Ethyl alcohol, 95% | 10.0 ml |
| Phenol, melted crystals | 5.0 ml |
| Distilled water | 95.0 ml |

Dissolve the basic fuchsin in the alcohol; the phenol in the water. Mix the two solutions. Let stand for several days before use.

ACID ALCOHOL

| | |
|---|---|
| Ethyl alcohol, 95% | 97 ml |
| Hydrochloric acid, concentrated | 3 ml |

METHYLENE BLUE COUNTERSTAIN

| | |
|---|---|
| Methylene blue | 0.3 g |
| Distilled water | 100.0 ml |

*Procedure:*
Heat fix on air dried smear. Flood entire slide with carbol fuchsin and heat slowly to the steaming point. Use low or intermittent heat to maintain steaming for 3 to 5 minutes. Cool. Do not allow stain to dry on the slide. Wash briefly with tap water and decolorize with acid alcohol until no more stain comes off. Wash with tap water and counterstain for 20 to 30 seconds. Wash, dry, and examine. Acid-fast organisms are red; the background and non-acid-fast organisms are blue.

## Sano Trichrome Method[3]

*Solutions Required:*
0.25% hematoxylin
0.5% HCl
Trichrome mixture
0.2% acetic acid
Alcohol
Xylol

*Procedure:*
1. Use slide fixed in 95% ethanol which is smeared with sediment of fluid originally fixed 1:1 with 40 to 70% ethanol.
2. Place in dilute hematoxylin (0.25%), 6 minutes.
3. Three dips in distilled water.
4. Six dips in 0.5% hydrochloric acid.
5. Place under running tap water (filtered), 6 minutes.
6. Place in Pollak's Trichrome mixture, 6 minutes.
7. Two dips in 0.2% acetic acid in distilled water.
8. Dehydrate through 95% and absolute alcohol followed by two changes of xylol.
9. Cover slip.

## Papanicolaou Staining[1]

*Preparation of Stain*
*Formula for EA 36, Equivalent to EA 50+*

| | |
|---|---|
| 1. Eosin Y | 10 g |
| 2. Bismarck Brown Y | 10 g |
| 3. Light green SF, Yellowish | 10 g |
| 4. Distilled water | 300 ml |
| 5. 95% Alcohol (ethyl) | 2000 ml |
| 6. Phosphotungstic acid | 4 g |
| 7. Saturated lithium carbonate solution (in distilled water) | 20 drops |

*Procedure:*
1. Stock Solution No. 1
   Prepare separate 10% solutions of each of the stains as follows:
   A. 10 g Eosin Y in 100 ml distilled water.
   B. 10 g Bismarck Brown Y in 100 ml distilled water.
   C. 10 g Light Green SF in 100 ml distilled water.
2. Mix (for 2000 ml stain):
   A. 50 ml Eosin Y stock No. 1.
   B. 10 ml Bismarck Brown Y stock No. 1.
   C. 5.5 ml Light Green SF stock No. 1.
3. Take mixture up to 2000 ml with 95% alcohol.

4. Add:
   A. 4 g phosphotungstic acid.
   B. 20 drops saturated lithium carbonate solution.
5. Mix well. Store solution in dark-brown, tightly capped bottles.
   *For Use:* Use full strength; filter before using.
   (+) EA-50 is the commercial preparation.

*Formula for OG 6*

| | |
|---|---|
| 1. Orange G crystals | 10 g |
| 2. Distilled water | 100 ml |
| 3. 95% Alcohol (ethyl) | 1000 ml |
| 4. Phosphotungstic acid | 0.15 g |

*Procedure:*

1. Stock Solution No. 1.
   —Prepare 10% aqueous solution as follows:
   10 g Orange G crystals in 100 ml distilled water.
   Shake well and allow to stand 1 week before using.
2. Stock Solution No. 2.
   —Orange G (0.5% solution): dilute 50 ml stock solution No. 1 up to 1000 ml with 95% alcohol.
3. Final solution for 1000 ml stain.
   A. 1000 ml stock solution No. 2.
   B. 0.15 g phosphotungstic acid.
   Mix well. Store in dark brown stoppered bottles.
   *For Use:* Use full strength; filter before using.

*Formula for Harris' Hematoxylin Without Acetic Acid*

| | |
|---|---|
| 1. Hematoxylin (dark crystals) | 8 g |
| 2. 95% alcohol (ethyl) | 80 ml |
| 3. Aluminum ammonium sulfate | 160 g |
| 4. Distilled water | 1600 ml |
| 5. Mercuric oxide | 6 g |

*Procedure:*

1. Dissolve aluminum ammonium sulfate in distilled water by heating.
2. Dissolve hematoxylin crystals in 95% alcohol.
3. Add hematoxylin solution to sulfate solution.
4. Bring mixture to 95°C.
5. Remove from flame and slowly add the mercuric oxide while stirring. Solution will be dark purple in color.
6. Immediately plunge into a cold water bath.
7. When cool, filter.
8. Store in dark brown bottles and let stand 48 hours.

*For Use:* Dilute the required amount with an equal part of distilled water and filter again.

*Procedure for Staining:*

1. The slide carrier is first placed in a staining dish containing 80% ethyl alcohol. Then the slides are removed from the fixative, appropriately identified with a diamond marking pencil, and placed immediately in the carriers. Slides may remain in the 80% alcohol for as long a time as is required for filling the carrier.
2. 70% ethyl alcohol—5 dips (8 to 10 seconds)
3. 50% ethyl alcohol—5 dips
4. Distilled water—5 dips
5. Harris' hematoxylin (without acetic acid)—6 minutes
6. Distilled water—5 dips
7. 0.5% aqueous solution of hydrochloric acid—3 to 5 dips (dip slowly—the number of dips depends on the strength of the hematoxylin)
8. Running tap water—6 minutes
9. 50% ethyl alcohol—5 dips
10. 70% ethyl alcohol—5 dips
11. 80% ethyl alcohol—5 dips
12. 95% ethyl alcohol—5 dips
13. Orange G (1½ minutes)
14. 95% ethyl alcohol—5 dips
15. 95% ethyl alcohol—5 dips
16. EA 65—1½ minutes
17. 95% ethyl alcohol—5 dips (dip slowly)
18. 95% ethyl alcohol—5 dips (dip slowly)
19. 95% ethyl alcohol—5 dips (dip slowly)
20. Absolute ethyl alcohol—5 dips (8 to 10 seconds)
21. Absolute ethyl alcohol—5 dips (dip slowly)
22. Equal parts of absolute ethyl alcohol and xylol—5 dips
23. Xylol—5 dips
24. Xylol—5 dips
25. Xylol—5 dips

26. Xylol—5 dips
27. Xylol—5 dips
28. Xylol—5 dips
29. Xylol—5 dips

The number of changes of xylol necessary for thorough dehydration and clearing depends on the number of slides processed. For a small number of slides, three or four changes may be adequate.

NOTE: The carriers should be lowered and removed gently from the solution. Vigorous agitation of the slide carriers in transferring them from one solution to another should be avoided in order to prevent washing the material from the slides.

Solutions may be used over a longer period of time if the slide carrier is rested on several thicknesses of paper toweling for a few seconds after removing it from the solutions in steps No. 8, 13, and 16. Smears should never be allowed to dry during any step of the staining process.

The hematoxylin solution should be filtered each day. The other stains and solutions should also be filtered or changed accordingly. When large numbers of slides are processed, the addition of stains may be necessary. Care in keeping the stains and the solutions free of sediment prevents cell contamination from one smear to another.

*Keep staining solutions covered when not in use.*

1. Koss LG. Diagnostic Cytology and Its Histopathologic Bases. 2nd Ed. Philadelphia, JB Lippincott Co, 1968, p 601.
2. Henry JG (ed). Clinical Diagnosis and Management by Laboratory Methods. Philadelphia, WB Saunders Co, 1979, p 1567.
3. Sano ME. Trichrome stain for tissue section, culture or smear. Am J Clin Path, *19*:898, 1949.

*Appendix B*

# Antibiotic Doses and Serum Levels

| Drug | Reference | Dose/Kg/Route | Serum Concentrations | | | | Comments/Indications |
|---|---|---|---|---|---|---|---|
| | | | Peak | | Low | | |
| | | | Time (hr) | μg/ml | Time (hr) | μg/ml | |
| Amikacin | (1) | 4.4 mg IM q6–8h | 1 | 13.3 | 6 | 2.6 | Expense deters common use. Usually administered tid or qid. Three-times-daily dosing has been recommended for foals. Its use should be restricted to infections requiring its use where m.o. such as many *Klebsiella* spp. are resistant to other antimicrobial agents. Potential nephrotoxicity. |
| | (1) | 4.4 mg IV q6–8h | ¼ | 30.3 | 6 | 1.55 | |
| | (1) | 6.6 mg IM q6–8h | 1 | 23 | 6 | ~5 | |
| | (1) | 6.6 mg IV q6–8h | ¼ | 61.2 | 6 | <4 | |
| | (2) | 7 mg IM q12h | | | | | |
| | (3) | 7 mg IV or IM q8hr | 1½ | 19.4±4.7* | 8 | 4.4±2.0 | |
| | (3) | 7 mg IV or IM q8hr | 1½ | 15.9±2.6* | 8 | 4.0±1.8 | |
| Amoxicillin | (4) | 2–7 mg IM q24h | ¼ | 10 | 8 | 0 | Coughs, bronchitis. Response in UK rated about 80% efficacy in respiratory infections. Oral dosing may be effective only against the most susceptible m.o., such as *Pasteurella, Streptococcus* spp., and non-β-lactamase-producing *Staphylococcus* spp. High doses advised. |
| | (4) | 4–12 mg PO q24h or q12h | 2 | 5 | | | |
| | (2) | 22 mg IM q6h | 4 | 2 | | | |
| Amoxicillin-trihydrate | (5) | 20–30 mg PO q6h | 2 | ~10 (30 mg dose) | 6 | ~1 | |
| Ampicillin Na | (6) | 15 mg IM q6h | ½ | 4.4–9.0 | 6 | .2 | Bronchopneumonia and generalized streptococcal infections. Long-term therapy is safe. Individual variation in peak levels. Mares' levels may be less than those in geldings. Serum levels lower in pregnant mares. |
| | (7) | 4.4 mg IM q6h | ½ | 2.5–9.2 | 6 | 0.3–3.4 | |
| | (7) | 11 mg IM q6h | ½ | 5.3–16.0 | 6 | 4.4–5.6 | |
| | (8) | 22 mg IM | ½ | 5.5–26 | | | |
| Ampicillin-trihydrate | (6) | 19 mg IM q12h | 8 | 1.24 | 12 | 1.0 | Low serum levels and relative expense limit its use. Combining it with Na ampicillin does not appear to significantly prolong effective serum concentrations of ampicillin. |
| | (7) | 11 mg IM q12h | 2 | 1.0–2.1 | 8 | 0.18–2.1 | |
| | (7) | 22 mg IM q12h | 2 | 2.42–3.2 | 8 | 2.42–3.2 | |
| Cefazolin | (9) | 11 mg IV or IM q12h | ¼ | 16.8 | | | Half-life after IM dosing approximately twice that after IV dosing. Effective against many gram-positive and some gram-negative m.o. |
| Cepharin | (10 and 11) | 20 mg IM q6h | ⅙ | 21–25 | 4 | .3 | Useful for treating infections caused by gram-positive β-lactamase-producing bacteria including *Staphylococcus aureus*. Dosage given is for 250 mg/ml drug concentration. Clearance in neonatal foals is almost twice that of adults. |
| | | | | | 6 | Not detectable | |
| Cephalothin (Na) | (2) | 18 mg IM or IV q6h | | | | | |

| | | | | | | | |
|---|---|---|---|---|---|---|---|
| Ceftiofur | (12) | 2.2 mg IM q24h<br>4.4 mgIM or IV q6hr | | | | | Only preliminary information is available now. Effective against many gram-positive and some gram-negative m.o. Third generation cephalosporin. No information yet on foals. |
| Chloramphenicol | (13) | 20 mg IV | ¼ | 11 ± 1.3 | 3 | ~1.0 | Used for treating pneumonia, including lung abscesses and pleuritis. It has been given for about 10 weeks (44 to 50 mg/kg PO q6h) using crushed dissolved tablets without problems. Its use is not recommended because of potential human health hazards and for legal reasons. Very rarely soft feces occur. Bitter taste makes treatment difficult and animals will not eat it. |
| | (13) | 40 mg IV | ¼ | ~20 | 5 | ~1.0 | |
| | (13) | 22 mg† IV | ½ | 21.5 | 4 | ~1.0 | |
| | (13) | 20 mg IM | 2–3 | ~ 1.0 | | | |
| | (14) | 22 mg† IM | ¼–½ | 11–12 | 5 | ~2.0 | |
| | (14) | 22 mg PO | 3 | 3.5 | 6 | <1.0 | |
| | (15) | 50 mg† IM q6h | | 32 ± 6.1 | 6 | 9.4 ± 1 | |
| | | | | | 8 | 6.5 | |
| | (15) | 50 mg‡ PO q6h | 1 | 66 ± 6.3 | 6 | 10.6 ± 1 | |
| | | | | | 8 | 4.3 ± 0.6 | |
| Erythromycin | (16) | 20 mg PO<br>25–30 mg PO q6–8h | 2 | 0.423 | 8 | 0.015 | It is used for treating pneumonia due to gram-positive m.o. Streptococci and *R. equi* have a low MIC. Very effective against *R. equi* infections especially when given with rifampin. High lung tissue/serum concentration ratio. Rarely, oral administration causes transient diarrhea. |
| | (16) | 5 mg IV q4–6h | | | | | |
| Gentamicin | (6) | 1.3 mg IM q8h | ¼ | 2.4 | 8 | .05 | It is used for treating pleuropneumonia and pneumonia. It is usually not used by itself except in rare cases where only gram-negative m.o. are isolated. It has been used for 4 wks duration (2.2 mg/kg IV q6h) without problems in mature horses. The IM dosing may cause local myositis especially during chronic use. Creatinine should be monitored. Potential ototoxicity and nephrotoxicity. Foals are more susceptible to nephrotoxicity than adult horses. Use q8h dose (2 mg/kg) in foals. It should be given very slowly IV. Use should be avoided if possible if there is neuromuscular weakness. When possible, monitor peak and trough levels to achieve appropriate dosage. Trough levels should be less than 2 μg/ml. |
| | (17) | 1.7 mg IM q6h | 1 | 5.2–16.0 | 8 | 0.5–0.7 | |
| | (17) | 4.4 mg IM q6h | ½ | 15–21 | 8 | 1.2–1.5 | |
| | | | | | 6 | 1.2 | |

| | | | | | | | |
|---|---|---|---|---|---|---|---|
| Isoniazid | (18) | 5–15 mg PO q12h | | | | | Despite its common use concurrent with penicillin for chronic infections and abscesses, there is no proof of its efficacy for any disease other than those of Mycobacterial origin. Potential hepatotoxicity. |
| Kanamycin | (6) | 5 mg IM q8h | 1 | 17.6–21.4 | 8 | 1.5 | Combined with penicillins for pleuritis and pneumonia. Its spectrum is less than Gentamicin's. Potential ototoxicity and nephrotoxicity. The latter is more common in foals than in adults. Use q8h in foals. |
| Metronidazole | (19) | 15–25 mg PO q6h | 15 mg 1–2<br>25 mg 1–2 | 8.4<br>12.6<br>(12–24 range) | 6<br>6 | 2.8<br>4.3 | Used for anaerobic infections. Oral dose usually used. Low dose adequate for more susceptible anaerobes and higher dose needed for more resistant strains. |
| | | 25 mg IV q6h | ½ | 26<br>(19–34 range) | 6 | 3 | |
| Moxalactam | | 22 mg IV q6h | | | | | Broad spectrum. Restrict use to specific cases. |
| Oxacillin | (20) | 25 mg IM q8–12h | ½ | 9.75 | 6<br>8<br>12 | 0.54<br>0.44<br>0.34 | Used for treating Staphylococcus aureus (MIC <.5 μg/ml) and other infections due to penicillinase-producing gram-positive bacteria. |
| Oxytetracycline | (6) | 5 mg IV q12h | ½ | 5–8 | 7 | 1.0 | Used for treating pneumonia and less frequently pleuritis. Relatively inexpensive. Dilute and administer slowly. Soft feces, and rarely severe diarrhea (more common with large doses in stressed horses). Phlebitis common. Horses may collapse with too-rapid IV dosing. |
| K Penicillin G | (6)<br>(6)<br>(6)<br>(6)<br>(6)<br>(6) | $10 \times 10^3$ U IM q6h<br>$20 \times 10^3$ U IM q6h<br>$40 \times 10^3$ U IM q6h<br>$20 \times 10^3$ U IV q6h<br>$60 \times 10^3$ U IV q6h<br>$200 \times 10^3$ U PO | 1<br>1<br>1<br>½<br>½<br>½ | 0.4<br>0.5<br>2.2<br>2.7–4.4<br>17.5–22.5<br>1.4 | 6<br>6<br>6<br>6<br>6<br>12 | 0.3<br>0.3<br>1.6<br>0<br>0.5<br>12 | Penicillin is commonly used for treating bronchopneumonia and pleuritis, often in conjunction with aminoglycosides in pleuritis or when there is a mixed gram-negative and gram-positive infection. IV doses should be used when high levels are needed. IM procaine penicillin probably adequate for most streptococci. Absorption varies with different oral forms. Rarely hives may occur, "Procaine reaction" (rapid respiration, excitement, incoordination). Salivary and mucus gland secretion occurs with high IV doses. Diarrhea sometimes occurs with oral dosing. IV dosing should be slow. |

| | | | | | | | |
|---|---|---|---|---|---|---|---|
| Phenoxymethyl penicillin (Penicillin V) | (21) | $110 \times 10^3$ U PO q8h | ½–1 | 2.38 ± 0.18 | 8 | >0.10 | |
| Na Penicillin G | (6) | $30 \times 10^3$ U IM q6h<br>IV q6h | ¼ | 6.1 | 6 | .65 | |
| Procaine penicillin G | (6) | $22 \times 10^3$ U IM q12h | 2 | 1.8 | 12 | .5 | |
| Rifampin | (22) | 5–10 mg PO q12h | 3–4 | 2.9 ± 0.4 | | | High doses IV may cause hemolysis, depression and sweating. IM route may cause soreness and sweating. Gram-negative m.o. MIC may exceed 10 μg/ml and lower dose (which suffices for most susceptible gram-positive m.o.) may be inadequate. It is usually used with another antibiotic to avoid development of resistance. The 5–10 mg dose is used with erythromycin for *R. equi* infections. Sweating and depression follow IV or IM administration; therefore it is usually administered orally. |
| Spectinomycin | (23) | 20 mg IM q8h | | | | | Insufficient data. Some practitioners use it for pneumonia. High lung serum concentration ratio. Local myositis. |
| Streptomycin | (24) | 5.5 mg IM | ½ | 2.3–15.5 | 12 | 1.59 | Not recommended due to poor spectrum, nephrotoxicity and ototoxicity. |
| Sulfamethazine | | See label. | | | | | Usually used concurrently with oxytetracycline and less commonly penicillin for treatment of pneumonia. There is good distribution in pleural fluid and tissues. One should ensure good hydration of the horse during its use. Occasionally trembling and "blowing" occur during or shortly after IV administration. |

| | | | | | | | |
|---|---|---|---|---|---|---|---|
| Ticarcillin | (25) | 44 mg IV q6h | ½ | 104.3 ± 6 | 6 | ~4 | IV dosing may increase % drug entering pleural fluid. Synergistic with aminoglycosides. Expensive. Clavulanic acid broadens the spectrum to include penicillinase-producing m.o. Ticarcillin is effective against most anaerobes. Use of ticarcillin plus clavulanic acid could replace the common practice of using an aminoglycoside plus penicillin plus metronidazole. Pain and recumbency may occur if drug is given IM to foals. Also, large volume makes IM impractical. Administer IV. |
| | (25) | 44 mg IM q8h | 2 | 28.3 ± 5.5 | 6 | >10 | |
| Ticarcillin plus clavulanic acid in adult horses | (26) | 50–100 mg IV q6h | | | | | |
| | (26) | 50 mg IM q6h§ | ½ | 87.6 ± 25.5 | 6 | 13.2 ± 3.7 | |
| | (26) | 50 mg IV q6h§ | $\frac{1}{12}$ | 277 ± 50 | 4 | 11.4 ± 3.6 | |
| | | IV‖ | $\frac{1}{12}$ | 7.5 ± 1.8 | 2 | <.35 | |
| | | IM‖ | ¼–½ | 2.8 ± .6 | 4 | .2 ± .1 | |
| | | | | | 4 | 24 | |
| Ticarcillin plus clavulanic acid in foals | (26) | 100 mg IV§ | $\frac{1}{12}$ | 362 ± 124 | 6 | 6.4 | |
| | (26) | 100 mg IM§ | ¼–½ | 72 | 6 | 23.2 | |
| | (26) | 50 mg IV§ | $\frac{1}{12}$ | 208 | 4 | 10.6 | |
| | | | | | 6 | <4.0 | |
| | (26) | 50 mg IM§ | 1 | 36 | 6 | 9.3 | |
| | (26) | High dose IV‖ | $\frac{1}{12}$ | 10.8 | 4 | <.2 | |
| | (26) | High dose IM‖ | ½ | 3.9 | 4 | .23 | |
| | (26) | Lower dose IV‖ | $\frac{1}{12}$ | 4.6 | 3 | <.2 | |
| Trimethoprim sulfonamide | (1) | 5.5 mg TMP (Trimethoprim) PO or in feed q12h | 1½ | ~2 | 6–7 | ~0.5 | It is used for treating bronchopneumonia and pleuritis. It has been administered over long time periods without complications. Broad spectrum. Occasional diarrhea may be severe. |
| | | 5.5 mg TMP PO or by the tube q12h or q8h | ⅓ | 3.2 | 6–7 | <0.5 | |
| | (1) | 5.5 mg TMP IV q12h | ½ | 7.5 | 6–7 | ~1.0 | Study in healthy neonates. Primary use against gram-positive bacteria. Pharmacokinetics for TMP similar in foals and adults but elimination of sulfa drugs is slower in foals. Although not significant, concentrations of both TMP and sulfa drug were higher in pony foals than in horse foals. |
| | (27) | 2.5 mg TMP IV and 12.5 mg SMZ IV q12 hrs | | | | | |
| Tylosin | (5) | 10 mg q8h | 4 | 1 | | | Insufficient data. Rarely used. |

* Sample not obtained prior to 1-1½ hours, therefore peak levels probably higher earlier. Studies on neonatal foals. In uremic foals, levels are higher and clearance delayed.

† = Succinate
‡ = Palmitate
§ = Ticarcillin levels
‖ = Clavulanic acid levels

Table adapted from Bristol Veterinary Handbook of Antimicrobial Therapy. 2nd Ed. D.E. Johnston, ed. Vet Learning Systems Co., Inc.

1. Orsini JA, Soma LR, Rourke JE, et al. Pharmacokinetics of amikacin in the horse. J Vet Pharmacol Ther, *8*:124, 1985.
2. Carter GK, Marten RJ. Septicemia in the neonatal foal. Comp Cont Ed, *8*:S256, 1986.
3. Adland-Davenport P, Brown MP, Robinson JD, et al. Pharmacokinetics of amikacin in critically ill neonatal foals treated for presumed or confirmed sepsis. Equine Vet J, *22*:18, 1990.
4. Yoeman GH. Amoxicillin: United Kingdom Clinical Field Trials. VM/SAC, *72* (special suppl):787, 1977.
5. Love D, Rose RJ, Martin ICA, et al. Serum levels of amoxycillin following its oral administration to Thoroughbred foals. Equine Vet J, *13*:53, 1981.
6. Knight HD. Antimicrobial agents used in the horse. Proceedings of 21st Annual Convention of American Association of Equine Practitioners, 1975, p 131.
7. Beech J, Kohn C, Leitch M, et al. Serum and synovial fluid levels of sodium ampicillin (totacillin) and ampicillin trihydrate (Polyflex) in horses. J Equine Med Surg, *3*:350, 1979.
8. Traver DS, Riviere JE. Ampicillin in mares: a comparison of intramuscular sodium ampicillin or sodium ampicillin-ampicillin trihydrate injection. Am J Vet Res, *43*:402, 1982.
9. Sams RA, Ruoff WW. Pharmacokinetics and bioavailability of cefazolin in horses. Am J Vet Res, *46*:348, 1985.
10. Brown MP, Gronwall R, Gossman TB, et al. Pharmacokinetics and body fluid and endometrial concentrations of cepharin in mares. Am J Vet Res, *47*:784, 1986.
11. Brown MP, Gronwall R, Gossman TB, et al. Pharmacokinetics and serum concentrations of cepharin in neonatal foals. Am J Vet Res, *48*:805, 1987.
12. Beachnau BA, Foly B. Unpublished data.
13. Pilloud M. Pharmacokinetics, plasma protein binding and dosage of chloramphenicol in cattle and horses. Res Vet Sci, *15*:231, 1973.
14. Davis LE, Neff CA, Baggot JO, et al. Pharmacokinetics of chloramphenicol in domesticated animals. Am J Vet Res, *33*:2259, 1972.
15. Oh-Ishi S. Blood concentration of chloramphenicol in horses after intramuscular or oral administration. Jpn J Vet Sci, *30*:25, 1968.
16. Prescott JF, Hoover DJ, Dohoo IR. Pharmacokinetics of erythromycin in foals and in adult horses. J Vet Pharmacol Ther, *6*:67, 1983.
17. Beech J, Kohn C, Leitch M, et al. Therapeutic use of gentamicin in horses: Concentrations in serum, urine and synovial fluid and evaluation of renal function. Am J Vet Res, *38*:1985, 1977.
18. Roberts MC, English PB. Antimicrobial chemotherapy in the horse: 11. The application of antimicrobial therapy. J Equine Med Surg, *3*:308, 1979.
19. Sweeney RW, Sweeney CR, Soma LR, et al. Pharmacokinetics of metronidazole given to horses by intravenous and oral routes. Am J Vet Res, *47*:1726, 1986.
20. Stover SM, Brown MP, Kelly RH, et al. Sodium oxacillin in the horse: serum synovial fluid, peritoneal fluid and urine concentrations after single dose intramuscular administration. Am J Vet Res, *42*:1824, 1981.
21. Schwark WS, Ducharme NG, Shin SJ, et al. Absorption and distribution patterns of oral phenoxymethyl penicillin (penicillin V) in the horse. Cornell Vet, *73*:314, 1983.
22. Burrows GE, MacAllister CG, Beckstrom DH, et al. Rifampin in the horse. Comparison of intravenous, intramuscular and oral administrations. Am J Vet Res, *46*:442, 1985.
23. Burrows GE. Pharmacotherapeutics of macrolides, lincomysin and spectinomycin. J Am Vet Med Assoc, *176*:1072, 1980.
24. Rollins LD, Teske RH, Condon RJ, et al. Serum penicillin and dihydrostreptomycin concentrations in horses after intramuscular administration of selected preparations containing these antibiotics. J Am Vet Med Assoc, *16*:490, 1972.
25. Sweeney CR, Soma LR, Beech J, et al. Pharmacokinetics of ticarcillin in the horse after intravenous and intramuscular administration. Am J Vet Res, *45*:1000, 1984.
26. Sweeney RW, Beech J, Simmons RD, et al. Pharmacokinetics of intravenously and intramuscularly administered ticarcillin and clavulanic acid in foals. Am J Vet Res, *49*:23, 1988.
27. Brown MP, McCartney JH, Gronwall R, et al. Pharmacokinetics of trimethoprim-sulfamethoxazole in two day old foals after a single intravenous injection. Equine Vet J, *22*:51, 1990.

# Index

Page numbers in *italics* indicate illustrations; numbers followed by "t" indicate tables.